T5-AGS-554

THE
SURGICAL DISEASES OF THE GENITO-URINARY ORGANS

BY

E. L. KEYES, A. M., M. D., LL. D.

Consulting Surgeon to the Bellevue, and the Skin and Cancer Hospitals; formerly Professor of Genito-Urinary Surgery, Syphilology, and Dermatology at the Bellevue Hospital Medical College, etc.

AND

E. L. KEYES, Jr., A. B., M. D., Ph. D.

Adjunct Professor of Genito-Urinary Surgery, New York Polyclinic Medical School and Hospital; Assistant Visiting Surgeon to St. Vincent's Hospital; Special Lecturer on Genito-Urinary Diseases, Georgetown University Medical School, etc.

SECOND EDITION, REVISED

WITH ONE HUNDRED AND SEVENTY-FOUR ILLUSTRATIONS IN THE TEXT AND TEN PLATES, EIGHT OF WHICH ARE COLOURED

NEW YORK AND LONDON
D. APPLETON AND COMPANY
1906

PRINTED AT THE APPLETON PRESS
NEW YORK, U. S. A.

PREFACE

Each year adds so much to the practice of medicine in these rapid days that a constant readjustment of the point of view is imperative for text-book as well as for practitioner, if they would keep abreast of the times. Hence a new edition of this work following so close upon our late revision. Already there has been a notable advance in the treatment of gonorrhea and in the pathology of prostatic hypertrophy. Renal decapsulation, the new star dimly discernible in 1902, has attained its greatest magnitude and begins to wane. The revision demanded in these subjects has been extended to other matters of minor import, which, it is hoped, will add to the value of this work.

E. L. Keyes,
E. L. Keyes, Jr.

109 East Thirty-Fourth Street,
New York City.

PREFACE

In September, 1867—thirty-five years ago—were written the first words of that book of which this volume is the legitimate grandchild. It was then entitled Genito-Urinary Diseases with Syphilis, and presented a group of maladies customarily associated in the daily experience of those practitioners who were being forced into specialism by the requirements of large cities. It was the first book in any language grouping these maladies. Indeed, the book was made a subject of adverse criticism on the ground that it arrogated to its authors a greater degree of special knowledge than the condition of the community at that time warranted.

In 1888, after the death of the senior author, Dr. William H. Van Buren, a total revision was made with slight change of title, and the tendency was to make it less venereal and more genito-urinary.

A second revision, more thorough even than the first, is now called for by the exaction of circumstances and the accumulation of experience general and personal. Syphilis has been entirely eliminated, since it is a genital disease only in its method of approach, not at all in its manner of expression. Thus this book has lived through three generations, both in its presentation and in its authors, the infusion of new blood saving it from the imputation of senectitude.

In order to insure facility and directness of expression, the subject-matter is presented in the first person, but that first person is as often the junior as the senior author.

The anatomical order followed in the two earlier editions has been abandoned. Venereal diseases, as such, having been shut out, it seems proper to relegate sexual and genital maladies to the second place, giving the surgical picture of urinary disorders the first and more prominent position, a position deserved alike by their relative gravity and their transcendent interest. Just as syphilis has grown away from true genito-urinary surgery, so have all the sexual psychoses naturally estranged themselves and sought shelter with the venereal specialist. They have therefore received but scant courtesy here.

Gonorrhea, however, is so intimately associated with all the inflammatory disorders of the genito-urinary tract, both in its physical expression as an acute disease and in the wide-reaching influence of its sequelæ, that its consideration has been greatly amplified and its course followed up far beyond the genito-urinary system (into the eye, the joints, etc.). This is essential in order to make the subject complete.

A conservative attitude has been adopted upon some important questions of surgical treatment, such, for instance, as ureteral catheterization, a subject not yet logically judged by experience nor sufficiently tried in the furnace of statistics.

We have adopted a certain classification of the inflammations of the posterior urethra, the bladder, and the kidney in the interest of clinical clearness; and while this may ultimately require modification, it avoids confusion and the multiplicity of descriptive detail.

No modification has been made in the treatment of hydrocele and varicocele. The simple methods originally advocated have been adhered to; but an attempt has been made to expound in a practical manner the pathogenesis of urethral stricture, extravasation of urine, and bacteriuria. The new surgical treatment of chronic Bright's disease, by stripping the kidney capsule, receives no notice in the text, since the evidence thus far accumulated is insufficient for trustworthy generalization.

For two very distinct improvements in surgical technic relating to the irrigation treatment of acute gonorrhea and the operative treatment of enlarged prostate we are indebted to our associate, Dr. Charles H. Chetwood.

The urine has been considered only from the surgical-clinical standpoint; and urinary antisepsis not theoretically, but according to the dictates of common sense.

The French metric system has been adopted; but it is not yet possible wholly to give up the minim, the grain, the dram, the ounce, etc.

The bibliography has been arranged to suit the requirements of the advanced student. To this end original work has in some cases been neglected in favour of more comprehensive recent publications.

E. L. Keyes,
E. L. Keyes, Jr.

109 East Thirty-fourth Street,
New York City.

PREFACE TO THE ORIGINAL TREATISE

The steady growth of the science and art of surgery has involved a corresponding increase in bulk of the text-books in which its principles and practice are set forth—an increase already suggestive of either a limit in bulk soon to be reached, or the omission or slurring over of special subjects. In this alternative the preparation of text-books on special subjects would seem to be the appropriate remedy.

The tendency of mankind to aggregate in large and constantly increasing cities has led to a corresponding tendency to the growth of specialists in the different departments of medicine and surgery; and the development in large cities of hospitals and schools, and opportunities for teaching, would seem to render them the natural repositories of accumulating experience and the sources of advancing knowledge. It is from city practice and hospital experience, therefore, that the materials for the preparation of text-books on special subjects would be naturally sought, and from these sources the substance of the present work has been mainly derived. Its object is to present to the student and general practitioner a succinct account of the nature and treatment of the diseases incident to the genito-urinary organs as they are encountered in private and hospital practice by those engaged in their daily and especial study. The literature of this department of surgery has been carefully studied with the purpose of reproducing every fact of *practical* value. It is hoped that the reader will recognise a conciseness in the grouping of these facts which will save him the necessity of reference to the numerous monographs and essays from which they have been collected.

On account of the general character of the work as a text-book, it has been impossible to refer very largely to personal authority and experience, and this has been for the most part avoided except in reference to mooted points and exceptional or noteworthy phenomena. The extent of the subject-matter treated of, and the necessity for compression, will be regarded, it is hoped, as a sufficient apology for terseness and directness of expression or defect in style, while the circumstance of joint-authorship will explain any lack of uniformity in manner throughout the work, of which the preparation for the press has devolved mainly upon the junior author.

The plan of the work is based upon an anatomical classification of the tissues and organs of which the diseases and deformities form the subjects of description. This necessitates some repetition and frequent reference to facts, cases, or illustrations already given, or to be given, in connection with other anatomical divisions of the genito-urinary tract. These references are usually made thus: (Nephralgia), (Plate XX), (Case 45), the page not being specified, as the constant appearance of signs scattered through a page tends to confuse the reader. No difficulty need be experienced in turning to these references promptly, as the parenthetical word, case, or plate may be found at once credited to its proper page in the general index at the end of the book, or in the index to plates, or list of cases, at its commencement.

The terms of measurement employed are uniformly English, with the exception of the centimetre and millimetre, which frequently occur in the text. These may be readily reduced to their equivalent in inches by computation from the subjoined table.[1]

The subject of syphilis is included, of necessity, in a treatise like the present. Opportunities for the observation and study of this disease on a large scale fall mainly to the share of the metropolitan hospital-surgeon and special practitioner. Although properly belonging to the department of Principles of Surgery, there is no disease falling within the limits of this work concerning which clear and correct ideas as to nature and treatment will, at the present time, so seriously influence success in practice.

Chapter VIII, Part II, on "Syphilitic Diseases of the Eye," has been kindly furnished, at the request of the authors, by Prof. H. D. Noyes, M. D., whose authority on this subject is undisputed.

They beg leave to thank Dr. Roosa for aid, both personally and through his excellent work "On Diseases of the Ear," in the preparation of Chapter IX, Part II, "On Syphilis of the Ear."

Acknowledgments are also due to Dr. Partridge and Dr. Morrison-Fiset, of the house-staff of the Charity Hospital, for kind assistance; and to Dr. L. A. Stimson for aid in many ways.

NEW YORK, *March, 1873.*

---

[1] 1 centimetre = 4·433 lines, or ·393708 inch;
1 millimetre = ·443 line, or ·03937 inch;
or, roughly, 1 millimetre equals half a line—about one twenty-fifth of an inch.

CONTENTS

PART I

DISEASES OF THE URINARY ORGANS, INCLUDING GONORRHEA

LIST OF PLATES AND TEXT ILLUSTRATIONS

THE SURGICAL DISEASES OF THE GENITO-URINARY ORGANS

PART I

DISEASES OF THE URINARY ORGANS, INCLUDING GONORRHEA

CHAPTER I

ANATOMY AND PHYSIOLOGY OF THE URETHRA—CURVE OF URETHRAL INSTRUMENTS—URETHRAL AND SEXUAL HYGIENE

ANATOMY OF THE URETHRA

The urethra is always a closed canal throughout its whole course, except when distended by some foreign substance. Commencing at the neck of the bladder, it tunnels the upper part of the prostate, perforates the triangular ligament, and terminates at the end of the penis. Its outer opening is known as the *meatus*, or the *meatus urinarius*. The urethra is divided naturally into two parts, the *anterior* and the *posterior urethra*, by the triangular ligament, the anterior urethra lying external to the anterior layer of that structure, and the posterior urethra being the continuation of the canal backward into the bladder. The anterior or spongy portion of the urethra is again subdivided into four parts, the navicular (or the fossa navicularis, Fig. 1), penile (Fig. 2), scrotal, and bulbo-perineal (or simply the bulb) (Guyon [1]). The posterior urethra is subdivided into the membranous and the prostatic portions. It is much more accurate to speak of a lesion, such as a foreign body or a stricture, as being at the peno-scrotal angle or in the bulb, than to say it lies at a depth of 4 or 6 inches, for not only does the length of the urethra vary according as the penis is erect or flaccid and in disease (hypertrophy of the prostate), but the urethral *length*, the urinary distance,[2] varies widely in different healthy individuals.

---

[1] Leçons cliniques, 1896, ii, 295.

[2] Keyes, Am. J. of Med. Sci., 1898, cxvi, 125.

The mucous membrane of the urethra consists of a layer of epithelium, of which the superficial cells are squamous in the navicular and prostatic regions and columnar elsewhere, on a connective-

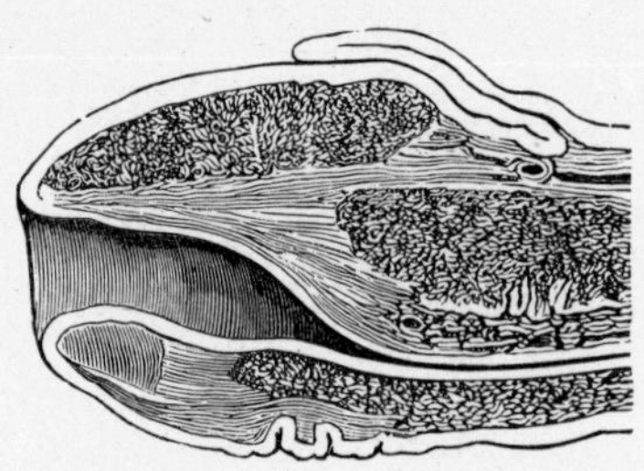

Fig. 1.—Cruveilhier.
Vertical section through glans and fossa navicularis.

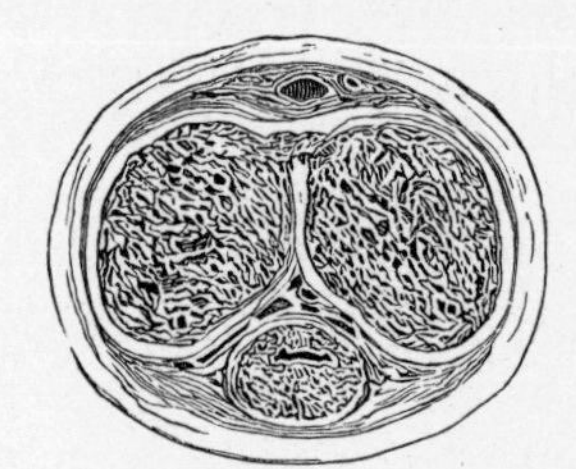

Fig. 2.—Cruveilhier.
Transverse section of penis.

tissue basement substance particularly rich in elastic fibres to allow for the great distensibility of the canal.

The Anterior Urethra.—In the anterior urethra the mucous membrane is surrounded, except in the fossa navicularis, by a very thin longitudinal layer of unstriped muscle-fibres (in direct continuity with the inner fibres of the prostate), and these are in turn surrounded by a circular layer of unstriped muscle. These circular fibres are so few around the spongy urethra that their very existence was denied by Sappey. These muscle-layers are so thin and weak that they have no clinical significance. (See Spasm of the Urethra.) Finally, the anterior urethra is surrounded from triangular ligament to meatus by the corpus spongiosum, except for the half-inch nearest the bladder, where the corpus spongiosum fails to cover the roof of the urethra and is enlarged below into the *bulb*.

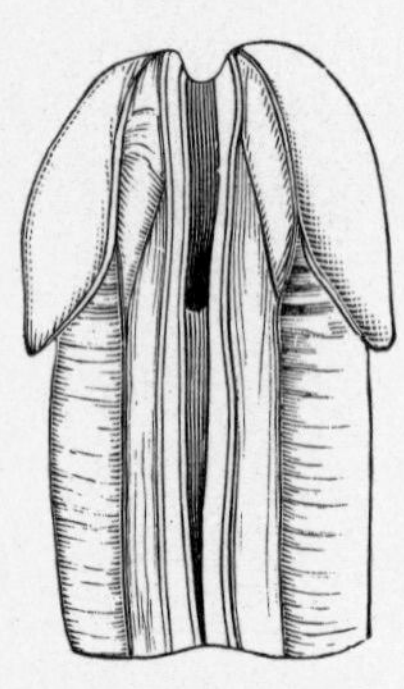

Fig. 3.—Cruveilhier.

Crypts and Glands.—In the roof of the fossa navicularis lies the *lacuna magna* (Fig. 3), a simple pocket in the mucous membrane with its orifice towards the meatus, and consequently open to entrap small instruments. This lacuna varies greatly in size in different persons, being sometimes entirely absent, and occasionally running as far back as the triangular ligament, forming the so-called double urethra (*q. v.*). A few other smaller lacunæ lie along the roof of the penile urethra. *The glands of the urethra*, to be distinguished from the lacunæ, are of the compound racemose type, of very small calibre, lined with a cylindrical epithelium. They lie chiefly on the roof of the urethra, are more numerous in its deeper parts, and, in many instances, pierce the sheath of the corpus spongiosum and extend for some distance within it—an important fact in relation to organic stricture of the canal, since these glands convey the products of urethral inflammation into the corpus spongiosum and so involve it in the subsequent cicatrization. *Cowper's glands* are two small, round, lobular bodies each about the size of a cherry-stone, lying just behind the bulb of the urethra in the transverso-urethral muscle between the layers of the triangular ligament. Their ducts are sometimes very long, but average a full inch, and open out of the floor of the bulbous urethra. Their fluid is supposed to aid in diluting the sperm.

The urethra has about the same sensitiveness in health as the conjunctiva. In the membranous urethra, however, sensibility is exaggerated. The colour of the membrane is pale pink. In rest its walls are in contact, obliterating the cavity of the canal, so that a cross-section presents a transverse slit instead of an opening (Figs. 154, 155).

The anterior urethra might well be called the *external urinary tract*, and the canals and reservoirs beyond the *internal urinary tract*, for the anterior urethra is in free communication with the surface of the body and harbours all the micro-organisms that may lie thereon. As a general thing it does this with perfect impunity. Its *flora* includes the bacillus coli communis, pyogenic streptococcus and staphylococci, and other less noxious germs without number. All of these flourish and multiply within it harmlessly enough unless the tissues have been already damaged by other agencies. Of these, trauma and the gonococcus stand first. The gonococcus is the only microbe pathogenic to the anterior urethra yet positively identified. That there are others, as yet unnamed, which do cause lower grades of urethral infection there can be no doubt; but, at best, they are relatively unimportant. Such bacteria as flourish normally in the anterior urethra, being constantly washed out by the urine, and entering only through the meatus (except under pathological conditions), are more numerous in the fossa navicularis, and the bacillus coli and the pyogenic cocci are usually found only in that region.

The Posterior Urethra.—The posterior urethra, extending from the anterior layer of the triangular ligament to the bladder, presents many notable points of contrast with the anterior urethra. The canal is no longer surrounded by erectile tissue, and, indeed, it could scarcely become erect, for whereas the anterior urethra is freely movable with the penis, the posterior urethra possesses a fixed curve—of which later. Moreover, the posterior urethra is, in its normal state, entirely free from the germs harboured by the anterior urethra; it is the lowest section of the aseptic internal urinary tract.

The posterior urethra is divided naturally into the membranous and the prostatic urethra.

The Membranous Urethra.—Of all parts of the canal the membranous urethra is the most fixed, running, as it does, from the aperture in the anterior layer of the triangular ligament to the aperture in the posterior layer. Its mucous membrane, though of a darker colour and much more sensitive, does not differ in structure from that of the anterior urethra. This in turn is surrounded by the thin layer of unstriped muscle derived from the prostate, but instead of being sheathed in the corpus spongiosum, it is embedded in the voluntary muscle that fills the space between the two layers of the triangular ligament. This muscle has had special names given to different portions of it by Guthrie, Müller, Wilson, and others, but it may be considered clinically as one muscle, the *constrictor* or *compressor urethræ*, the *cut-off* muscle, the external or voluntary sphincter of the bladder. The last term best expresses its function. It is the muscle by which the outflow of urine from the bladder is voluntarily opposed. If a catheter is introduced through it no voluntary effort of the individual is able to arrest the stream of urine. Indeed, inhibition of this muscle is the chief act of the will in voluntary urination. It may, however, suffer from spasm, and so not only prevent urination, but also present a serious obstacle to the introduction of instruments. This is spasmodic stricture (*q. v.*).

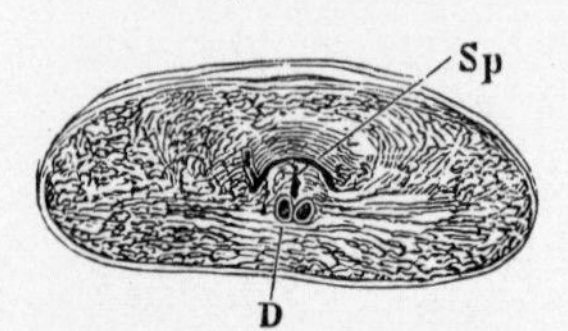

FIG. 4.—CRUVEILHIER.
Transverse section of centre of prostate: *D*, ejaculatory ducts; *Sp*, sinus pocularis.

The Prostatic Urethra.—The prostatic urethra tunnels the prostate, sometimes barely covered by that organ above, sometimes deeply embedded in it (Fig. 4). It is fixed only where it joins the membranous urethra. It is fusiform in shape, being closed internally by the internal or involuntary sphincter of the bladder. Into it the ducts of the sexual organs empty. It is lined by squamous epithelium like that of the bladder, and is liable to great deformity and obstruction by hypertrophy of the prostate gland. Beyond this it requires no description here. The detail of its anatomy belongs to the prostate rather than to the urethra, and is therefore better classified under that title.

Length.—The length of the urethra, varying as it does in different individuals and in the same individual with erection of the penis and hypertrophy of the prostate, may be set down as averaging 20.5 cm. ($8\frac{1}{4}$ inches),[1] and varying in different normal individuals

[1] Keyes, *loc. cit.*

from 18 to 23 cm. ($7\frac{1}{4}$ to $8\frac{3}{4}$ inches). The posterior urethra is usually 5.5 cm. ($2\frac{1}{4}$ inches) long—2.5 cm. (1 inch) to the membranous portion, 3 cm. ($1\frac{1}{4}$ inches) to the prostatic—and the anterior urethra 15 cm. (6 inches) long, subdivided as follows: 2.5 cm. (1 inch) to the navicular region, 6.25 cm. ($2\frac{1}{2}$ inches) to the penile, 3 cm. ($1\frac{1}{4}$ inches) to the scrotal, and 3 cm. ($1\frac{1}{4}$ inches) to the bubo-perineal.

Diameter.—The diameter of the normal urethra (Fig. 5) varies even more than the length—it has been estimated at from two to six lines. A fair average is not larger than 0.75 cm. (0.3 inch)—about No. 27 French scale. But, whatever its size, the urethra is not a tube of uniform calibre from end to end. It has naturally four points of physiological narrowing: the first at the meatus; the second at the peno-navicular junction; the third beginning about half an inch back of this, and becoming most pronounced at about the peno-scrotal junction. The fourth and fifth constrictions are the voluntary sphincter—namely, the entire membranous urethra—and the internal orifice of the prostatic urethra. Of these five narrow points, three, it will be observed, are organic and situated in the anterior urethra, while the other two are muscular and situated in the posterior urethra. The muscular constrictions are widely dilatable, and the calibre of the canal is determined by the meatus, normally the narrowest point. Hence, *the calibre of the urethra is the calibre of its normal meatus* —a rule of great importance in the dilatation of the urethra, and which will be explained farther on. (See Stricture of the Meatus.) The peno-navicular and peno-scrotal constrictions are usually mere irregularities in the canal, besides which there are often lesser contractions at various points, making the urethra, when distended, not a smooth, evenly calibrated tube, but a very irregular one. The three chief *dilatations* of the normal canal are the fossa navicularis (so called from its supposed resemblance to a boat), which is situated just inside the meatus; the bulbous urethra, occupying a position immediately in front of the triangular ligament; and the prostatic urethra (prostatic sinus, Fig. 5). Of these the second is the largest.

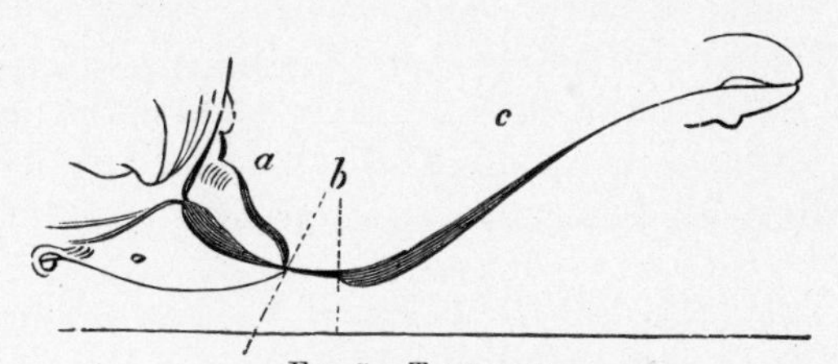

Fig. 5.—Thompson.
a, *b*, and *c* represent the prostatic, membranous, and spongy portions of the urethra.

Curve.—In relation to these variations of calibre Guyon's observations upon the relative qualities of the urethral roof and floor are of interest far more from a practical than from a theoretical point of view.[1] His observations may be classified as follows:

I. The roof of the urethra (when the penis is erect) forms an uninterrupted curve from the fossa navicularis to the bladder.

II. All the variations of calibre, except the fossa navicularis, are produced at the expense of the floor, which is, in consequence, very irregular.[2]

III. The mucous membrane of the roof is more closely adherent to the subjacent structures than that of the floor.

IV. The mucous membrane of the floor of the urethra is much more elastic than that of the roof.

Therefore, not only is the floor of the urethra more irregular than the roof, but its irregularities may be increased with much greater facility by any object introduced into the canal, as well as by disease. In other words, instruments, especially if small and rigid, may, with their points, furrow the floor of the urethra until, finally, they become pocketed (usually in the bulb), and so are brought to a full stop, while an instrument whose point impinges always on the roof avoids these obstructions and glides easily into the bladder. Therefore this eminent French surgeon has termed the roof the surgical wall of the urethra—the wall, namely, which is the guide to the instrument in entering the bladder. That fistulæ and false passages always occur in the floor and lateral walls, never (practically) in the roof, and that the orifice of a stricture is usually nearer the roof than the floor—these two facts make the roof the surgical wall in disease even more than in health.

THE CURVE OF URETHRAL INSTRUMENTS

From these considerations it follows that *the curve of the urethra is the curve of its roof*. Now the entire anterior urethra is freely movable with the penis, and can be made to assume any curve. Not so the posterior canal. The membranous urethra, bound tightly at its extremities by the two layers of the triangular ligament, is the real fixed point of the urethra, and runs at a distance of from 1 to 2 cm. ($\frac{2}{5}$ to $\frac{4}{5}$ inch) below the symphysis pubis. In front of this the bulbous urethra tends slightly upward because of the tension of the suspensory ligament and of the skin and fascia, while a similar elevation is given to the pros-

---

[1] *Op. cit.*, ii, 309 *et seq.*

[2] Though not absolutely accurate, these two observations are clinically correct.

tatic urethra behind by the pubo-prostatic ligaments and the anterior fibres of the levator ani muscles. Thus is formed the so-called fixed curve of the urethra—not a true fixed curve, for by depression of the bulbous and the prostatic urethra to the level of the membranous portion it can be, and often is, transformed into a straight line, as when a sound is pushed home until its shaft is in line with the patient's body, or when straight metal instruments are introduced. (This latter proceeding, sometimes difficult, often painful, is never absolutely necessary.) The curve varies slightly with different persons, and in the same person at different periods of life, being shorter and sharper in the child, longer in the old man. A distended bladder or an enlarged prostate lengthens the curve.

The proper average curve, as recognised by Sir Charles Bell and insisted on by Sir Henry Thompson—the one which will mathematically accord with the greatest number of urethræ—is that of a circle 8.125 cm. in diameter; and the proper length of arc of such a circle, to represent the subpubic curve, is that subtended by a chord 6.875 cm. long.[1] An instrument made with a short curve of this sort will readily

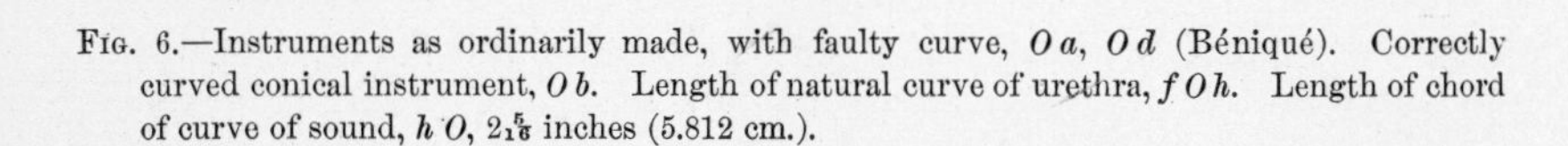

FIG. 6.—Instruments as ordinarily made, with faulty curve, *O a*, *O d* (Béniqué). Correctly curved conical instrument, *O b*. Length of natural curve of urethra, *f O h*. Length of chord of curve of sound, *h O*, $2\frac{5}{16}$ inches (5.812 cm.).

find its way through the normal urethra into the bladder without the employment of any force. It is very desirable that instruments in-

[1] In the winter of 1852–'53, assisted by the late Dr. Isaacs, I made a series of careful experiments upon sections of frozen subjects, as well as by injecting the urethra with numerous substances afterward carefully cutting out the casts. I found the average curve to be identical with the one given above.—VAN BUREN.

tended for habitual use should be so constructed,[1] inasmuch as many of the difficulties of catheterism are due to a defective curve in the instrument employed. The defect most frequently encountered is too great straightness of the last half inch—a deviation of the curve at its most important point. In an instrument properly made (Fig. 6) it will be found that a tangent to the axis of the curve *at its extremity* will intersect the projected axis of the shaft at a little less than a right angle (*n k h*). If the curve comprised only a quarter of the circle, the tangent would meet the projected shaft at a right angle (*m g h*); but instruments made a little longer, as they are usually found, invariably have the *last part of the curve* tilted off into a faulty direction, as shown in Fig. 6, making the angle between a tangent to the axis of the curve at this point and the projected axis of the shaft obtuse (*l j h*), and falling within the right angle.

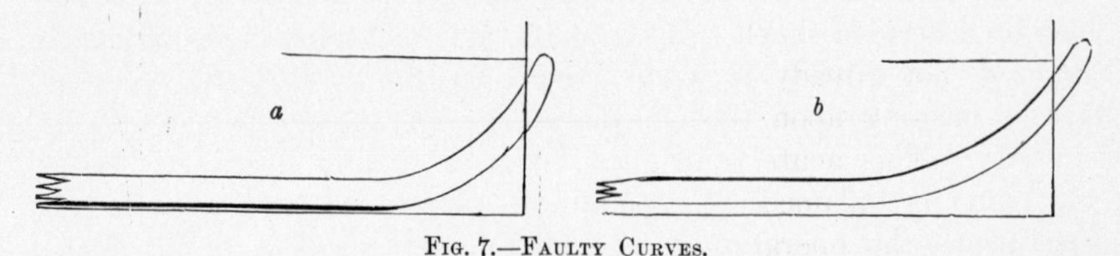

Fig. 7.—Faulty Curves.

Fig. 7, *a* and *b*, represent faulty curves, still occasionally encountered in instruments. Fig. 8 shows the correct curve.

It is better to prolong the curve around the circle, and even to slightly *decrease* that of the terminal quarter of an inch, as instruments so made cling more tenaciously to the roof of the canal, and the point is, for all practical purposes, still at right angles to the shaft, and 4.375 cm. from it. A knowledge of this relative position and direction of the point is of great importance in difficult catheterism. A moderately short curve is as good as a long one, provided it is accurate; indeed better, for when the instrument is made with the full length of curve, $\frac{3}{10}$ of the circle, its point is so far from the shaft that it is sure to wabble when it encounters an obstruction. This objection is all the more applicable to the Béniqué instrument (Fig. 6, *dho*) on account of its having a posterior as well as an anterior curve. This wabbling is not of

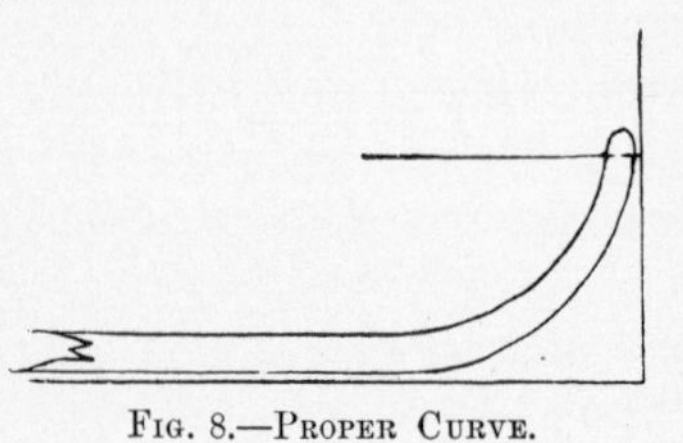

Fig. 8.—Proper Curve.

[1] An instrument destined for habitual use *by the patient* is sometimes made half an inch short in the curve, on account of the greater facility of its introduction through the pendulous urethra.

serious importance in the healthy canal, but it is very distracting to the surgeon when a tight stricture is to be entered. Here the short conical point, at right angles to the shaft, is vastly superior on account of steadiness, and is equally certain to follow the urethral curve accurately.

PHYSIOLOGY OF THE URETHRA

Sensibility.—Under normal conditions the sensibility of the anterior urethra is slight, although it is exquisitely sensitive when inflamed. The prostatic urethra is practically insensitive, while the membranous portion of the canal is always somewhat sensitive. Indeed, the first passage of an instrument through this part of the urethra of a nervous individual is attended not only by pain but also by a decided shock. He becomes pale and nauseated, may even faint, if not already in a recumbent position; while the recorded deaths ensuing upon this simple maneuvre, though few, attest its severity. This acute sensibility becomes rapidly deadened, unless the canal is inflamed by repeated soundings, so that after a few repetitions the operation is attended by no shock and but little, if any pain.

This urethral shock is an important element in many cases of so-called urinary fever, yet rarely the sole cause of death, but often contributory by its reflex action upon enfeebled kidneys, and usually tingeing the frankly septic cases with a neurotic element not otherwise to be explained. Moreover, it contributes to the elucidation of the mystery of urethral neuralgia and urethral spasm, and is doubtless concerned in the explanation of the fact that the form of septicemia known as urinary fever, so common after injury to the deeper portions of the canal—namely, the bulbous and the membranous urethra—becomes less and less to be feared the farther forward the injury, and is unheard of when the trauma affects only the balanitic portion of the canal.

Mobility.—The *muscles* of the penis and urethra are thrown into action only during urination or erection and emission, and their functions are therefore more fitly described under these titles. A few words concerning the cut-off muscle may not be amiss in this place. Besides its most important function of preventing the urine from escaping from the bladder by an effort of the will and of cutting off the stream, it presents several interesting physiological characteristics. It has been stated that the urethra in front of the cut-off muscle swarms with bacteria, while all beyond is germ-free. This is so not because the muscle presents an impassable barrier, for it does not. When violently contracted it doubtless does form an insurmountable barrier to bacterial invasion, but its periods of contraction, like those of the external sphincter ani—to which it bears a close resemblance—are comparatively infrequent and of short duration. Its normal tone, however, is sufficient to make the channel a narrow and difficult one, readily cleansed of any chance invader by the periodical outflow of urine. This irrigation is only of secondary importance, for no infection occurs by this route when the stream of urine is diverted through a suprapubic fistula; but the rapid multiplication of bacteria in the anterior urethra under these circumstances demands an occasional flushing of the canal to check the increase of its prolific population. It is suggestive, moreover, that the cut-off muscle surrounds the most sensitive part of the urethra. Hence the cause of spasm in this muscle, whether acute from some local or general shock, or chronic as a specific evidence of a neurotic habit, is not far to seek.

URETHRAL AND SEXUAL HYGIENE

Before passing to the morbid conditions of the urethra its hygiene in health and in disease demands consideration.

In order that the urethra may be in a healthful state, able to get well if diseased, and then to remain well, two points must be observed. They comprise fully the hygiene of the canal. They are:

(1) That the urine be non-irritating in character.

(2) That sexual excitability be quieted.

(1) Urine, to be non-irritating, must be normal, faintly acid, or neutral, free from sharp crystals, and not too concentrated. Hence measures tending to bring the fluid to this state are hygienic. These include general hygiene of the skin, stomach, muscles, lungs, etc., but also in many cases (especially where the subject is of gouty habit) certain dietetic precautions. The latter consist in the avoidance of all alcoholic fluids, especially sweet fermented wines and malt liquors. New ale is particularly harmful. All of these substances tend to create sharp crystals of uric acid in the urine as well as to concentrate and acidify it. From this cause alone inflammation of the urethra may spring. Lemon-juice is also somewhat irritating to the urethra, as are, to a mild degree, all the condiments—salt, pepper, mustard—and, it is said, asparagus. In inflamed conditions of the canal, general hygiene prescribes rest.

(2) The quieting of sexual excitability is an object not less important, but far more difficult to accomplish. No part of the body can be in perfect health unless its function is being regularly

and satisfactorily performed. This is seen in stomach, brain, muscle, and excretory duct. For example, when all the urine escapes from the urethra, through a large fistula in the perineum, the fore part of the canal contracts and becomes hyperesthetic.

The urethra, however, only performs the function of a sexual canal at longer or shorter intervals. If there were no erotic fancies, the urethra would never be called upon to participate in the sexual function, and the latter would have no influence over its health or its disease. In the eunuch the hygiene of the urethra undoubtedly does not include the sexual problem.

If, then, the individual be absolutely pure in thought, word, and deed; if he never has or has had an erotic fancy, direct or remote, then his urethra would be a urinary canal, and its hygiene would be simple. But absolute purity is not a common attribute of man, as any one who has the honesty to accept facts must confess, and the rule that every male adult has more or less strong sexual longings and necessities must be admitted. Hence is established the rule, borne out daily and hourly by intelligent study of the parts concerned, both in health and disease, that the urethra is not in the best conditions for health unless the sexual needs are attended to. There is no possible means of accomplishing this result except marriage. Fornication is always irregular, unnatural, often excessive, and therefore is harmful and worse than nothing, looked at merely from a worldly point of view. Masturbation is degrading, and affects the general health of the individual by ruining his *morale*. Nature's safety-valve, involuntary ejaculation during sleep, is inefficient. Marriage only allows healthy, natural, unstimulated sexual relations, and accomplishes the first necessity of urethral hygiene—namely, sexual quietude. Hence the value of marriage as a curative agent in morbid conditions of the urethra, especially if there be any nervous element in the case—an element almost invariably present in some degree.

In all conditions of acute inflammation, sexual intercourse must be, of course, absolutely interdicted. Excessive indulgence is bad at any time, but worst of all is stimulation without relief. This state is, unhappily, a common one among the unmarried men of large cities. Such individuals, looking at suggestive pictures, reading exciting books, taking part in impure conversation, become ripe subjects for nervous disease of an obscure sort, not only of the urethra but of the whole body. In fact, this undue stimulation, without appropriate relief, is far more often the cause of hypochondria, melancholy, and functional perversion, than is the masturbation to which the public generally ascribe it. Nor can such an individual, by any plan of fornication, escape the evil consequences to which stimulated but ungratified desire exposes him. Marriage with a pure woman may right him—rarely anything short of this. Hence, when a case presents itself where marriage is impossible, or if the patient be already unhappily married, there is but one course left to advise, and that is absolute continence and an effort at purity of thought, with a strict avoidance of all possible temptations to erotic thought or act, whether entering through the mind, the eye, or the ear—whether actual or implied, direct or remote. Could such a patient imitate the heroic example of St. Augustine—a record of which that honest father of the Church has left behind—he would control the hygiene of his urethra, and doubtless save himself much distress in life.

CHAPTER II

MALFORMATIONS OF THE URETHRA

The urethra is subject to arrest and error of development, but is not often seriously deformed. Among curiosities of deformity may be mentioned abnormal position of the meatus on the side of the glans penis; termination of the ejaculatory ducts in a separate canal, running along the dorsum of the penis and opening behind the glans[1] (gonorrhea of this canal has been noted); and termination of the urethra in the groin.[2] Perkowsky [3] found in a well-formed penis, besides the healthy urethra, a second canal opening at the base of the glans above the meatus, and affected with gonorrhea. He split this subcutaneous canal to the symphysis, where it terminated in a blind pouch. Luxardo [4] describes a gonorrheal patient who had three openings at the end of the penis. One gave exit to semen only. The two lower ones appeared to communicate, and both had gonorrhea. E. B. Ward [5] reports three brothers, each with three openings to the urethra, but he does not state whether they communicated, or that one was not a seminal duct. Englisch [6] has reported several cases similar to Perkowsky's. Le Fort [7] has collected and classified the different varieties of fistula of the penis and the so-called double urethra, and shows that the second urethra is always a blind pouch, usually a prolongation of the lacuna magna. In fact, double urethra does not exist, except with double penis.

All these deformities, dependent upon excessive and unnatural development, are exceedingly rare. Deformities caused by a defect of development are more common. Either the canal is obstructed or it is not closed in. In the former case the junctions among the

---

[1] Cruveilhier, Traité d'anatomie descriptive, Paris, 1865, vol. ii, fasc. 1.
[2] Haller, quoted by Pitha, Krankheiten der männlichen Geschlechtsorgane, 1864.
[3] Centralbl. f. Chir., Nr. 50, 1883, 816.
[4] L'Union médicale, No. 54, 1883, 663.
[5] New York Med. Record, September 1, 1883, 251.
[6] Internat. Centralbl. f. d. Phys. u. Path. d. Harn. u. Sex. Org., 1892, iii, 327.
[7] Guyon's Annales, 1896, xiv, 624, 792, 912, and 1095.

various parts of which the canal is formed are incomplete (atresia—congenital stricture); in the latter the closure of the walls is defective (hypospadias—epispadias).

Atresia.—Atresia, commonest at the meatus, may occur at any part of the canal. Indeed, the entire urethra may be replaced by a fibrous cord. The prostatic urethra is never obstructed.[1]

The obstruction is usually but a thin membrane which may be punctured and the orifice kept patent until it heals, after which no further trouble need be anticipated. If, however, the urethra is imperforate for some distance, it may be punctured with a small trocar, but only after the internal segment has been accurately located by external urethrotomy, or, if the membranous urethra is also involved, by suprapubic cystotomy. In these cases the urachus often remains patent, and the patient urinates through it. Removal of the urethral obstruction is soon followed by closure of the urachus. Englisch [2] has furnished a contribution to this subject. The stricture liable to ensue upon puncture of a diaphragm or of a band must be combated by the usual methods. Major surgical procedures are best delayed, if possible, until the patient has attained his sixth or eighth year. Guyon [3] and Demarquay [4] have collated interesting cases. Demarquay's puncture through a band without preliminary perineal opening is too blind a proceeding to be approved.

Congenital Stricture.—Congenital stricture, usually of the meatus, is so common, and has such a direct bearing upon the treatment of the so-called organic stricture, that it will be considered in that connection.

Dilatation of the Urethra.—Bokay [5] has collected 14 cases of congenital urethral diverticula, only 3 of which were due to stricture.

HYPOSPADIAS

Hypospadias is that form of imperfect development of the urethra in which the canal terminates in an opening in its lower wall instead of extending to its normal termination in the end of

[1] Mercier's *valvule de la vessie,* which he claimed to be a common cause of obstruction at the neck of the bladder, appears to have been either contracture of the vesical neck or hypertrophy of the prostate. Guyon, once a stanch supporter of the *valvule* theory, has so far modified his opinion as to admit that he has seen the valve demonstrated post mortem only six times, and has known it to cause symptoms but once. (*Op. cit.,* iii, 151.)

[2] Arch. f. Kinderheilk., 1881, ii, 85 and 291.

[3] Des vices de conformation de l'urètre chez l'homme, etc. Thèse de Paris, 1863.

[4] Maladies chirurgicales du pénis, 1877, p. 581.

[5] Dermatolog. Zeitschr., 1900, vii, 721.

the glans penis. There are three degrees of hypospadias: 1. *balanitic hypospadias*, in which the urethra opens on the lower surface of the glans or at the peno-balanitic junction; 2, *penile hypospadias* (peno-scrotal and scrotal hypospadias), in which the canal opens on the under surface of the penile urethra, or more often at the peno-scrotal angle; and (3) *perineal hypospadias*, in which the urethra terminates in front of the triangular ligament and opens in the perineum. Thus hypospadias always occurs in front of the cut-off muscle, and, no matter how extensive it may be, the patient always has control over the escape of urine.

Hypospadias at the peno-scrotal angle is more common than the perineal variety, and most frequent of all is hypospadias confined to the glans penis or to its immediate vicinity. That part of the urethra lying between a hypospadial opening and the meatus is usually absent or impervious, but may be patulous for a short distance in front of the opening on the floor of the urethra, or even up to the meatus. Hypospadias, as commonly encountered in practice, consists in an absence of the frenum preputii and a flaring open of the meatus inferiorly, or an opening in the floor of the canal within a few lines of the natural meatus, the position of which latter is usually marked more or less perfectly in its usual site. The glans penis may be bifid. The urethral orifice in hypospadias is small as a rule. With penile hypospadias there is usually some downward curvature of the penis, and not infrequently adhesion of the penis to the scrotum. The under surfaces of the corpora cavernosa are not developed, the fibrous sheath of the penis is thickened and too short beneath, so that the condition may be called one of permanent physiological chordee. The penis, freed of all cutaneous and urethral attachments, cannot be straightened until the fibrous sheaths of both corpora have been transversely incised beneath, and sometimes not then until the fibrous septum has been incised. The penis, usually small, is sometimes completely buried in the scrotum. With perineal (sometimes called scrotal) hypospadias the scrotum is bifid, and the penis is usually very imperfectly developed, imperforate, and looks like a large clitoris. The bifid scrotum passes very well for a vulva, and in this way some of the so-called hermaphrodites are formed, the true sex perhaps only being discovered after adult age is reached.

Etiology.—Hypospadias is usually regarded as a simple arrest of development in a portion of the lower wall of the urethra, its lateral halves failing to unite in the median line. In favour of this view are the manifest hereditary tendency to this deformity seen in some cases, and the fact that at two months the embryo has hypospadias normally. The scrotum has not yet united, and if natural development ceases here the last degree of hypospadias results. It may be urged that this theory does not explain the incurvation of the penis, nor its adhesion to the scrotum, nor the scar-like contracted appearance of the orifice. To explain these facts Kaufmann[1] advances the theory that hypospadias and epispadias are examples of congenital fistula dependent upon imperfect union of the penile and the balanitic urethra. These two portions of the canal, it is known, are developed separately, and if imperfectly approximated atresia at the peno-balanitic junction may result. Now Kaufmann supposes that the urine secreted by the fetus may break either through the obstruction, leaving congenital fistula, or through the floor of the canal, producing hypospadias, or through its roof, thus causing epispadias. Even supposing that this theory explains incurvation and adhesion (which it does after a fashion), it can scarcely explain malposition of the urethra in epispadias, or exstrophy of the bladder, with non-union of the symphysis pubis—phenomena so closely related to epispadias that no theory which does not elucidate them can be invoked to account for the urethral deformity. And why, moreover, does not the urine find a free vent through the urachus as it does when the urethra remains closed? In short, Kaufmann's theory, though ingenious, is insufficient.

Symptoms.—Balanitic hypospadias is unimportant; many patients have it without being aware of the fact, while the greatest inconvenience it produces is a slight imperfection in erection and a dribbling at the end of urination. With penile or perineal hypospadias, however, the patient may be forced to urinate in a squatting posture to keep from wetting himself, erection may be very imperfect, and there may be impotence from inability to throw the semen into the vagina. An associated inconvenience is the necessity of enlarging the contracted meatus, in order to introduce dilating instruments, in case of stricture.

Treatment.—For *balanitic hypospadias* no treatment is actually necessary unless a meatotomy to permit the introduction of instruments into the urethra. Kaufmann suggests that a triangular skin-flap be sutured into the orifice to maintain its calibre, but I have found this unnecessary. If, however, the patient demands that his urethral orifice be brought forward to its natural position, one of two operations may be selected. The accepted method is that of Duplay:[2] if the glans is deeply furrowed the edges of the furrow are simply denuded of epithelium and sutured together. Usually,

---

[1] Deutsche Chirurgie, L. a., 60. [2] Arch. gén. de méd., 1874, mai et juin.

though, the groove must be deepened by one vertical or two lateral diverging incisions. The edges are sutured over a small (12 French) soft-rubber catheter, and both the sutures and the instrument removed at the end of the week. After the wound has healed firmly, the new balanitic urethra is united to the penile portion of the canal

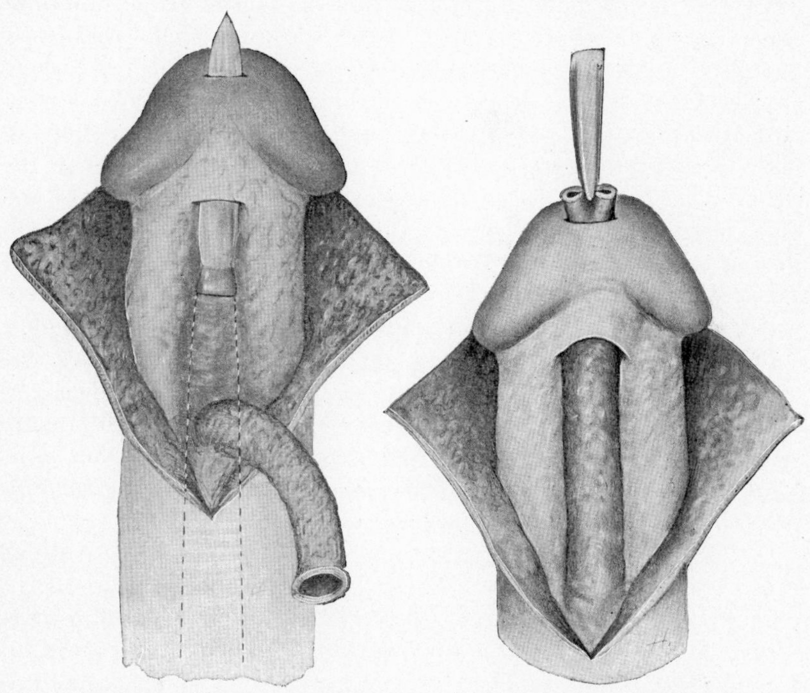

Fig. 9.—Beck's Operation for Balanitic Hypospadias.
Liberation of the urethra—puncture of the glans.

Fig. 10.—Beck's Operation for Balanitic Hypospadias.
The urethra drawn through the glans.

by freshening the edges and by direct suture, preferably over a retained catheter, or after an external perineal urethrotomy to divert the stream of urine from the wound. Recently Beck[1] has cured three cases by freeing the urethra, bringing it forward and suturing it to an orifice punched through the glans (Fig. 9). The urethra must be freed well back and sutured to the apex of the glans to prevent incurvation (Figs. 9, 10, and 11). This is a much simpler expedient than Duplay's, and is commendable, since the formation of a fistula—which is the bane of the older operation—is avoided, and the sutures usually hold.

[1] N. Y. Med. J., 1898, lxvii, 148; *ibid.*, 1900, lxxii, 969.

For *penile hypospadias* the operations are many and various. Certain preliminary steps are necessary in almost all cases.

First, the penis must be freed from its scrotal adhesions. If these are slight, a transverse incision through the peno-scrotal frenum will, when sutured in a longitudinal direction, suffice to free the organ. But if the penis is deeply buried in the scrotum the integument of the former must be derived from the latter with regard only to covering in the penis; the scrotum will, by virtue of its looseness, adapt itself to the loss of almost any amount of skin.

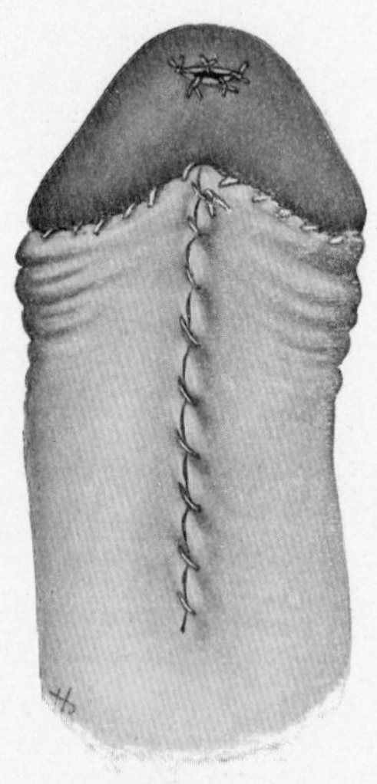

Fig. 11.—Beck's Operation for Balanitic Hypospadias. Suture.

Secondly, the incurvation of the body of the penis often demands attention. This may be corrected through the liberating incision. A transverse incision is carefully made through the whole thickness of the sheath of the corpora cavernosa on its under surface, care being taken to avoid the erectile tissue. This is usually sufficient to permit straightening the penis. If not, the intercavernous septum may require division down to the dorsum. Then the penis is forcibly straightened and snugly bandaged about a slight splint in an overextended position to prevent recontracture. I can vouch from personal experience for the satisfactory results obtainable by this somewhat violent procedure. If the penis is kept straight until entirely healed it may be anticipated that subsequent erections will be complete and direct.

Finally comes the most delicate part of the treatment—the extension, namely, of the urethra to its proper length. This is done in two stages: First, the new urethra is built, and then it is joined to the old canal. Great ingenuity has been displayed in the formation of the new canal. The operation of Duplay is preferred by most surgeons, though the methods of Thiersch [1] (an adaptation of his operation for epispadias), Dieffenbach,[2] Dolbeau,[3] Laurent,[4] and Van Hook [5] also deserve mention. In each of these the lining membrane of the new canal is derived, in one way or another, by flaps turned in

---

[1] Arch. für Heilk., 1868, x, 20.
[2] Gaz. méd. de Paris, 1837, 156.
[3] De l'épispadias . . . et son traitement, Paris, 1861.
[4] Bull. de l'acad. de méd. belg., 1895, iv, ix, 685.
[5] *Cf.* Mayo, J. Am. Med. Ass'n, 1901, xxxvi, 1157.

from the adjoining regions. That each has been devised to supplement the older ones is an evidence—to which the surgeon who has tried any will certainly testify—of how rarely they succeed and how utterly baffling they all are. A more recent operation, based upon an entirely different principle, promises so well that I venture to refer the reader seeking for details of the earlier operations to the original monographs or to any of the current text-books, while I describe only this one of Nové-Josserand,[1] prefacing that the restoration of the urethra, whatever the method employed, should not be attempted until the wounds made in straightening the penis have entirely healed.

Through a transverse incision 2 cm. long and just in front of the hypospadic meatus, a stout probe is introduced and passed forward along the under surface of the penis, in the subcutaneous connective tissue, until it reaches the base of the glans, elevating the skin from the entire under surface of the penis. The anterior orifice of the canal is then formed by slitting up the under surface of the glans, or by puncturing it with a trocar. To obtain an epithelial lining for this canal—and herein consists the originality of the operation—an Ollier[2] skin-graft, 4 cm. wide and considerably longer than the intended canal, is taken from the inner side of the thigh, where there are no hairs, and wrapped, inside out, around a woven catheter, 21 French in size, and held in place by a ligature at each end and one or two sutures, all of 00 catgut. (Rochet[3] has improved the operation by employing, instead of the Ollier graft, a flap taken from the scrotum, with its base at the abnormal urethral orifice. This device eliminates the fistula between the old urethra and the new (Figs. 12, 13).) The catheter thus covered is then inserted into the canal, and when the graft is in place the anterior ligature is cut and removed, and the edge of the graft sutured to the glans penis. The catheter is then cut off short so that each end barely protrudes from the canal, and a snug dressing is applied with the penis held in the erect position. A retained catheter is used to draw off the urine. (In the Rochet operation the catheter around which the graft is wrapped is used as a retained catheter.) On the eighth day the posterior ligature is cut and the sound removed. Five days later the daily passage of sounds is

---

[1] Lyon méd., 1897, lxxxiv, 237, and Revue de chir., 1898, xviii, 333.

[2] The Ollier graft, the only one, as far as I know, yet used for this operation, differs from the Thiersch graft only in that it is made as thick as possible without including any of the subcutaneous tissue, instead of—as in the Thiersch method—as thin as possible.

[3] Guyon's Annales, 1900, xviii, 648.

begun, and this is continued for two or three weeks to prevent contracture of the graft.

This operation has been performed three times, twice by Nové-Josserand and upon one patient after Duplay's method had been tried and had failed. The first operation was a success, but a 15

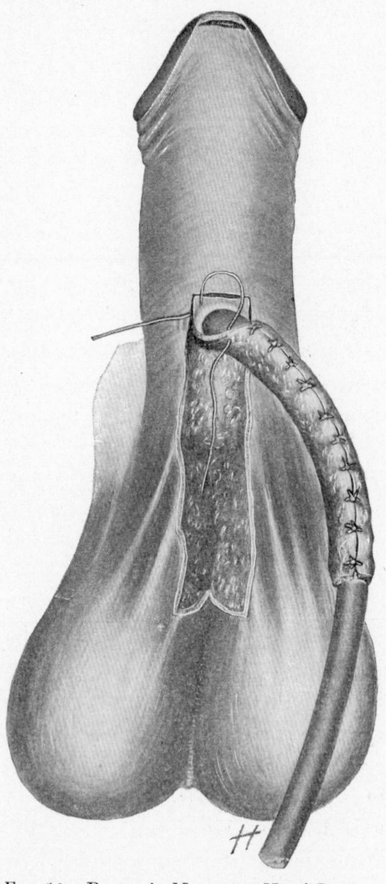

FIG. 12.—ROCHET'S MODIFIED NOVÉ-JOSSERAND OPERATION FOR HYPOSPADIAS.

The flaps are cut, the catheter introduced, the scrotal flap sutured around it.

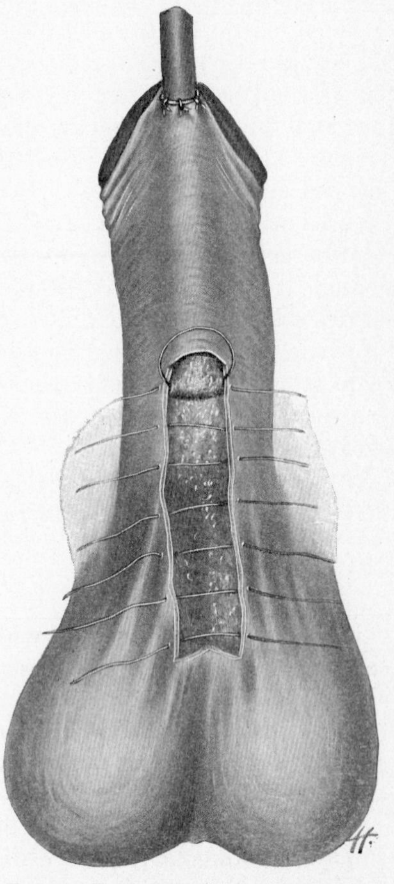

FIG. 13.—ROCHET'S MODIFIED NOVÉ-JOSSERAND OPERATION FOR HYPOSPADIAS.

The final sutures.

French catheter had been used, and the surgeon, being dissatisfied with the calibre of the resultant canal, simply repeated the operation, using a larger catheter. Tuffier [1] has also operated successfully. No failure has been reported.

[1] Guyon's Annales, 1899, xvii, 370.

The canal produced by this operation is devoid of a corpus spongiosum, and will therefore always allow some dribbling after ejaculation or emission; but this annoyance is slight compared to that of a peno-scrotal hypospadias.

After the formation of the new canal there still remains the most difficult task of all—namely, the junction of the natural and the artificial portions of the urethra. (This is not required in the Rochet operation.) This, the simplest in the chain of operations, is the one most likely to fail, for the urine tends to infiltrate the suture line and thus to perpetuate the fistula. The operative steps are simple. The adjoining extremities of the new and the old canal are denuded and sutured together over a small soft-rubber catheter (12 French) with silver wire or silk. The catheter is retained in place —with the usual precautions (p. 210)—and all the urine drawn through it until union is complete, after which both catheter and sutures are removed. If union is incomplete because of urinary infiltration, the fistula must be allowed to heal perfectly before it is again attacked by the same method, or, if small, its complete occlusion may be encouraged by injections of peroxid of hydrogen (p. 130).

For *perineal hypospadias* the same treatment is indicated as for the penile or peno-scrotal deformities.

EPISPADIAS

Epispadias (*επι, above*; *σπαζω, I separate*) is a fissure of the superior wall of the urethra with ectopia of the canal (Guyon). It is extremely rare. According to Baron[1] epispadias occurs once for 150 cases of hypospadias, but Marshall did not find a single case of epispadias in examining 60,000 conscripts.[2] The epispadias may be balanitic or penile, or the urethra may be entirely laid open. This complete epispadias is almost always accompanied by exstrophy of the bladder, and will be considered in that connection. A case of complete epispadias, without exstrophy, is figured by Dolbeau.[3] The epispadiac orifice is large, and sometimes the finger may even be passed through it into the bladder. The prepuce forms a knob of loose tissue below the glans. The penis is short and thick, or small and more or less deviated. It is usually adherent to the

---

[1] Dolbeau, *op. cit.*, p. 11.

[2] Englisch (Bull. méd., Paris, 1895, ix, 153) has reported a case of complete separation of the penis into lateral halves, each corpus cavernosum forming a penis by itself, and the urethra opening between them.

[3] *Op. cit.*, Plate III.

scrotum, sometimes practically buried in it. The pubic bones may be separated even when there is no exstrophy of the bladder, and there may be hernia of that organ without exstrophy.

Etiology.—The observations made upon the etiology of hypospadias apply equally well to this condition. Epispadias is certainly an arrest of development in the upper wall of the urethra, but it is still a matter of hypothesis how the urethra gets above the united corpora cavernosa; for even when the genital buds which are to form the corpora cavernosa are still separate at the fortieth day of fetal life, the urethra is beneath them. However, the fact remains that the urethra gets above the corpora cavernosa and fails to unite in its upper wall, the corpora cavernosa effecting their faulty union none the less. With exstrophy of the bladder, where the lower portion of the abdominal wall is lacking and the pubic bones do not come together, it is easier to understand how the roof of the urethra may be wanting throughout.

Symptoms.—The symptoms consist in the functional derangement of micturition, erection, and emission, as in hypospadias; but it is to be noted that incontinence of urine, which never complicates hypospadias, is usually the main feature of severe cases of epispadias, and this cries out for operation more loudly and incessantly than even the most aggravated symptoms of hypospadias. Unfortunately, it is precisely here where operations are most in demand that they are most difficult.

Treatment.—For the milder cases, uncomplicated by the loss of sphincter power, the counsel to bear their woes patiently is a good one. The methods hitherto employed to relieve this condition—even the favoured procedures of Thiersch and Duplay—are tedious and fraught with failures. Thiersch estimates the minimum of time required for the different stages of his operation at three months and a half—a sufficiently dreary prospect. In view, however, of the success of the Nové-Josserand operation for hypospadias, I should be tempted to try it for simple penile epispadias. In addition to the changes obviously necessary to adapt the operation to epispadias it would be necessary to divert the stream of urine by ureteral catheterism, and it might seem advisable to connect the new and the old urethra by continuing the graft into the outer extremity of the epispadic urethra previously denuded. I see no reason why the Nové-Josserand operation should not succeed when thus applied to the upper surface of the penis as well as it has undoubtedly succeeded on the opposite side of that organ. The unsatisfactory plastic operations of Thiersch and Duplay need not delay us.

When the sphincter is lost it cannot be replaced. If there is exstrophy of the bladder, that deformity requires attention (p. 336). Without exstrophy the Nové-Josserand operation might succeed; but probably a modification of one of the urinals adapted to the more severe deformity will give the patient greater comfort than any operation, unless it be Maydl's (p. 498).

The complicating adhesions, torsion or flexion of the penis, must be dealt with here, as in hypospadias, by liberating incisions of the skin and the sheaths of the cavernous bodies.

CHAPTER III

CATHETERS AND CATHETERIZATION

Catheterization, broadly speaking, is the introduction of an instrument through the urethra into the bladder; strictly speaking, however, catheterization is the introduction of a *catheter*—viz., that particular kind of a hollow instrument which, having an opening at each end, is used to introduce fluids into, or evacuate them from, the bladder or upper urinary organs.

A *sound*, on the contrary, is an imperforate urethral instrument, and has no connection with the introduction or evacuation of fluids.[1] A *bougie* is a flexible sound.

Scales.—The scale for grading the calibre of urethral instruments was first accurately fixed in France, where two scales are at present in use—the Charrière (commonly known as the French scale) and the Béniqué. Other scales are the English and the American.

Of late years the tendency in this country, as well as in England, has been to adopt the French scale as the most convenient, while in France itself there is a tendency to replace the old French (Charrière) by the new Béniqué scale. Although Dr. Van Buren, senior author of the first edition of this work, was very tenacious of the American scale—which indeed was born in his office—the almost universal adoption of the French scale since his time has led me, in subsequent editions, to drop the American in favour of the French scale.

The French (Charrière) scale indicates diameters in $\frac{1}{3}$ mm. No. 1 has a diameter of $\frac{1}{3}$ mm., No. 2 a diameter of $\frac{2}{3}$ mm., and so on. From this scale, therefore, the diameter of an instrument may be determined by dividing its number by 3. A No. 30 sound has a diameter of 30 mm. $\div$ 3 = 10 mm.

The Béniqué scale indicates diameters in $\frac{1}{6}$ mm. It numbers in-

[1] To the French all urethral instruments are *sondes*, and the verb *sonder* means to catheterize in the broadest sense.

struments twice as high, therefore, as the Charrière. A No. 30 French sound is a No. 60 Béniqué. $B. + F. \times 2.$

The American scale indicates diameters in $\frac{1}{2}$ mm. Thus its numbers are $\frac{2}{3}$ as high as the French. $30\ F. = 60\ B. = 20\ A.$ $A. = F. (1 - \frac{1}{3}) = \frac{2}{3}\ F.$

The English scale follows no rule, but its numbers are generally about 2 less than the American. Thus, $30\ F. = 60\ B. = 20\ A. = 18\ E.$ $E. = A. - 2 = \frac{2}{3}\ F. - 2.$

The best scale-plate I know of is the one furnished with a triangular slot so marked as to give the sizes in the English, American, and French numbers for any instrument, and also marked off in inches and millimetres upon one edge (Fig. 14). It is essential to the surgeon's armamentarium in the state of confusion in numbering urethral instruments which still prevails in this country.

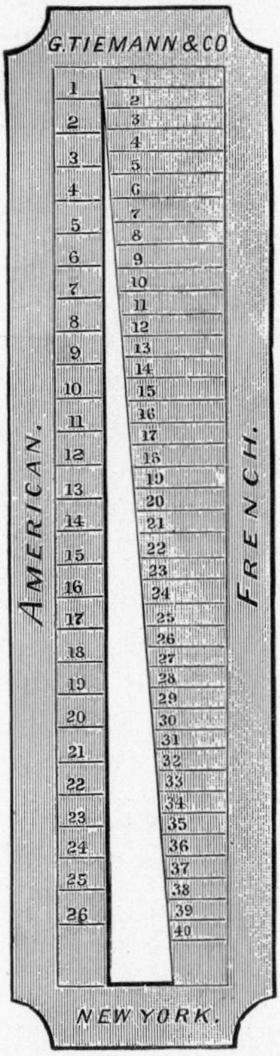

Fig. 14.

The Instrument.—Rigid urethral instruments are made of silver or of nickeled steel. Flexible ones are of rubber or of woven silk coated with wax or varnish: these woven instruments are less flexible than the rubber ones. There are also small whalebone instruments, which on account of their tenuity are called filiform.

The *qualities* essential to a good urethral instrument are:

1. Smoothness,
2. Sterilizability, and
3. Durability.

For sounds external smoothness suffices. For catheters the eye should be depressed so as not to scrape the mucous membrane, and the interior must be smooth and free from pockets so as to submit readily to mechanical cleansing. Not only, therefore, should it be as smooth inside as outside, but also its lumen should terminate in the eye and not in a pocket beyond the eye, wherefore the ordinary catheter, with its eye a little distance from the tip, should have a solid end.

The sterilization of catheters is most effectively and conveniently accomplished by boiling. Metal, rubber, and whalebone instruments all may be boiled satisfactorily. The only instrument that rebels is the woven one. This is the one point of inferiority in that excellent class of instruments, and it bids fair to be soon overcome. Several French makers have already attained the ideal. Their woven instruments may be boiled with impunity. No doubt others will soon follow the example set.

The durability of catheters is essential from an economic point of view, and in order to minimize their liability to become rough or to break off in the bladder. Woven catheters are the least durable, and are likely to stick together in warm weather, unless kept segregated and in a cool place, or covered with French chalk.

Detailed descriptions of the various urethral instruments are deferred to those chapters which explain their uses.

Preparation of the Instrument.—To be ready for use in the urethra an instrument must be smooth, clean, and slippery. Metal instruments are, moreover, usually better borne when warmed.

Smoothness.—This most essential quality has already been noted. It is a quality of the instrument itself, not of its preparation. When an instrument has lost its smoothness it must be discarded. Neither the most careful asepsis nor the most generous lubrication will atone for such a fault.

Cleansing.—The tendency of surgical cleanliness at the present day is to lay less and less stress upon destruction of microbes *in situ* by fire and poison and more and more upon their elimination, together with their toxins, as ordinary dirt, by generous washings and scrubbings; and it is tacitly conceded that sterilizers and drugs shall be used only where scrubbing and washing cannot reach. The genito-urinary surgeon cannot afford to fall behind in this esthetic and scientific advance. Now more than ever before must he be scrupulously clean in his person, his appointments, and his instruments no less. Every instrument should be made to shine both inside and outside immediately after as well as before using. A rubbing down with hot soap and water and drying with a clean towel in some cases will actually fulfil all the requirements of asepsis for a smooth sound; and for a catheter this need only be supplemented by a thorough irrigation, best accomplished by one who has running water at his command by slipping the end of the catheter on to the faucet and allowing the water to run through it for three minutes. For some cases, I repeat, this will suffice; but such asepsis is not adequate for all cases. We have no right to run an avoidable risk. *To insure the absolute sterility of a catheter it should be boiled for fifteen minutes.*[1] This is an ideal method of sterilizing rubber, whalebone, and the best woven instruments. For the woven instru-

[1] Albarran has shown that this suffices to sterilize an instrument already clean, but that half an hour is required to sterilize a dirty instrument.

ments that cannot be boiled, Elsberg's method of catgut sterilization may be employed—i. e., the instrument is boiled in a supersaturated solution of ammonium sulphate, and rinsed clean in sterile water. For metal instruments, however, neither method is ideal. There are two more convenient ways of cleansing them:

1. Pass the instrument slowly through the flame of a Bunsen burner or an alcohol lamp, allowing each part of it to remain long enough in the flame for the evaporation of the water of condensation that appears as it grows warm. Then cool it rapidly by plunging into cold sterile water,[1] or—

2. Pour a few drops of alcohol over the instrument. Be sure that it is entirely covered with the fluid and that there is no drip. Then light the alcohol and let it burn out. This method has its dangers for the carpet.

Many compound instruments—e. g., certain cystoscopes—may not be boiled and must, therefore, be submitted to some chemical cleansing process, of which Janet's formaldehyd method [2] is the best. All of the newer instruments may be boiled.

Lubrication.—The object of lubricating a urethral instrument is *not to make the instrument slippery, but to let it slip through the meatus.* A small dab on each lip of the meatus is all that is needed, and this is best applied, not by greasing the whole shaft of the instrument, but by transferring a bit of lubricant to its tip and with it smearing the lips of the meatus.

There is a great variety of lubricants. Vaselin is practically aseptic, though theoretically susceptible of contamination. It is greasy and unirritating. It has the disadvantage of being insoluble in water, sticking to the instrument, and in cystoscopy of obscuring the field. Olive-oil is not so good as vaselin. Glycerin is not sufficiently greasy. Preferable to any of these is Bangs's solution of Iceland moss sold under the name of lubrichondrin. Guyon uses a mixture of equal parts of water, glycerin, and soap powder. White uses a 33% solution of boro-glycerid.

Preparation of the Patient.—The anterior urethra swarms with germs, and while these are not necessarily pathogenic to the more sensitive mucous membranes beyond, they are likely to be so, and it is by no means impossible in practice to introduce these germs into the bladder on an instrument previously aseptic. Even so, no

---

[1] It is not essential, in the ordinary office manipulations, that the handle of a sound should be aseptic; the handle as well as the surgeon's hands need only be clean in the ordinary sense. Hence the instrument may be manipulated in the flame by holding its handle.

[2] Guyon's Annales, 1896, xiv, 122.

harm may come of it; the microbes may be expelled by the bladder quite as the bacilli of tuberculosis and of typhoid fever may be passed off from a healthy kidney through a healthy bladder without determining any local infection. But let the instrumentation be forced, bruising the delicate mucous membrane, or let there be other predisposing causes of cystitis (which see) at work, and the chances are that the surgeon will rue the day he trusted to the cleanliness of his catheter and took no account of where he used it, or how. Not only does the anterior urethra contain pyogenic bacteria, but these cannot be dislodged from it. The preliminary irrigations in which so many surgeons indulge are futile in principle, though they may succeed in some degree. The experience of years makes me absolutely certain that a preliminary cleansing of the urethra is a useless refinement, unless it is acutely or specifically inflamed, in which case catheterization is practically prohibited (p. 119). *The success of catheterization depends first and above all upon the gentleness and dexterity of the manipulation, and secondarily upon subsequent antisepsis* in order to atone for the necessary defects in preliminary asepsis. The details of this operation are given below.

Technic of Catheterization.—The introduction of a sound, staff, or catheter into the bladder is generally spoken of as catheterization. The use of the staff or sound is sometimes denominated sounding. The maneuvre in either case is the same. Given a canal of certain dimensions and curvature, and an instrument to fit, the problem is to introduce the latter into the former. Nothing is easier, although to perform the operation perfectly is less simple than would at first appear. No amount of instruction, no volumes of directions, can teach the student how to pass the sound. He must learn by doing it first upon the dead then upon the living body. Some suggestions may, however, be given.

Always make the patient lie on his back, with his head on a pillow, his legs slightly separated, his body relaxed, his fears quieted, and himself as comfortable as possible. Both hands should be practised in introducing the sound, and the surgeon should keep his elbow supported during most of the operation, in order that his hand may be more steady. If the right hand is used, the surgeon places himself at the patient's left, and *vice versa*.

To explore the canal, a simple, blunt, steel instrument of medium size (20 French) is selected, and properly warmed. The penis, with foreskin drawn back, is gently encircled by the fingers and thumb of one hand, the instrument held lightly with the tips of three fingers and the thumb of the other. The shaft of the instrument is held over the fold of the groin, its handle nearly in contact with the skin, from which latter (the integument, first of the groin and then of the abdomen) it is not to be removed until the point of the instrument is about to enter the fixed portion of the urethra (membranous). The instrument, at first held along the groin, with point

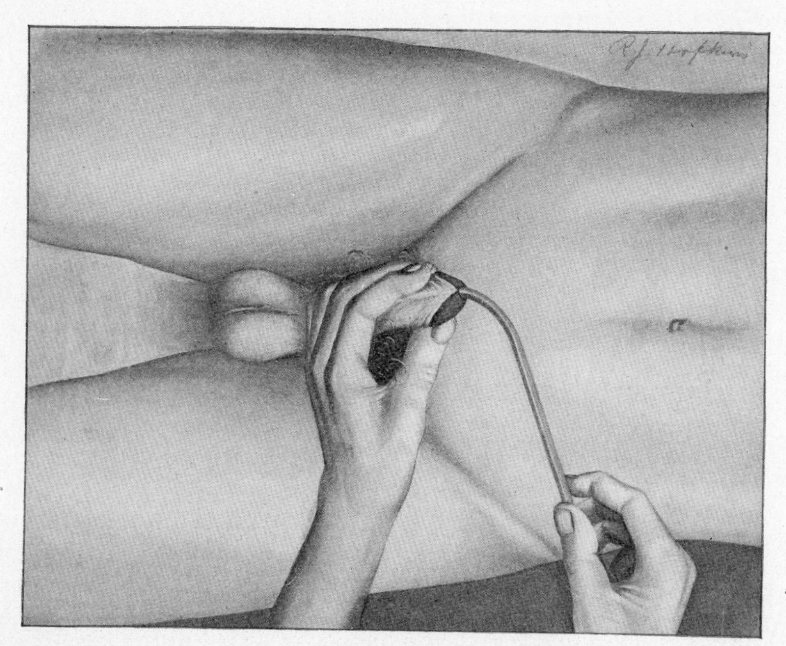

Fig. 15.

high and handle low (Fig. 15), is introduced at the meatus previously lubricated, and the penis moulded up over it. It is not pushed into the urethra, but the urethra is made to swallow the instrument, as it were. When the curve—and perhaps an inch of the shaft—has disappeared within the meatus, the handle of the instrument is swept around over the surface of the belly, so as to lie exactly over the linea alba, parallel with it, and still close to the integument (Fig. 16). The whole shaft of the instrument is now to be gently pressed towards the feet, being still kept close to and parallel with the surface of the belly (the penis, meanwhile, being lightly grasped behind the corona glandis and held steady). The point of the instrument should be followed with the little finger of the hand which manages the penis, and, when it gets fairly past the peno-scrotal angle, the whole scrotum, with the testicles and penis, should be largely seized with the hand and pressed against the pubis, with slight upward traction. The point may now be felt to settle down and adapt itself to the subpubic curve, after which the weight of the instrument, properly directed, should carry it into the bladder.

As soon as the curve lies well against the symphysis, the scrotum, testicles, and penis should be dropped; the hand which held them takes the instrument, steadies it in the median line, and gradually carries the shaft away from the abdomen (Fig. 17), making the handle describe the arc of a circle, and depressing the shaft between the thighs until it lies nearly in the same plane with them. No pushing movement should be imparted to the instrument during this time. The handle is made to describe the arc of a circle, and in a healthy urethra the point cannot go astray. While the instrument is being depressed between the thighs, the free hand is employed in pressing down upon the mons veneris and the root of the penis (Fig. 18), to stretch the suspensory ligament—a point of importance to the easy introduction of an instrument, and one which

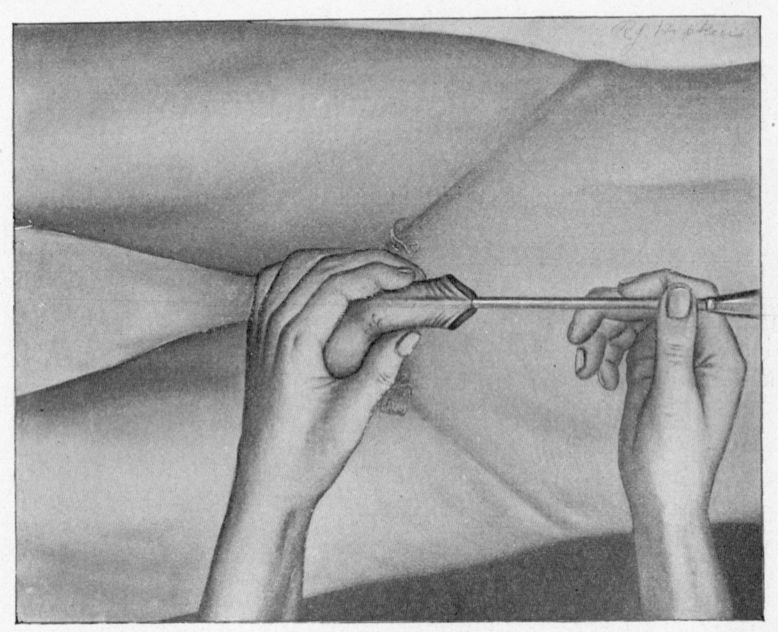

Fig. 16.

supplies to the short curve all the advantages claimed for the longer Béniqué curve. When the instrument is in the bladder, its point may be moved freely from side to side by rotating the handle.

The instrument should be withdrawn with the same deliberation and care with which it is introduced. No traction is needed. The motions used in introduction are simply reversed. The handle of the instrument is lightly caught, and without traction made to describe the arc of a circle until it touches the abdomen over the linea alba. It is then carried around to the groin, and, by a tilting motion, unhooked from the urethra, ending exactly where it commenced along the groin, the handle low, the point high.

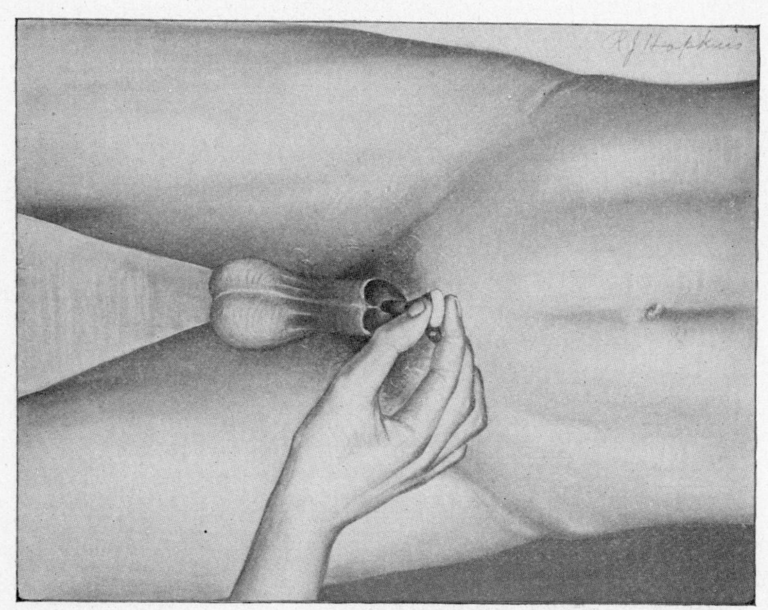

Fig. 17.

The first principle of instrumentation in the urethra is to avoid the use of force. Even in a healthy subject, sometimes, the beak of the instrument will become arrested by pocketing in the floor of the urethra. It is to avoid this that upward traction on the scrotum and penis is made, whereby the beak of the instrument is held in contact with the roof of the urethra, the surgical wall, until it gently slides of its own weight into the bulb and impinges against the triangular ligament. Here the beak of the instrument naturally sinks into the sinus of the bulb, and ceases to advance. Now it is that the operator, by pressing downward the mons veneris, tilts the instrument so that its beak touches the roof of the canal, and slides gently into the membranous urethra, the cut-off muscle relaxing before it. But often the beak is not so readily liberated. That it is still caught in the bulb may be known by the bulging out of its curve in the perineum as the shaft is being depressed between the thighs, and by the rebound of the handle when liberated. The obstacle is overcome by gently maneuvring the point of the instrument, by partial withdrawal and reintroduction, or by slight depression of the beak, then lifting it over the obstacle with a finger in the perineum, at the same time pulling up the point of the instrument to make it sweep the roof of the canal. This will generally render the introduction of a finger into the rectum unnecessary. The dangerous *tour de maître* [1] should never be tried, nor any force used in the manipulations at this point, as a false passage is easily made here and under these very circumstances. The depression of the handle of the instrument alone is capable of exerting enormous power. The sound represents a lever of the first order, and the surgeon has the long arm.

With a little patience a suitable instrument will always pass into the bladder unless there is stricture. When the point has

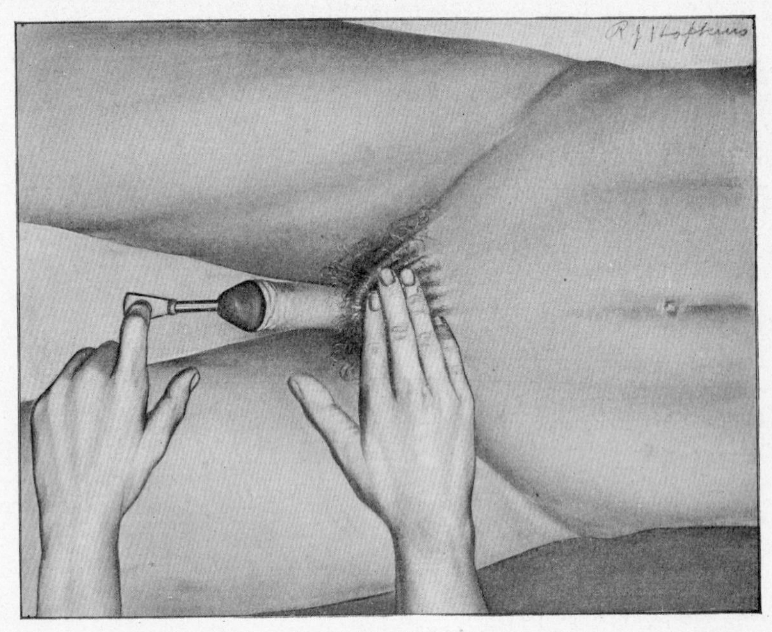

Fig. 18.

traversed the membranous urethra it must continue on freely if the prostate is normal. The so-called spasm of the neck of the bladder does not exist as an obstruction to the passage of instruments.

Instruments small enough to engage in the sinuses of Morgagni

[1] The *tour de maître* consists in introducing a sound with the shaft between the patient's legs until the point is arrested at the bulb; then the handle is rapidly made to describe a semicircle until it reaches a vertical position, when it is at once depressed between the thighs. This is brilliant but dangerous.

are not used in the healthy canal. Instrumentation in morbid conditions will be detailed in connection with the different diseases requiring it.

A *silver catheter* is introduced in the same manner as the sound. In using *soft instruments* without a stylet the penis is slightly pulled upon, so as to efface any circular wrinkles, and the instrument is pushed straight onward into the bladder. If it is arrested, partial withdrawal and rotation during the next forward movement will cause it to pass. One occasionally encounters a spasm of the cut-off muscle that resists prolonged firm pressure by a rubber instrument.

The sensation experienced by a healthy urethra is that of hot points pricking the canal along the part being traversed by the foreign body. As the instrument enters the membranous urethra, a desire to urinate begins to be felt, which increases as the prostate and the neck of the bladder become distended by the instrument, so that the patient sometimes believes the urine is flowing away, in spite of the surgeon's assertions and his own observation to the contrary. Nausea, and even syncope, may occur as the instrument distends the prostate, especially on the first introduction in sensitive young people. Occasionally distention of the prostatic sinus produces a partial erection.

If the patient faints, the instrument should be withdrawn at once and the legs elevated, while the head is hung over the edge of the lounge upon which he lies. The facility with which this may be done, if necessary, is one of the reasons for placing the patient on his back for his first catheterization.

The more serious *complications* of catheterization, such as false passages, urethral fever, etc., will be considered in the succeeding chapters. Ordinarily speaking, none of these complications need be expected to follow the gentle passage of a clean instrument into a urethra which is neither inflamed nor lacerated; but in order to avert the possibility of cystitis or chill it is safe to *terminate every catheterization or sounding by an instillation along the whole urethra of a few drops of silver-nitrate solution* (1:1,500), unless some other solution is used as a part of the treatment, or the temper of the urethra is well known (p. 218).

CHAPTER IV

URETHRAL WOUNDS AND FOREIGN BODIES

The urethra may be wounded by traumatism from within or from without. External wounds only concern us here. Internal wounds, whether produced by foreign bodies or by instrumentation, such as false passages, internal urethrotomy, etc., find more appropriate exposition under their respective titles.

WOUNDS FROM WITHOUT

Punctured Wounds.—The prognosis of a punctured wound of the urethra is generally good. For simple punctured wounds a single irrigation of the wound and the urethra with an antiseptic solution, e. g., permanganate of potash, 1 : 4,000, followed by careful catheterization for each urinary act during the first one to three days, should result in a cure. If the puncture is merely the central point of a laceration or a contusion of the canal, the treatment must be carried out as laid down for these conditions. Complicating suppuration, infiltration, or fistula requires appropriate treatment, as indicated below.

Incised Wounds.—Clean-cut wounds are very rare in the perineum; they usually implicate the penile urethra, the corpus spongiosum, and often some portion of the corpora cavernosa. The *complications* to be feared are periurethritis (infiltration of urine) with prolonged suppuration and secondary gangrene, traumatic stricture, and fistula. Wounds in the scrotal region are most likely to be followed by severe inflammation, while obstinate fistula is the usual complication of wounds of the penile urethra. The prognosis of stricture, on the other hand, depends on the extent rather than on the situation of the lesion. Stricture does not follow longitudinal wounds of the urethra, but results rapidly from any transverse or oblique wound. When the urethra is completely severed, the cut ends—especially the proximal one—retract within the corpus spongiosum to such an extent that it may be difficult to bring them together again.

Treatment.—Immediate suture is the first indication. It may usually be performed under local anesthesia. If the gaping is slight, satisfactory approximation may be obtained by silk sutures inserted into the skin, the corpus cavernosum, and the deeper part of the mucous membrane without touching the epithelial surface, the wound having been cleansed by copious irrigation. If the wound gaps widely, or the urethra is completely divided, buried catgut sutures or skin-grafting may be employed with intermittent catheterization, or the retained catheter, as in rupture of the urethra (see below).

RUPTURE OF THE URETHRA

This includes all contused and lacerated wounds of the canal inflicted from without, and is by far the most common urethral injury, the lesion usually involving the bulb, rarely the pendulous, and still more rarely the posterior urethra.

Etiology.—1. *The pendulous urethra* is practically safe from injury except during erection; but in that condition it is liable not only to extensive injury, as in fracture of the penis and breaking a chordee, but also, as Guyon insists, to slight tears by bruising during coitus—injuries which, though scarcely noted at the time, may have dire consequences.

2. *Rupture of the bulb* is usually the result of direct violence—falling astride of a beam or some such hard object (in 82%—Kaufmann), a kick upon the perineum, or the jolting of a rider onto the pommel of his saddle.

3. *The posterior urethra* is torn only with fracture, dislocation or severe strain of the pelvis, or, exceptionally, by excessive direct violence. The membranous urethra is commonly involved, being torn with the triangular ligament, while the prostatic urethra is spared in all but the most extensive fractures.

The *mechanism* of rupture of the bulb has provoked much dispute. When the force is applied obliquely, the canal is crushed against the ischio-pubic rami; when from in front, as, for instance, in a fall with the body bent forward, the impact is against the front of the pubes (Oberst, Terrillon); while in certain cases, where the force is applied directly from below, the urethra is probably torn at the sharp edge of the subpubic ligament (Ollier and Poncet). It is upon the truth of this last fact that differences of opinion persist.

Morbid Anatomy.—The trauma which ruptures the urethra generally spares the surrounding soft parts. As the injury is usually the work of a blunt implement, the skin and the muscles are not torn, and the superficial aspect is, frequently enough, that of a mere bruise or abrasion.

The canal itself may be merely bruised, or more or less completely torn asunder. In the posterior urethra complete laceration is the rule, the canal being broken, as it were, in the grip of the triangular ligament. In the bulb complete laceration through part of the circumference of the canal is the rule; but the roof is usually spared—a point of considerable importance in subsequent catheterization. In the anterior urethra the milder injuries consist in mere interstitial hemorrhage [1]—contusion, as it were—of the corpus spongiosum, with perhaps slight lacerations of the mucous membrane or of the sheath of the spongy body.

Symptoms.—The cardinal symptoms of injury to the urethra are pain, tenderness, bleeding, interference with urination, and tumefaction.

The *pain* is sharp and occurs at the moment of rupture. It may be the only symptom of interstitial rupture due to a jar to the erect penis. As it abates rapidly the patient may pay but little attention to it, though even a slight injury may lay the foundation for traumatic stricture. The pain recurs with each act of urination for a longer or shorter time, according to the gravity of the injury and the temperament of the person. *Tenderness* exists primarily at the point of injury and later in the course of inflammation.

Bleeding from the meatus is a constant symptom. It is lacking only in the rare cases in which the mucous membrane is uninjured (see above). It occurs quite independent of urination (urethrorrhagia), its quantity not indicating the severity of the lesion. The unbroken skin usually prevents external (perineal) hemorrhage, though a hematoma of some size is not unusual. Hematuria combined with urethrorrhagia indicates an injury to the posterior urethra.

The *disturbance of urination* varies from the hesitancy excited by the pain of the milder cases to complete retention. This latter, indeed, is the usual condition, and is due to contraction of the lacerated urethra and to spasm of the cut-off muscle, rarely to hema-

[1] The possibility of this condition, as well as its clinical importance, has been warmly debated. In a recent article (Presse méd., 1898, i, 250) Baron sums up the evidence at hand, and shows that a simple contusion, without any break in the mucous membrane, may perfectly well be the starting-point for traumatic stricture. I believe that this occurs when there is enough mucous membranous abrasion to allow a slight contact of urine with the bruised tissue. I think a trauma to produce stricture yields at least a trace of blood (it may be minute) in the urine at first.

toma of the corpus spongiosum or to clots in the urethra. If the retention is not speedily relieved it is increased by the congestion and inflammation about the wound.

Tumefaction, primarily the effect of hemorrhage, secondarily of urinary infiltration and suppuration, follows the fascial spaces. The tumour after injury to the pendulous urethra is usually a circumscribed one within the corpus spongiosum, but may follow the course of a perineal infiltration and extend throughout the scrotum and penis. Effusions within the triangular ligament are retained there to form a tense perineal tumour, which may burst either forward or backward, while injury to the prostatic urethra leads to infiltration of the recto-vesical space. (See Urinary Infiltration.)

Diagnosis.—The diagnosis of the extent of injury is not easy. Immediate interference with urination, which always follows complete rupture, may be caused by spasm or by retained clots. Catheterization, impossible if there is complete rupture, may fail even in milder cases. (See Treatment.) It is sufficient, however, for practical purposes, to diagnose the severity of the case according to the symptoms, as indicated below. Diagnosis of the position of the injury may be made with a fair amount of accuracy from its etiology, the location of the tenderness and tumour, and the presence or absence of hematuria. The presence of urethrorrhagia, while establishing the existence of rupture of the urethra, does not exclude rupture of the bladder; but a positive diagnosis of the latter condition is usually practicable. (See Rupture of the Bladder.)

Course and Prognosis.—Guyon's classification is convenient as offering the most precise indications for treatment. It is as follows:

1. *Mild injuries to the pendulous urethra*, in which the trauma is succeeded by a sharp pain, slight bleeding, and a few painful urinary acts, are not likely to be followed by any serious consequences, except traumatic stricture, which is almost inevitable.

2. *Moderately severe injuries to the pendulous urethra* are characterized by free bleeding, painful and impeded urination, and a hematoma of some size. The chief danger here lies in infiltration and periurethral suppuration.

3. In the *severe injuries* and in most *perineal cases* complete retention is the prominent symptom. It can rarely be relieved otherwise than by external urethrotomy.

In any case traumatic stricture may be predicted—a condition formidable both in its rapidity of onset and its rebelliousness to treatment. (See Stricture.)

The mortality from rupture of the urethra is low. Terrillon

records 12 deaths in 170 cases, chiefly from uremia, septicemia, and hemorrhage.

Treatment.—1. For *mild injuries to the pendulous urethra* expectant treatment should be employed. Rest in bed, free purgation, and the internal administration of urotropin should be supplemented by a gentle injection twice a day of 3 to 5 c. c. of silver-nitrate solution (1: 2,000) or protargol (1: 1,000) into the anterior urethra. Catheterization is unnecessary and absolutely contraindicated. Extravasation or suppuration must be met by prompt incision (p. 234). Three days after the symptoms have subsided the patient may be pronounced free from all dangers except stricture, against which he must be warned, and for which treatment is to be instituted on its appearance. The contraction usually begins within six weeks of the time of injury.

Perineal rupture, however mild, demands immediate external section to avert deep resilient stricture.

2. *Moderately severe anterior injuries* represent, in a general way, slight lacerations, in which one may hope to avoid infiltration by keeping the urethra cleansed, as above, and preventing any contact of the urine with the wound. A small (Nos. 7 to 15 French) rubber or elbowed catheter should be used. The latter is the better instrument, as it can be made to force the cut-off muscle and to hug with its tip the uninjured roof of the canal. The catheter should be introduced every six hours and each catheterization followed by a nitrate-of-silver or protargol wash.

3. *Perineal ruptures* and all *severe injuries to the pendulous urethra* call for immediate external urethrotomy and suture. Palliative measures, such as suprapubic aspiration (p. 209), catheterization, or the retained catheter (p. 210) cannot save the day. Aspiration may be useful to relieve the distention of the bladder and thus to gain time, but the retained catheter is worse than useless. It serves only to invite infiltration, while repeated catheterization is impossible as soon as congestion sets in. On the other hand, perineal section relieves the retention at once and for all time, while suture of the divided ends of the urethra affords the surest means of preventing resilient traumatic stricture. While opinions may vary as to whether stricture can be absolutely prevented by this operation—and I believe that in some cases it can—there can be no doubt but that the scar after operation is far less retractile, and either will cause no trouble or will prove amenable to treatment by sounds.

The *operation* varies only in its details from the ordinary external urethrotomy (p. 201). With the patient in the lithotomy position, but without a staff in the urethra, the median perineal incision is carried down to the hematoma, which may be plainly felt. This is freely opened up and the clots evacuated by irrigation with warm saline solution through the wound itself and the anterior urethra. A medium-sized sound is introduced gently into the anterior urethra until its tip appears in the wound. Then a systematic search is made for the proximal segment, which may be identified in recent cases by profuse oozing from the bulb (Cabot). If this cannot be found it may be necessary to resort to retrograde catheterization (p. 206), though, if the operation is done under local anesthesia (a valuable precaution for just such an emergency), I have found it easy to induce the patient to urinate; in fact, it is sometimes impossible to restrain him, and thus the proximal end of the urethra is located. The torn ends of the urethra are trimmed away and all crushed tissue removed. This trimming need not be very radical, for the urethral wall, surrounded by the vascular corpus spongiosum, possesses great vitality. With three or four sutures of the finest catgut the severed ends are then approximated, the sutures being passed through the corpus spongiosum—thereby checking the oozing from the erectile tissue—close to, but without including, the mucous membrane. (If from loss of tissue the ends cannot be approximated, a graft may be inserted, as after excision of stricture.) A soft-rubber catheter is then fastened into the urethra and the perineal wound lightly packed, since suture of the perineum would but invite infiltration.

FOREIGN BODIES, INCLUDING STONE

Foreign bodies may enter the urethra at either extremity or may develop in and about the canal.

From without: { Fragments of surgical instruments. Substances introduced by the intoxicated, insane, or sexually perverted.

From within: { Renal or vesical calculi, or any substance which might form a nucleus for such calculi (p. 429).

Originating in or about the canal. } Stone: { Formed about a foreign body, or in an ulcerated spot, pocket, or fistula.

Foreign Bodies.—The most varied substances are found in the urethra,[1] introduced by the patient under the influence of that perverted and depraved sexual instinct which affects the male of all ages who gives up his mind to impure thoughts and whose sexual necessities are not gratified.

[1] *Cf.* Poulet. Foreign Bodies (translation). New York, 1880, p. 110.

Seeds, stones, beads, beans, peas, nails, pins, needles, hair-pins, slate-pencils, portions of glass, wax, cork, and a host of other substances, are thus introduced into the meatus, and, slipping beyond the reach of the fingers, are not infrequently swallowed by the urethra. Broken catheters and bougies, especially in cases of stricture, and instruments left *à demeure*, if not well fastened may slip past the meatus and travel towards the bladder. Their constant tendency is to slip persistently onward, not because of any urethral suction or peristalsis, but merely because they are introduced blunt end first, and consequently, unless quite round, the outer end is likely to be the sharper. Therefore every erection or effort at extraction, if it move the foreign body at all, pushes it inward. Rounded bodies, such as beans or pebbles, lie in the natural pouches of the canal (fossa navicularis, bulbous urethra) or become arrested by stricture.

If foreign bodies are not removed, one of three consequences follows: 1. They travel on into the bladder and form a nucleus for stone there; or, 2. Stone forms around them in the urethra; or, 3. They cause the urethra to inflame, bring on retention of urine, and finally either become encysted or ulcerate their way out, leaving behind fistula and ultimately stricture.

Treatment.—If the body be long and soft (catheter, piece of wood), it may be transfixed with a stout needle through the floor of the urethra and the canal pushed back over it, like a glove over a finger, as far as possible, when it may be transfixed again, and so urged forward until it reaches the meatus; otherwise the long urethral forceps, the ingenious scoop of Leroy d'Etiolle for small round bodies, or the urethral lithotrite, may be used. For this purpose I have successfully employed[1] the Thompson stricture divulsor, opening it after passing the foreign body, and finding the latter between the blades on closing the instrument. In manipulating with any ordinary forceps, if the finger on the outside can detect and get behind the foreign body, nothing should divert the surgeon from keeping up pressure at that point in order to prevent his instrument from pushing the offending substance still deeper into the canal.

If the foreign body lies behind a stricture, the latter must be cut or rapidly dilated (continuous dilatation), to allow the passage of an instrument suitable for extraction.

Pins and needles may be extracted through the floor of the canal if their blunt ends can be steadied. To remove a hat-pin its point is pushed through the urethral floor and its shaft drawn out until the head can be turned so as to extrude through the meatus. I have

[1] N. Y. Med. Record, March 6 and May 1, 1875.

extracted a pin with Thompson's divulsor, and Dieffenbach removed one from the membranous urethra by pushing it with his finger in the rectum until the point protruded through the perineum, and then forcibly extracting it.

All other manipulations failing, perineal section will reveal the position of the object and permit extraction. The penile or the scrotal urethra should never be excised for fear of fistula in the one case, infiltration in the other.

Urethral Calculi.—A stone descending from the kidney or the bladder may be caught in the prostatic, the bulbous, or the navicular urethra, or behind a stricture; or it may form about an impacted foreign body, or on any ulcerated spot or fistula. It assumes the shape of that part of the canal or cavity in which it lies. Voillemier describes a set of six calculi filling the anterior urethra, and Blasius mentions a periurethral pocket containing eighty stones. As a rule, however, but one is found.

Symptoms.—If the calculus comes from the bladder the onset of symptoms is sudden. As it enters the urethra during urination the flow stops suddenly, while a sharp pain is felt. A second effort may extrude it from the canal or only impact it more firmly, or it may fall back into the bladder and remain a vesical calculus. Once impacted it may cause complete retention, or, more commonly, dysuria.

If, on the other hand, the stone forms *in situ* the onset of symptoms is insidious. First, there is slight gleet and some difficulty in urination. The gleet becomes slowly worse, and finally periurethritis occurs, which goes on to extensive suppuration and fistulization. The obstruction to urination is not complete.

Periurethral calculi may remain latent for a long time, until they obtrude upon the lumen of the urethra or excite suppuration in the pocket within which they lie.

Diagnosis.—A sharp attack of urethral colic is unmistakable, but the less acute conditions just described simulate stricture of the urethra; indeed, stricture and stone often coexist. The mistake is not a vital one, however, for any attempt at dilatation will produce a grating sound characteristic of stone, and the calculus may be felt between the instrument and the finger externally.

Treatment.—In acute cases an attempt may be made to push the stone back into the bladder if it has not passed the membranous urethra; or, if it has passed, the anterior urethra may be distended with olive-oil and the stone worked forward to the meatus, whence it may be extracted by crushing or by meatotomy. These failing, the meatus may be pinched and the patient encouraged to urinate; when the canal is fully distended the meatus is released and the stone expelled by the gush of urine. The urethral lithotrite is a dangerous instrument and of doubtful utility. The scoops and forceps of Collin and Leroy d'Etiolle, though ingenious, are never at hand at the right moment. I have extracted a stone with Thompson's divulsor. When all these methods fail external urethrotomy succeeds.

Chronic cases of urethral calculus call for external urethrotomy to remove the stone, to excise the pocket in which it lies, and to divide or excise the stricture which is usually present.

Infiltration, abscess, and fistula are considered in another section.

CHAPTER V

URETHRAL CHILL

The term *urinary fever* is commonly bestowed upon any continuous febrile condition occurring in the course of an inflammation in the urinary organs or resulting from an operation upon them, while the term *urethral chill* or *fever* is restricted to the more acute cases usually attributable to urethral instrumentation. Both terms are misleading from a scientific point of view, since they give no clew to the real nature of the disturbance, and, indeed, group under one title several conditions of widely different natures; and yet, clinically speaking, they represent a set of well-defined phenomena, and they will doubtless always find a place in the clinician's vocabulary. Urinary fever will interest us later; our present concern is urethral chill. This term includes three conditions, any one of which may prove fatal. They are:

1. Shock to the whole nervous system;
2. Shock to the kidneys, inducing uremia; and
3. Toxemia, septicemia, or pyemia.

The first two conditions deserve the title *urethral shock* or chill, while the last is urinary fever or chill, properly speaking, since the toxic elements are derived from the urine.

Etiology.—That urethral chill does not occur more constantly under similar conditions is the mystery. The majority of patients escape, whether the urine is infected or not, whether the wound or the trauma be great or small. The same patient may have a chill one day, and escape it after an exactly similar operation on the next. The simple gentle passage of a small, soft bougie may give rise to it, while violent divulsion or urethrotomy, performed a day or two afterward, may evoke no reaction; and again, after divulsion, which has been negative, the passage of a steel sound may produce a chill. Nor is it instrumentation only which is the exciting cause, since patients suffering from stricture, upon whom no instruments have ever been used, have well-marked exacerbations of chill and fever in connection with renal and bladder disease, and these patients cease to have chills (which they usually call dumb ague) after the use of instruments in their urethræ has dilated the strictures. Other patients have no chill until dilatation has reached a certain limit, after which every effort to pass an instrument of a larger size is liable to be followed by urethral fever. The extent of injury bears no relation to the amount of fever that will follow. The gentle passage of a smooth sound may cause speedy death, while extensive wounds and lacerations of the canal are often absolutely innocuous, and that, too, when the urine is manifestly purulent, even ammoniacal. I have had a number of cases where the passage of any instrument effecting even very moderate dilatation, without bringing blood, would be followed by chill, and yet divulsion, tearing the urethra, and opening the tissues freely, did not occasion the customary chill and fever. Moreover, the position of the injury inflicted by the instrument is of importance. At and near the meatus the most serious injuries do not give rise to chill, though decomposed urine pass freely over the raw surface. The danger increases in proportion to the depth at which the injury is inflicted. Nor does a wound seem at all necessary, since cases are on record where death, following rapidly upon the introduction of a smooth instrument, has failed to reveal on autopsy any lesion of the canal. Here shock and reflex action (Banks) arresting kidney secretion would seem to be the immediate cause of death. The chill may come on before the instrument has been withdrawn from the urethra, but usually it does not follow for some hours, and generally not until after urine has flowed through the canal. In rapidly fatal cases, old and often advanced kidney disease, or at least intense kidney hyperemia, is found on autopsy; but in some cases the kidneys have been pronounced normal.[1] Even in these latter there has usually been suppression of urine; but simple suppression of urine does not often kill in one or two days, and, to solve the problem in these cases, we are forced to fall back upon the effects of shock. The French school, championed by Guyon,[2] stoutly maintains that the entire range of cases is septic; but the experience of many observers confirms the belief that, although most are of a mixed type, in which the element of sepsis predominates, there are also purely nervous and purely renal cases. How sharply the posterior urethra resents the first introduction of an instrument—the sudden faintness, even complete syncope—attests its sensitiveness and its power of reacting upon the whole economy; while the wholesome apprehension of sup-

[1] *Cf.* Velpeau, Leçons orales de clin. chir., etc., 1841, p. 326.

[2] Cong. franç. de chir., 1892, vi, 77 ; Leçons clin., 1896, ii, 135 *et seq.*

pression of urine felt by every genito-urinary surgeon after an operation upon the deep urethra and bladder speaks for the close reflex connection between the extremes of the internal urinary tract.

The predisposing causes of urethral chill are therefore: 1, urinary infection; 2, disease of the kidneys; and 3, a susceptibility to shock impossible always to foresee or to prevent. The efficient cause is shock to the deep urethra, or abrasion, laceration, or inflammation, permitting the absorption of bacteria or their toxic products from the urine, the urethra, or both.

Symptoms.—No two cases present exactly the same picture, the symptoms of shock, uremia, and sepsis intermingling variously, sometimes one predominating, sometimes another; but they can usually be classed in one of the following types:

1. *Urethral Shock.*—Mild urethral shock is often seen typically upon the first passage of an instrument. The patient, usually of a nervous type, fearful of all manipulation, complains of great pain from the unobstructed and gentle introduction of a sound into his bladder. Immediately he feels faint and nauseated; he may vomit or faint away; his skin is cold, pale, and dry, his pulse weak, rapid, or irregular. He may have a slight chill, and as the attack passes the skin becomes flushed and moist. Such a paroxysm lasts but a few moments. Exceptionally, the collapse and chill are unduly severe and prolonged, anuria is complete, and the patient dies of shock in a few hours; or the fatal issue may be delayed some days, the suppression of urine continuing and the patient dying of uremia with acute congestion of the kidneys. In this last class of cases it is probable that the acute renal congestion is grafted upon a chronic nephritis which, up to that time, may have passed unnoticed. That this prolonged suppression may occur from the effect of urethral shock on normal kidneys has not been disproved.

2. *Acute Urethral Fever.*—Sir Henry Thompson's[1] classical description I here transcribe:

The patient has undergone his first urethral instrumentation—the gentle and bloodless dilatation of a urethral stricture: then, "some three or four hours afterward, the patient wants to pass water, and feels, in doing so, a smarting sensation which, after all, is the natural consequence of passing any instrument through the urethra whether healthy or diseased. Soon after, it may be a few minutes, or an hour, or even more, the patient suddenly feels a cold chill through his back, thence invading the whole system, so

[1] Dis. of Urin. Org., 8th Edit., 1888, p. 180.

that his teeth chatter involuntarily, and all his limbs tremble so much that it is obvious to a bystander that he is the subject of a convulsive shudder which he cannot control, affecting the voluntary muscles. The patient's look is haggard, he becomes grayish in tint, dark beneath the eyes, the expression of his face is altered, his breathing is hurried, and the voice changed. The attack varies greatly in intensity in different cases and circumstances. Such a patient is, of course, sent to bed at once, if not already occupying one, that hot bottles and warm coverings may be applied; and the bed itself shakes with the rigor, if the fit is severe. He now begins to complain of severe pains in his head, back, and limbs; there may be an attack of vomiting or of purging, although these are not so common. The temperature if taken now is high, and rising rapidly reaches nearly 104 degrees or passes it, sometimes to 105 degrees. In half an hour, perhaps, more commonly an hour or more, the pale and contracted features become red, then flushed, the mouth is dry, he asks for a drink, and with an oppressive sense of heat he is eager to throw off the coverings which have been heaped upon him. His pains are now severe and his temperature at its maximum; the pulse is rapid, hard, and vibrating. There gradually appears a little glistening in the dry, cutaneous surface, the commencing dew of gentle perspiration which quickly becomes profuse from the now soft, relaxed, and reddened skin, with sensible relief to pain and feverish heat. The respiration becomes slower and fuller, and the patient is tranquil, passive, exhausted in appearance as he lies on his back sweating at every pore. Then the pulse slowly grows less rapid, is soft and full, temperature diminishes, thirst continues, and he passes a little urine dark in tint. After six, twelve, or eighteen hours, the signs of fever disappear, leaving him more or less weak, and he is convalescent the next day or the following one."

Such is the typical attack—sharp, intense, transient. It doubtless indicates the sudden spread of some toxin through the system; but—more than that—it represents the equation between the trauma and the urethral susceptibility. For this chill is too severe to be comparable to any other septic phenomenon of so ephemeral a nature, and, moreover, it seems to depend rather upon the location of the lesion than upon the septic materials present (see above). Yet what we do know quite definitely is the proper preventive treatment for this condition, and this is a knowledge not to be exchanged for many theoretical data.

Treatment.—The best treatment for urethral chill is prophylaxis. The five essentials of prophylaxis are:

1. Gentleness in manipulation;

2. Nitrate-of-silver irrigation of the urethra and bladder at the end of every operation;
3. Efficient drainage—according to the nature of the case;
4. Urinary antisepsis and dilution; and
5. Stimulation of the kidneys and other emunctories.

The first two points have already been noticed (p. 28). The third and fourth (and second) sound the surgeon's warning, "For pus—antisepsis, drainage, and irrigation." Antisepsis and irrigation are achieved by local washings and, at the same time, by rendering the natural irrigating fluid—the urine—as unirritating, as plentiful, and as antiseptic as possible. Copious draughts of diuretic mineral waters, and the administration of urotropin (0.5 to 1.5 grammes *t. i. d.*), or salol (2 to 3 grammes a day in divided doses), fulfil this latter indication, while drainage is established according to the requirements of the case. The final requisite is fulfilled by the diuretic mineral waters and urotropin (a valuable renal stimulant), together with a warm bath and a cathartic before any operation upon the urinary tract.

Practically speaking, therefore, the patient must be prepared for every formal operation upon his urinary organs by a course of two days' administration of urotropin (0.5 gramme *t. i. d.*) and a diuretic water (Suwannee, Stafford, Poland, Bethesda), a warm bath and a cathartic, and some attempt must be made by daily irrigations of the bladder to render his urine as sweet as possible (see Cystitis); while, if the patient suffers from cystitis or pyelitis, or threatens to become septic or uremic, the same course of treatment is to be instituted, and drainage established, if necessary, through the loin, the perineum, or the retained catheter. (See Cystitis, Pyelitis.) Quiet and rest in bed are beneficial. Anesthesia exerts no effect on urethral chill, except in so far as ether is a tax on damaged kidneys, and cocain more toxic in the deep urethra than elsewhere.

For urethral shock or chill, when it has once set in, rest in bed, a hot foot-bath, fluid diet, and urinary dilution and antisepsis usually suffice; but if the attack is a rapidly pernicious one, morphin, hot-air baths, the hot pack, stimulants, and cups to the loins constitute the treatment. The suggestions of Gouley and Long as to the prophylactic value of the tincture of the chlorid of iron and of 2-minim doses of Fleming's tincture of aconite I cannot indorse by any personally favourable experience, while quinin has given no satisfaction at my hands. The sodio-salicylate of theobromin seems to be of service only in chronic cases, and the benefit of venesection and infusion in uremia must not be lost sight of.

CHAPTER VI

ACUTE INFLAMMATIONS OF THE URETHRA

Inflammations of the urethra, like those of other mucous membranes, are catarrhal in character and yield pus, which pus, flowing out at the meatus or mingling in the urine, constitutes their most salient feature.

The main, and for practical clinical purposes the only notable urethral inflammation is gonorrhea and its long train of sequences; but before approaching this subject it may be as well to clear the field a little of certain minor maladies, to get them out of the way. They are traumatic urethritis, urethritis *ab ingestis*, diathetic urethritis, and the mild discharges attending ulcerations within the urethra—i. e., chancroid, chancre, tubercle, herpes, syphilitic deposits.

Polypi and warts will be touched upon when dealing with chronic anterior urethritis, and the pseudo-gonorrheal inflammations will be considered in connection with the diagnosis of that malady.

TRAUMATIC URETHRITIS

This is an inflamed condition of the urethral mucous membrane following injury, chemical or mechanical. It ranges through various degrees of intensity according to the severity and continuance of the provoking causes.

These causes are *wounds of the urethra* by instruments, more especially crushing or bruising injuries. Bending the penis when erect, as in tempestuous and badly directed coitus, may be followed by mild urethritis (sometimes ushered in by hemorrhage and followed by traumatic stricture).

A foreign body in the urethra, such as retained stone, may give rise to a mild discharge. Hallé and Wassermann have attempted to explain urethritis following moderate and aseptic traumatism on the ground that minor organisms existing normally in the urethra become capable of exciting suppuration when the soil is prepared for them by the concomitant action of trauma.

Rough catheterism, à fortiori if the instrument be dirty, may produce urethritis, and the suppuration habitually attending instruments left *à demeure* in the urethra is too well known to require more than a statement of the fact.

Caustic injections of any kind act as traumatic causes of urethritis. Some urethras are very sensitive to the action of solutions of corrosive sublimate and carbolic acid, and much more so to the minutest dilutions of formalin, all of which substances, used as sterilizers of instruments, sometimes provoke the very mischief they would avoid.

Treatment.—The treatment of these inflammations is very simple. The cause (retained catheter, stone, etc.) being removed, the malady disappears spontaneously or under an alkaline diuretic, perhaps aided by a mild irrigation or an astringent injection (p. 125). Special care in urethral antisepsis is called for in the management of even very mild bruising injuries in order to heal them as quickly as possible, for the proneness of traumatic stricture to follow such injuries should never be overlooked.

URETHRITIS AB INGESTIS

Certain substances taken into the stomach may occasionally produce a mild urethritis. Among these alcohol holds a high rank. Excessive potations, notably of beer or champagne, or prolonged excesses of alcohol in any form, will occasionally, without other cause, produce urethral discharge. As an adjuvant to sexual excess the influence of alcohol is paramount, more particularly if there be already a pre-existing patch of chronic inflammation anywhere along the urethra. Cantharides, arsenic, purgative mineral waters, iodid of potassium, turpentine, asparagus, have all been accused of lighting up mild urethral inflammation, but the rarity of such attacks makes their consideration trivial, and the whole subject may be dismissed with the words *Causa sublata, tollitur effectus.* The effect of lochial and leucorrheal discharges and of the menstrual flow as etiological factors of urethral inflammation will be referred to when considering gonorrhea (p. 67).

DIATHETIC URETHRITIS

A gouty urethritis is accepted honestly in England and among old gentlemen in our large cities, and a strumous urethritis has been mentioned; but as essential maladies both are a refinement of diagnosis. Surely the gouty old gentleman with a fibrotic prostate and densely acid urine suffers from more surface discharge because of his gout, and treatment of the latter may be essential to his recovery. Rheumatic subjects also are often catarrhal all along their various mucous membranes, and the remains of their gonorrheal inflammations are on that account the more difficult of removal. Strumous subjects sometimes get into a condition of granular urethritis following gonorrhea. In such cases the entire canal is thickened and velvety and cod-liver oil is helpful.

There are also well-observed instances of the appearance of a discharge from the urethra upon the subsidence of an arthritic eruption upon the skin, and Desnos [1] alludes to the sudden appearance of a spontaneous urethral discharge during the course of the grip, believing it due to small prostatic abscesses bursting into the urethra. These diathetic agencies are then surely concomitant factors, if not essential causes, of primary urethral inflammation, and for the benefit of obstinate and protracted cases of relapsing chronic urethritis it is well for the surgeon to bear the fact in mind. From his knowledge the therapeutic deductions become obvious.

Herpetic and Eruptive Urethritis.—That an attack of ordinary vesicular herpes may occur within the urethra is well known although not common. I have seen a group or two of vesicles outside and a mild urethral discharge, with smarting on urination, coinciding with the attack and disappearing spontaneously with it. Alternating attacks, one outside the next inside, have also been observed. Eczematous subjects sometimes suffer from a mild discharge coincident with a new outcrop of cutaneous eruption upon or near the genitals, or with the sudden disappearance of the outside eruption. I have also distinctly noted an attack of gleet accompanying the development of a patch of tubercular syphilid upon the outside of the penis and disappearing under the use of mixed antisyphilitic medication by the mouth. Bassereau and Bumstead speak of cases of muco-purulent urethral flow coming on with the first appearance or with a relapse of secondary syphilitic eruptions, the cause of which was the development of syphilitic mucous patches upon the urethral mucous membrane. I have several times seen a patch of tubercular syphilid involve the urinary meatus and occasion a slight discharge. I have also seen relapsing gummatous ulceration of the urethra.

Syphilitic Urethritis.—*Syphilitic chancre* not infrequently involves one lip of the urinary meatus, more often perhaps the entire circumference, stiffening it, thickening the lips, and being more or less eroded and ulcerated down into the canal of the urethra. The

---

[1] Traité élémentaire des maladies des voies urinaires, 2de éd., 1898, Paris, p. 93.

discharge in these cases is very slight, but the sore lasts many weeks. Concomitant symptoms—inguinal adenopathy, finally an eruption—clinch the diagnosis. The urethral inflammation is only an epiphenomenon.

A mistake, however, may arise when the chancre is situated at some distance within the urethra. The discharge in such event is slight, the incubation period between sexual contact and commencing discharge has been usually long (unless, unhappily, there be double infection), the gleet is more or less streaked with blood. But care will detect the enemy, and usually a hard lump of varying size, most often about that of a pea, may be plainly felt from the outside through the skin, and the endoscope easily clears up the diagnosis by disclosing a gray or livid, bleeding, exulcerated erosion. I have seen two of these through the endoscopic tube, one at a distance of about 2 inches from the meatus. How the virus reached this spot without infecting the outside is not clear, but the fact remains.

Chancroid.—Chancroid, in my personal experience, rarely gets very far into the urethra. It does involve the meatus, and thence by extension works backward into the canal and may even perforate its floor, leaving ultimate fistula; but I have not known it to arise *de novo* within the urethra except by extension from the meatus, where it may be seen. That such ulceration is possible in the inside of the urethra, however, is attested by the recorded case of Duncan, who inoculated his own urethra by transporting into it some chancroidal pus, and was rewarded by getting urethral chancroid with double bubo.[1] Ricord has figured a case of deep urethral chancroid with chancroidal-looking ulcerations of the bladder; but tubercular ulceration has been suggested to explain this unusual case, and in my opinion such a presumption is well founded.

Tubercular Urethritis.—That tubercular ulceration occurs within the urethra *de novo*, or except in connection with the very common prostatic ulceration, I have no knowledge. It is possible, perhaps, but not probable. When cancer involves the deep urethra, the part played in the drama by the mild accompanying urethritis is too subordinate to be billed.

GONORRHEA

Gonorrheal Cellulitis and Lymphangitis

It may be as well here, before taking up the main urethral inflammation, gonorrhea, to dispose also of two of its modest complica-

[1] Cours des maladies syphilitiques. Petit Radel, 1812.

tions, since they are in no way directly implicated in the one grand feature—urethral discharge. I refer to lymphangitis and adenitis. Balanitis and posthitis also often complicate gonorrheal inflammation, but will be considered in their appropriate section (p. 658).

Cellulitis.—A mild cellulitis not very infrequently complicates acute gonorrheal anterior urethritis. When the inflammation runs high and the discharge of pus is profuse the foreskin will sometimes swell acutely, becoming hot, edematous, red, and tender, and this cutaneous inflammation may extend backward and involve the entire integument of the penis. Periurethral abscess, and even follicular abscess about the urethra, may be attended by a similar inflammatory quasi-erysipelatous condition of the skin. This is a superficial dermatitis and cellulitis. It is generally confined to the prepuce and causes only a little uneasiness with temporary phimosis; but sometimes, when the whole penis is involved, there are chilly sensations and considerable fever.

Treatment.—A little lead-and-opium wash upon lint or gauze inside of a wrap of gutta-percha tissue quickly reduces the milder cases. More severe attacks call for rest in bed with a continuance of the same wraps or the application of ichthyol. This treatment, aided by saline laxatives, gets the better of the attack. Cutaneous abscess is the rarest of sequences, but when threatened calls for prompt and very liberal incision. An indication for the knife is a porky, doughy, brawny condition of the integument like that felt in phlegmonous erysipelas. The inguinal glands become sympathetically engorged.

Lymphangitis.—With this inflammation, or independent of it, the lymphatic trunks may become implicated during suppurative urethral inflammation. Fournier[1] has made an exhaustive study of the various forms of lymphangitis accompanying gonorrhea. There is an indolent variety in which no pain is felt (except occasionally during erection), and no external sign attracts the patient's attention; but the examining finger detects indurated cords under the skin, the dorsal trunk being most marked. The feel of these cords is exactly similar to that of the same vessels in the lymphangitis of infecting chancre. If there be also perilymphangitis, red streaks are to be seen upon the sides or the back of the penis, and the corded lymphatics are hard and knotty. Several trunks may be matted together. Sometimes they are tender. The inguinal glands are often tense, the prepuce edematous.

---

[1] Nouv. dict. de méd. et de chir. prat., p. 185.

Treatment consists of wet dressings under oil silk or gutta-percha tissue, possibly aided by hot hip-baths and ichthyol locally, with laxatives. Occasionally abscesses form along the course of the hard cords. These should be opened early, as the pus is liable to burrow and may denude a considerable extent of the penis.

A hard edema of the prepuce may be left behind by these various forms of lymphangitis, especially marked in the neighborhood of the frenum and perhaps giving rise to phimosis or to partial paraphimosis. Lymphangitis may leave the lymphatic trunks in a varicose condition (Ricord), or lymphatic fistula may result, usually requiring excision for its cure.

The way is now open for approaching the most common of all genito-urinary disorders—gonorrhea, a malady scoffed at by the light-brained, hot-blooded younger members of the community, but deserving grave consideration from serious minds, since its ultimate results are far-reaching and potential. In its train are found ascending pyelitis, of which I have seen some desperately acute examples, fatal general infection, fatal peritonitis from seminal, vesicular, or periprostatic suppuration with extensive burrowing abscesses.

Add to this the ocular and articular complications, the far-reaching influence of the disease upon the uterus and its adnexa, the sterility to which it gives rise in both sexes, and the untold surgery it furnishes the gynecologist, and gonorrhea rises in dignity from its putrid source and becomes an object worthy of serious study for every conscientious surgeon and physician.

GONORRHEA

Of all the affections encountered by the genito-urinary surgeon specific urethral inflammation is the most common. Furthermore, it is the most venereal of all venereal diseases, since it is the commonest malady acquired during the copulative act.

A most respectable antiquity is given to gonorrhea by the fifteenth chapter of Leviticus, although it is contended that the discharge known to the Jewish law-giver was a simple urethritis, and that gonorrhea did not appear until later (according to Astruc[1] in the year 1545–'46).

All inflammations of the urethra are characterized by a discharge of pus or of muco-pus from the meatus, and the best guide for treatment is the grade of inflammation in a given case, an inflammation of a certain intensity often requiring the same treatment whether

[1] De morbis venereis. Paris, 1736.

it has sprung from a specific organism or from a chemical or a mechanical irritation.

Modern science, however, has solved the question of specific *versus* simple urethritis by the discovery of the gonococcus of Neisser, a living germ that has established its claim to be considered the active, virulent cause of true specific gonorrhea.

The term gonorrhea is etymologically inaccurate, indicating, as it does, a flow of semen (*γονος*); but usage has secured to it a precise signification even among the laity (almost to the exclusion of the old Saxon term clap). Urethritis signifies simply inflammation of the urethra, consequently gonorrhea is urethritis. But the converse does not hold good, and although without the microscope it is impossible to pronounce with certainty upon the nature of many cases of urethral inflammation, yet it is essential to retain the two terms, calling that gonorrhea which is caused by the gonococcus and has been unmistakably derived from an individual of the other sex with a gonorrhea, and reserving the term urethritis for all inflammatory urethral discharges having other origins. This latter precaution is of the utmost importance to the student and young practitioner. It is better that a hundred guilty should escape than that one innocent person should be accused. Experience proves beyond a doubt that a high urethral inflammation attended by an abundant discharge and presenting absolutely no clinical features to differentiate it from a gonorrhea—unless the microscope solves the doubt —may be acquired by a healthy young lover from his equally healthy mistress, by a young husband from his wife, or may be produced by applying a chemical irritant to the urethra. These cases are of undoubted authenticity, and it becomes the surgeon's duty to hesitate long before asserting the infidelity of a man or a woman, and thus, perhaps, accusing the innocent and destroying the harmony of a family. It is proper to state that a healthy man may get a urethritis from a woman who has none (may give himself the gonorrhea, as Ricord puts it) far more easily than a woman can get a discharge from a healthy man, unless, of course, great mechanical violence be used, as in rape.

The Cause of Gonorrhea.—Gonorrhea may be acquired from any person having it by the mere contact of the discharge with the mucous membrane of the urethra.[1] It is not necessary that the surface should be abraded; mere contact is sufficient without any sexual act. The infectious agent is the gonococcus.

---

[1] Other mucous membranes are liable to become infected, but to a less degree, excepting the conjunctiva, which is even more sensitive than the urethra.

PLATE I

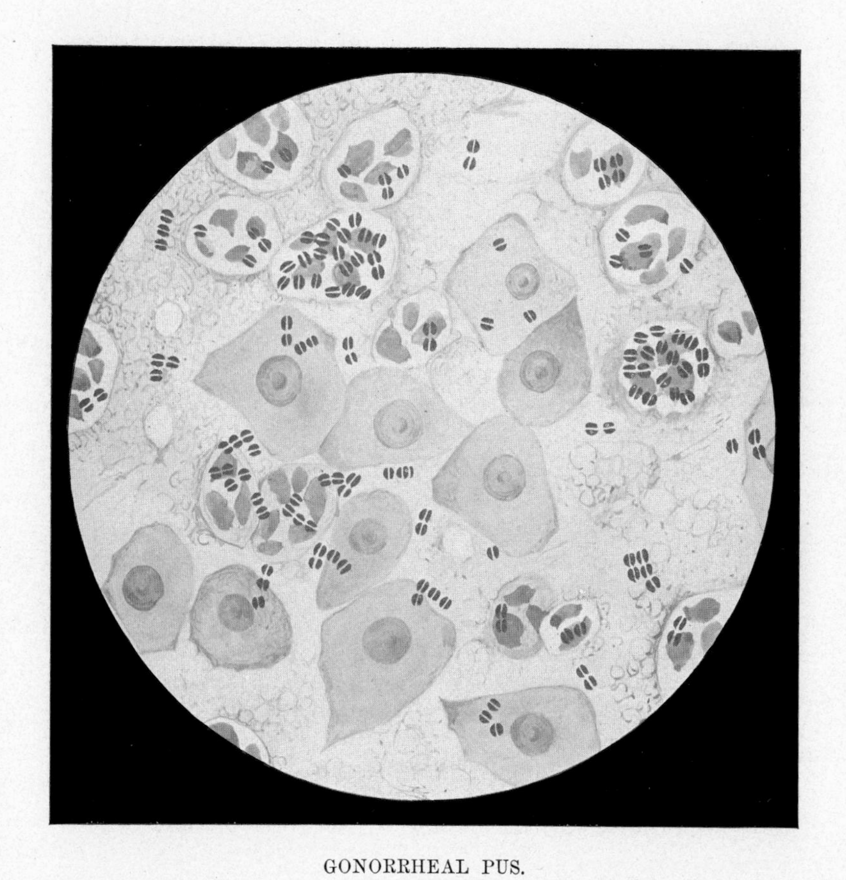

GONORRHEAL PUS.

First stain: Gentian violet solution. Microscopic enlargement, 2,000 diameters.

The Gonococcus

The discussion upon the very existence of a virulent gonorrhea has been active of late years. Ricord did not believe strictly in it, thinking that one could give himself a gonorrhea. Bumstead decided against it. The German school declared the inflammation to possess no virus *sui generis*, and matters were rapidly approaching a position that would make untenable the assumption of any difference between gonorrhea and urethritis, when Neisser claimed to have discovered the essential causative element of gonorrhea to be a peculiar vegetable parasite which he likened to sarcina and christened *gonococcus*. This announcement naturally challenged controversy, and there has been no stint of investigation.[1] Pure cultures of the vegetable organism have been difficult to obtain, and much confusion in the long discussion to which this question has given rise is due to the fact that there are other cocci, diplococci much like the gonococcus, which may be found normally in the urethra. Indeed, a similar organism has been found in the normal secretions of other membranes (mouth) and even in the pus of an acute abscess.

Lustgarten and Mannaberg[2] have made an admirable study of the micro-organisms found normally in the healthy urethra. Some of them are pathogenic, and capable in co-operation with the gonococcus of intensifying the mischief occasioned by the latter and of modifying the clinical picture. Rovsing[3] has contributed an excellent chapter upon the same subject in his book on cystitis, and Petit and Wassermann[4] and H. Heiman[5] have added precision to our knowledge.

But in spite of other microbes and other secretions, the specificity of gonorrheal pus is splendidly demonstrated by Welander,[6] who inoculated the male urethra five times without success, using pus containing small bacilli and derived from putrid balanitis; sev-

---

[1] Among the ablest articles may be instanced: A. Neisser, Ueber eine der Gonorrhoeae eigenthümliche Mikrococcusform, Centralbl. f. d. medicin. Wissenschaften, Nr. 28, 1879, which introduces the gonococcus to the world; Ernst Bumm, Der Mikroorganismus der gonorrhoischen Schleimhaut-Erkrankungen, Wiesbaden, 1885; Bosc, from the historical standpoint, Le Gonocoque, Thèse de Montpellier, 1893, and in every particular the masterly essay of Marcel Sée, Le Gonocoque, Paris, 1896, p. 354; and a contribution upon successful cultures from Cases of Arthritis, etc., by Hugh H. Young, J. of Cut. and Gen.-Urin. Dis., 1900, xviii, 240.

[2] Vierteljahresschrift f. Derm. u. Syph., 1887, S. 905.

[3] Berlin, 1890. A. Hirschwald, S. 60.

[4] Guyon's Annales, 1891, ix, 378.

[5] N. Y. Med. Record, June, 1895, p. 769.

[6] Cited in Thesis of Bosc from Gaz. méd. de Paris, 1884, p. 267.

eral times with vaginal secretions containing a variety of microbes; three times with vaginal secretions containing several rounded and bacillary microbic forms; three times from a putrid and purulent vaginal flow containing moving bacilli; three times with *vaginal secretion* containing *no gonococci* from women whose urethras *did contain these microbes*, and then he gave a typical gonorrhea to these last three subjects by inoculating them with the above-mentioned *urethral pus from the same women, which pus did contain gonococci.* What more is needed? Surely there is justification in the modern French retort to Ricord's famous recipe for catching a gonorrhea—the answer being "*La plus belle femme du monde ne peut donner que ce qu'elle a*" (Sée).

The gonococcus, then, is the cause of gonorrhea, and is always found in the infectious discharge: not in all the secretions of an infected person, as Welander's experiments show, but only in the infectious secretions—urethral, prostatic, etc. An accurate diagnosis of the presence or the absence of the gonococcus is therefore absolutely essential to the comprehension of urethritis.

The discussion of the presence or the absence of the gonococcus in the individual, i. e., the person's infectiousness, is taken up elsewhere (p. 64). We are only interested here in the discovery of the specific coccus in a suspected secretion. The problem is: given a drop of pus, does it contain gonococci? There are two methods of investigation, viz., by the microscope and by cultures. The former suffices in any acute case and for any purulent discharge from which the gonococci have not been driven by treatment. But in obscure and chronic cases cultivation must be resorted to before the specific microbe can be declared absent.

Microscopic Examination.—The gonococcus may be stained with the familiar anilin dyes, such as methyl violet, gentian violet, and fuchsin. For purposes of study a minute drop of pus may be spread between two cover-glasses and dried, fixed, and stained in the usual manner (see below). Examined under an oil-immersion lens (magnifying 2,000 diameters), the gonococcus then presents the following characteristics (Plate I):

1. It is a diplococcus. Each individual of a pair is D-shaped (coffee-bean shaped) with the flat (or slightly concave) border opposed to its fellow, so that the couple form an ovoid made up of two separate hemispheres. The length of the pair averages about 1.25 μ (Bumm), and the interspace is about half as wide as either segment. Yet such is the divergence of size in the gonococcus that the figures of no two observers agree exactly.

2. The diplococci are found grouped in pairs, fours, and other

PLATE II

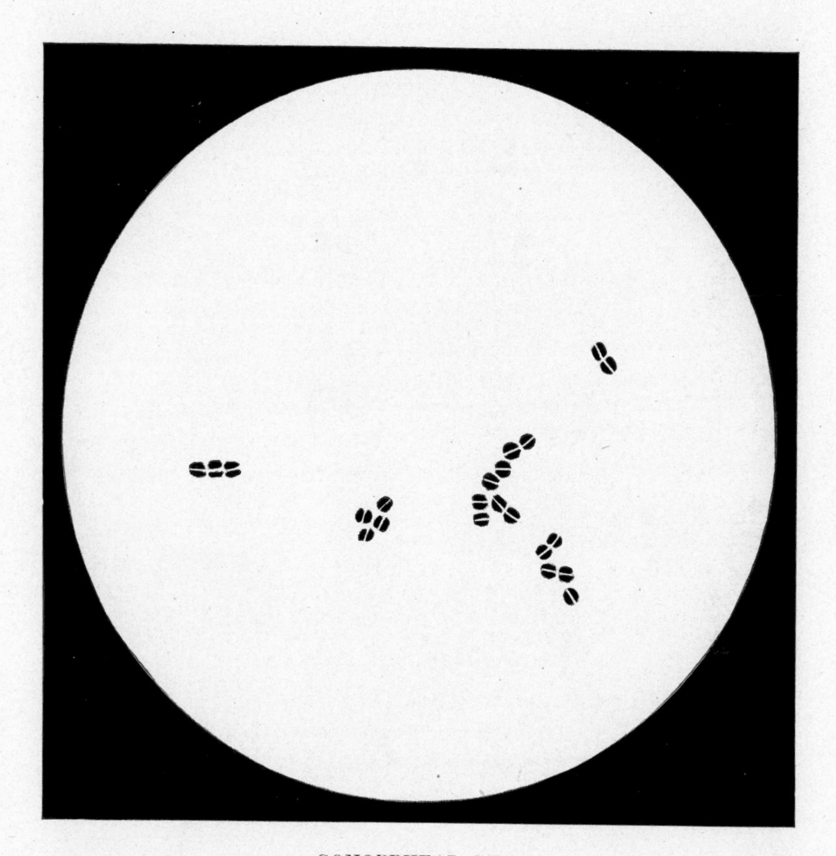

GONORRHEAL PUS.

Gram stain after washing with alcohol. Cells and gonococci decolorized and pseudo-gonococci stained black.

multiples of two, showing a tendency to rectangular disposition, in marked contrast to the irregular massing of staphylococci and the linear arrangement of streptococci. This characteristic grouping is due to the fact that the multiplication of gonococci occurs by fissure at right angles to the central interspace.

3. The gonococcus, when it occurs in pus, is found both within and without the pus and the epithelial cells.[1] Indeed, the most characteristic groups are met with inside the cells. The extracellular gonococci may be scattered or irregularly grouped, but the intracellular specimens present a greater regularity of arrangement. Without being mathematically distributed, there is still a certain symmetry in the grouping, an absence of jumbling, which the observer soon learns to appreciate at a glance and which the plates attempt to reproduce.

Such are the characteristics of the gonococcus. It is a double D diplococcus occurring intracellularly and in typical groups. But these characteristics are sometimes shared by other bacteria met with in urethral pus. We must look further for a distinguishing feature. This we find in the reaction of the gonococcus to the Gram stain.

Gram Reaction.—Gonococci do not take "the Gram." This means that if these cocci are stained first with an anilin dye and then with Gram's reagent (see below) the resultant stain may be washed from them, from the cells, from many other bacteria, but *not from pseudo-gonococci*, i. e., those microbes which, under the microscope, resemble true gonococci. Hence, when the Gram stain is applied, a thorough washing with alcohol leaves the cells and gonococci colourless, while the pseudo-gonococci stand out in bold relief, stained darkly by the combined colour of the anilin dye and the Gram stain (Plate II).

In order to make the effect of the Gram stain more apparent, it is customary to restain the cells and gonococci with a contrasting colour, in order that the true gonococci may be visible for direct comparison with the false (Plate III).

Preparation of the Specimen.—From what has been said in the preceding paragraphs, it is clear that recognition of the gonococcus depends upon the proper preparation of the specimen—the proper performance of the Gram test—and while I cannot say that

---

[1] I have never been able to ascertain any relation between the intracellular or the extracellular position of the gonococci and the grade or the stage of the inflammation. Every specimen contains gonococci both inside and outside the cells, and in no definite proportion.

the test is complicated, it is delicate, and, like so many other laboratory methods that appear entirely simple when one is familiar with them, it does not succeed at the hands of the beginner. Hence every practitioner is by no means competent to perform and interpret the Gram stain; but any one who can smear a cover-glass and focus a microscope may become competent by practice.

I shall not attempt to describe the methods of others, but only the one that I have employed for over two years. For the development of this method I am indebted to Dr. Chetwood.

I. *The Smear.*—A very small drop of the pus to be examined is placed upon a clean cover-glass. Upon this another cover-glass is dropped, the two pressed together and slid apart. This leaves each covered with a thin film of pus (the thinner the better). Each is then dried by evaporation at a gentle heat and fixed by rapidly passing it three or four times through the flame of a spirit-lamp or a Bunsen burner.

II. *The First Stain.*—One of the films is now covered with the following solution: [1]

Saturated alcoholic solution of gentian violet........	1 part
2% carbolated water	9 parts.

This is left on for thirty seconds, the excess washed off with water (no water must be used if the Gram stain is to be employed—see below), the glass dried in the flame, mounted in Canada balsam, and examined with the oil-immersion lens. If no bacteria with the morphological characteristics of gonococci are seen after a careful examination, it is a waste of time to employ the Gram. But if what appear to be true gonococci are found, the Gram test is applied to the other cover-glass. The Fraenkel-Ehrlich stain is applied for thirty seconds, as above described, but this time the excess of solution must be shaken from the specimen. *No water nor alcohol* may be applied at this juncture. The cover-glass is immediately floated "butter-side down" on a dish of Gram's solution.

III. *The Gram.*—Gram's solution is made up as follows:

Iodin.......................................	1 part
Potassium iodid.............................	2 parts
Distilled water.............................	300 parts.

[1] Fraenkel's modification of Ehrlich's gentian-violet solution. This solution has the advantage of resisting decomposition. It may be kept in stock for six months at a time without suffering any deterioration.

PLATE III

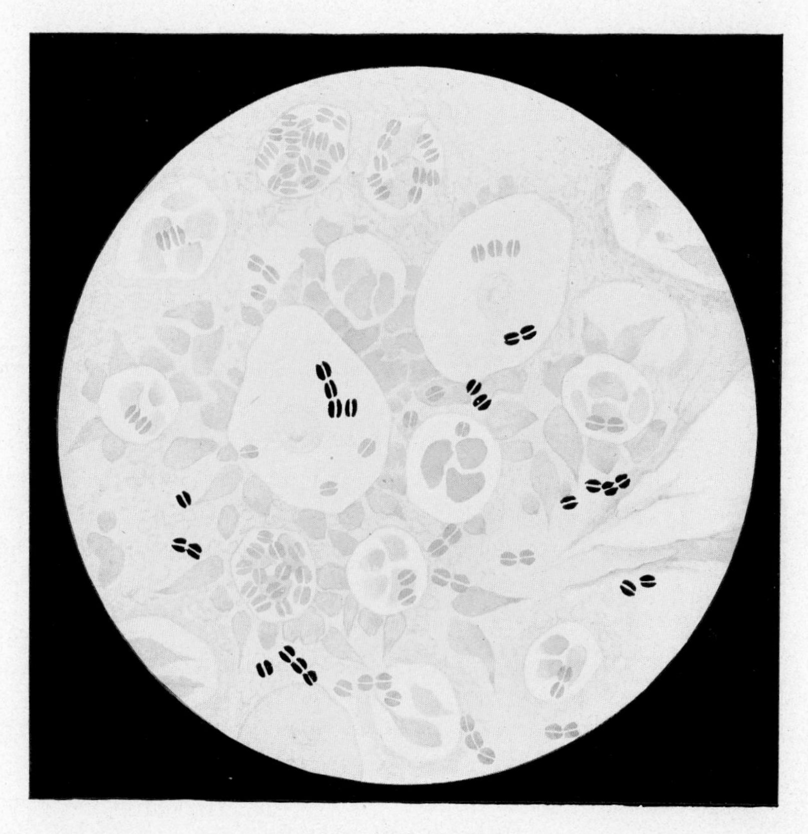

GONORRHEAL PUS.

Contrast stain: Bismarck brown. Cells and gonococci take the brown stain, while the pseudo-gonococci remain black.

The cover-glass is allowed to float upon this for four or five minutes.

IV. *The Alcohol.*—As soon as the cover-glass is removed from the Gram solution it should be washed with alcohol until all the stain has, apparently, been removed from it, and it presents much the same pearly white appearance as before the staining was begun. This requires a half minute to a minute.

V. *The Water.*—It is absolutely essential that up to this time no water shall have touched the film. Now the alcohol is washed away in running water, the film is roughly dried and submitted to the second or contrast stain.

VI. *The Contrast Stain.*—After using various more or less satisfactory counter-stains I now employ only the following:

Carbolic acid	2 parts
Saturated aqueous solution of Bismarck brown.....	98 parts.

If the decolourized smear is covered with this solution for four or five minutes and then rinsed in water it acquires a light-brown tint and, under the microscope, the cells and gonococci appear yellowish and in marked contrast to the deep purple, almost black pseudo-gonococci. A more prolonged staining with the brown gives the gonococci a deeper colour, which is not so readily distinguished from that of the pseudo-gonococci.

Such is the technic of staining the gonococcus, which may be employed by any one having an elementary familiarity with medical microscopy, and which may be depended upon to furnish accurate results when once one has familiarized himself with it. But let me repeat: its positive evidence is final; its negative evidence—its failure to find gonococci—is only final when the urethral discharge is free and has not been influenced by any local treatment. Otherwise the suspected pus must be submitted to the test of culture.

Finally, emphasis must be placed on the use of 95% alcohol for decolourizing, and the avoidance of water in every stage of the operation until after decolourization.

Gonococcus Culture.—Since the cultivation of the gonococcus requires laboratory facilities and considerable technical skill, it should not be undertaken by any but an expert bacteriologist. The detailed studies of Dr. Henry Heiman explain the methods to be employed.[1]

The necessity of employing this test before pronouncing a patient finally cleansed of his gonococci is insisted upon in another place.

[1] Med. Record, 1895, xlvii, 746; *ibid.*, 1896, l, 887; *ibid.*, 1898, liii, 80.

GONORRHEAL URETHRITIS

Morbid Anatomy.—The most accurate data we possess in reference to the invasion of the urethral tissues by the gonococcus are those published by Finger, Gohn, and Schlagenhaufer.[1] These authors inoculated the urethræ of criminals condemned to death, and were able, by means of immediate post-mortem examination, to investigate the various stages of invasion of the tissues by the specific microbe. Thirty-eight hours after inoculation the gonococci had only just begun to effect an entrance between the epithelial cells. The lacunæ of Morgagni were crowded with the cocci, diapedesis had begun, and intracellular gonococci were found among the few leukocytes on the surface of the epithelium. At the end of three days[2] the inflammatory process was well under way. The surface of the mucous membrane was covered with pus, the epithelium infiltrated by bacteria from one side and by leukocytes from the other. The inflammation showed four striking characteristics, viz.: 1. The pavement epithelium of the fossa navicularis, although swollen with leukocytes, resisted the invasion of the gonococci almost absolutely. 2. The cylindrical epithelium of the penile urethra was generally invaded. 3. This invasion was most marked about the crypts and glands, which were packed with pus and gonococci; and 4. The subepithelial connective tissue, though showing every evidence of inflammation, contained few gonococci, except in the neighbourhood of the crypts and glands and in all places not covered by epithelium.

These conclusions—viz., that squamous epithelium is especially resistant to gonococcal invasion, and that the urethral inflammation is habitually confined to the epithelium and is sharpest about the crypts and glands—are generally accepted.

The importance of *gono-toxin*, the virus of the gonococcus, in producing the inflammatory reaction has not been definitely determined. Our knowledge of the subject is summed up by Christmas.[3]

Symptoms.—True gonorrhea requires no idiosyncrasy, no ale nor champagne, no excess, no weakened condition of the urethra for its development, but simply the contact of the gonococcus with the mucous membrane of the urethra, a contact usually effected through intercourse with a woman having a gonorrheal discharge. Here, after a period of perfect rest, lasting habitually from three to five

[1] Arch. f. Derm. u. Syph., 1894, xxviii, 277.

[2] Since the average period of incubation is rather longer than this, the rapid onset in these experimental cases may be attributed to the massive infection.

[3] Ann. de l'Institut Pasteur, 1900, xiv, 331.

days, the urethral disturbance commences and runs the given course of virulent specific gonorrhea.

Incubation of Gonorrhea.—The incubation or hatching time—the period that elapses between suspicious contact and the first appearance of discharge—varies from one to fourteen days. The earlier authors recognised longer incubation periods. But I confess to some suspicion of inaccuracy in reference to those cases on the subjoined list that give a story of more than ten days' incubation. Experimental inoculation produces a discharge on the second, third, fourth, or fifth day; but it has been my experience that the shorter incubations are clinically due to the association of sexual strain or of simple urethritis with the gonococcus. Several of the cases noted below have begun with a light discharge on the second day which did not assume a purulent and specific character until two or three days later. Such a condition may be expected to occur most often in the damaged urethra of the *roué;* hence the relatively large number of short invasions among recurrences as compared with first attacks. In fact, an uncomplicated gonorrheal infection of the virgin urethra has an incubation period of from three to ten days.

Length of Incubation[1]

Day.	First Attack.	Recurrence.
1	0	2 cases.
2	2 cases.	12 "
3	2 "	15 "
4	3 "	13 "
5	11 "	10 "
6	6 "	4 "
7	4 "	10 "
8	1 case.	2 "
9	1 "	1 case.
10	1 "	4 cases.
11	1 "	1 case.
12	1 "	0
13	1 "	0
14	0	2 cases.
Total	34	76

Average incubation of 34 primary attacks, 6 days.

Average incubation of 76 secondary attacks, 4.88 days.

Of the primary attacks, 20% appeared before the fifth day; 61% on the fifth, sixth, and seventh.

Of the secondary attacks, 55% appeared before the fifth day; 31% on the fifth, sixth, and seventh.

[1] I have included in this list only those cases in which the incubation period was unmistakable and the disease absolutely characteristic—microscopically, clinically, or both.

The Acute Stage.—A tickling, teasing, itchy irritation is felt at the orifice of the urethra. The lips of the meatus are found adherent or a bluish sticky discharge is seen between them. A slight stinging is felt on urination. The lips of the meatus now swell slightly and redden. The quantity of discharge increases and it becomes opaline, then purulent. The meatus feels hot and sore. The pain on urination increases.

After the fifth day from its first appearance the discharge has become very much more copious (if unrestrained). It gets thick and purulent and soon acquires a greenish colour from slight admixture with blood, which latter may appear in little streaks.

Under the microscope the discharge is seen to contain at first pavement epithelium, mucous filaments, a few pus cells containing gonococci, and many gonococci outside of the cells. As the pus increases the epithelium diminishes and red blood cells appear, while the gonococci constantly increase in number within and without the cells. Finally, as the discharge thins down, epithelial cells reappear, while the pus cells and gonococci steadily diminish and finally disappear altogether. In the chronic gleety discharge gonococci may still sometimes be found and sometimes not. When the discharge recurs in relapse the pus cells again appear, but contain very few gonococci, these being for the most part free in the fluid and attached to the outside of the epithelial cells (Legrain [1]).

During erection the mucous membrane may be cracked, perhaps occasioning considerable hemorrhage. Pain is now felt all along the pendulous urethra, and the canal is sensitive to pressure. Irradiating pains may be complained of in the groins, testicles, perineum, cord, and back. Involuntary seminal discharges at night are sometimes brought on by the local irritation, and these ejaculations may be exceedingly painful. The urethral mucous membrane becomes thickened by the inflammation, and the stream of urine is consequently small, forked, or dribbling. Retention may come on, possibly from spasmodic muscular contraction or by extension of the inflammation backward, causing sudden congestion of the prostate (Thompson)—a condition recognised by rectal examination. But retention with gonorrhea is the rarest of complications, unless the patient continues to drink hard or has a rather tight stricture before he acquires the disease.

As the inflammation increases the prepuce may become edematous, occasioning phimosis or paraphimosis; or, if the prepuce be

---

[1] Archiv. de physiologie, 15 août, 1887.

naturally tight, the inflammation may extend into the balano-preputial cavity and light up balanitis.

Chordee.—Erections at this time become painful, threatening chordee. This indicates that the inflammation has extended beyond the free surface of the mucous membrane, and has included the delicate meshes of the erectile tissue of the corpus spongiosum. As a rule, the acuter the urethral inflammation the greater the liability to chordee. In actual chordee more or less of the areolar structure of the corpus spongiosum is obliterated by the effusion of plastic lymph, while other portions lose their distensibility. This condition may implicate a longer or a shorter distance of the urethra, sometimes almost all the pendulous portion. Consequently complete distention of the areolæ of the corpus spongiosum does not occur, and the urethra is too short for the erect corpora cavernosa, and bends the penis downward like a bow during erection, the urethra being the cord to the bow. If the corpora cavernosa become inflamed and the corpus spongiosum escapes, the arching is in the opposite direction. This takes place sometimes, but very rarely. A sort of spurious chordee, upward or lateral, may be caused by inflammation of the lymphatics along the dorsum or the side of the penis. In chordee great pain is felt from the stretching of the inflamed erectile tissue. This is measurably relieved by bending the penis so as to increase the bow, thus slackening the string; and it passes off entirely as erection disappears. Chordee is most frequent during the night and towards morning. It may render sleep impossible. The point of greatest curvature is situated anywhere along the pendulous urethra, most frequently near the glans penis. The pernicious practice of breaking the chordee—viz., roughly straightening the penis when erect—gives rise to a hemorrhage which may become excessive and be the starting-point of organic stricture.

The Decline.—After the disease has continued at its height for several weeks, the pain on urination ceases, the discharge becomes more watery, chordee infrequent. The discharge finally diminishes to a drop in the morning, the meatus again sticks together, and the patient is presently well, unless the inflammation is perpetuated behind a stricture or in the prostatic urethra.

During all the local, surface, inflammatory disturbance there is no constitutional sympathy. Feverishness means complication, although nervous individuals commonly complain of a real or fancied sense of prostration during the continuance of the discharge.

The Cure of Gonorrhea

"May I get married?" The frequency with which the sufferer from gonorrhea presents himself with this question on his lips is a sad commentary upon the levity of youth. Yet it is a question which the practitioner is frequently—nay, commonly—called upon to answer. And upon the correctness of that answer the happiness of a household often depends. An error on the side of overcaution —forbidding a man to marry when he has a perfect right to do so —is only less heinous from the patient's point of view than the permission to marry before the danger of infection has passed. On the one hand there is the prospect of moral despair for both parties, on the other the certainty of infection of the innocent with all its train of physical woes and the possible discovery of the guilty partner, with results that need not be dwelt upon.

And unhappily the question is not an easy one to answer. So difficult is it indeed that scarcely any two authorities agree as to the criteria upon which the answer shall be based. Against the genial vagueness of the light-hearted practitioner, himself a rounder and a *roué*, who proclaims that one is free from danger as soon as he is down to his customary morning drop, we may oppose the Spartan severity of those few authorities who assert that once a gonorrheic always a gonorrheic, once infected always infectious.

The broad-minded adviser will avoid either extreme. He will seek a middle course. Knowing full well that the majority of men who have had gonorrhea become and remain absolutely sound and clean, and recognising also that while most of those who exhibit the traditional morning drop are undoubtedly infectious, there remains an important minority that cannot impart its disease, under whatever stress of sexual excitement. These are practical facts commonly encountered. We need not concern ourselves with those rare cases of alleged marital infection ten or twenty years after a cured gonorrhea. By their very nature such cases are open to a suspicion of that symptom common to all venereal disease, viz., lying; and against them I can advance the experience of thirty-five years, during which I have advised countless patients to marry, with no disastrous consequences so far as I know, and all will recognise the probability that such an error would rebound forcibly enough upon its perpetrator. Such being the case, I am willing to assert the possibility of determining in any given instance that infection may or may not occur.[1]

[1] While the *diagnosis* may thus always be definite, the *prognosis* must remain indefinite. I can tell a man that he is or is not now infectious, but if he is now infec-

When does the gonorrheic patient cease to be in danger of infecting the woman with whom he cohabits? Not until the gonococci have been entirely eliminated from him. The gonococcus is the sole infectious agent. If it is present there is danger; if not there is none. But to find the gonococcus is no easy matter. Its presence may be *suspected* on account of the symptoms the patient presents—and this clinical evidence was all we had to go by until within a few years—or it may be *proved* by the evidence which bacteriology has at last evoked.

Clinical Evidence.—The clinical evidence of the presence or the absence of gonococci, which has been for so many centuries the surgeon's only criterion, is overshadowed nowadays by recent advances in bacteriology; to such an extent, indeed, that the signs and symptoms of the disease scarcely figure in the surgeon's estimation. Yet the bacteriologist is by no means infallible, and it is absolutely essential that the clinical evidence should accord before science is allowed to conclude that a patient is clean.

The notable clinical evidence of the presence of gonococci is pus, and in view of the prevalence of gonorrhea it is a general rule that *whenever there is pus anywhere in the genital or the urinary tract the presence of gonococci may be suspected, and conversely when the whole tract is proved free from pus the presence of gonococci may be denied.*[1]

Clinically speaking, a great many classes of cases may be ruled out at once. Thus, gonorrhea of the kidney is very rare and never occurs except in conjunction with gonorrhea of the lower urinary passages. Similarly the history of suppuration due to hypertrophied prostate, stone, tubercle, or tumour is usually such as to rule out gonorrhea. But the cases which come for a diagnosis on this point may be divided into three classes:

First, those who having had gonorrhea continue to have pus in the urine or are subject to relapses at every indiscretion, be it sexual or alcoholic.

Secondly, those who, having had gonorrhea, whether they allege a continuance of the discharge or not, are not subject to relapses, no matter how much sexual and alcoholic dissipation they indulge in.

Thirdly, those who, after a gonorrhea, have no longer a discharge or any other symptom, and show perfectly sparkling urine.

---

tious I cannot tell, with any certainty, when he will become clean. That is a matter of relative immunity, severity of lesion, faithfulness to treatment, and a thousand other details, differing for every case.

[1] With the single exception that the patient may have just been infected and may still be in the incubation period.

Of the first class the majority are still infectious; of the second class the majority are no longer infectious; while all who continue in the third class for a month are certainly free from gonococci and from all danger. For these last, then, the clinical diagnosis suffices; for the others there is only a probability from which the experienced surgeon may often reach an assured conclusion one way or another, but a probability which always deserves to be confirmed by scientific tests.

Bacteriological Evidence.—Here there is such a disparity of opinion as almost to shake one's faith. It is customary to excite a urethral discharge by an orgy of drink, of copulation, or of both, or by irritating the urethra by the passage of a full-sized sound or by the instillation of a strong solution (1% to 10%) of silver nitrate. The discharge is then examined for gonococci by cover-glass or by culture. Of these various methods none impresses me favourably. Such of them as are not of unsavoury morality have the distinct disadvantage of making a well man—a man supposedly well, at least—ill, and are, I believe, quite unnecessary.

I have obtained entire satisfaction by an opposite method. Instead of stirring up the gonococci, and the patient as well, I have submitted all the discharges to a practised bacteriologist. I employ three sterilized centrifuge tubes. One is filled with the first drops of urine passed by the patient, another with some of the "second flow" of urine, and a third with the secretion expressed from the prostate and vesicles. These three tubes are centrifuged and the sediments submitted to cover-glass and culture examinations. In every case the result has been accurate. The only precautions required to insure success are:

1. Sterilized tubes into which the urine is passed directly.
2. Immediate examination.
3. The application of the culture as well as of the staining tests (p. 59).
4. A bacteriologist thoroughly conversant with the delicate technic of cultivating the gonococcus.

With these precautions accuracy is assured, as fully, at least, as by any other method, and with the concurrence of the clinical evidence it is absolute—given an expert clinician and an expert scientist.

Diagnosis of Gonorrheal Urethritis

In the acute stage it is necessary to distinguish urethral gonorrhea from simple urethritis, while in the chronic stage the distinction between true relapsing gonorrhea and simple recurring urethritis is, if anything, more important still. In either case, the ultimate conclusion must rest with the discovery of the gonococcus; but there are many signs to guide the experienced practitioner, straws that show which way the wind blows, and a knowledge of these will, in many cases, suggest a brilliant diagnosis and cure, even without the aid of bacteriology.

Acute Simple Urethritis and Gonorrhea.—When a patient presents himself complaining of having contracted a gonorrhea, an inspection of his penis will often confirm or refute this opinion. If the lips of the meatus are red and swollen, exuding a creamy discharge, there can scarcely be a doubt of the specific nature of the infection. But *unless the urethral orifice is greatly swollen—unless there is ardor and chordee—an examination of the discharge is necessary to differentiate true gonorrhea from simple urethritis.* It may be that the gonorrheal inflammation is not yet well under way, or that there is chronic gonorrhea, of which this is an exacerbation, or, on the other hand, the whole matter may be a mere sexual strain. In either case the discharge may be slight or profuse, watery or creamy. The microscope and "the Gram" are required for an immediate decision, to save the surgeon from the possibility of an erroneous diagnosis and to afford the patient the advantages of immediate local treatment.

I fear not every one will accept the statement that non-gonorrheal urethritis can simulate the true specific inflammation; but I have seen cases that went through a very fierce attack and proved exceptionally unmanageable by permanganate irrigations, although the patients denied any sexual act for many weeks before the beginning of their attacks, while repeated microscopical examinations revealed no gonococcus in the discharge. In many other cases the acuteness of the onset gave every promise of a true gonorrhea, but the negative microscopic evidence was confirmed by the rapid subsidence of the inflammation under a course of treatment that never could have conquered the gonococcus. It is the relative frequency of such inflammations of the urethra that supports the quack and deludes the unwary. In view of the Protean nature of acute pseudo-gonorrheal urethritis, a few paragraphs may be profitably devoted to it here.

Acute Pseudo-gonorrheal Urethritis (bastard gonorrhea) may occur without any sexual contact whatever. I have known a sharp case to occur after a very severe sunburn, and I recall another, only a trifle less severe, in which the discharge came upon a robust and healthy man while camping in the woods, and was attributable to no cause. Such cases are, however, rare; as a rule, there has been sexual intercourse a-plenty. Indeed, excess, whether sexual or alcoholic, is so commonly an exciting cause that the patient himself readily recognises the milder form of the disease as a strain. The immunity to simple urethritis of married men who remain true to their vows shows how necessary some illicit excitement is. Although the patient is always ready to attribute his troubles to some leukorrheal or menstrual discharge of his partner, I confess that I doubt very much whether these have anything to do with the matter. Certainly newly married men do not often acquire simple urethritis, though they are not famed for their respect for the menstrual epoch nor for their sexual moderation.

But there is another and more important side to the picture. The predisposing cause of simple urethritis usually exists in the patient himself. It may be local or general—i. e., urethral or constitutional. A sharp attack of simple urethritis has been known to occur in a virgin urethra; but I believe, nevertheless, that a urethral past—a history of previous gonorrhea—is an important etiological factor. Of no less importance is the patient's diathesis. Severe simple urethritis is most commonly seen in patients of the soft, flabby, lymphatic type. Such men are liable to catarrh of any of their mucous membranes, and the urethra forms no exception. In brief, the exciting cause of simple urethritis is some external influence, almost always sexual excess; the scars of previous inflammations prepare the urethral soil, and a lymphatic, catarrhal habit makes the patient an easy victim to such an inflammation. Thus, if the excess is sufficient, there may be simple urethritis without any predisposing cause; but the attack will be light and transitory, while a slighter strain in a fit subject may well light up a sharp inflammation.

The course of non-specific urethritis depends upon the state of the urethra, the patient's general health, and the treatment. Its natural tendency is to get well promptly, and failure to do this is due either to continued excess (alcoholic or sexual), or to the damaged condition of the urethra, or to some personal idiosyncrasy, or to the local treatment. Wine and women must, therefore, be absolutely and immediately forbidden—though later mild alcoholic or sexual stimulation may prove beneficial—and the surgeon must decide, according to the evidence at hand, whether the discharge is being kept up by the state of the urethra or by the treatment. When a patient comes with a gonorrhea which he controls by a protargol injection thrice a day and a dash of permanganate after each urination, stopping his treatment will usually cure his disease; on the other hand, a history of repeated protracted attacks will suggest recurrent urethritis and demand appropriate treatment (p. 92). Any individual catarrhal predisposition that may exist will militate against a cure by any treatment, and may sometimes require a change of climate (p. 137) to overcome it.

Relapsing Gonorrhea and Recurring Urethritis.—The predisposing cause of these two conditions is the same, viz., a damaged urethra. If the case is a true gonorrhea, gonococci still exist in the discharge; if a recurring urethritis they do not; but beyond this the clinical symptoms are much the same. There is a long history of repeated attacks of urethral discharge; often enough the patient will confess that for many years he has never been well for six months at a time; there has been some stickiness of the meatus, or a morning drop. The occasional exacerbations to which such a patient is subject do not much concern him. If gonococci still inhabit his canal he has become relatively immune to them. The worst of his attacks is but a week or two of purulent discharge without any notable swelling of the meatus or chordee, and unless he is neurotic, or subject to relapsing swelled testicle, he takes a very light-hearted view of the situation. Forgetful of the sorrows of his initial attack, he proclaims that a "dose" is no worse than a cold in the head, and, acting accordingly, he spreads infection broadcast throughout the community, all the while enticing his young friends to a fate that has lost its terrors for him.

To decide whether such a man harbours gonococci or not requires the microscope and "the Gram"; or, if his troubles are quiescent, prostatic massage, the centrifuge, and cultivation of the gonococci. And definite knowledge on this point is essential both for a decision as regards matrimony and for the direction of treatment—if, perchance, he really wishes to get well. Gonococci being absent, the case may be attacked boldly. There is little danger of lighting up an acute prostatitis or epididymitis, and gentleness is practised only out of respect for the tenderness of the urethra—a respect to be observed always. The sound is introduced in search of a possible stricture; the discharge is treated by astringent instillations of nitrate of silver, thallin sulphate, or protargol, unless its profuseness calls for irrigations of permanganate of potash, or nitrate, or protargol. But if gonococci are present, the mildest measures are more likely to succeed. The sound will irritate; the epididymis must be watched; perhaps rectal irrigations or a vacation from all treatment will be required before the disease can be finally conquered. In short, this is the most tenacious type of chronic urethritis, and must be treated as such.

Course of the Disease and Complications

For purposes of clinical description and methodical treatment urethral inflammation (whether gonorrheal or other) must be distinguished as anterior and posterior and as acute and chronic in the anterior and posterior localities, since the treatment, notably the mechanical topical treatment, varies greatly with the locality. The general internal treatment, on the other hand, is not so essentially modified either by the intensity of the inflammation or the region upon which it manifests itself, being for all areas a proper balance between balsamics, alkalies, diluents, rest, and anodynes as required. Therefore the malady may be rationally presented here, as in a clinical study, all surface inflammations being considered together.

Acute Anterior Urethritis

Morbid Anatomy.—Gonorrhea, the type of this inflammation, commences at the meatus and travels slowly backward. By the eighth day all the anterior urethra has become invaded. Its surface is congested, without polish, and covered with little bare spots like those seen in balanitis where the epithelium has exfoliated. There is no ulceration. These lesions tend to become localized at the bulb, in the fossa navicularis, or at some intermediary point where there may have been much chordee.

The gonococcus first gains lodgment upon the soft epithelium just within the meatus, rapidly multiplies and penetrates between the cells into the deeper epithelial layers, into the foramina and the ducts of the mucous glands, and into the subepithelial tissues. The minute foreign bodies act like the stings of so many countless nettles, and Nature enters at once into a fierce contest to get rid of the enemy.

Hence the inflammation and the running together of myriads of leukocytes which, possessing themselves of the microbic enemy, float them out to the surface of the mucous membrane and thence to the meatus, where they appear in a stream of creamy pus.

The pus is really Nature's method of cure—a method unfortunately slow, and when left to itself painful and not without its complications.

This bird's-eye view of the situation makes it at once clear why local treatment by injection and irrigation is so tardily effective, even when the agent employed is deadly to the gonococcus, unless it be set to work while all the gonococci are upon the surface and within easy reach of the destructive agent. When the microbes have worked their way beneath the surface, which they seem to accomplish in a few hours to a greater or less extent, and each hour to penetrate more deeply, they become shut in and protected from the action of any germicide locally employed against them, and it is only by repeated and prolonged irrigation that they can be finally mastered. To expect to destroy them by one or two injections, however powerful in a germicidal way, is as sensible as to expect to drain a swamp with a broom.

A moment's contemplation of this idea intensifies one's appreciation of the truth of the fact that in an acute gonorrheal case local treatment to be promptly effective must be commenced very early—certainly within twenty-four hours of the appearance of the discharge. Every hour later makes the prompt efficiency of local germicidal treatment less brilliantly effective.

A thorough conviction about this rapidity of penetration of the bacteria is most valuable to the surgeon.

In three autopsies of cases of acute gonorrhea produced by inoculation,[1] it is shown that the pavement epithelium of the anterior urethra somewhat opposes the penetration of the gonococci, which, thirty-eight hours after inoculation, are found in groups upon the cells and commencing to penetrate between them.

It is through the foramina and foraminulæ of Morgagni and the ducts of the urethral follicles and of the glands of Littré that the germs find readiest entrance to the subepithelial tissues, and even as early as the thirty-eighth hour a certain number of leukocytes, having devoured some of the advance guard of the enemy, reach the surface and are found in the discharge, notably in the mouths of the foramina of Morgagni.

However, the germs soon get beneath the surface, and are there protected from the action of parasiticides even better than they are in laboratorial cultures.

And it has been found that antiseptics applied even for two minutes are not able to sterilize cultures. Finger made such experiments with permanganate of potash 1: 10,000 to 1: 1,000, carbolic acid 1: 10,000 to 1: 1,000, corrosive sublimate with salt 1: 100,000 to 1: 5,000, nitrate of silver 1: 2,000 to 1: 1,000, and all failed; a failure ascribed to the fact that the cultures cover themselves with an albuminous coagulation when in contact with these antiseptics, and in this way the central portions of the culture remain protected.

Symptoms.—The symptoms of anterior urethritis are the same as those of gonorrhea. Repetition is unnecessary. When the inflammation is traumatic, chemical, or of any non-virulent variety,

---

[1] Cited by Sée, p. 117, from Finger, Gohn, Schlagenhaufer.

the discharge varies in intensity even down to a moderate seropurulent oozing of short duration with little else to stamp the catarrhal character of the attack or to render it worthy of the qualification acute. The only point of prime importance is this: Does the discharge contain true gonococci, or not? If so, it is a gonorrhea and should be treated with unrelenting zeal; if not, temporizing with it is justifiable.

For treatment, see page 119.

POSTERIOR URETHRITIS

When urethral inflammation passes the hole in the triangular ligament and enters the membranous urethra posterior urethritis exists. It was formerly believed by every one that the membranous urethra is the natural terminus of many, perhaps of most gonorrheas; but there is no reasonable reason why the gonococcus should stop at the bulb. It doubtless always travels backward into the membranous urethra, but there finds an uncongenial home, for this relatively narrow portion of the canal is not luxuriously furnished with mucous glands to harbour the gonococci, and is swept fiercely by the outflowing torrent of urine, all of these conditions being unfavourable for a lodgment of the invading foe. But in a certain proportion of cases the gonococcus effects a lodgment beyond the membranous urethra and reaches the prostatic sinus, the neck of the bladder, even the bladder itself, and the inflammation occasionally mounts to the kidney; or the invasion may be propagated downward through the ejaculatory ducts into the seminal vesicle and the epididymis on one or both sides.

In this way we have as true evidences of posterior urethritis, and therefore logically to be considered as part of the urethral inflammatory picture, prostatitis, follicular and parenchymatous, acute urethrocystitis or gonorrheal cystitis, and seminal vesiculitis with or without an accompanying prostatorrhea or urethrorrhea; and all of these maladies must here receive a few words of description in their acute and in their chronic aspects.

ACUTE POSTERIOR URETHRITIS

Acute posterior urethritis is practically always gonorrheal in origin. This is obviously true when the gonococcus has worked its way backward through the membranous urethra; but it is generally none the less true in those very common instances of acute posterior urethritis following unwonted alcoholic potations, prolonged sexual excess, local violence (bicycle); for in these cases the immediately active factor in lighting up what seems to be an acute spontaneous posterior urethritis (without accompanying anterior urethritis) is, as a rule, only an adjuvant, the real underlying etiological factor being a previous condition of mild latent posterior urethritis left behind by a former gonorrhea and kindled into sudden activity by the new provocation. The same remark holds good of the more or less acute posterior urethritis so often accompanying urethral stricture; unless, haply, the stricture owes its origin to traumatism and not to gonorrhea.

That acute inflammation of the virgin posterior urethra may occasionally occur from prolonged, repeated, excessive sexual strain or masturbation is possible, but nearly phenomenal in its rarity. Prostatorrhea and subacute inflammatory conditions are more likely to result from these causes.

The posterior urethra may also become acutely inflamed in connection with enlarged prostate, from local traumatism, retained stone, tubercle, cancer, etc.; but these non-specific inflammations of the posterior urethra soon assume a chronic character or go on to abscess formation. In either case they, together with the acuter forms of follicular and parenchymatous prostatitis and prostatorrhea, all belong to the group of maladies classed as chronic posterior urethritis. They will be considered later.

For present purposes, then, acute posterior urethritis is really gonorrheal urethrocystitis, and when well pronounced it is nothing less than gonorrheal cystitis. Yet there are grades in the extent of area invaded by the inflammation and in its individual intensity.

The prostatic sinus becomes engorged as the acute inflammation invades it. Its follicles grow edematous and yield pus, the prostate sometimes congests in its substance and swells, causing reflex spasm of the cut-off muscles and retention of urine, perhaps necessitating the use of a catheter. With this there is usually a diminution of the anterior urethral discharge, and generally more or less urinary urgency and precipitancy. A finger in the rectum detects some heat and engorgement of the prostate, which may throb so that the patient's pulse may be counted by the rectal finger. Possibly the intensity of the inflammation now expends itself upon the substance of the prostate, and multiple small abscesses form in that organ, or one large abscess; or again the course may be downward into the seminal vesicle, yielding acute catarrhal inflammation there, possibly abscess, or the epididymis may inflame—even (very rarely) suppurate.

The more usual course, however, for acute posterior urethritis is for the inflammation to remain upon the surface of the mucous membrane, in the membranous urethra and the prostate, or to travel backward into the bladder, localizing itself about the neck and yielding often the fiercest symptoms of urinary urgency and insistence, true gonorrheal cystitis, and finally simmering down to a chronic posterior urethritis.

For treatment, see page 131.

GONORRHEAL CYSTITIS

This malady when acute is a specific urethrocystitis—an acute posterior urethritis legitimately prolonged. It is, strictly, for clinical purposes, a malady of the urethra. When it has lasted long uncontrolled, and resulted in contracture of the vesical neck, it leaves the category of urethral maladies and becomes a true cystitis—a disease of the bladder and not of the urethra—to be controlled by operative measures and not by medicines and local applications (p. 317).

Etiology.—Fortunately some co-operative cause over and above a simple gonorrhea is usually required to yield gonorrheal cystitis, and these causes are well known and for the most part easily avoided. The narrow membranous urethra, with its intermittent urinary torrent, is the natural guardian of the bladder, just as the contracted vesical mouths of the ureters are the guardians of the kidneys, protecting the latter from many an ascending invasion of bacterial hordes.

A common adjuvant cause of gonorrheal cystitis is the use of a strong injection in the anterior urethra, notably if forced too deeply into the canal. Any instrument passed beyond the membranous urethra is another potent agent for evil, *à fortiori* if the instrument be large or roughly used, since a traumatism of the mucous membrane is the best possible preparation of the soil for invasion, and the instrument itself is quite liable to carry in the gonococcal seed.

For the same reason—preparing the soil for invasion by bringing the blood to it and congesting it—potent factors for evil are sexual excitement with or without attempt at intercourse during the existence of an anterior gonorrheal urethritis even when the latter is well on the decline, active physical exertion, dancing, running, tennis, horseback or bicycle exercise, etc., and, finally, the use and notably the abuse of liquor, since this congests the urethra and renders the urine dense and acrid.

Anything that locally bruises the parts (even serious constipation), anything that renders the urine dense and overacid, anything that congests the prostatic sinus, even erotic thoughts, must be set down as a legitimate contributing cause to the lighting up of gonorrheal cystitis, provided always the gonococcus be at hand to avail itself of its opportunity. These last-named causes alone may produce non-specific urethrocystitis, but only when there is some other co-operative agent, such as stricture, prostatic disease, active anterior urethritis (not gonococcal), and the like.

Gonorrheal cystitis, in the natural course of events, is not to be expected before the third week of a gonorrhea, but it may be brought on very much earlier by efficient co-operative causes. Gonorrheal cystitis, as a rule, confines itself to the posterior urethra and the bladder area just within the neck. It practically never, or very rarely, involves the entire mucous lining of the bladder. In my opinion such an involvement does not commonly occur unless the prolonged duration of acute gonorrheal cystitis leads to the chronic form with contraction of the vesical neck—a surgical condition to be considered elsewhere.

Finally, in those rare cases in which violent, virulent gonorrheal cystitis mounts during the acute stage to the kidney, the specific pyelo-nephritis there set up becomes a general systemic malady and needs little consideration in this section, which deals only with the urethral mucous membrane, its maladies and complications.

Symptoms.—From a little teasing urinary frequency, with urgency and insistence, felt at first only by day and relieved upon lying down, the urinary call may become fierce and uncontrollable night and day even to the point of incontinence. Emptying the bladder does not relieve urinary desire. Straining and tenesmus come on mechanically, aggravating the already existing inflammation, and this in all grades of intensity in different cases. In sharp attacks the urine is always tinged with blood from the excoriated vesical neck, and pure blood in a small stream or in drops not infrequently follows the urinary act.

Meantime the anterior urethral discharge, if present before the onset of the acute posterior urethritis, has become greatly reduced, perhaps it has ceased entirely, and the patient, deceived by this ostrich-act, congratulates himself that at least this enemy (his discharge) has been vanquished. Vain hope! The gonococcus still lurks in the anterior urethra, and a return of the anterior discharge may be expected as the bladder symptoms subside.

There is moderate suprapubic and sometimes perineal or rectal pain, weight, and pressure. The prostate may congest and swell. If so, the urinary stream will be small and there may be retention, complete or partial, notwithstanding intense urinary desire and tenesmus.

The urine is commonly acid in gonorrheal cystitis and full of free pus. It is often tinged with blood whether passed in one, two, or three portions, but the blood is most marked in the third portion. The pus is evenly distributed throughout the urinary specimens, and is not found in gouts and shreds and chunks of stringy muco-pus, with ammonio-magnesian phosphate and bacteria, as in the ammoniacal urine of chronic cystitis.

The general symptoms attending acute posterior urethrocystitis are often seemingly disproportionate. There may be considerable suppuration and perhaps even urinary urgency without notable constitutional reaction of any kind, while on the other hand, even with superficial inflammation, there may be chilly feelings followed by active fever and great mental depression.

Uncontrolled by treatment this malady may run on to the permanent detriment of the bladder, yielding a weakness of that organ, which persists indefinitely, due to contracture of the vesical neck, or even perpetuating itself as chronic general cystitis. Active treatment, on the other hand, usually controls it with comparative ease, leaving the bladder sound. Gonorrheal cystitis may last only a few hours, while its results may last a lifetime.

For treatment, see page 139.

CHAPTER VII

CHRONIC URETHRITIS AND PROSTATITIS

CHRONIC ANTERIOR URETHRITIS

THIS malady is a chronic catarrhal state of the mucous lining of the pendulous urethra. As a rule it is the sequence of a gonorrhea, the canal being left in a subacute catarrhal condition upon the subsidence of the acute inflammation.

ETIOLOGY

A gonorrhea, well handled in a healthy subject, should leave the mucous membrane of the urethra sound after recovery, but if the inflammation has penetrated deeply beneath the mucous membrane and been protracted there, and notably if the patient be of the catarrhal, gouty, or strumous type, or if there shall have been follicular abscess, or if stricture shall have formed, or warts or polypi—then chronic anterior urethritis is the result.

In debilitated, gouty, and strumous subjects, particularly if such be dyspeptic, with dense acid urine, and notably if they be masturbators or indulge in sexual excess, or subject themselves to prolonged sexual excitement without relief—such subjects, in connection with the posterior urethritis (which these causes are liable to occasion), also suffer sometimes from moderate chronic anterior urethritis without antecedent gonorrhea.

A congenital or a traumatic stricture may be a cause, as may urethral chancre or chancroid, polyp, or a crop of so-called venereal warts (papillomatous urethritis).

For treatment, see page 127.

Papillomatous Urethritis.—An admirable study of this condition has been made by Oberländer.[1] He does not believe that pointed warts under the prepuce or in the urethra are due to gonorrheal infection, yet he does consider them contagious. The urethral discharge in papillomatous urethritis is light in quality, and chronic

[1] Sajous's Annual, 1888, ii, 212, from Vierteljahresschrift f. Derm u. Syph.

from the first. Individual peculiarity Oberländer believes to play an important *rôle*.

The papillomata are exactly like subpreputial warts, varying greatly in size. Oberländer considers that papillomatous urethritis is only a more pronounced stage of the hypertrophic urethritis that sometimes follows gonorrhea. In this I differ with him, having often seen urethral warts, either a few near the meatus or many sprinkled along deeper in the canal, while the general mucous membrane was soft and pliable, and in no sense the seat of hypertrophic urethritis.

The malady may last indefinitely, individual warts disappearing to be replaced by others. Oberländer cites a case of warts in the urethra of a patient who had had a discharge for twenty years.

Warts are not easily inspected through the urethroscopic tube, as they bleed upon the slightest touch. When they are not visible at the meatus a diagnosis may be made by urethroscopy or by inserting a bulbous bougie of fair size and not bullet-shaped, but with shouldered acorn tip. This being deeply introduced is pulled out against resisting pressure made by the thumb and finger upon and along the integument underlying the urethra just in front of the shoulder of the instrument. Upon this shoulder when withdrawn will be found some typical chunks of warty material, and hemorrhage from the urethra will follow.

Polypi.—Polypi (Fig. 19) are also found occasionally but very rarely in the urethra—oval, elongated, pedunculated masses made up of more or less fibrous and connective tissue, and covered with smooth mucous membrane. They are of varying lengths up to $\frac{3}{4}$ inch (Thompson), and have been observed in the fossa navicularis, occasionally in the pendulous urethra, and in the sinus of the prostate. They do not bleed on contact with an exploring instrument, their only symptom being a slight urethral discharge and perhaps diminution in the size of the urinary stream, with some real or fancied urethral neuralgia.

True polypi are exceedingly rare in the male urethra.

Other Tumours.—Cavernous angiomata and cysts have been observed in the urethral walls. They are mentioned only as curiosities, and might occasion a minute discharge.

For treatment of papillomatous urethritis, see page 128.

Morbid Anatomy

In chronic anterior urethritis there are congested, sometimes even semi-excoriated or frankly granular patches anywhere or everywhere along the pendulous urethra; but, by election, in the second and third inches of the canal, and in the sinus of the bulb. When there is congestion at the bulb one may confidently infer that it extends backward into the membranous urethra or beyond (posterior urethritis). The urethral wall is often thickened, as evinced by the

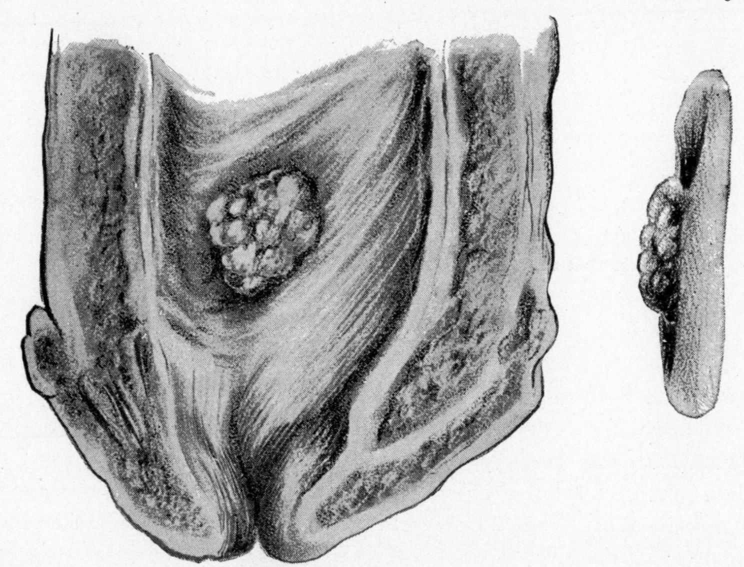

FIG. 19.—URETHRAL POLYPUS.

greater rigidity and the lack of suppleness and elasticity of the canal as it closes in upon the end of the urethroscopic tube during withdrawal. The colour of these patches is no longer the pale, boiled-salmon tint of the healthy urethra, but varies through many shades of brilliant red to dull, livid, purplish tints deprived of the customary urethral polish (from loss or alteration of epithelium), sometimes arborized with little blood-vessels, and often bleeding as the end of the tube is being withdrawn from the canal. The urethral follicles are dilated or occluded, perhaps occasionally oozing a drop of pus in severe cases, or the lesions may be quite superficial. There may, of course, be positive stricture, granular upon its surface, or with congested and granular patches behind it. This stricture the bulbous bougie will readily detect.

If there be urethral chancre as a cause for the sero-purulent gleety discharge it may generally be felt upon the outside as a palpable lump, and the urethroscope will plainly show the ulcer, while the discharge, although moderate, is often slightly bloody.

If there be polyp the urethroscope will make the diagnosis.

If there be multiple pointed condylomata (so-called venereal warts) one or more may usually be seen at or just within the meatus by distending it with the thumb and finger, while those more deeply seated may be detected by the urethroscope.

The Urethroscope.—The urethroscopes upon which I rely are two, both electric in their illumination—that of Leiter, which has long been before the profession and needs no special description here, and that of my associate Dr. Chetwood. In the country, where electric equipment is hard to keep in repair—and it will get out of order—the simple Klotz tube (Fig. 20) and head-mirror for re-

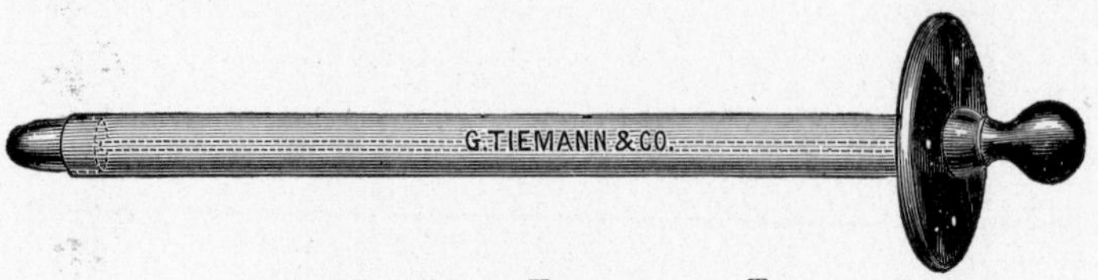

Fig. 20.—Klotz's Urethroscopic Tube.

flected lamp or sunlight will answer all purposes. In city practice electric illumination is more convenient and more brilliant.

There are two types of electric illumination, indirect from an external lamp—and perhaps the most excellent of this variety is the Otis urethroscope—and direct illumination, the lamp being within the canal; and the most convenient of these, in my opinion, is the instrument of Dr. Chetwood.

There are many other excellent urethroscopes in the market, and the selection of this or that model is a matter of personal preference.

Brown's urethral speculum (Fig. 21) is an instrument of considerable merit for some examinations, as is also its prototype, the old-

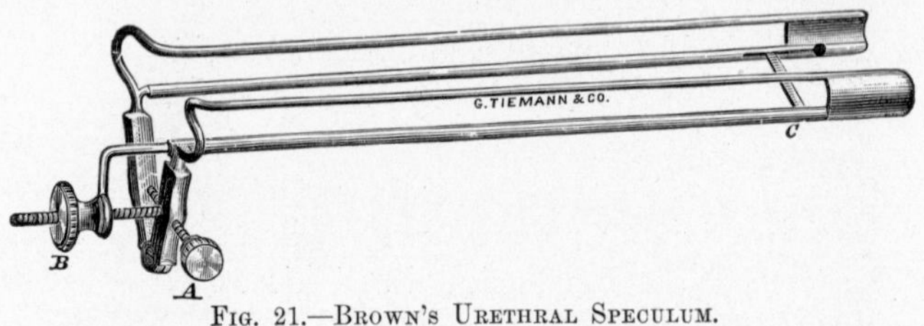

Fig. 21.—Brown's Urethral Speculum.

fashioned wire urethral speculum (Fig. 22 *a*) for use at the meatus and for the tissues just within.

It may be added here that to look into a urethroscope and to interpret what is seen are two very different matters. It requires an educated eye to see anything intelligently through this instrument, just as through the microscope.

The Chetwood urethroscope (Fig. 22) is an application of the

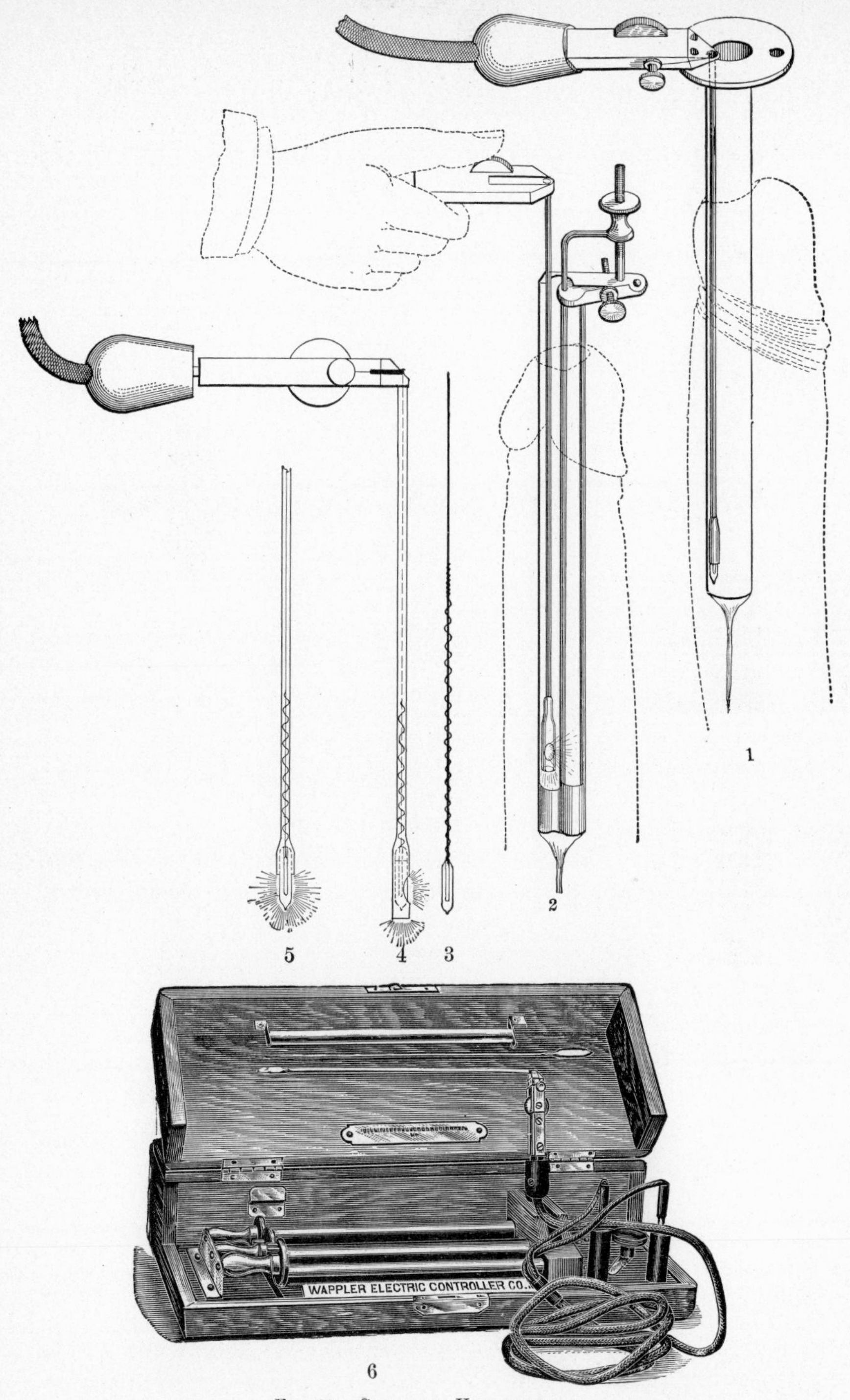

Fig. 22.—Chetwood Urethroscope.

1, instrument in use with endoscopic tube; 2, same, with wire speculum in place of tube; 3, Mignon incandescent lamp; 4, protected lamp used in wire speculum to avoid burning the urethra; 5, unprotected lamp; 6, apparatus complete, with battery; dimensions, 10 in. × $5\frac{1}{2}$ in. × $2\frac{1}{4}$ in.

principle of direct illumination by a minute incandescent lamp carried down within the tube to its end. The lamp is so small that it is practically cold, and does not heat the tube nor burn the urethra, nor get in the way of instruments. Dr. Chetwood has also adapted his lamp to Brown's urethral speculum, a manifest aid in many cases. The various parts of the instrument as depicted explain themselves. The endoscopic tube should always be as large as the urethra will readily admit without discomfort, to insure a large field for inspection.

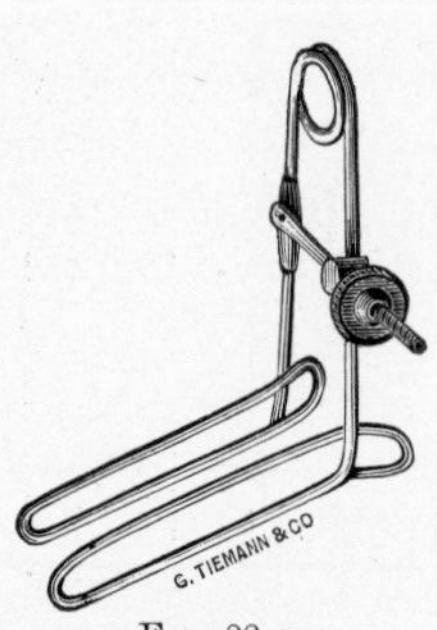

FIG. 22 *a*.
WIRE MEATUS SPECULUM.

The tube must always be introduced very gently with its end protected by an obturator, and the lubricant employed should be one without any grease in its composition and must be perfectly soluble in water. Lubrichondrin in sterilized tubes meets these conditions, or a drop or two of glycerin and water will serve in an emergency. The tube is introduced to the sinus of the bulb, the obturator removed, and the urethra inspected while the tube is slowly withdrawn.

SYMPTOMS

The one and only objective symptom is a persistent muco-purulent or frankly purulent gleet, more or less intense, and habitually worse in the early morning on rising. There are usually no subjective symptoms, but there may be tickling, itching sensations, or occasional neuralgic pains along the canal—only this and nothing more; but this little disturbance often torments the patient to the verge of distraction, and he is intensely importunate to be rid of it. The same patient with a chronic posterior urethritis, all the discharge flowing backward into his bladder, will complain little or not at all if he have no subjective symptoms, but the persistent pearly drop at the meatus, which he can see, drives him to despair, and is often rated as a malady only just short of cancer. Consequently it becomes a serious matter worthy of respectful consideration.

DIAGNOSIS

The diagnosis of urethral discharges covers a differentiation upon two questions: First, what is the lesion in the anterior urethra? Secondly, is there also posterior urethritis?

The first point can be decided by the gentle use of the bulbous bougie and by inspection through the urethroscope. Yet it is well to emphasize the fact here that these exploring instruments should not be introduced into the urethra when the discharge is abundant, though chronic and technically a purulent gleet. The traumatism likely to be occasioned in such cases by improper instrumentation may greatly intensify the inflammation and lead to folliculitis, abscess, stricture, and the like.

Therefore, in chronic anterior urethritis, when the discharge is abundant, the grade of the inflammation and the abundance and quality of the discharge must be first reduced by general and local treatment (irrigation and injection) before the bulbous bougie or the endoscopic tube be called into use for a finer definition of the ultimate lesion—stricture, granular spot, chronic suppurating follicle, polyp, wart—keeping up the discharge.

When the discharge is reasonably moderate two simple means may always be used to decide whether all the pus comes from the anterior urethra or some of it also from the posterior part of the canal.

Two-glass Test.—The first of these means is to cause the patient to urinate into two glasses. The first glass, to contain about two ounces, will hold the washings of the entire urethra, anterior and posterior. The second, if cloudy with pus, either shows sufficient posterior urethritis to have furnished pus enough to tinge the entire vesical contents by flowing backward into the bladder, or indicates that the source of pus supply is above the vesical neck, in the bladder, ureter, or kidney, in which case the first flow is usually but little more purulent than the second.

If, however, the second urinary flow is perfectly clear it does not necessarily exclude the participation of the posterior urethra in the catarrhal process, because the first urinary gush washes the posterior as well as the anterior urethra.

But if the anterior urethra down to the bulb be washed out with a hot boric-acid solution, introduced through a small, soft-rubber catheter, and the first urinary gush is still full of pus, the presumption that this pus comes from the posterior urethra becomes a conviction.

Injection Test.—The second means of differentiation consists in using an injection capable of permanently colouring the anterior urethral shreds. The one I prefer is the permanganate of zinc, about 1:500.

If the patient, not having previously urinated, be told to inject his urethra with an ordinary blunt-nozzled syringe and to retain the injection in the canal for about twenty seconds, and then, half an hour or more later, to present himself for examination, it will be found, if he have chronic anterior urethritis, that some of the urethral shreds will be coloured brown, plainly indicating that the patches yielding these soft scabs have been bathed in the colouring solution, and consequently must have been in the anterior urethra.

The bulbous bougie may now be used, and upon its shoulder on withdrawal will be found other coloured clots of pus which had adhered to the urethral wall and had not been washed away by the escaping stream of urine, a further evidence that the anterior urethral wall is in a damaged condition.

Finally, when the urethroscope is used, and the back part of the sinus of the bulb is found livid in colour (perhaps bleeding) up to the hole in the triangular ligament, then it may be confidently assumed that over and above the anterior urethritis posterior urethritis also exists.

Shreds (Tripperfäden).—The trained eye comes to recognise a certain individuality in urethral shreds as passed in the first urinary gush. There are five main varieties, any one of which may exist alone or all together. They are: small granular flakes, threads, the tadpole shred, angular pieces, cottony shreds, and for the most part may be safely interpreted as follows, whether occurring in company with free pus and bacteria in the urine or not.

The small granular flakes, a sort of urethral dust, are usually made up of pavement epithelium and more or less pus cells intermingled. They generally come from the anterior urethra, are not very heavy, and settle slowly in the glass.

The threads look like bits of cotton thread. They are very white, of greatly varying length, dense in structure, and settle at once. They are composed of a dense aggregation of pus cells, and if the gonococcus be contained in them it can be detected by careful double staining. They come from the anterior urethra.

The tadpole shred is a similar white thread with a globular head. It has the same general characteristics, and settles at once. It means that a small exulcerated or granular spot or an ulcerated follicle exists yielding the pus that constitutes the head of the tadpole, the rest of the shred forming as usual along an inflamed line of urethra or in a fold of mucous membrane. Such shreds often come from the deeper parts of the urethra.

The angular broken pieces of irregular size (not threads) are usually an indication of chronic inflammation (often stricture) at the hole in the triangular ligament, and of chronic inflammation in the membranous urethra behind. They settle quickly and are little masses of pus.

The fleecy, cottony, filmy shreds often seen single and alone in otherwise nearly or absolutely clear urine come from the prostatic sinus about the colliculus seminalis. This filmy mass floats a long time in the urine, and sometimes rises to the top instead of settling to the bottom, sometimes dissolving in the urine. Microscopically it is found to be thin, striated mucus entangling in its meshes leukocytes, prostatic round cells, squamous epithelia, sometimes sympexions, and rarely a stray spermatozoön or a few crystals of oxalate of lime, with possibly some bacteria, but seldom, if ever, gonococci.

For treatment, see page 125.

CHRONIC POSTERIOR URETHRITIS, INCLUDING THE INFLAMMATIONS OF THE PROSTATE GLAND

It is convenient to group under chronic posterior urethritis all the inflammations of the prostate, since however widely these latter may diverge in the acuteness, intensity, or importance of their symptoms from the comparatively benign (though intractable) aspect that chronic posterior urethritis commonly presents, nevertheless the urethral inflammation is, clinically, the *fons et origo* of every one of them. The inflammation begins and ends in the posterior urethra, and is in a great majority of cases of gonorrheal origin.

These various inflammations may be classed as follows:

1. Chronic non-specific posterior urethritis.
2. Chronic gonorrheal posterior urethritis.
3. Acute parenchymatous prostatitis.
4. Chronic parenchymatous prostatitis.
5. Periprostatitis, acute and chronic.

The human imagination has not sufficient breadth to grasp such a group of inflammations collectively. They must be treated separately and consecutively; yet be it understood they are all phases of one general condition, viz., chronic gonorrhea, and it requires the keenest diagnostic acumen to differentiate them one from the other. In order to set each in as striking opposition to its neighbour as possible, I shall endeavour to render my descriptions as brief as consistent with clearness, and shall close the description with a *résumé* of the clinical varieties of the disease in order to sketch in outline the usual clinical pictures resulting from the various combinations of lesions described below.

Chronic Non-specific Posterior Urethritis

Simple (non-specific) chronic posterior urethritis, or surface prostatitis, might be termed a secondary inflammation. Its underlying cause is always some other disease. It is usually a direct consequence of gonorrheal posterior urethritis, from which it can only be distinguished by the absence of gonococci from the discharges.

It is also encountered under the form of recurring urethritis (p. 69), and is then often associated with some prostatorrhea (p. 95). Again, it is met with—and under a more acute form—as the result of slight injuries, usually at the hands of the surgeon. It is a negligible phenomenon in many cases of stricture. It may be due to habitual sexual excess. Finally, it occurs in the hypertrophied prostate, and is an epiphenomenon in prostatic tuberculosis and cancer.

All these forms of the inflammation, while varying in degree, are comparable in their morbid anatomy and symptoms to the gonorrheal process. The only variety sufficiently characteristic to delay us is that form of simple urethritis, or surface prostatitis, as it is more appropriately termed in this connection, which occurs in the hypertrophied prostate. This inflammation is commonly due to instrumentation, and when once it has set in, the vulnerable condition of the prostate makes of this simple trouble a malady even less amenable to treatment than the notoriously intractable chronic gonorrheal inflammations of the unhypertrophied gland. Moreover, in its tendency to complications, this simple inflammation, instead of exhibiting a benign aspect, shows a virulence exactly comparable to that of the specific disease.

Chronic Gonorrheal Posterior Urethritis

This is chronic gonorrhea. The German school has a tendency to exaggerate the importance of chronic anterior urethritis. Many American authors have insisted upon the importance of stricture, which is a special form of chronic *anterior* urethritis. But it has been my experience that chronic gonorrhea, with its cardinal symptom, viz., gleet, is nothing more nor less than chronic posterior urethritis. There is, practically, always some anterior urethritis, whence the gleety discharge; but to insist solely upon that discharge, and to relegate the inflammation of the posterior urethra to a position of secondary importance, while making every effort to cure the inflammation of the anterior canal, is a position unwarranted by science and unsupported by practice, for the anterior urethra is a comparatively smooth canal. Every urination flushes its deepest crevices. Unless there is stricture, or follicular abscess, or papillomatous growth—and a careful examination of a series of patients will convince the surgeon how relatively infrequent these conditions are—the urethral walls present few lodging places for the gonococcus once the acute inflammatory stage is past.

But in the posterior urethra all is different. Posterior urethritis is synonymous with surface and follicular prostatitis. The canal is here nothing more than a tunnel through the thousand-mouthed, succulent prostate. The gonococci once established in the ducts of the prostatic glands—and they are not slow so to establish themselves—are not swept by the urinary stream, and are all but inaccessible to the surgeon's irrigations. This is pure theory, but practice bears it out. The recognised tenacity of all prostatic inflammations, the futility of anterior injections to cure these cases, the evil wrought by sounds, which only irritate the sensitive prostate, and the presence, in practically every case, of pus in the second flow of urine, prove, I believe, the importance of posterior urethritis. I feel justified in asserting, therefore, that with a few exceptions, among which stricture is the most important, chronic gonorrhea is posterior urethritis.

Morbid Anatomy.—The essential lesion in chronic posterior urethritis is a catarrhal inflammation of the mucous membrane of the prostatic urethra, the prostatic glands, and the orifices (at least) of the ejaculatory ducts. Thus the inflammation may easily spread in several directions—viz., up the seminal canals to produce vesiculitis and epididymitis, deep into the prostate to produce parenchymatous prostatitis, forward into the bulb to produce gleet or perhaps to light up an acute urethritis, and backward into the bladder to set up cystitis or contracture of the neck (p. 317). It is to some one or more of these complications that the symptoms are due. Yet the essential underlying lesion is usually found in the prostatic urethra.

Symptoms.—Chronic gonorrheal posterior urethritis is commonly encountered towards the end of an acute attack of the disease. It is characterized by but two symptoms. There is pus in both urinary flows (p. 83)—rarely only in the first—and there is more or less gleety discharge; a morning drop or a fairly free flow, varying from day to day, and dependent upon the degree of inflammation of the anterior canal. Be it clearly understood, gleet almost invariably accompanies posterior urethritis; but local treatment may stop the gleet by curing the inflammation of the anterior urethra without so much as affecting the posterior inflammation. Any stoppage of discharge will be hailed by the patient with delight as evidence of a cure; but so long as the urine is hazy with pus the surgeon must recognise that the enemy is only repulsed, not conquered.

Beyond this there is usually nothing. Prostate and vesicles feel normal to rectal touch, though the expressed contents of either may be found to contain pus and gonococci. There may be prostatic neuralgia. There are often some symptoms of parenchymatous prostatitis, even though no enlargement of the gland can be detected.

Acute Parenchymatous Prostatitis—Prostatic Abscess

An acute inflammation of the prostate may occur at any time in the course of a posterior urethritis, or may be induced by trauma even though the urethra is not permanently inflamed. When occurring in the course of a gonorrheal posterior urethritis it is due to some indiscretion, sexual excitement, alcoholic excess, or the passage of instruments; even exposure to cold or undue fatigue may induce it.

The initial symptom is usually a sharp chill immediately followed (perhaps preceded) by an increasing sense of heat and weight in the perineum, a frequent desire to urinate, with a sensation of burning during the act and an acute pain at its termination. Defecation is almost equally painful. The fever runs high and is irregular; there may be a succession of chills; the prostration, loss of appetite, and constipation are marked. In fact, the patient is the subject of an acute septicemia which terminates either in resolution or in abscess formation—usually the latter—and the abscess, in turn, bursts into one or more of the neighbouring viscera, or is evacuated by the surgeon. An infrequent complication is gonococcus pyemia (p. 145).

As the tension of the abscess increases the local symptoms are intensified. The dysuria becomes continuous and frightfully painful, the soreness radiating in all directions, and if the prostate becomes so swollen as to obstruct the urethra, retention adds its miseries.

Rectal examination may well be exquisitely painful. It reveals an enormously enlarged, hot, throbbing prostate. An abscess is distinguishable as an edematous or a frankly softened and fluctuating area amid the surrounding, hot, hardened prostatic mass. A deeply seated abscess cannot be distinguished by rectal touch.

As the disease progresses the suppurating foci, be they few or many, usually fuse into an extensive cavity, generally situated towards the rectal surface of the gland and in one or other lateral lobe. The abscess habitually opens through the urethra spontaneously during an effort at urination or defecation, or is accidentally opened by a catheter introduced to relieve retention, or during exploration with a sound or a searcher. Once opened it discharges intermittently during the intervals of urination in jets, or with the urinary stream only, for the cut-off muscle usually keeps the pus from flowing away constantly from the meatus. If the abscess has been small, recovery is prompt; if large, the drainage is often imperfect, and the grave responsibilities remain of a chronic, persisting granulating cavity, and of possible pyemia or infiltration of urine. Again, the spontaneous opening may have been small, and when the tension is relieved it may close, forcing the pus to find another means of exit, and giving rise to an abscess cavity with multiple openings.

Petit and Erichsen have both recorded a direct opening of prostatic abscess into the bladder. I have observed this on one occasion.

Rupture of prostatic abscess into the rectum is another spontaneous effort at cure on the part of Nature. Such rupture can only occur after the rectum has been sealed to the prostate by preliminary inflammation of the connective tissue between them. Under these circumstances all goes well, but if such adhesions default, as they very well may, the result is diffuse cellular periprostatitis or periprostatic abscess.

An accumulation of pus within the prostate may take two routes instead of one, and burst into the rectum as well as into the urethra, eventually leaving urethro-rectal fistula, through which intestinal gas and fecal material may invade the urethra. I have seen this occur. Spontaneous closure of such fistulæ is possible.

Chronic Parenchymatous Prostatitis

Chronic parenchymatous prostatitis may follow an acute inflammation, but its onset is usually insidious, not attributable to any cause, nor characterized by any special symptoms. Indeed, there is doubtless a diffuse inflammation of the prostate gland that never shows any symptoms, except those mentioned above as characteristic of chronic posterior urethritis. And conversely there may be a slight parenchymatous prostatitis, producing the symptoms of that disease without its one physical sign—which is an enlargement of the prostate quite comparable to the lateral enlargement of the hypertrophied gland. The prostate swells within its capsule, often to the size of a small orange, perhaps unevenly, one lobe being involved to a greater extent than the other—sometimes in an irregular, nodular manner. The exploring finger in the rectum at once strikes against this mass, which encroaches upon the cavity of the gut and is hot, tense, and sensitive in proportion to the acuteness of the symptoms.

While it is possible for parenchymatous prostatitis to give no evidence of its existence other than the physical signs, there are certain characteristic subjective symptoms that appear and disappear as the inflammation varies in intensity. These symptoms are vague, and are described differently by different patients. Some complain of an irritation, as though there was a ball in the rectum, and may demand a purgative under the mistaken impression that clearing the lower bowel will relieve the discomfort. Pressure upon the perineum by the finger or in sitting may be painful, and there is a subjective sensation of pain, heat, throbbing, or weight in the perineum and lower belly, penis, and scrotum, with, perhaps, constant pain running along the urethra to the head of the penis. There may also be pain in the back, down the thighs, and perhaps in the feet. These symptoms are all due to the tension of the swollen prostate within its capsule.

Periprostatitis

Chronic periprostatitis is the direct extension of some inflammation of the prostate to the connective tissue about the gland. This inflammation results in the formation of masses of inflammatory tissue about the prostate. They give no symptoms. I have seen a case of diffuse chronic pericystitis and periprostatitis diagnosed as cancer of the prostate.

Acute periprostatitis—i. e., periprostatic cellulitis or abscess—usually results from a prostatic purulent focus pointing downward; but wounds through the rectum may occasion it, abscess of the seminal vesicle may be its cause, it may be a complication of cancer or of tubercle of the prostate or of the base of the bladder near the neck, and it may owe its origin to a suppuration of one of the lymphatic glands lying between the prostate and the rectum (Lannelongue [1]).

Such accumulations are diffused in the meshes of the connective tissue about the prostate. The symptoms are, in the main, those of prostatic abscess, but are less intense and run a slower course. A general diffuse inflammatory edema is easily appreciated by rectal touch, blotting out the limits of the prostate, and more boggy in some places than in others, perhaps frankly fluctuating at a given point.

This collection, following the line of least resistance forward into the perineum and the ischio-rectal fossa, generally opens into the urethra or the rectum, sometimes into the ischio-rectal fossa, or even through the perineum; sometimes, not uncommonly (21 times in 115 cases reported by Ségond), both through the rectum and the urethra. Before doing this it has usually given rise to urinary retention, and afterward to all the inconveniences of a urethro-rectal fistula, urine passing into the rectum each time the bladder is emptied, and gas and fecal matter finding their way, from time to time, into the urethra. Such a fistula does not often close spontaneously, because it is usually a long tract with a chronic abscess cavity situated along its route. Sometimes this cavity becomes very extensive, dissecting up the rectum more or less, and perhaps occa-

[1] Bull. de la soc. de chir., 1878, iv, 600.

sioning quite a formidable retrovesical abscess pouch, or running into the ischio-rectal fossa, there to give rise to all the symptoms of abscess of that region.

If the pus burrows forward into the perineum it may occasion considerable mischief following along towards the corpus cavernosum, or even laying it bare (Demarquay). It has been known to go through the obturator foramen (Tillaux), and even to follow the connective-tissue plane about the spermatic cord and to point in the inguinal canal, or to get into the space of Retzius, to appear at the umbilicus, to pass by the sciatic notch (Guyon), or to burst through the posterior vesico-rectal *cul-de-sac* into the peritoneal cavity, or even, circumventing the bladder, to mount in front of the abdomen in the sheath of the rectus up to the ribs (Desnos, referring to Curtis)—all very rare, but still possible culminations of periprostatic suppuration. As Guyon has put it, every connective-tissue plane in communication with the retroprostatic layer is a route open to suppuration.

When such long burrowing courses are followed it is usual for several spontaneous perforations to occur *en route*.

As may be inferred from what has just been written, the course, duration, and termination of periprostatic suppuration are all open to wide variation, and may call for expert surgery.

In discussing these points Desnos [1] refers to the limit of cure as being twelve days and fifteen months, and in 114 observations, cure 70 times, persistence 10, death 34—of which latter 11 were due to a cause foreign to the prostatic malady.

Phlebitis, pyemia, and peritonitis may at any time complicate periprostatic suppuration.

Clinical Varieties of Posterior Urethritis

All cases of posterior urethritis may be classed as follows:

1. Mild cases.
2. Intractable cases.
3. Relapsing cases.
4. Irritable cases.
5. Neurotic cases.

1. Mild Cases.
2. Intractable Cases. } —Although most chronic inflammations of the posterior urethra are mild in the sense that their symptoms are not annoying, few of them are mild in responding promptly to treatment. And so it is that many a man does not much care

[1] Traité élém. des mal. des voies urin., 2de éd., 1898, 327.

whether he has a posterior urethritis or not, so long as it remains symptomatically mild. But to the conscientious surgeon nothing is more exasperating than those cases that persist in hanging fire in spite of his best efforts to cure them. Cases that are rapidly curable are those in which the prostate is not hypertrophied, the inflammation not gonorrheal, and the patient docile; conversely, an intractable patient, a gonorrheal inflammation, and a hypertrophied prostate are elements that tend to make the inflammation resist all treatment. Another feature that militates against a cure is the existence of such complications as parenchymatous prostatitis, periprostatitis, vesiculitis, and epididymitis. The battle with these conditions is often tedious to the last degree, and it is small wonder that the surgeon's judgment and the patient's endurance should fail, as they so often do during the long months that may be required before a cure is reached.

3. **Relapsing Cases.**—Every case of chronic urethritis has some little tendency to relapse after a cure has apparently been effected. But certain urethræ show a tendency in this respect little less than maddening. Perhaps the patient will have been carried successfully through an acute gonorrhea by the irrigation treatment when an unexpected outbreak of the disease in the deep urethra disappoints surgeon and patient alike. Or a chronic case may have gradually yielded to methodical treatment only to burst out afresh at the slightest provocation. Those cases that relapse year after year are often more annoying to the surgeon than to the patient. It is especially provoking when a patient leaves town with all the evidences of a cure to have him wire from the first station he stops at that his discharge is in full blast. To avoid this mishap it is absolutely essential to know, before declaring a patient cured, that his prostate no longer harbours gonococci. This fact ascertained, the surgeon may at least prophesy that if a relapse does occur, it will only be a light non-specific inflammation that will subside in a few days without local treatment.

A peculiar feature of the relapse is that it may act more or less like a new infection. The inflammation spreads throughout the urethra in a few hours, due, apparently, to a reinfection by the gonococci that had seemingly lost their virulence.

The cause of relapse may be a collection of pus in some gland or follicle, urethral or prostatic, or a local irritation due to alcohol, to sexual excess, to a cold in the head, or to excess in the local treatment. But the great predisposing cause is the catarrhal habit, whether natural to the patient or induced by overmuch work or dissipation. Without this any of the exciting causes may light up a relapse; but with it relapses occur and recur on the slightest provocation or on no provocation whatever, defying local treatment and demanding hygiene and tonics to effect a cure.

4. **Irritable Cases.**—Some urethræ are so sensitive that local treatment is next to impossible, whether because of the pain and spasm it evokes, or because an outburst of acute inflammation in the neck of the bladder, the prostate, the vesicle, or the epididymis follows every attempt at local treatment and every indiscretion on the part of the patient. This local irritability, while in a sense peculiar to the individual, is usually the result of a habitual disregard of the rules of prudence. The patient is either a hard drinker, or addicted to sexual excess, or overworked and overworried, or—and this alternative is, unfortunately, not a rare one—he has been irritated by local treatment. An appreciation of this fact will help to direct the treatment of such cases.

5. **Neurotic Cases.**—The neuroses of the prostate are not habitually due to antecedent gonorrhea of that organ, and it is only exceptionally that one encounters evidence of neurosis while the inflammation still continues. The neurotic taint adds many and various symptoms to those of the inflammation, and protracts the patient's miseries even after his prostate has apparently returned to its normal state.

This consideration of the prostatic inflammations has insensibly brought about a digression from the clinical plan proposed—namely, to consider all the urethral, suppurative, and catarrhal maladies together. It would seem natural here to take up a consideration of the maladies of the seminal vesicle associated with gonorrhea, with urethral discharge, and with evidences of prostatitis. But before doing this it is better to dispose of mucous discharges from the urethra and then through prostatorrhea, again to approach the seminal vesicles, and to terminate the study with follicular urethral abscess, periurethritis, and cowperitis, bringing up with the treatment of everything at the end to avoid repetition.

URETHRORRHEA

This term has for the most part a negative significance, and is only useful in that it may be employed to designate a mucoid flow from the urethra, not purulent, not prostatic, not seminal. It is a pellucid, sticky drop—or a number of drops, indeed, sometimes a flow—which sticks the lips of the meatus together; and on separation of these the glue-like fluid of blue-white colour is seen. When caught upon the finger and rubbed against the thumb this drop is tenacious, and strings out as the thumb and finger are separated, feeling soapy as they are again rubbed together; or, on the other hand, the drop may be quite watery and thin, but it is always somewhat sticky and never has a seminal odour. This flow when abundant stiffens, but does not stain the linen, and it may come away in greater quantity during straining effort, as at stool, during exercise, or after micturition. If the discharge be due to surface urethral congestion it is quite watery, clear, and only slightly sticky. When the secretion of the glands of Littré and Cowper is mixed with it or constitutes its main bulk, it is thick, cohesive, and tenacious. Patients generally think that it is spermatic fluid. The microscope shows it to be composed of single flat epithelial cells and clusters of the same, mucous corpuscles, films of striated mucus, granular *débris* of various kinds, no pus threads (unless there be also a patch of chronic anterior granular urethritis, which is quite possible as a concomitant), no prostatic bodies, no spermatozoa, no lecithin bodies, no Böttcher's [1] crystals.

The causes of this affection are prolonged, ungratified sexual desire, constant impurity of thought, a sort of mental masturbation through the imagination, often indulged in by weak-minded youths, as well as by old men who are regretfully conscious that they are getting beyond the potential stage of sexuality. Another cause is delayed orgasm during intercourse or withdrawal before emission, pernicious practices which occasion sexual strain. Masturbation if excessive, or too much natural sexual exercise under the stimulus of mental provocation—all these and the like, being a violence to the various urethral mucous glands and to the circulation of the urethra by prolonged, sustained, excessive nervous tension, lead to passive congestion and lack of tone in the circulation of the urethra and in its mucous glands and follicles, and thus occasion an excess of mucous secretion all along the line, together with more or less desquamation of pavement epithelium—and this is the malady and the whole of it.

The natural beading of the meatus during intense sexual excitement is physiological. It is equivalent to the watering of the mouth when one is hungry and smells appetizing food.

Whether it is fair also to denominate urethrorrhea that form of mucous oozing following chronic anterior urethritis in some cases, notably in the strumous, gouty, and debilitated, after the pus and shreds have disappeared, may be questioned; but it is much the same thing, being a mucoid oozing from congested surfaces which are not

[1] The fluid must be examined in substance. It cannot be recovered by the pipette from a specimen of urine since the latter totally dissolves it.

inflamed enough to yield pus, and it gets well, not by local treatment, which indeed may maintain and prolong it, but by improved general health, change of air, etc., with lapse of time. I well remember such a case, which came to me thirty years ago, a solicitous young man who had been under continuous treatment for a year at the hands of one of New York's most noted surgeons without avail. I stopped all treatment and sent him to Bermuda. The vessel had not been twenty-four hours out of port before his mucoid drop diminished notably. It promptly disappeared and never returned.

Many a time a little, final mucoid drop of this sort is entertained for weeks or months by excess in local treatment due to unnecessary solicitude on the part of the patient and inordinate zeal on the part of the surgeon.

But the true urethrorrhea, be it due to whatever cause among those enumerated, gets slowly better upon doing away with the continued action of that cause—be it lust, masturbation, excess, or what not which has occasioned it—and by insisting on urethral and general hygiene aided, perhaps, by monobromid of camphor 30 centigrammes 3 times a day, if erections be insistent, and such tonics as seem indicated, notably iron and strychnin. A minute dose of atropin, sufficient to dry the mouth slightly, assists. I think it also somewhat dries the urethral and prostatic secretion. Massage of the urethra by the passage of a large steel sound every two or three days through the anterior canal, or by the double-current cold-water metallic sound (Winternitz) with iced water, is sometimes helpful, with perhaps a light injection of the non-alcoholic fluid extract of hydrastis 8%, or claret and water 50%, once or twice a day. Strong injections irritate, and any injection may do as much harm as good, notably in those self-centred cases where morbid introspection is the salient feature of the malady. Here anything that keeps the patient's mind upon his genitals harms him, and any local treatment may be mischievous. A cold morning douche to the external genitals has a tonic effect. The patient's mind must be disabused of his morbid fancies. Horseback exercise is helpful, unless there be also chronic prostatitis, when it might do harm.

For treatment, see page 140.

PROSTATORRHEA

This malady may occur alone, in which case it is not inflammatory, not a prostatitis—with which it is almost universally confounded, nor yet a urethritis—but a sexual malady, and, like urethrorrhea, due to some form of sexual strain.

But prostatorrhea may very well be engrafted upon an already existing surface or follicular prostatitis, and in the declining stages of the latter may form part of the picture—or a person with prostatorrhea may get chronic follicular prostatitis as a sequence of gonorrhea—but the point is that true prostatorrhea is a local sexual weakness due to strain and not a sequence of local inflammation.

Chronic spermato-cystitis is distinctly a sequence of gonorrheal inflammation after the latter has invaded the prostatic sinus, and this vesiculitis may yield some of the symptoms of prostatorrhea; indeed, the two may also coexist. So that, clinically speaking, a true case of uncomplicated prostatorrhea is very rare, since it is likely to be affiliated on the one hand with chronic inflammatory follicular prostatitis, and on the other with chronic seminal vesiculitis. It may also be associated with urethrorrhea, and share some of the symptoms of the latter.

Sturgis[1] has made an admirable study of the malady, differentiating its individuality in a very concise manner.

Prostatorrhea is a sexual weakness due to strain or sexual perversion of some sort. It is a local lack of tone due to deteriorated nerve force from prolonged nervous tension, and is not an inflammation.

It consists in an intermittent discharge from the meatus of thin, white milky fluid of acid reaction, sometimes neutral, not sticky, soapy, nor cohesive to the feel, and when uncomplicated containing no pus cells, spermatozoa, or leukocytes. It does, as a rule, contain prostatic bodies (sympexions), cubic and pyramidal epithelia, and upon the addition of a 1% solution of phosphate of ammonia, a drop of which may be added to a portion of the discharge upon a microscopic slide, it does produce the peculiar star-like angular collection of pointed and crossed buck-saw crystals known by the name of Böttcher, not found in any secretion from any portion of the genito-urinary tract except the prostate. It contains also clumps of lecithin granules.

This distinguishing mark is notable, but unfortunately there may be a combination of prostatorrhea and chronic spermato-cystitis; and then sometimes the Böttcher's crystals are found in the discharge expressed from the meatus without the addition of the ammonia solution, because the secretion of the inflamed vesicles is alkaline.

The prostatic secretion smells like semen on account of the lecithin which it contains. It is acid in reaction in the normal state,

---

[1] N. Y. J. Cut. and Gen.-Urin. Dis., 1898, xvi, 263.

but Lohnstein,[1] recording recently his 542 examinations of the prostatic secretion, carefully obtained by massage from the prostates of 80 patients, noted certain variations from Fürbringer's dictum as to the reaction of the normal secretion. For even in these pathological states the fluid was 404 times (75%) acid, 30 times (5%) neutral, 108 times (20%) alkaline; but it was not always the same in the same patient, being in 5 cases alternately acid and neutral, in 8 neutral and alkaline, and in 15 acid and alkaline, while the proportion of moving spermatozoa was equally great in both cases. This mixture of spermatic elements in the fluid would, however, indicate either that Lohnstein was dealing with cases of spermatocystitis as well as of prostatitis, or that his massage included the vesicles as well as the prostate.

These investigations, however, establish the fact that the secretion in prostatitis is generally acid, as the fluid of the vesicles alone is known to be feebly alkaline. Fürbringer says of these vesicular and testicular fluids that they become easily alkaline.

This, then, being the quality of the fluid—acid, thin, watery, white (opalescent)—the question is, Does prostatorrhea ever occur as a distinct malady independent of prostatitis or spermato-cystitis? In my opinion, although possible it is very rare—so rare as a distinct malady that it may be almost disregarded, being better considered as an associate symptom sometimes with urethrorrhea, sometimes with prostatitis, sometimes with chronic spermato-cystitis.

Symptoms.—In a true case—always a masturbator or one given to perverted or excessive sexual exercise, most often a neurotic or neurasthenic subject—the patient finds a whitish, thin, watery drop at the meatus, and notices that the same is extruded in greater quantity at stool, and sometimes after urination.

He believes this to be a seminal loss, and is on that account excessively despondent. He is likely to have obscure neuralgic sensations along his urethra, a feeling as if a cold, occasionally a hot, drop were trickling along the canal at odd times. There may be a little vesical irritability not noticed by a man in health, for *raro mingitur castus* is as true now as of old. Every physical and functional evidence of sexual lack of tone may be present. The penis may be long, cold, and flabby, blue at the glans penis, notably about the corona glandis. The testicles may be flabby, soft, neuralgic, or at least oversensitive to handling. There may be pain in the back, radiating down the thighs or in the perineum, and various other reflex pains. There may be dyspeptic symptoms, a white tongue, a soft

---

[1] Guyon's Annales, 1900, xviii, 1188.

rapid pulse, dilated pupils, cold, moist palms, headache, tendency to mild vertigo, loss of memory, inability to concentrate the attention or to sustain prolonged mental effort, as in study or even in reading. With this there may be premature ejaculation during intercourse, and excessive sexual desire with diminished power—possibly functional impotence due largely to solicitude and to neurotic causes.

The patient may be melancholic and despondent to the verge of mania, incapable of consolation; and this all the more if with his prostatorrhea he has spermato-cystitis, a perfectly possible combination. In fact, all the evidences of the so-called sexual neurasthenia may be present in any or every combination.

But it is not a fact that true spermatorrhea alone or true chronic spermato-cystitis alone necessarily gives rise to these symptoms of despondency, sexual incompetence, or precipitate ejaculation, for a considerable number of patients have both spermatorrhea and spermato-cystitis, and are not subjectively conscious of it, unless by the physical signs of pain and local discomfort to which the inflamed vesicles give rise. I have again and again found spermatozoa constantly in the urine of patients being examined for another malady, and have not communicated my information to them because the seminal loss occasioned no symptoms whatsoever, and I preferred not to arouse the attention and fix it on this very delicate sexual centre. Yet the combination of prostatorrhea with spermato-cystitis is more likely to be associated with this train of symptoms than is either malady alone, and I ascribe this to the fact that in these cases there is often a combination of inflammatory action with sexual exhaustion; and that the patient, usually a neurotic, is unable to withstand the combination. The symptoms are neurotic rather than physical. They occur in neurotics who have no local disease, neither prostatorrhea nor spermatorrhea, and conversely, patients with prostatorrhea and with spermatorrhea may be entirely devoid of this combination of symptoms.

It is proper, however, to note the frequent combination of the symptoms with the maladies, and the fact that the cure of the local symptoms may and often does greatly improve the neurotic state, probably by calming the mind and doing good by the process of suggestion.

In true uncomplicated prostatorrhea the prostate is not necessarily sensitive, either subjectively to the patient or to rectal touch; but as prostatorrhea is often a part of the general picture in which another malady (prostatitis, spermato-cystitis) is concerned, the prostate may be subjectively and objectively excessively sensitive where there is true prostatorrhea.

The malady is of long duration, but is always capable of betterment, often of entire cure.

For treatment, see page 140.

SPERMATO-CYSTITIS

Spermato-cystitis, inflammation of the seminal vesicles, is a result, early or late, of posterior urethritis, and as such is almost always of gonorrheal origin.

There is, however, a very chronic form of vesicular dilatation (usually bilateral),[1] due to masturbation, to sexual irregularity, to excess, or to prolonged, ungratified desire. This occurs particularly in neurotic subjects, and is accompanied by prostatorrhea, with or without a little chronic surface or follicular prostatitis. These patients are often afflicted with sexual neurasthenia and complain of so-called spermatorrhea.

The frequency of spermato-cystitis as a complication of gonorrhea is a matter in much dispute, and cannot be determined until our methods of diagnosis become more refined. This is due to the fact that in a certain indefinite proportion of cases of gonorrheal posterior urethritis, and in all cases of epididymitis, there is subacute spermato-cystitis. This passes unrecognised, as it yields no especial symptoms, calls for no particular treatment, and subsides spontaneously with the disappearance of the greater malady which it complicates.

Therefore Von Petersen's estimate of the relative frequency of the complication (14%) must be considered much too low.

Spermato-cystitis may be acute or chronic, and in either case may run a mild or a severe course. The mild cases, whether acute or chronic, yield no symptoms other than those of the prostatitis which they accompany; and while such cases may be recognised by careful examination (see Diagnosis) they require no treatment. But the contrary is true if the symptoms become intense.

Acute Spermato-cystitis

In mild cases there are no symptoms, except the objective one of moderate distention of the vesicle with extra sensitiveness, recognised by rectal touch.

Severe cases may be accompanied by considerable fever, and have for local symptoms pain in the perineum, anus, rectum, or hip.

---

[1] Old men with enlarged prostates very commonly have also largely dilated vesicles, which are in a more or less definite condition of chronic inflammation. These are some of the patients that get good temporary results from orchidectomy.

This pain is of an aching, a throbbing, or a burning character, and is increased by urination (which is urgent and frequent) and by defecation. There may be partial priapism, and emissions may be painful and frequent, the semen bloody. The urine contains free pus, usually a little blood and shreds, as in acute prostatitis, the shreds often entrapping sympexions or spermatozoa, and free spermatozoa may also be found. There may be epididymitis.

Chronic Spermato-cystitis

Octave Guelliot restricts the symptoms of chronic spermato-cystitis to those of a not infrequent complication—i. e., recurrent epididymitis. This is far too narrow a view, but it emphasizes an undoubted fact—namely, that chronic inflammation in a vesicle is often entirely overlooked, being dominated perhaps by a more obvious disorder in the testicle, or oftener shrouded by and mistaken for prostatitis.

Symptoms.—The symptoms of chronic seminal vesiculitis are often definite, and evince themselves in one or more of the following three ways:

1. Pain, often with more or less vesical irritability and functional sexual disturbance.
2. Gleet, pyuria, pyosperm or hemosperm.
3. Recurrent epididymitis.

The pain is usually neuralgic in character, and resembles the pain of chronic prostatitis or of urethral neuralgia; or it may be reflected to various regions, notably the testicle, where it may manifest itself as a neuralgia more or less intense. Pain may exist in the back, low down, may radiate down the sciatic nerves, or along the front of the thigh (more marked if the testicles and cord be sensitive). Pain in the hip, said to be pathognomonic, but often absent, has led to confounding this malady with hip disease. Defecation may be painful and may leave a dull aching sensation high up within the rectum, which may come on spontaneously at night, awaking the patient. It recalls fissure pain.

Ejaculation, often unsatisfactory, may be painful, and is generally premature. There may be feeble erection and functional impotence from lack of desire; but desire is usually increased, while capacity is lessened. Nocturnal emissions may be frequent, the sperm may be bloody or chocolate-coloured; there may be symptoms of cystitis, even retention.

As in prostatitis, there may be slight but obstinate urethral discharge. The pus in the urine or semen shows macroscopic and microscopic characteristics distinguishing it from pus from the prostate.

(See Diagnosis.) Occasionally, however, the pyuria is intermittent or remittent, resembling the urine of pyelo-nephritis rather than that of prostatitis. If the blood mixed with semen comes from the vesicle they are intermingled, if from the prostate it occurs in streaks.

Epididymitis may be the sole symptom worthy of attention. Melancholia, depression of spirits, and all the symptoms of sexual neurasthenia (see Prostatorrhea) may be also present, notably in neurotic and oxaluric patients.

The physical signs of spermato-cystitis are essential to the diagnosis.

Diagnosis.—The symptoms are so variable and so nondescript, including as they do many of the symptoms of posterior urethritis, prostatitis, prostatorrhea, and even neurasthenia, that careful examination of the vesicles and of their secretion may be necessary before an accurate diagnosis of the malady is possible. In every case of gleet or of persistent urethral or perineal pain the vesicles require examination, since they may be the chief or the sole seat of the disorder. A history of hemosperm, priapism, seminal colic, or recurrent epididymitis strengthens this probability that the vesicle is the *corpus delicti*.

Rectal Examination.—The vesicles like the prostate are reached by the finger in the rectum. The procedure has already been described.[1] Suffice it to say that the normal vesicles cannot be felt unless overdistended. If inflamed, the finger passing up over and beyond the prostate meets with no resistance in the middle line, but laterally, instead of slipping around the corner of the prostatic lobe, it meets a prolongation of this lobe upward and outward in the shape of a boggy, tense, or soft, fluctuating, elongated, sausage-like tumour, often exquisitely sensitive, and always more or less tender. The tip of the finger cannot reach the upper limit of the vesicle. Indeed, in some cases it can scarcely reach the lower part of it. A full bladder and counterpressure on the lower abdominal wall are aids in examination. The surgeon need not hesitate to crowd his finger into the rectum as far as it will go, but he should fear the exhibition of any roughness, for it is easy by too much pressure still further to inflame a vesicle not yet quite out of the acute stage, and to bring on active symptoms of irritation of the neck of the bladder (cystitis) or acute epididymitis, bloody emissions, aggravation of urethral discharge, etc.

Two questions arise here: Are all enlarged vesicles inflamed?

---

[1] The rubber-tissue finger-stall does not interfere with the exploration, protects the surgeon's finger for other surgical work, and possesses an esthetic advantage.

Are all inflamed vesicles enlarged? To both the answer is negative. An enlarged vesicle may be inflamed, or tubercular (p. 787), or cancerous (p. 791), or cystic (p. 790), and an inflamed vesicle, though not obviously enlarged, may be sensitive—a sensation of pain or of sickening—to pressure; or rough pressure upon it may set up an epididymitis, evidence enough.

In doubtful cases, when the vesicle is not enlarged, the diagnosis is rarely of any clinical importance, but may be made by an examination of the contents of the vesicle obtained in the following manner:

Method of obtaining the Contents of the Vesicle.—The patient passes his urine, and if the strictest care is aimed at, the urethra and bladder are next washed clean and the latter left full of boric-acid solution. The prostate is then thoroughly massaged by the finger in the rectum and the bladder partly emptied, to wash away the contents of the prostatic sinus.

Now the finger is introduced into the rectum as high as possible over the suspected vesicle, pressed with gentle firmness against it, and then brought slowly downward with a zigzag motion, and the maneuvre repeated several times. If the pressure be too severe an epididymitis may result, if too slight nothing will be expressed. The just mean can only be acquired by practice. The bladder is then emptied and the fluid centrifuged and examined. If pus and bacteria are present over and above the spermatozoa and spermatic cells there is spermato-cystitis. The pus so obtained may contain gonococci, a sufficient explanation for some of those cases of relapsing posterior urethritis which appropriate irrigation treatment fails to cure radically.

Prognosis.—The prognosis of spermato-cystitis, as it ordinarily occurs in connection with gonorrheal posterior urethritis, is, as a rule, excellent, because the implication of the vesicle is most often ignored, needs no especial treatment, and takes care of itself. To this rule, however, there are three classes of exceptions:

1. The cases which persist in chronic catarrh with dilatation, giving rise to a variety of symptoms, including recurring epididymitis.

2. Cases of latent gonorrheal spermato-cystitis, in which although the posterior urethra is apparently well, and pus and shreds have disappeared from the urine, gonococci still lurk in the vesicles. In such cases the first intercourse or nocturnal emission may infect the patient and renew the urethritis, or discharge may relapse a few days after giving up local treatment and without the intervention of any new cause. This condition of affairs, while not common, does undoubtedly exist.

Abscess of the Seminal Vesicle

3. Occasionally the inflammation goes on to abscess of the seminal vesicle, the ejaculatory duct becoming occluded. Such abscess, while giving rise to the symptoms of acute prostatic abscess (p. 88)—being differentiated from it as to position by the rectal touch—may burst into the peritoneum, or, infiltrating the perivesicular and periprostatic connective tissue, go on to post-vesicular ischio-rectal, or pelvic abscess (p. 90).

Such abscesses usually point spontaneously into the bladder or the rectum. Very exceptionally a fatal peritonitis or a burrowing periprostatic abscess may result (p. 91).

For treatment of spermato-cystitis, see page 141.

SPERMATORRHEA

Improved methods of modern diagnosis, aided by a broadened common sense, justify the surgeon, I believe, in dismissing spermatorrhea from the catalogue of diseases. There is no such disease as spermatorrhea. The alleged malady is a fetich created largely by Lallemand—a fetich to which its morbid worshippers, young and old, bow down throughout the community morning, noon, and night, offering to it the incense of their distorted erotic fancies.

Spermatorrhea exists surely as a symptom, but not as a malady. As well call cough or pain a disease.

Spermatorrhea is the intermittent or constant involuntary escape of seminal elements (spermatozoa) without orgasm, and not in nocturnal emissions. This escape occurs during the urinary act, during defecation or rectal straining, sometimes during jolting exercise, sometimes in slight constant discharge mingled with prostatic and follicular secretions. It means that the ejaculatory duct is patulous, either atonic and relaxed, or catarrhal.

The duct may be atonic and relaxed and even catarrhal from the debility of age when there is enlarged prostate. Sometimes it becomes relaxed during the weakness following prolonged fever (typhoid). Sometimes it is relaxed by the congestion and strain of masturbation, or more often by excessive and prolonged sexual excitement without relief, aided by erotic fancies and imaginings, but in such instances a prostatorrhea or a spermato-cystitis is the malady that gives the symptoms, and not the escape or loss of semen.

I have known men having sexual intercourse nearly every night of their lives for years, and often more than once in a night, who had no single symptom of any sexual malady, and surely, if an excessive expenditure of seminal fluid were in itself capable of producing symptoms, these individuals should have shown some sign of these symptoms.

I have known every symptom attributed to spermatorrhea to occur in individuals who had no seminal loss whatsoever, voluntary or involuntary.

Finally, I have repeatedly found seminal elements constantly in the urine of vigorous men, ignorant of the fact, perfectly healthy in a sexual sense, and absolutely devoid of any of the alleged symptoms of the bugbear.

Therefore, while spermatorrhea as a symptom is a valuable factor in diagnosis—indicating atony or catarrh of the ejaculatory ducts, and, usually, spermato-cystitis—yet I cannot consider it a malady, since the loss of semen *per se* does not occasion symptoms. It is only a part of the picture in other maladies, maladies that have already been described. Where it occurs essentially without the concomitance of a definite malady it does not cause symptoms, does not interfere with bodily or sexual health, does not threaten life nor entail any consequences, and it may be and should be wholly disregarded.

I think it is time for the self-respecting genito-urinary surgeon to leave the ranks of quackery and to disabuse the public of false ideas on this subject.

ASSOCIATE COMPLICATIONS OF GONORRHEA

To complete the clinical picture of those maladies directly associated with and capable by their continuance of maintaining urethral discharge, there remain to be considered folliculitis, periurethral abscess, and cowperitis.

FOLLICULITIS

This is an inflammation of one of the urethral follicles. The cause is surface inflammation of the urethra, most commonly gonorrhea, although the inflammation of a follicle behind a stricture is far from uncommon.

Doubtless many of the urethral follicles are inflamed during the course of a gonorrhea without giving rise to any symptoms referable directly to them. This is certainly the case whenever there is chordee. But such general superficial implication of the follicles and their ducts takes care of itself and may be clinically ignored.

Normal and Morbid Anatomy.—A short enumeration of the pores of the urethral mucous membrane may not be out of place here. There are in the urethra a large number of minute openings (pores).

These have been called, the larger, the foramina; the smaller, the foraminulæ of Morgagni. The larger ones do not seem to be at all glandular, but reduplications, infoldings in pouch form, of the mucous membrane; yet they are lined in their depths by cylindrical and not by pavement epithelium. The smallest are said to have true glandular structure.

These foraminulæ dot the roof of the urethra, and at about two inches back from the meatus there is a little group of small ones upon the floor. They are also occasionally found upon the lateral walls.

The big lacuna, the lacuna magna, opening upon the roof of the urethra near the proximal end of the fossa navicularis, is well known to any one using filiform instruments, for the advancing tip of which the lacunal mouth is an efficient trap.

Besides these larger openings there are smaller ones along the urethra communicating with ordinary mucous glands much like those found upon other mucous membranes. These are quite superficial, and do not penetrate deeply.

Finally come the glands of Littré. They exist all along the urethra, and are rather large racemose glands situated deeply among the muscular fibres surrounding the urethra. Their ducts point forward in the pendulous urethra, like the foraminulæ and the ducts of the mucous glands; but in the membranous urethra, where they are quite abundant, they open at right angles to the mucous membrane, and here their ducts are rather long, the glands being situated among the muscular fibres of the membranous urethra, and being necessarily squeezed when this muscle contracts. These glands of Littré, indeed, are only so many minute glands of Cowper. Their secretion is alkaline and tenacious, and they are sexual rather than ordinary mucous glands.

Finally, the glands of Cowper are situated in the perineum beneath the floor of the urethra between the two layers of the triangular ligament. They are grape-like in structure and of considerable size, with long ducts leading forward and emptying upon the floor of the urethra at the back part of the bulb. These also are sexual glands, not simple mucous glands.

Now a follicle or a lacuna anywhere along the urethra may become the seat of inflammation which has invaded it by creeping in through the mouth of the duct.

The lacuna magna (Fig. 3) has a wide mouth. Sometimes there are two wide-mouthed lacunæ on the roof. When the lacuna magna inflames, its mouth never becomes occluded, and the process remains a surface one and gets well, or persists sometimes as a chronic inflammation after the remainder of the urethra has recovered from its gonorrheal attack. Phillips[1] has called especial attention to this.

Other wide-mouthed foramina behave in the same manner, but their ducts, being relatively small, easily become occluded by the swelling which the inflammation causes, and we have at once all the conditions for follicular abscess and for periurethral inflammation. These abscesses may occur anywhere along the urethra, but there seem to be points of election, one on each side of the frenum in the floor of the urethra, and another at about 2 inches back, frequently upon the roof. But a follicle may occasionally suppurate anywhere, perhaps burrowing forward through the tissue of the glans penis and opening alongside the meatus (paraurethral fistula).

But little of importance has been added to our knowledge of these follicular abscesses since the study made of them by Hardy.[2] He likened these small tumours to wens of the scalp on account of their round shot-like feel, and believed that there were two special lacunæ most prone to involvement, one on each side of the frenum in the floor of the urethra.

Etiology.—The cause of lacunal and follicular inflammation is primarily surface urethral inflammation, usually gonorrhea, assisted by some such adjuvant as increased intensity of the disease from drinking, prolonged erection and the like, or occasioned by direct violence (too strong injection, rough use of instruments).

Symptoms.—The symptoms are local pain (worse during erection) and a hard, shot-like body under the integument, at first not adherent and often not very tender upon handling. If the tumour appears beside the frenum, it may be felt, when not very acute, like a hard pea, with a little fibrous string extending from it to the mucous membrane, this string being the obliterated duct of the little gland.

These follicular indolent tumours vary from the size of a pinhead to that of a pea or a bean. They commonly resolve. If pus forms, a route for its escape is usually opened by ulceration either towards the urethral surface or externally into the tissues, forming periurethral abscess, or externally through a previously adherent integument.

When the discharge is inward, the abscess may remain with hard walls as a chronic suppurating pouch for months or years, filling up and becoming prominent from time to time, and maintaining a moderate gleet, subject to exacerbations, but always palpable be-

---

[1] Maladies des voies urinaires. Paris, 1860.

[2] Mémoires sur les abcès blennorrhagiques. Paris, 1864.

tween the attacks as a small, insensitive, shot-like lump. Sometimes the abscess points both ways, and urethral fistula results.

For treatment, see page 129.

PERIURETHRAL ABSCESS

Periurethral abscess is generally the result of the extension of follicular or lacunal suppuration, although it may originate spontaneously. It may occur anywhere along the canal, and is distinguishable from the follicular inflammation by its acuteness and size. Such a central inflammation beneath the frenum bulges on each side, and somewhat resembles the double follicular abscess of that region; indeed, it may have originated in one of the follicles of Morgagni situated there.

It is entirely possible that one of the glands of Littré in the membranous urethra might suppurate, but this is rare, and we have no especial symptomatology.

For treatment, see page 129.

COWPERITIS

This is a folliculitis on a large scale, and its causes and symptoms are much the same as those already detailed for folliculitis of the anterior urethra, of course intensified in all respects and differing in the position of the swelling.

Cowper's glands are really a sexual annex. Their alkaline, tenacious fluid pours out during sexual excitement to lubricate the urethra and to facilitate the ejaculation of the sperm.

Urethrorrhea, which has been already considered (p. 93), is largely a functional weakness of Cowper's glands due to prolonged sexual strain, but this is not cowperitis.

Etiology.—The causes of cowperitis, like those of folliculitis, are primarily gonorrhea or inflammation behind a stricture, aided by too strong an injection, an irrigation, or the use of an instrument; but it may arise spontaneously, or occur after horseback-riding, dancing, bicycling, prolonged erection during gonorrhea, etc. Its date of occurrence is usually during the fourth week of a gonorrhea or thereabouts; or, more rarely, at any time during a chronic urethritis of the anterior urethra, since the ducts open upon the floor of the bulbous urethra, and these are the natural doors for microbic invasion.

Symptoms.—During an acute gonorrhea attention is called to Cowper's glands by vague discomfort in the perineum, amounting perhaps to positive pain. These perineal pains, however, may be reflex from the urethra or from the prostate. It is necessary to place the patient in the lithotomy position and to palpate the perineum. If acute cowperitis be present, the position of the gland on one or the other side of the raphe, usually the left, will be excessively sensitive to pressure. There may be no lump nor tumour, for the inflammation usually aborts spontaneously, and does not get past the congestive stage. Indeed, the malady is not habitually recognised unless the surgeon takes the trouble to palpate the perineum.

If the inflammation does not subside, an oval, hard tumour, as large as a small nut, presently shows itself on one side of the raphe, its larger diameter being antero-posterior and its blunt end turned towards the anus.

This lump behaves much like the other follicular abscesses of the urethra. It may long remain tender and hard; it may go on unceasingly to increase in size, finally forming a definite abscess over which the perineal integument adheres. It may point within through its own duct and then subside and get well, for the long duct, starting in the bulb and directed forward, does not invite urinary leakage backward. Indeed, in the not uncommon event of a double opening, one through the duct into the urethra and the other by ulceration through the skin, although there is urethral fistula, as proved by injecting the sinus from without, there is habitually no escape of urine from within through the fistulous canal.

Of course, during this abscess formation, sitting, standing, walking, even pressure of the clothing, all cause local pain. The swelling mechanically pressing upon the urethra makes urination painful, the stream small. Retention of urine does not seem to occur. The function of the rectum is not interfered with.

The course of the acute malady is rather rapid. The congestive stage, if resolution is to be the termination, is over in less than a week, and suppuration generally established in ten or twelve days, if at all. Resolution is possible, after there has been a distinct tumour, and appears to be the rule (Critzmann).

For treatment, see page 131.

Chronic Cowperitis

Chronic cowperitis is less common than the acute form. It manifests itself by a viscid gleet, worse in the morning, the urine containing a very long, thick shred from Cowper's duct entrapping cuboid and cylindrical epithelia, mixed with striated mucus, pus, detritus, and bacteria, perhaps gonococci.

Perineal palpation establishes the diagnosis by a feeling of greater resistance at the site of the gland than elsewhere in the perineum. The thickened area is very slightly sensitive to pressure. These features differentiate chronic cowperitis from chronic posterior urethritis.

Pericowperitis.—Pericowperitis occurs in the acute form of the malady, more especially if the abscess bursts through the skin of the perineum, or, burrowing forward, points near the peno-scrotal angle. In chronic cowperitis, however, it is a constant accessory phenomenon, either as a thickening of tissue about the chronically inflamed gland or as a chronic suppurating process, the pus slowly burrowing and opening spontaneously through the integument of the perineum. Such opening often communicates with the urethra, but does not habitually give exit to urine.

Diagnosis.—The only possibility of error in diagnosis lies in confounding ordinary perineal urinary abscess with suppuration of one of Cowper's glands—yet the distinction is usually easy. The perineal urinary abscess is habitually an accompaniment of stricture, or follows upon local external violence to the perineum. Except after excessive external violence the course is generally less rapid than that of cowperitis, and the urinary abscess is quite often central, the suppuration in cowperitis always commencing on one side. However, the distinction towards the end is often difficult, perhaps impossible; but this is not of practical importance as the treatment is identical.

Cowper's glands occasionally develop *retention cysts* by the occlusion of their ducts, especially in infants (Englisch), primary tuberculous degeneration (Critzmann), and primary carcinoma as a result of chronic inflammation (Kaufmann). J. Englisch, of Vienna, has made thorough studies of this subject, the results of which are embodied in a number of monographs.[1] Gubler cites as a curiosity a syphilitic gummy tumour of the perineum which occupied the exact position of Cowper's gland.

Prognosis.—The prognosis of acute cowperitis is the best. It habitually gets well without difficulty or delay. Abscess, of course, aggravates the prognosis, but this also habitually recovers under a spontaneous or a surgical opening, without fistula. In chronic cowperitis the prognosis is far more grave as to the local conditions, which may perpetuate themselves indefinitely in the form of fistula and its various attending complications, calling ultimately for a free use of the knife for its cure.

For treatment of cowperitis, see page 131.

[1] Wien. med. Jahrbüch., 1883, p. 269; Jahrbücher d. k. k. Gesellschaft d. Aerzte in Wien, 1883, p. 397; Wien. med. Wochenschrift, 1886, xxxvi, 1105; Centralbl. f. d. Krank. d. Harn u. Sex. Org., 1897, viii, 341.

CHAPTER VIII

THE TREATMENT OF URETHRAL INFLAMMATIONS AND THEIR IMMEDIATE COMPLICATIONS

THE METHODIC TREATMENT

The methodic treatment of urethral inflammation is the rational application of the general hygienic, external, and medicinal measures suitable to inflammatory conditions of the urethral membrane. Such measures apply equally to the management of all forms of urethral discharge, being based upon the quantity and quality of the discharge and the grade of the inflammatory action rather than upon the cause or the nature, specific or otherwise, of the flow.

The hygienic and dietetic part of the treatment is of the utmost importance. If disregarded, the best-directed efforts may miscarry. Many cases of simple urethritis require little else than hygienic and dietetic treatment, which may be epitomized as follows:

Cleanliness.—The parts should be washed as often as required, soap and warm water being as good as an antiseptic solution and more readily at hand. The discharge should be kept from smearing the underclothing by one of the following methods: When the foreskin is long a little absorbent cotton may be tucked into its orifice, and renewed after each urinary act. The glans penis is thrust through a slit in the centre of a small square of gauze until the slit lies snugly behind the corona glandis. Thus held in place the gauze is folded forward over the glans penis, covered by replacing the foreskin, and left puckered up and long enough to protrude in a bunch for a scant inch in front of the preputial orifice. An apron of old cotton or linen doubled is fastened to a string about the waist or pinned to a suspensory bandage, and the entire genitalia wrapped up in this, or a triangular diaper of gauze doubled may be made to envelop the penis and its folds pinned to a suspending band. Finally, one of the various penis suspensory bags furnished by the shops, preferably of cloth, may be employed, the bottom to be kept supplied with renewed portions of absorbent cotton; or a piece of toilet paper may be wrapped about the penis and twisted at the end—any device to keep the discharge from defiling the person or the clothing, for this discharge in gonorrhea is most virulent (besides its nastiness), and any moisture exuding from the urethral meatus should be regarded with grave suspicion. Indeed, during the first interview each patient individually should be cautioned to make it a routine custom to wash the hands carefully after every handling of his organs, fearing inoculation of the eyes and that dreadful complication—gonorrheal conjunctivitis.

It is a proper precaution to urge the patient during an acute gonorrhea to wear a snug suspensory bandage as a preventive of epididymitis. This protects the testicles from injury and exposure, and assists in retaining dressings when required.

Diet.—The food should be bland and partaken in moderation in all acute conditions of urethral inflammation. All wines, liquors, champagne, beer, strong black coffee, acids, spices (including ginger-ale), condiments, sauces, rich and indigestible foods, are to be interdicted. Vegetables, milk and bread, fish, and a little white meat (rather than red) make the best diet—but all this is for the acuter stages only. There comes a time, after the malady grows chronic, when the diet must be made generous, when coffee is rather helpful than otherwise, and a small quantity of wine or whisky positively beneficial, with plenty of meat and good cheer.

I remember a striking lesson I once received in this line. A big, sturdy, free-living clubman appeared with a rousing gonorrhea. His customary tipple was two bottles of brandy a week. I put him at once upon a penitential diet. He did very well, and presently his acute symptoms subsided, and I struggled for weeks and weeks with his gleet—in vain, for he maintained his abstinence honestly. Finally he disappeared, and I bemoaned him as a failure at my hands. Some months later he turned up upon another matter, and I asked him what had become of that everlasting gleet. "Oh!" he said—searching to recall the facts—"yes, I got tired of treatment, so I went off on a spree the night after I last saw you and drank a whole bottle of brandy. The next morning my discharge had ceased, and I have been well ever since and continue my brandy as of old."

Rest.—Physical repose is desirable, sometimes essential, in acute cases with much chordee and a tendency to epididymitis or to bladder implication, but it may fail. I have seen a boy put to bed, fed on milk, alkaline drinks, and balsams, and his urethra not touched by any local treatment, and yet have the fiercest kind of an attack culminating in double suppurating epididymitis. And again I have seen a fat, middle-aged man with a sluggish but most pronounced chronic posterior urethritis get perfectly well so that all pus disappeared from the urine, by horseback exercise alone, after the failure of months of all sorts of internal treatment with local instillations and irrigations. No rule can govern this matter. It is a question of individual acumen and surgical judgment.

Sexual Hygiene.—During the acute stage again absolute continence is essential, and this should be extended at least two weeks after the cessation of all discharge, with the avoidance of anything liable to induce sexual excitement—association with women, racy books and pictures, erotic thoughts *et id genus omne*; but here again in the remote chronic stage—after repeated microscopical tests shall have demonstrated the absence of gonococci, even if there be shreds containing leukocytes—a return to sexual life may be the shortest and surest method of cure for the remaining mucoid sweating from the meatus which torments the patient and fills him with hypochondriacal fears. But to urge a patient with even the least suspicion of a discharge to marry is a grave responsibility—of the gravest, for it may involve contamination of an innocent victim (p. 64). Recognition of this fact is the safeguard from error.

Diluents.—Diluent drinks like the bland (non-mineral) natural waters, milk, buttermilk, plain hydrant water, or well water in abundance are desirable and effective in conditions of acute discharge, because they dilute the naturally acrid and irritating urine, and when the latter is made balsamic by medication they repeat the physiological retrojection the more often, with the double effect of mechanically cleansing the excoriated surface from its accumulated pus and medicating that surface with the balsamic solution.

But here again common sense must temper routine practice. In acute gonorrheal cystitis and in very acute posterior urethritis more harm may be done by the muscular straining attending the frequent repetition of the urinary act than is atoned for by any amount of dilution of the urine.

The drugs that may be effectively exploited to combat urethral inflammation belong to five orders:

I. Urinary antiseptics.

II. Alkalies.

III. Demulcents.

IV. Anodynes.

V. Balsamics and astringents.

I. Urinary Antiseptics

Urinary antiseptics, such as the ammonio-formaldehyd preparations (urotropin), methylene blue, salol, benzoic acid and the benzoates, boric acid and the borates, have little influence upon urethral inflammation. Theoretically they ought to be of paramount importance, since suppuration is a process always associated with, indeed caused by, germs of one sort or another; but practically these substances, so valuable in suppurative conditions of the urinary tract above the vesical neck (p. 372), are nearly useless below that point, whether because their bactericidal efficiency is slight, or because their sojourn in contact with the inflamed urethral wall is limited, or because the bacteria are shielded from the antiseptic action of the medicated urine by the tissues in which they lie, I shall not discuss, my belief being that each of these reasons has a share in accounting for their inefficiency. The value of urotropin and of methylene blue in gonorrhea has been vaunted. In my opinion it is slight, so slight that it does not deserve more than experimental consideration.

II. Alkalies

The virtue of alkalies in the treatment of urethral inflammations depends rather upon the condition of the urine than upon the grade of the inflammation. The urine, normally acid and often dense, is, *ipso facto*, harmful except in so far as it washes the urethra, and the alkali is negatively a very good thing, but good only when required to counteract acidity. In other words, there is no specific action whatsoever in the alkalies. They do not in the least control suppuration. If one had two burned hands, and placed one of them in vinegar and water and the other in a watery solution of bicarbonate of soda, he would doubtless prefer the sensations experienced in the hand immersed in the mild alkali, and so it is with the urethra.

Patients having normally bland, alkaline, dilute urine, and there are many such, stand in no need of alkalies, and, indeed, may occasionally be injured by them, by indigestion, or by having the urine rendered too alkaline—depositing perhaps phosphatic dust, itself a mechanical irritant, or by increasing the activity of the bladder contraction in acute gonorrheal cystitis.

When, however, the urine is brown, dense, overacid, *a fortiori* if it contains uric-acid crystals which, whirled along in the escaping torrent, act as a sand-blast upon the sensitive urethra, in such cases an alkali is balm indeed, and often alone quite capable of affording material comfort.

But there are certain conditions to its use even in these cases, a routine employment indicating carelessness or incompetence on the part of the surgeon. These conditions are easily formulated. When the urine is acid an alkali is indicated. If the urine be also dense a diuretic alkali is called for; if light (sp. gr. 1.015 or thereabouts), the diuretic quality is not needed. If the urine be alkaline then no alkaline medicine is needed, for dilution, if required, can be produced by other means.

Bicarbonate of soda is the mildest of the alkalies. Its chief virtue is that it aids digestion, while the other alkalies impede digestion more or less. Dose, 0.50 to 1.00 gramme. It is often prescribed under the form of soda mints, two with, or better between, meals.

Sweet spirits of nitre (spts. etheris nitrosi) is notable for its anodyne rather than its alkaline properties. It is chiefly employed for the slight irritation of the bladder so common in women.

Potassium citrate, Potassium acetate, Liquor potassæ.—These three salts are employed more than any others as urinary alkalinizers. The citrate is the most efficient as an alkali, but irritates some stomachs, the liquor the most anodyne, the acetate the most diuretic. Therefore the liquor is most useful in acute cases, and the citrate in chronic cases. The acetate is a stronger diuretic than the citrate, but I have found it also more irritant to the stomach. The dose of each drug is about 0.5 gramme in a considerable quantity of water. The disagreeable taste of the liquor is well disguised by sirup of cinnamon.

Bromid of potash acts as an alkali and is sometimes efficient in controlling the smarting upon urination. Alkalies produce the greatest effect relative to the size of the dose, if administered towards the end of the second hour after eating.

III. Demulcents

Demulcents are much less used now than formerly, but occasionally are comforting when combined with an alkali. To this class belong flax-seed tea, gum water and elm-bark water, the various teas of fluid extracts made from buchu, pareira brava, uva ursi, triticum repens, and corn-silk.

IV. Anodynes

Anodynes are called for to moderate pain on urination, and for this bromid of potassium or the tincture or fluid extract of hyoscyamus generally suffices. A favourite old-fashioned prescription is:

℞	Liq. potassæ..............	5.00–25.00	grammes	ʒ ij–vj
	Tr. hyoscyami............	15.00–35.00	"	℥ ss–j
	Syr. cinnam........q. s. ad	100.00	"	℥ iij.

M.

Sig.—Teaspoonful in water two hours after each meal.

For intense *chordee* lupulin in doses of 2 to 4 grammes taken upon retiring is sometimes effective, or a similar dose of the bromid of potassium. The coal-tar preparations are of decided value for this condition. Acetanilid, antipyrin, phenalgen, in 30 centigrammes to gramme doses on retiring—perhaps aided by codeia. In the intense dysuria of acute gonorrheal cystitis, codeia, McMunn's elixir, and morphin are indicated in doses large enough to obtain the desired effect—accompanied always by a laxative.

Hot water is of value in various ways. When the pain on urination is intense it may be somewhat moderated by immersing the penis in very hot water and urinating into it. Prolonged soaking of the penis, just before retiring, in water as hot as can be borne, will often prevent or moderate chordee during the night.

A *hot hip bath* is full of comfort for the patient with any form of acute prostatic, vesical, or seminal vesicular inflammation. Such a bath may be repeated every few hours. It should be short, not lasting more than five minutes. The temperature of the water to begin with should be near 104° F., and after the patient is in the bath more hot water should be added until the temperature of the bath is as high as the patient can tolerate.

Iced water is useful when the penis is erect and in chordee, but not when the penis is relaxed before retiring, as this rather encourages erection later in the night. In chordee the patient naturally urinates at once, if he can, and then by pouring iced water over his turgid and unruly member, or by placing it alongside a cold piece of metal, he strives to reduce it to subjection. To break a chordee is to invite stricture.

V. Balsamics and Astringents

Balsamics and astringents, last to be named, are first in efficacy for the management of urethral discharges by internal medicinal means. In the order of their usefulness they may, perhaps, be rated as follows: Oil of yellow sandal-wood, balsam of copaiba, cubeb, oil of wintergreen, eucalyptol, matico, pichi, spirits of turpentine, tincture of cantharides, tincture of the chlorid of iron—and finally tonics of all sorts, and particularly cod-liver oil for mild chronic discharges in broken-down subjects. The types among the balsams are sandal-wood oil and copaiba—the others are less useful.

These balsams are of great value in the treatment of every form of suppuration originating in the urethral membrane, but to be of service they must be digested comfortably. It is like giving cod-liver oil for pulmonary tuberculosis, a medicine which sometimes takes away what little appetite the poor patient has, and is itself vomited. Under such circumstances cod-liver oil would do more good if rubbed upon the boots. And so it is with balsams; if they upset the stomach they do not benefit the urethral catarrh. If sandal-wood oil in small quantity gives a man so severe a pain in his back that he can neither exercise nor sleep, and if copaiba in moderate dose so upsets his stomach that he is constantly semi-nauseated, or if he easily gets copaibal erythema, he certainly cannot derive proper advantage from these drugs, and it is folly to push them. But, on the other hand, when the balsams agree they are exceedingly helpful, and their dose may be pushed with advantage up to the limit of satisfactory digestion.

Sandal-wood Oil.—The preparation made from yellow sandalwood is probably better than that made from the red, but both have merit. The oil, however, is expensive, and often adulterated. Modern fastidiousness demands that it be prescribed at meal times in capsules, and the markets are flooded with these, soft and hard, containing 5 and 10 minims, and in all sorts of combinations with other balsams and with salol, with pepsin, etc. Generally, however, it is better, if a huntsman be after reasonably large game, to shoot with a rifle rather than with a shot-gun.[1]

The dose of sandal-wood oil to do any good should be at least 0.5 gramme (8 minims) 3 times a day, and it may be pushed to 2 grammes (30 minims) 4 times a day. Rarely, however, is so much required, and even the lowest dose sometimes upsets digestion or gives the distressing pain in the back, which calls for a halt and a diminution in dose or a change of drug. The warm urine is redolent of sandal-wood.

If a liquid be preferred to a capsule the alkali and balsam are easily combined.

℞	Potass. citrat............	5.00–25.00	grammes	ʒ ij–vj
	Ol. santal...............	15.00–25.00	"	ʒ iv–vj
	Syr. acaciæ	50.00	"	℥ j
	Aquæ menth. pip. q. s. ad	100.00	"	℥ iij.

M. Shake.

Sig.—Teaspoonful in water two hours after eating.

Copaiba may be prescribed instead of sandal-wood oil in this combination late rather than early in the disease, and a little fluid extract of hyoscyamus or deodorized tincture of opium if required.

[1] I cannot but recall here the graceful words of a charming lecturer upon dermatology. I heard them in Paris, in my student days of 1866. "Gentlemen, you all remember well that famous sirup of Monsieur ——, in which iodin, iron, arsenic, mercury, and potash give themselves a rendezvous in the same bottle, and seem to make the learned professor say: 'La nature, plus forte que moi, saura bien choisir celui qui lui conviendra! . . .'"

This dose is easier to take than the time-honoured Lafayette mixture—Heaven knows why that warrior allowed his name to become attached to such a compound!—and the citrate of potash seems to do better work than the nitre and the liquor potassæ of that mixture. Bicarbonate of soda may substitute the citrate of potash when a diuretic effect is not desired, and wintergreen or liquorice flavours be substituted for the mint.

Copaiba more than sandal-wood oil, however, demands the capsular form of administration. Its dose also varies from 0.5 to 2 grammes. Less than 0.5 gramme (8 minims) does no good, and that quantity often nauseates, sometimes occasions diarrhea.

Copaibal erythema consists in the appearance of closely aggregated, slightly elevated, red blotches scattered over the whole trunk. They itch and are hot and tingling, like urticaria—features distinguishing this eruption from roseola, with which the timid are prone to confound it. It is easily cured by a discontinuance of the drug, an alkaline laxative, a few warm baths containing some bicarbonate of soda (3 ounces to 60 gallons), dusting the body with powdered talcum, and applying twice a day—

℞ Acidi carbolici.................. 5.00 grammes ʒ j
Spts. rect...................... 150.00 " ℥ v
Aquæ ....q. s. ad 250.00 " ℥ viij.
M.
Sig.—Lotion.

Or,

℞ Menthol .... 3.00 grammes ʒ j
Spts. rect...................... 50.00 " ℥ jss
Aquæ.......................ad 100.00 " ℥ iij.
M.
Sig.—Lotion.

When copaibal erythema appears, the patient feels ill, has fever, etc., and the discharge diminishes greatly or ceases. But it returns as the eruption fades. The eruption does not mean that the drug must be given up entirely, but only that it must be considerably reduced in quantity.

The headache and giddiness, and the urticaria caused by copaiba need only be mentioned. They are due to indigestion.

Cubeb is a stimulant as well as a balsamic. It agrees with most stomachs, but in large dose sometimes irritates the neck of the bladder slightly. Hence it is more applicable to the declining than to the advancing stage of urethral inflammation. The powder is always spoken of, but rarely given in this country. The dose is one or two teaspoonfuls in sweetened water. The fluid extract is better, in half-teaspoon- to teaspoonful doses hot, the oleoresin in capsules, perhaps best in the dose of 0.5 to 1 gramme (8 to 15 minims) (1 to 2 capsules).

Wintergreen oil, or its synthetic substitute the salicylate of methyl, in 0.75 gramme (10-minim) capsules, 1 or more at a dose, seems helpful in some cases of subacute or chronic posterior urethritis, particularly if the prostate be engorged, and especially in rheumatic subjects, and *eucalyptol* in 5-minim capsules, 1 or 2 at a dose, if there be much debility and headache, especially for chronic malarial cases. *Matico* seems a sort of a fancy, and is generally used in combination with something else, while *pichi*, at one time fashionable and seemingly astringent, appears to have been lost in the shuffle of late years. By ringing the changes upon these various drugs, all of which possess some degree of merit, the requirements of every case may be reached in any stage of urethral inflammation.

Towards the end of the attack, in the remote gleety stage, the *oil of turpentine* has a place as a stimulating balsamic in 5-minim capsules, 1 to 3 at a dose, and the tincture of *cantharides* for the same conditions in from 0.05 to 0.25 gramme (1- to 5-minim) doses. Too much cantharides is, of course, irritating.

Fluid extract of *kava-kava* in 0.5- to 2-gramme doses is suitable, and apparently sometimes helpful towards the end of a gleet.

The *tincture of the chlorid of iron* has a certain value for atonic cases, especially in very chronic mild posterior urethritis, in doses of from 0.5 to 1 gramme well diluted. Its effect upon the teeth and its constipating tendency must be remembered.

Tonics and *cod-liver oil* find their proper place along general lines of indication, with change of habitat, sea air, etc.

The balsamic remedies have been found ineffective when administered locally. They undergo a change in passing through the kidney. Most of them give an especial odour to the urine.

The excreted urine exercises a local action [1] upon the inflamed surface of the urethra, consequently the balsams are useless in female gonorrhea, unless the urethra or bladder be involved.

[1] As has been proved when large fistula in the floor of the urethra permitted the urine to be turned off, the part behind the opening getting well first, and the anterior urethra being subsequently cured by injection with the patient's own urine, freshly passed and full of modified copaiba. I do not know that this has been demonstrated except for copaiba; and yet, strangely enough, Steinschneider and Schaeffer (cited by Sée) found that the urine of patients who had taken copaiba or salicylate of soda did not show bactericidal qualities—while iodid of potassium possessed more merit in this respect—which only goes to prove that, for practical purposes, the conclusions of the bedside are sometimes wiser than those of the laboratory.

LOCAL TREATMENT

Local measures are employed in the treatment of gonorrhea both in its acute and in its chronic stage. Indeed, for chronic gonorrhea local treatment is almost our sole resource. And although there is still a wide divergence of opinion as to the propriety of interfering locally with an acutely inflamed urethra—some preferring treatment wholly by internal measures, others employing local treatment, but only when the disease has spent its force, and others still depending chiefly upon local measures at all stages—it is not worth while to argue the case; the facts will carry the day in the end.

Let me, therefore, speak in favour of local treatment, but with the following provisos for acute cases:

1. Local treatment must always be associated with the methodic measures already detailed.

2. In exceptional instances all local treatment does harm; hence it should be discontinued unless it does good promptly.

3. The patient must keep constantly under observation.

4. The surgeon, recognizing that he is combating one of the fiercest local inflammations to which mankind is liable, must always proceed with caution and the greatest gentleness.

Local Treatment of Acute Anterior Urethritis, Gonorrheal and Simple

I shall describe the only two methods that have achieved success in my hands, placing first the method of *argyrol injections*, in favour of which I am relinquishing an older friend, *the Janet method.*

Argyrol Injection.—In order to control acute gonorrhea by this treatment the urethra must be kept constantly bathed in argyrol for at least two weeks in severe cases. To this end the injections must be administered every three or four hours (even during the night, if possible), each time following this method:

Method.—Having filled a quarter-ounce, blunt-nozzle urethral syringe (Fig. 27) with a 10% solution of argyrol, the patient urinates, and then, placing the nozzle of the syringe within the lips of the meatus and compressing these upon it, slowly presses the piston home and injects the solution. Then withdrawing the syringe and pinching the lips of the meatus together, he retains the injection five (in severe cases ten) minutes by the watch. In order to keep himself clean, he must wear a "gonorrhea bag" and must be supplied with a 1:500 solution of corrosive sublimate, a drop or two of which removes the black stains of argyrol as if by magic.

The effect of this treatment is to keep the urethra constantly bathed in argyrol, for the injected fluid almost always forces its way into the bladder so that the next urination is a retrojection.

Under this course the discharge rapidly diminishes, and at the end of two weeks, earlier in mild cases, the number of injections may be reduced to three, and then to two, a day, and a mild astringent injection of zinc or zinc and lead (p. 126) taken once or twice a day. This treatment is continued, depending more and more upon the astringent, less and less upon the argyrol, until the inflammation is checked, the urine becoming free from pus and so remaining, or else it proves obstinate and persists as a mild catarrh.

Then is the time to change to some other form of treatment. I usually begin by daily instillations (p. 133) of protargol, beginning at 1 : 200 and running to 1 : 20, or even higher concentrations if the method suits. If this fails to produce marked improvement within a week, try irrigation (p. 122) of the bladder with permanganate of potash (1 : 4,000), or a combination of permanganate of potash (1 : 4,000) and nitrate of silver (1 : 20,000), or protargol (1 : 5,000); or try instillations of nitrate of silver (1 : 1,000 and stronger). In the meanwhile palpate prostate and vesicles, and, if these are inflamed, institute appropriate treatment by massage and rectal douche (p. 131). If by these means the patient is not soon cured, he passes into a condition of chronic posterior urethritis, and should be treated accordingly (p. 131). Argyrol is of no particular value in chronic gonorrhea.

The Janet Method.—The purpose of this plan of treatment is to wash the urethra with large quantities of a weak solution of potassium permanganate. This is chemically and mechanically more irritating than argyrol, and cannot therefore be employed so freely.

Method.—The instruments required are a suspended tank capable of holding a quart of fluid, with rubber tube attached, a set of two-way nozzles of different sizes (Fig. 23), some small, soft-rubber catheters (15 to 20 French), and the scissors shut-off.[1]

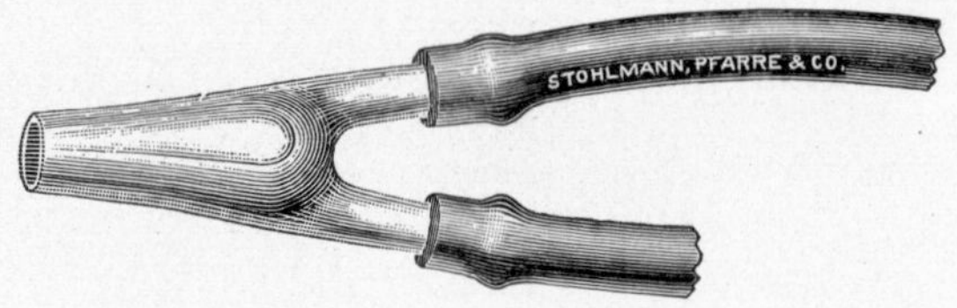

FIG. 23.—CHETWOOD'S TWO-WAY URETHRAL NOZZLE.

The alternating shut-off instrument clasps the rubber tubes attached to the nozzle, and by a scissors-like motion (Fig. 25), impeding the outflow as the fluid enters the urethra, distends the canal

[1] The special nozzles and shut-off are not essential, since Janet uses only a glass nozzle with protecting collar, which is applied and then withdrawn from the meatus; but this method is relatively clumsy and permits splashing.

(Fig. 26), and impeding the inflow when the urethra is full, allows the canal to empty itself. A proper distention of the urethra is secured by raising the reservoir 2 or 3 feet. Such elevation will not force the membranous urethra.

A hot 1: 6,000 solution of potassium permanganate is now made by crushing and dissolving 3 one-grain tablets in a quart of water at 110° F. (for the solution does not keep, and should be made fresh daily). This is poured into the tank, which is raised to a height of 3 feet, nozzle and scissors are attached, the patient (having urinated) stands, holding a wide basin to catch the outflow. The anterior urethra is irrigated by filling the nozzle with solution (Fig. 25), introducing it within the meatus, then slowly opening the scissors until the urethra is filled, then closing them until it is empty, and so proceeding to and fro until the tank is empty. After the first two or three treatments the strength of the solution is increased to 1: 4,000; beyond this it is unnecessary to go.

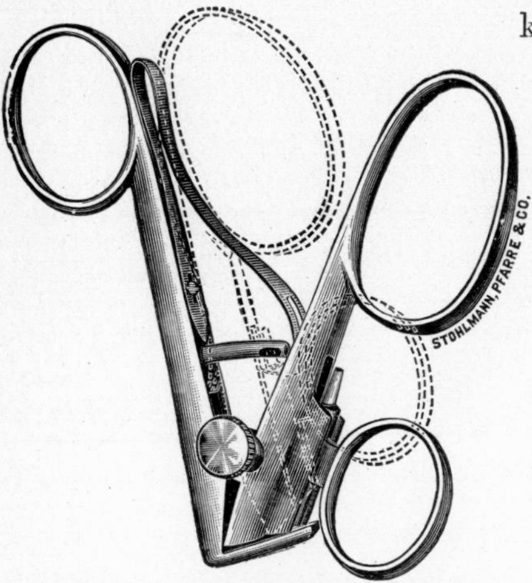

Fig. 24.—Chetwood's Scissors Shut-off.

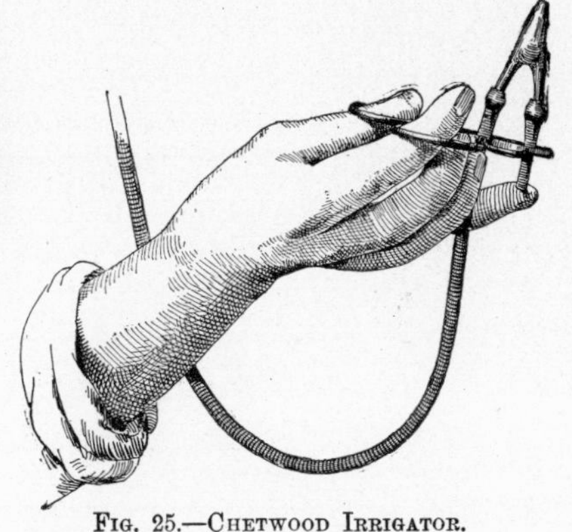

Fig. 25.—Chetwood Irrigator.
Filling the tube with fluid before applying it to the meatus.

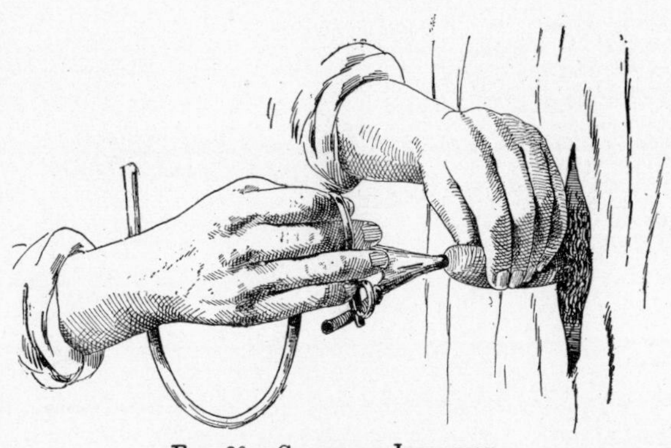

Fig. 26.—Chetwood Irrigator.
The fluid entering the urethra.

To irrigate the posterior urethra two methods are available:

1. Introduce a soft-rubber catheter, boiled and lubricated, into the urethra until it reaches the bladder, a fact indicated by the outflow of a few drops of urine. As soon as these appear withdraw the catheter a half inch or more so that its eye rests in the posterior urethra. Now inject, by means of tank or hand syringe, as much as the bladder will hold (from 200 to 500 c.c.) of 1:4,000 permanganate solution heated to about 110° F. This washes the posterior urethra as it flows in, and again when, after withdrawal of the catheter, the patient urinates it out.

2. The whole urethra may be irrigated without a catheter by forcing the cut-off muscle. This is not always an easy task (indeed, with some hypersensitive urethras it is impossible), and, in order to accomplish it, the patient had best be made to assume a reclining position, relaxing all his muscles. It is also useful at first—when the patient is unaccustomed to the treatment and likely to resist instinctively—to anesthetize the anterior urethra by an injection of 1:200 cocain solution. In most instances, a few treatments by this method suffice to tame the urethra, after which the cocain may be omitted and the injection administered with the patient sitting or standing up.

The irrigation may be administered from a tank hung 4 to 6 feet above the level of the bladder, but it is often easier, besides being safer, to employ a large piston syringe, with heavy, blunt nozzle to fit the meatus. In using this, however, the utmost delicacy of pressure must be employed, since excessive force excites a contraction of the cut-off muscle and only frustrates its own purpose. Holding the syringe in his right hand, the surgeon inserts its nozzle into the meatus, and with his left hand crowds the glans penis tightly around it, so that no drop of fluid shall leak out, and gently depresses the piston; the anterior urethra is readily distended, and then a sense of increased resistance announces that the barrier of the cut-off muscle has been reached. Gently and cautiously the pressure on the piston is increased and the patient instructed to breathe hard and deep in order to distract his attention, or else to pretend he is urinating in order actually to open the muscle. Gradually and by little jumps the muscle gives way, and it is amusing to feel the record of its unwilling submission transmitted by the fluid to the piston, though annoying if, as sometimes happens, it suddenly, and for no apparent reason, shuts down and refuses to admit any more fluid. When the syringe is empty it is refilled and a second and a third injection made until the bladder is full. The necessity of refilling the hand syringe is its one disadvantage as compared with the tank; but this is outweighed by the advantage of controlling pressure at will and adapting it to the needs of the case.

In selecting the method of washing the posterior urethra suitable for a given case several points are to be considered. In an acute case of gonorrhea the pressure necessary to force the cut-off muscle is calculated to bruise the inflamed urethral wall more than the gentle passage of a soft-rubber catheter, and, accordingly, an untimely epididymitis is more to be feared from forced injection. In chronic cases, moreover, while one need not fear the testicle, there is little to choose in efficacy between the two methods; and yet the catheter is a shade safer and a good deal easier to manage, so my usual preference remains with the catheter. Yet I have seen chronic cases that are apparently benefited by the searching effect of the forced injection, which drives the antiseptic fluid into all the wrinkles of the urethral wall while at the same time applying hydrostatic massage. It is well, therefore, always to bear in mind this possibility and to test the efficacy of forced injection if the catheter fails.

If Treatment is begun at the Onset of the Disease.—If the patient is seen at the onset, within three days of the beginning of his discharge, anterior irrigation alone (no forgetting the internal administration of sandal-wood oil) may suffice. If the discharge be free, the urethra should be irrigated twice a day, otherwise only once, for the first few days. Within four days of the beginning of treatment the discharge ought to be well under control. In favourable cases it will have ceased entirely; in any case it should be slight. Now we look for evidence of posterior urethritis. As a matter of routine, before irrigation the patient urinates in two glasses. Any slightest turbidity of the second flow (even if the discharge is profuse), any uneasiness in the perineum, any pain at the neck of the bladder during urination, is evidence of posterior urethritis. To establish this fact the anterior urethra is fully irrigated. The patient is then made to urinate, and the first flow now contains the washings of the posterior urethra only; if it is hazy there is posterior urethritis. As soon as the existence of this complication is ascertained—or, I might say, as soon as it is suspected, for it is far safer to err on the side of overcaution—the posterior irrigations are begun, the anterior canal being always washed first as long as there is any evidence of anterior urethritis. Thus we go well into the second week with daily anterior and posterior irrigations. If the case is progressing satisfactorily the discharge will have ceased completely, the patient will exhibit no symptoms whatever, and the urine will grow clearer daily. In the declining stage the treatment is the same as that with argyrol.

Choice of Treatment.—For *simple urethritis* it matters little whether argyrol or permanganate is employed; the inflammation is readily controllable by either.

For acute gonorrhea, I believe argyrol is usually the more efficacious, although one occasionally meets with a case that does better under permanganate. Indeed, the latter controls the discharge much more quickly (being more astringent), but it permits the inflammation to run into a chronic state more often, I think, than does argyrol. Minor points to be considered are, on the one hand, the dirtiness of argyrol; on the other hand, the necessity of returning daily for permanganate irrigations, though, even when injections are employed, it is necessary to see the patient often, in order to observe the progress of the disease and to keep him faithful to treatment. *Indeed, no "abortive" treatment can succeed unless the patient carries out faithfully its every detail while respecting the restrictions and taking the "balsam and alkali" of the methodic treatment.* In fact, I object to calling these treatments "abortive," for, at my hands—I confess it in face of the admirable results so frequently reported nowadays —they do not abort gonorrhea. They do control the disease just as mercury controls syphilis, and this I take to be their title to our respect. They keep the gonorrheic clean, they prevent chordee, cystitis and epididymitis, and sometimes they shorten the attack very considerably; but this is not to be counted upon. A virgin gonorrhea I am well satisfied to cure in six weeks. Secondary attacks may often be cured much more quickly, unless the urethra bears the scars of previous battles. But a cure of true gonorrhea in two weeks is altogether exceptional. It does occur, but usually—to employ a bull—only when there are no gonococci present.

Prognosis.—The advantages of the abortive treatment of gonorrhea are twofold, viz., the abolition of symptoms (discharge, chordee, dysuria, etc.) and the curtailment of the attack. The former is almost certain, the latter only probable. Against these advantages may be set the trouble and expense of the treatment, which count not a little, for the patient must be absolutely faithful; untimely remission of an irrigation may postpone the cure for days. Yet the strongest argument is that, of all the patients who have returned for the treatment of a new attack, not one has hesitated in preferring to be treated this way a second time.

The best results will be obtained with patients who, having had a previous attack, are in good general health and free from any chronic lesion or tendency to simple urethritis. Such cases are curable in three or four weeks.

Other Methods of Local Treatment.—Excepting the two just outlined, I know no commendable local treatment for acute gonorrhea. Protargol, argonin, mercurol, corrosive sublimate, and a host of others, have been employed and favourably reported upon. But they are all irritating to the urethra when employed strong enough and often enough to destroy the gonococcus, and, although each one may succeed in selected cases, their failures have merited the contempt of that great body of practitioners who deny the efficacy of all forms of local treatment in the early stages of gonorrhea.

Local Treatment of the declining Stage of Gonorrhea in the Anterior Urethra, and of all Subacute and Chronic Cases of Anterior Urethritis, whether Simple or following as a Sequence upon Gonorrhea.

Here irrigations are no longer necessary. The urethra may be more conveniently treated by injections, which the patient himself may apply.

In using injections upon himself the patient must be dispossessed of the idea that he needs a strong injection. He will generally, if he has suffered long, demand a strong lotion to kill the disease, and in such case may be gently reminded that, while a club in the hands of an athlete would doubtless be able to kill a mosquito upon his nose, still, to advise its employment for that purpose would be of doubtful propriety. More effect will be obtained by using an injection just strong enough to be of definite service than by using one as strong as the urethra will tolerate.

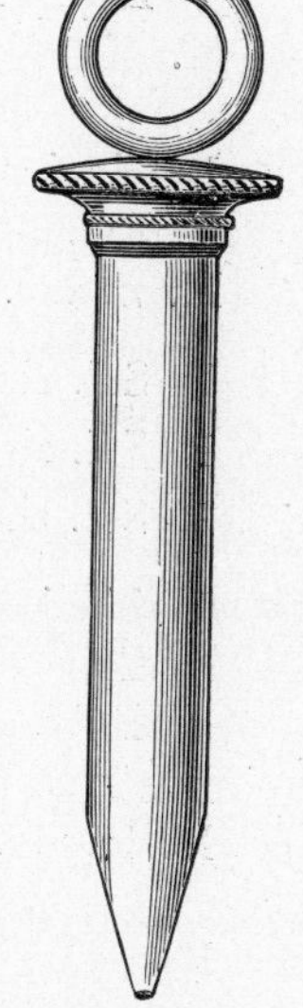
Fig. 27.

Another precaution, never to be forgotten, is that a discharge, at first checked by injections, may come to be perpetuated by them. This is especially likely to occur in mild simple urethritis. The patient checks his discharge by an injection, but if he omits it for a day or two a morning drop reappears to frighten him into renewed reliance upon it. Thus he will continue indefinitely, until the surgeon persuades him to let himself alone for a week or so, and his cure is accomplished.

The Method.—*To inject* the urethra several things must be remembered. Air must be expelled from the syringe. The solution must never be very cold—if warmed each time it is all the better; or, better still, the solution may be prescribed in twice the required concentration, to be diluted with an equal amount of hot water. No force should ever be used in making an injection, and too much fluid must not be forced in. Neglect of these last two precautions is responsible for many a case of posterior urethritis and many a swelled testicle. Only sufficient fluid to distend the anterior urethra moderately should be used.

The syringe should have a blunt nozzle (Fig. 27). It may be of vulcanite, or of glass, or may have a soft-rubber or cork tip. It should hold not less than 7.5 c. c. and not more than 12 c. c. The piston should run very smoothly, not in jerks. Injection should be made by slowly depressing the piston while crowding the blunt nozzle into the meatus, and the fluid should be retained by holding the nozzle there, or by pressure of thumb and finger as the syringe is being withdrawn. The fluid should never be restrained from penetrating too deeply by making perineal pressure with the finger. An astringent injection should be retained in the urethra for fifteen seconds, a bactericidal injection much longer.

Among injections—and their name is legion—the following are useful. The first ones are soothing—more or less—the next astringent, and the last antiseptic:

Soothing Injections

℞ Sol. cocain hydrochlorat.............................. 2%.

℞ Sol. extr. fl. hydrastis—non-alcoholic............ 4% to 8%.

℞ Morphiæ acetat.................... 00.20 grammes gr. iij
Liq. plumbi subacetat. dil........ad 100.00 " ℥ iij.
M.

Astringent Injections

℞ Zinci sulph................ 00.10–00.40 grammes gr. ii–vj
Liq. plumbi subacetat. dil..ad 100.00 " ℥ iij.
M. Shake.

℞ Sol. zinci sulph.............................. 1% to 4%.

℞ Sol. zinci permanganat................ 1 : 4,000 to 1 : 1,000.

℞ Sol. zinci sulphocarbolat....................... 0.5% to 1%.

℞ Zinci sulph............... 00.20–00.40 grammes gr. iij–vj
Bismuth subnitrat., } āā 4.00 " ʒ j
Pulv. acaciæ, }
Aquæ...............ad 100.00 " ℥ iij.
M. Shake.

Antiseptic Injections

℞ Sol. protargol................................ 0.25% to 1%.

℞ Sol. potass. permanganat..................... 1 : 4,000.

℞ Sol. argyrol................................ 2% to 10%.

With these may be met the indications of any case, from the most mild irritative urethritis up to the most tenacious chronic anterior urethritis; not that the injection will always cure—far from it—but it meets the indications and often renders valuable service.

The soothing injections are the least important. An astringent injection will reduce congestion, and pain with it, quite satisfactorily, unless the pain be neuralgic, in which case no injection serves.

The antiseptic injections are more serviceable as adjuvants to the irrigation treatment than when used alone. Indeed, in the declining and the chronic stages injections should be employed chiefly for the purpose of controlling the discharge and thereby keeping the patient clean. If perchance they also succeed in effecting a cure, so much the better. But in most cases a cure cannot be expected from them alone. They only hold the inflammation of the anterior urethra in abeyance, while the posterior urethra, which is almost always the real centre of trouble, is attacked by other measures or intrusted to the healing agency of time.

The Local Treatment of Chronic Anterior Urethritis

When astringent injections added to proper internal and hygienic means fail, and there is no stricture, follicular abscess, granulation, nor polyp, the light application of a 10% solution of nitrate of silver through the urethroscope upon the congested and granular surfaces may be made twice a week with advantage, or a few drops of a solution of nitrate of silver, 1 : 500 even up to 1 : 100, trickled along the canal with the deep urethral syringe at intervals of two to four days. This sometimes starts the reparative process, the astringent injection being kept up between times.

Massage of the urethra I have not found of any value, except such as is afforded by the gentle introduction of a warmed, full-sized double taper steel sound (Fig. 13) perhaps twice or three times a week, preferably just before an irrigation or an instillation. This stimulates circulation and empties the lacunæ and follicles of accumulated pus. If stricture exists it must be overdilated (p. 216) or cut.

I have found the steel sound admirably adapted by its solidity and smoothness to the needs of those cases that required stretching (and they are the ones that no longer harbour gonococci, whose urine is practically clear of free pus, and whose posterior urethræ are not irritable), while those chronic purulent cases that require irrigation bear stretching so ill that I have never seen the indication for the use of Kollmann's dilators (p. 197), nor have the results of this method of treatment at the hands of others shaken my unbelief.

It must be borne in mind that an astringent injection, especially if strong, is capable of maintaining enough surface congestion to keep up a discharge.

Treatment of Urethral Polyp

When a polyp is located by the urethroscope it must be removed by the urethral forceps or, preferably, by the wire snare (Fig. 28),

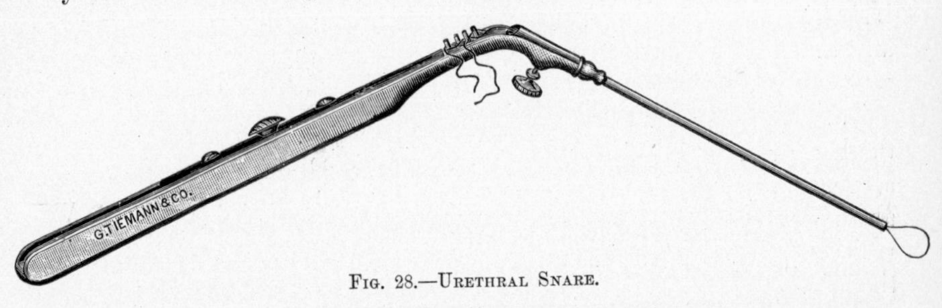

Fig. 28.—Urethral Snare.

or by the urethral curette (Fig. 29), after cocainizing the urethra, lightly cauterizing the raw surface later with a little fused nitrate of

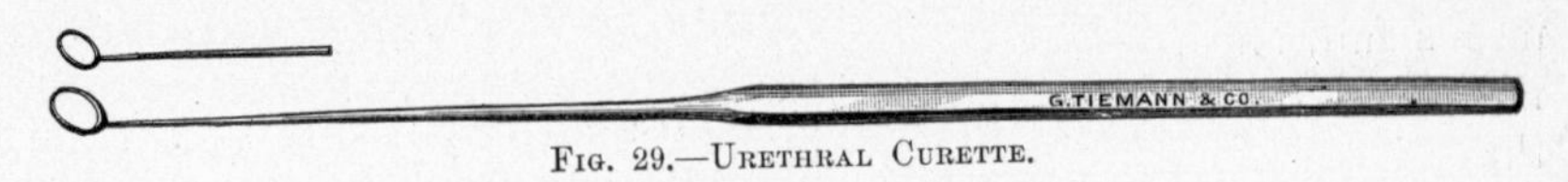

Fig. 29.—Urethral Curette.

silver upon the end of a long probe—all through the urethroscopic tube.

Treatment of Papillomatous Urethritis

The removal of urethral warts may also be accomplished by the snare or the curette, but when growths are numerous and large, lining the urethra, these instruments are too slow, abundant hemorrhage interfering with the work. In such case nothing is better than Oberländer's device, which I have used several times with admirable effect. Cocainize the urethra. Then by the aid of a tube place a large, tightly made cotton tampon behind and another in front, or in the midst, of the condylomatous mass, upon tampon holders (applicators). Now, keep the tube in place, straighten out the urethra, and by rubbing the two tampons back and forth upon each other the soft masses are disintegrated and come away in shreds among the blood-clots. Replace the old tampons with new ones as they become softened by the blood. The amount of friction and the length of the sitting are matters of personal judgment. The blood, at first free, soon ceases to flow. The frictions may be repeated once a week until all the papillomata have been removed, a soothing injection being employed between times. Finally, a few caustic applications upon the points from which the papillomata spring and a course of cod-liver oil with 10-drop doses 3 times a day of the tincture of thuja occidentalis perfect the cure.

Treatment of Folliculitis

An abscess of a follicle discharging within the urethra through an inadequate opening, or the chronic suppuration of a sinus of Morgagni may be detected by its pus-oozing point as seen through the urethroscope. The choice of treatment in such case lies between

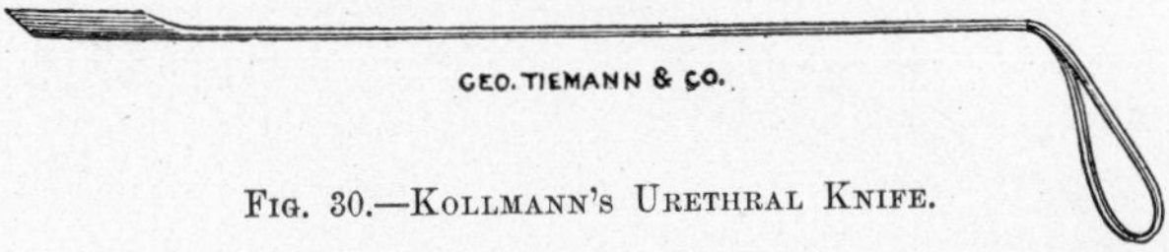

Fig. 30.—Kollmann's Urethral Knife.

an incision with (preferably) Kollmann's urethral knife (Fig. 30) alone, or the injection of the sac or the sinus by means of a pipette or the filiform urethral syringe (Fig. 31) with a couple of drops of the 25% ethereal solution of the peroxid of hydrogen, or by both means combined. The injected solution softens and disintegrates the inflammatory exudation, and leads to closure by contraction of the follicular cavity. The injection may have to be repeated several

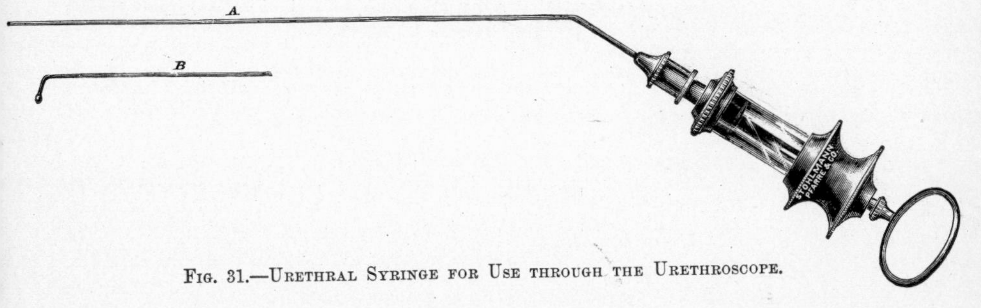

Fig. 31.—Urethral Syringe for Use through the Urethroscope.

times at intervals of a few days, the urethra meantime being irrigated or injected mildly.

All manipulations within the urethra by tubes and instruments should be made carefully and with definite intervals of rest between the applications. Zeal is to be discouraged. The more haste the less speed.

Treatment of Periurethral Abscess and of Folliculitis opening Externally, or both Externally and Internally (Acute Fistula)

All pus formations about the urethra, whether diffuse or contained within a follicular sac, are treated during the acute inflammatory stage on general surgical principles—by rest, protection from friction and injury, moist weak bichlorid or mild carbolized wet dressing under gutta-percha tissue. Incision should not be made too hastily nor until the formation of pus is pronounced, for resolution often occurs in follicular cases when suppuration seems inevitable. Ichthyol, pure or diluted, seems sometimes to favour resolution. When fluctuation is manifest an attempt should be made with a wire speculum to make an opening from within through the mucous membrane, thereby averting threatened fistula, for the abscess cavity may be better treated afterward from within than from without. This applies to follicular abscess—pus within a sac. When suppuration is diffuse under the skin a cutaneous incision is required, and frequently there will be no subsequent urinary leakage and the abscess may be treated along ordinary surgical lines.

When the abscess has discharged or has been opened, outside or inside, or both, the best results may be confidently expected from the use of pyrozone—the 25% ethereal solution of the peroxid of hydrogen, using a fine-drawn, rubber-capped, glass pipette (Fig. 32) with bent extremity.

By means of this instrument, aided if need be by a wire urethral speculum, a few drops of the solution are thrown into the abscess cavity to destroy the unhealthy granulations. This is repeated after

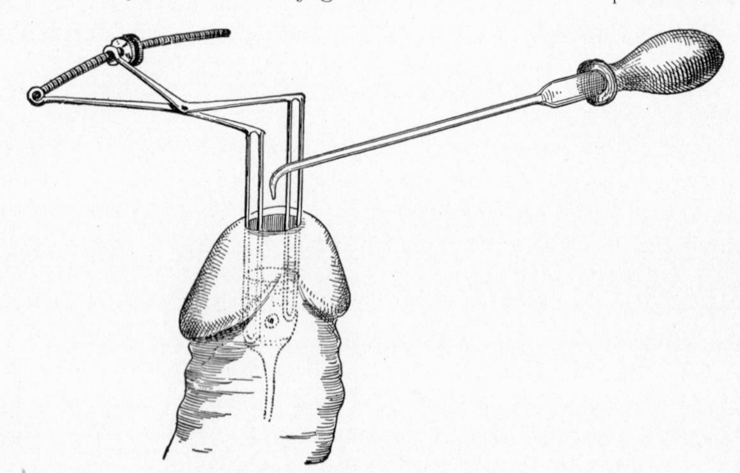

Fig. 32.—Injection of Urethral Fistula.

a couple of days, and then a milder solution (5%) is injected daily, then every second day, until the cavity has filled and healed or the fistula has closed. This treatment should be applied from within the urethra, the internal orifice of the abscess or of the sinus being enlarged for that purpose, if necessary.

If the case is more chronic from the start and the little shot-like or pea-like bodies remain under the skin refusing to suppurate actively, these little tumours may be cut out through a cutaneous incision. Frequently there is not sufficient communication with the urethra to permit the escape of urine, and the cut heals like a simple incision.

Treatment of Cowperitis

Hot hip baths, absolute rest, poultices, laxatives, and diluents, perhaps leeches, meet all indications in the earlier period of cowperitis. No instrumentation is allowable unless exacted by retention of urine. Resolution even when despaired of may occur, and the knife is not to be thought of until fluctuation is manifest. When a cut is made it should be ample so as to reach by drainage all the various branched pouches of the gland. The abscess cavity must be well stuffed with iodoform gauze to force granulation and closure from the bottom, on pain of leaving a chronic fistula.

When fistula persists after a trial of the pyrozone treatment suggested for folliculitis (p. 130) the only method of cure is to dissect out the entire tract and the granulo-spongy remains of the gland (Englisch).

LOCAL TREATMENT OF POSTERIOR URETHRITIS

This is encompassed by irrigations, instillations, hot baths, douches, and massage.

In a general way it may be said that most cases of very active acute posterior urethritis also implicate or threaten to implicate the neck of the bladder, the prostate, and the vesicles; and therefore they call for repeated very hot hip baths and rest in bed in order to avoid these complications or to meet their requirements, while chronic posterior urethritis does better under hot rectal douche, massage, and perineal counter-irritation.

The Rectal Douche.—The hot rectal douche is very conveniently administered by means of the Chetwood glass rectal tube (Fig. 33), a modification of the Tuttle and Kemp tubes devised for the same purpose.

The figure illustrates the mechanism. The hot water from a fountain-syringe enters the smaller inlet tube, thence flows into an outside sealed chamber from which there is no escape except through the small perforations near the end of the outside enveloping tube. The water flows back again through the central dark tube, which is larger than the combined holes of exit in the external tube. In spite of this facility of exit the water does not flow out of the rectum so readily as it flows in, and every patient has to learn for himself how to manipulate the end of the tube in order to favour the outflow of the hot water, on pain of giving himself an injection—no very serious matter.

Some patients prefer to sit upon the edge of a chair, the buttocks slightly projecting and the outflow being received into a foot-bath on the floor. Others prefer to get upon all-fours. Most patients soon learn to work the apparatus, controlling the inflow when the outflow ceases, and manipulating the end of the tube without withdrawal. Occasionally a man whose fingers are all thumbs, or whose rectum is hyperesthetic, cannot manage it and has to give it up.

The tube is introduced into the rectum about half its length, and generally two quarts of water, at a temperature (in the bag)

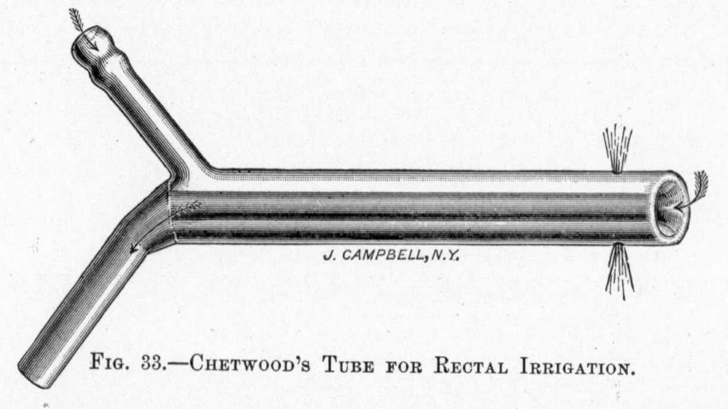

FIG. 33.—CHETWOOD'S TUBE FOR RECTAL IRRIGATION.

of 110° to 120° F., are employed, about ten to fifteen minutes being required for the douche according to the dexterity of the patient.

It is better to use this douche at night just before retiring and to continue it several weeks. Then after rest for a week it may often be resumed with renewed good effect. It is indicated in all local chronic inflammatory and neuralgic conditions of the posterior urethra, the prostate, and vesicles, and has largely replaced the need of that more disagreeable alternative, prostatic massage.

Sometimes in hemorrhoidal conditions, and with oversensitive rectums, the tube does more harm than the heat does good, but this is very rare.

Cold water may be used through this tube in neurotic, neuralgic, and neurasthenic conditions, but generally the hot douche does more good; its effect is sometimes surprisingly prompt and satisfactory.

Massage.—The more chronic the posterior urethritis, the more neuralgic its type, the deeper the inflammation of the gland, the greater is the need for something more than surface applications to the prostatic sinus and douches to the rectum. This need is met by prostatic massage. The patient cannot do this for himself, but a trained nurse may be taught to do it effectively, the only trouble being a tendency to exercise too much pressure and so to bruise the parts, turning a chronic into an acute inflammation. For massage of the prostate the patient bends forward nearly to a right angle at the hips, holding the knees stiff. The masseur, covering his finger with a thin rubber stall and lubricating it well, inserts it into the rectum, and mapping out the prostate by the sense of touch with gentle pressure and lateral sweeps of the finger, practises the maneuvre of massage during from one to three minutes.

Massage of the prostate, if gentle enough, may be performed daily with good effect. *The use of sounds* is to be deprecated in all forms of posterior urethritis, unless, of course, due to stricture of the membranous urethra, or sometimes where the neuralgic element runs high. In the latter the pressure and internal massage of the sound may do much good.

I have derived no advantage from the application of electricity or of ointments to the prostate per rectum.

Irrigation and Instillation.—*Irrigations* of the deep urethra have been already described (p. 122). They are most serviceable when the discharge is profuse and the inflammation chronic, while instillations are of use to check an acute inflammation or to moderate a mild chronic one.

Instillations are perhaps the most effective means of controlling chronic posterior urethral discharge, and they have also a definite value in chronic anterior urethritis. They are administered by means of the deep urethral syringe (Fig. 34), the long nozzle of

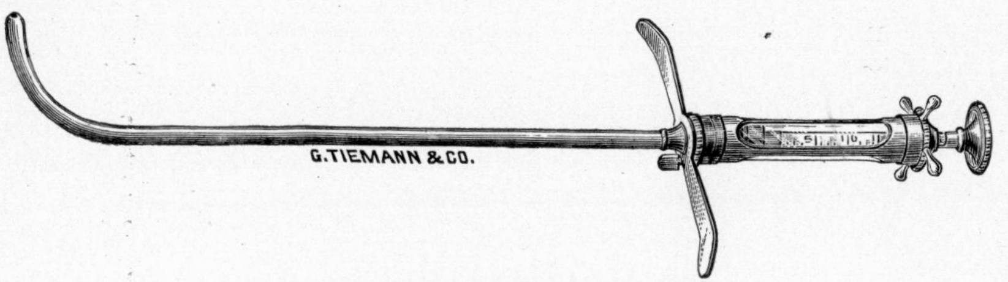

FIG. 34.—KEYES'S INSTILLATION SYRINGE.

which is made of silver with a minute central lumen terminating at the tip of the curve. The syringe part is like a large hypodermic syringe with minims graded on the piston. This syringe is made in one piece, and is cleanly. Its lumen does not corrode, its curve facilitates introduction, the wings indicate the position of the tip and facilitate slow and even depression of the piston. This syringe has been evolved out of the Ultzmann, upon which it is a distinct improvement.

For *anterior instillation* the tip of the syringe, properly lubricated, is introduced into the sinus of the bulb, where a few drops of the solution are deposited. These drops follow the instrument upon its withdrawal, appearing at the meatus and medicating the entire length of the anterior urethra.

For *posterior instillation* the tip of the syringe is inserted well into but not through the membranous urethra. Then the piston is depressed and 20 minims of solution instilled. This flows backward, bathes the posterior sinus, and flows over into the bladder. When the instrument is withdrawn none of the injection appears at the meatus.

In making instillations the bladder should be empty.

Solutions Employed.—The substances most useful for application by instillation are sulphate of thallin, nitrate of silver, protargol, sulphate of copper, glycerol of tannin, and ichthyol.

Sulphate of Thallin.—This astringent, antiseptic, and sedative drug makes a light, straw-coloured, saturated solution at 20% strength. It is best kept in a yellow bottle, but even then it darkens gradually, until it becomes of a rich brown colour, a change which does not lessen the efficiency of the drug.

It is used at 3% strength to commence with, and from that raised to 6% and 12% if it suits. In mild posterior urethritis, especially of the hyperesthetic sort, it often acts like a charm, immediately reducing discharge, and being followed, after the first mild sensation of warmth and smarting, by positive comfort.

It is a good injection to begin with in any case where there is doubt as to the amount of reaction that will follow any local treatment, and it is curative in simple posterior urethritis. To control gonorrheal urethritis, however, stronger applications are necessary.

Sulphate of Copper.—This may be suitably kept in a 10% solution in glycerin to be diluted in water as required. It is generally used in a strength of 1:500 to start with, increased slowly to 1:100 or 1:50 or higher. It burns very little. It is much more suitable for use in the posterior than in the anterior urethra, for what reason I know not. In mild catarrhal posterior urethritis following thallin it often renders distinct service as a mild astringent. It is of no especial value in gonorrheal cases.

Nitrate of Silver.—This drug takes the highest rank in the treatment of chronic posterior urethritis and in acute gonorrheal cystitis. The first effect of an instillation is an immediate sense of heat and smarting in the deep urethra, accompanied by a call to empty the bladder, which may be imperative, even though the patient has just urinated. When this call is responded to the urine is hot and burning and slight tenesmus follows the act. The next urination is less urgent and painful, and presently order is restored, a sense of comfort and of local anesthesia ensues, and the call to urinate is postponed beyond the habitual limit if the nitrate agrees. Discharge also is promptly checked, or moderated, in successful cases. Nitrate instillations, if very weak (1: 2,000), may sometimes be repeated daily, but generally it is better to make them strong enough to be felt (1: 1,000 or much stronger), and to repeat in forty-eight or seventy-two hours. The strength of the application may be slowly increased up to 1: 50 or higher, and in some cases of neuralgia without prostatorrhea even as high as 5%. It is not wise to use the nitrate stronger than 5% for fear of its caustic action. Even that strength often produces a temporary intense irritability of the bladder with bloody urine. Occasionally the injection induces priapism with pollution the night after its use.

Protargol.—This is a proteid silver salt discovered by Eichengrün and introduced by Neisser, Nogues, and Desnos.

It is less irritating than the nitrate, and may be used much stronger. Three-per-cent solutions sometimes cause considerable and intense urinary stress. Protargol makes a thickish viscid mixture, and calls for a little wider calibration in the syringe employed, and the quantity used is generally greater, 2 to 6 c. c. being thrown in at a single instillation.

The best effects from protargol are obtained in chronic cases, with large instillations commencing at 0.5% and working up as high as 10%. I have used it effectively as high as 40% in one case.

The solution should be freshly made as required for use at each application. The urgent desire to urinate that it occasions is sometimes irresistible, occasionally lasting a couple of days. Other cases tolerate the drug better. The intensity of dysuria does not necessarily increase proportionately to the increase in strength of the solution, but the patient should not be treated brutally, and strong solutions should not be resorted to unless weaker ones fail. All irritation should be allowed to subside before a new protargol instillation is attempted.

In chronic urethritis, even when not gonorrheal, protargol is sometimes a very effective agent. In the congestions existing behind old strictures it has undoubted advantage following the insertion of the sound, and its property of not coagulating albumin permits it to penetrate deeply into the tissues and makes it especially useful in chronic parenchymatous prostatitis.

Ichthyol instillation is occasionally helpful in old chronic posterior urethritis after other means fail. It is well to begin mildly at 2% or 3%, and push, if well borne, even to 20%.

Glycerol of Tannin, diluted from 1 to 5 times with water, is an excellent tonic astringent for instillation in some cases, but it is less useful than the others.

Résumé of the Treatment of Posterior Urethritis

As I have said in another place, chronic gonorrhea is posterior urethritis, and the description of the treatment of posterior urethritis will, accordingly, be adapted to embrace that great multitude of cases whose only symptom is gleet, whether that gleet be due to simple or to gonorrheal posterior urethritis, prostatitis, periprostatitis, or to vesiculitis.

The first requisite is a thorough diagnosis. Inspection of the urine and palpation of the urethra will rule out grave lesions of the anterior canal (any doubts about stricture are set at rest by the first passage of an instrument). Rectal palpation reveals the presence or absence of parenchymatous prostatitis, periprostatitis, and vesiculitis.

Having thus made an accurate diagnosis, a rational treatment may be instituted. The rules of diet, urethral hygiene, and systemic medication must always be enforced, with a few restrictions. The patient must often be prepared to undergo a long course of treatment, and while the local treatment is the actual efficient agent in his cure, he can expect no advantage from this unless he keep himself in as healthy and robust a condition as possible. Hence it is more than ever essential at this stage of the disease that the balsamic administered be entirely compatible with the patient's digestion. When the inflammation has lasted several months, it is often quite useless—the patient's urine being neither too dense nor too acid—to administer any balsamic or alkali. At this stage tonics are far more likely to do good, and, in some of these cases, the stimulation of a little alcohol, which is so deleterious in the early days, may be distinctly beneficial. Simple urethritis may sometimes be cured by alcohol alone, a fact that always gains wide circulation among the patient's friends and encourages them to disastrous efforts in that direction.

Simple Urethritis.—To return to the local treatment: for non-specific posterior urethritis thallin sulphate and silver nitrate are the best local remedies, with an occasional exception in favour of protargol, potassium permanganate, and copper sulphate.

Mild Gonorrheal Posterior Urethritis.—This inflammation usually yields to irrigations of permanganate, beginning at 1:8,000 or 1:6,000, and repeated daily at 1:4,000. Protargol by instillation or irrigation may do better, while in some cases I have often found the admixture of silver nitrate (about 1: 20,000) with the permanganate irrigation the most efficient.

Intractable Posterior Urethritis.—This may be said to exist when the inflammation does not yield in the course of a few weeks to the treatment just mentioned. Such cases are usually complicated by parenchymatous prostatitis, by vesiculitis, or by contracture of the neck of the bladder. One of three courses of treatment is likely to prove efficacious, viz., rectal douche and prostatic massage, hygiene and tonics, or perineal cystotomy.

The douche and massage properly belong to the treatment of parenchymatous prostatitis and of vesiculitis (see below); but the douche is applicable to these cases as well, since there is always a slight implication of the prostatic parenchyma or of the vesicle. The effect of the douche may not be immediately visible to the patient, but several weeks of this treatment, combined with appropriate irrigation, will often work a great change in the patient's urine, even though the individual treatments have no visible effect.

At this stage of the disease it may be advantageous to drop the balsamic and to administer a tonic in its place. And it may be proper to encourage the playing of tennis or of golf. I have even known horseback-riding to effect a cure, in spite of, or perhaps because of, the contusion of the prostate thus incurred. But this is a matter to be decided differently for each case. (I believe bicycles and railroad trains are always injurious.) In selecting a form of exercise the patient's habits, taste, and constitution must all be considered, and the results of the exercise closely watched. If he returns refreshed and exhilarated, the treatment suits him, even though it produce no change in his local symptoms. On the other hand, I have known a desperately chronic case cured by local treatment, rest in bed, and diuresis by mineral waters.

There remain a few cases that none of the above measures can cure. Their proper course is to go away for several weeks to an unaccustomed climate, taking with them an injection (anterior or posterior) to check the discharge. I have seen patients cured when all other means had failed by simply crossing the Atlantic and returning on the same ship, or by a trip to the Adirondacks or to Asheville. They return either entirely cured or in such good condition that it is only a matter of a few weeks of local treatment before they are well.

Finally, the last resort is operation. If there are symptoms of contracture of the neck of the bladder (p. 317) perineal section with drainage is required, and the same treatment may be efficacious in mere chronic posterior urethritis; but it should be reserved absolutely until every other method of treatment has failed. Again, when there is recurring epididymitis, nothing cures that complication, and with it the posterior urethritis, so surely as vasectomy (p. 729). Tying off the vas in these cases acts quite as an acute epididymitis sometimes does. The inflammation seems to expend its force in the epididymis—I know no explanation of the fact—and with the resolution of the inflammation there, whether spontaneous or by ligature of the duct, the posterior urethritis disappears.

Parenchymatous Prostatitis.—The treatment of parenchymatous prostatitis is that of posterior urethritis, as detailed above, with special attention to the local treatment per rectum. I have derived no benefit from the application of ointments or from electricity by this route, and confine my efforts to douches and massage. The hot douche is applicable to all cases, the cold douche to neurotic cases, massage never to acute cases and only to those chronic cases that are not benefited by the douche.

PERIPROSTATITIS, if chronic, is best treated by massage and douche together.

Abscess, Prostatic and Periprostatic (see p. 140).

Irritable and Relapsing Cases.—These are often only made worse by local treatment. Hygiene and tonics are our weapons here. Urotropin seems beneficial in a few of these cases.

Neuralgic Cases.—Neuralgic cases demand the patience of Job. Some do well under tonics and hygiene; others under nitrate of silver; others under rectal douche, hot or cold, under massage, or under vibratory percussion.

Harmful Treatment.—Finally, I have found certain methods of treatment harmful, and as several of them are constantly employed, I venture to record my objections, although I know that many experienced practitioners will disagree with my conclusions. When convinced of error it will be a pleasure to change my opinion.

1. Sounds and dilators I object to absolutely. The massage and pressure of these instruments are beneficial in chronic anterior urethritis almost always, in prostatic hyperesthesia and congestion often, in simple posterior urethritis rarely, in gonorrheal posterior urethritis never.

2. Urethroscopy I object to on the same ground. The mechanical injury wrought by these instruments outweighs all the benefits they bestow.

3. The use of large rubber catheters or of woven instruments is harmful in the same way, but to a less degree.

4. Forced retrojection—forcing the cut-off muscle by the weight of a column of water—is not necessarily harmful, but I believe that

in acute cases it does harm fully as often as good. In some cases with a tendency to spasm of the cut-off it is quite impracticable. In acute cases and in many chronic ones there is a very real danger of lighting up an epididymitis by this treatment. Yet I have occasionally found it useful in sluggish chronic cases, the gentle massage of the column of fluid acting as a stimulant.

TREATMENT OF GONORRHEAL CYSTITIS

Like any other acute cystitis the gonorrheal inflammation calls for attitude (rest), alkali (bicarbonate of soda or liquor potassæ), anodyne (repeated hot hip baths about 104° to 110° F., opium suppository—watery extract 3 to 6 centigrammes with extract of belladonna 1 to 2 centigrammes repeated every few hours, if required). Many light cases, however, go about without much distress, often terminating spontaneously in a few days, and being only troublesome by day.

The question always arises in gonorrheal cystitis when to begin local treatment of the neck of the bladder. If improvement commences promptly under general treatment and is progressive, as is often the case, the patient may be spared the possible danger of complication incident to instrumentation in the urethra. But in any case when the symptoms progress rapidly it is allowable to call in local means very early in the endeavour to destroy the gonococcus. These means are permanganate-of-potash irrigation and nitrate-of-silver instillation.

The former has many advocates, and sometimes seems to do very well; personally, I rather prefer the latter.[1] In a mild case the strength of silver nitrate may be 1: 500, 20 drops being instilled, while the bladder is empty. In very acute cases I do not hesitate, after first giving the patient a morphin or phosphate-of-codein hypodermic injection, to instil at once a 2% solution of nitrate of silver, and if the effect be good, as is generally the case after the first pain is over, to repeat that instillation or a stronger one once a day for 3 or 4 days, then rest a few days and renew the course if required.

The effect of this expedient is sometimes startling, and the slight risk of epididymitis assumed is as nothing compared to the possible horrors of prolonged chronic gonorrheal cystitis with contracture of the vesical neck, a condition only properly overcome by perineal section.

---

[1] In my second edition of The Venereal Diseases (1900, p. 94), Dr. Chetwood's milder views on this subject have been allowed to preponderate.

When in gonorrheal cystitis the impetus of the disease is arrested, then permanganate of potash or mild nitrate of silver 1:10,000 to 1:2,000, or protargol 0.25% to 1%, aided now by balsams and diluents is very useful. The last-named cannot be employed during acute gonorrheal cystitis for mechanical reasons.

TREATMENT OF PROSTATIC AND PERIPROSTATIC ABSCESS

Rest in bed and hot hip baths are essential. Fournier counsels the early application of 15 or 20 leeches to the perineum. Hot poultices to the perineum are comforting and helpful. Hot enemata may be employed to evacuate the rectum. Anodynes and laxatives must be used, and perhaps the catheter, a soft one by preference (tied in rather than too frequently introduced). Aspiration may be required. When pus is suspected, as indicated by persistence and intensification of symptoms, chill, mild urinary sepsis, etc., careful examination of the prostate should be made from time to time by the finger in the rectum. When fluctuation or aspiration reveals pus, it may become a nice question to decide whether (1) to let it burst by the urethra, if it seems to be small, central, and near the surface of the prostatic sinus; (2) if there be multiple small foci, to make a perineal incision to cut down the bladder neck and prostatic lobe and to insert a tube to cure retention, to ward off sepsis, and to prevent thrombus of the prostatic veins; (3) to open by the simplest of all routes, through the rectal wall (and this is best, if there be adhesion and the pus is pointing towards the rectal cavity), or (4) to open by a free prerectal incision of the perineum, a most admirable method in case of an extensive collection of pus, and particularly for periprostatic suppuration. Positive rules in any of these directions would be unwise. Surgical tact must be the guide; all things considered, the median perineal incision is preferable in case of doubt.

TREATMENT OF URETHRORRHEA AND PROSTATORRHEA

These two maladies, as they produce a flow from the urethra, are often treated like cases of chronic urethritis. This is an error. Sometimes the patient feels better under a soothing or an astringent injection (p. 126). In neurotic subjects, thallin or nitrate of silver applied to the prostatic sinus by instillation (2 drops of a 5% solution), or touching the swollen verumontanum with a little fused nitrate of silver upon a long probe through the urethroscope may be of service. An occasional steel sound or a cold-water sound adds tone to the urethral circulation, and massage of the prostate helps, perhaps, a little; but tonics, cod-liver oil, local cold-water douche, horseback exercise, a pure mind, and absolute sexual continence or matrimony of a proper kind (p. 112)—these things must be relied upon to effect a cure, and in the right-minded they will do so. The sexual pervert in this condition is all but hopeless.

If, as is often the case, prostatitis or spermato-cystitis complicates prostatorrhea—and they may well do so—the treatment of the complication greatly helps the prostatorrhea.

TREATMENT OF ACUTE SPERMATO-CYSTITIS

In treating acute spermato-cystitis it must be remembered that the malady is often so mild as to yield no symptoms, and to subside spontaneously. Doubtless in every case of gonorrheal epididymitis there is coincident acute vesiculitis of that side, but it gives no sign, and is only discovered by rectal exploration. When the symptoms do manifest themselves, however, the malady is treated like acute prostatitis, by rest, bodily and sexual, alkaline diluents, light diet, laxatives, anodynes, sitz baths (rarely by the rectal tube for acute cases), possibly even by perineal leeches. Opium suppositories, monobromid of camphor, antipyrin, and heavy doses of potassium bromid are employed for nocturnal priapism and pollution.

Rectal examination is to be avoided, and the vesicle must never be stripped for fear of producing one of three things: priapism with bloody emissions, acute urethro-cystitis, or epididymitis. The only object of rectal examination is to detect abscess of the vesicle early, and to incise it opportunely. Such abscess may be afforded a rectal opening, but strong advocacy of the perineal route has been made (Guelliot,[1] Collan [2]). There is no danger of ultimate fistula. Nature habitually opens the abscess into the rectum, and the surgeon may anticipate her choice with a tenotomy knife or a sharp-curved bistoury partly wound with adhesive plaster introduced flat upon the finger through the rectal sphincter. No anesthesia is required. A hot enema or a rectal douche twice daily perfects the cure if the incision has been ample.

If the abscess is not detected soon enough and bursts into the bladder, both that viscus and the rectum must receive repeated hot

---

[1] Presse méd., 1898, i, 193.

[2] Ueber Spermato-cystitis Gonorrhoica. Leipzig. 1894, S. 65.

irrigation—mildly disinfectant—until the abscess cavity has healed and the flow of pus ceased.

TREATMENT OF CHRONIC SPERMATO-CYSTITIS

This malady is so involved with other affections, prostatorrhea, prostatitis, sexual neurasthenia, and so often associated with a life of sexual riot of one sort or another, that it is difficult to portray or to differentiate, and it forms the richest possible field for the unscrupulous practitioner.

The cause for continuance of symptoms must be discovered and stopped or all effort will prove futile; masturbation and sexual strain, notably ungratified sexual desire, must be absolutely prohibited. Almost invariably one of these factors has been a co-operating cause of the symptoms, because we often find chronic seminal vesiculitis with practically no *symptoms of a neurotic or neurasthenic kind.* Constipation and straining at stool should be interdicted. Bicycle or even horseback-riding is inadvisable in severe cases.

Diet, exercise, and air must be studiously regulated and the mind properly occupied, for morbid introspection is fatal to the success of treatment. General massage, cold hip baths, cold douches, or sponging of loins, back, and genitals in the morning, a course of cold drip sheet, the cold-water psychrophore or the rectal tube, employing very hot and very cold water in alternating courses—all these have their places and their uses as adjuvants.

Sexual hygiene is most important, and matrimony in appropriate cases a positive specific—often alone effecting a cure.

Among medicines iron, cod-liver oil, hypophosphites, and strychnin are the standard tonics. If local irritability be marked, 30 centigrammes of monobromid of camphor or 12 of valerianate of zinc, or 30 of asafetida 3 times daily, may be comforting, or 0.5 milligramme of sulphate of atropin 3 times a day.

No benefit may be expected from ichthyol or iodoform suppositories, and instillations of the prostatic sinus are not reliable. The two most commendable methods are massage of the vesicles and rectal douching with very hot water with the Chetwood tube (p. 131). The latter expedient possesses two great advantages. In the first place, it may be used daily by the patient, to the saving of his pocket and the increase of his self-respect; and in the second place, it is often more efficient than massage, for I have observed a number of cures by its use after massage at most competent hands had failed. Inexpert massage is attended by constant danger of lighting up epididymitis, a risk that does not seem to attach to the tube.

The vesicle is stripped by introducing the finger just as far as it can possibly be pushed above the upper corner of the prostate upon one side, and then the peanut-shaped, distended body of the vesicle, moderately palpated by the pulp of the finger, is slowly pressed upon by withdrawing the finger and making very moderate lateral movements. The instruments devised to strip the vesicles are more brutal than the finger and not to be recommended, although they may do the work more decently and more thoroughly. I constructed probably the first of these about thirty years ago, long before the modern furor for treating vesiculitis had been dreamed of. It consisted of a double rubber balloon introduced collapsed, then inflated and withdrawn. It did not long survive the injury it occasioned.

There is something very wonderful about the effect produced upon some minds (and upon some bodies, for that matter) by the introduction of a finger into the rectum. How else shall we explain the pretensions of the school of orificial surgery, never better exemplified than by that delightful and now classical story of the quack at Bath, England, who discovered that all the ills of the flesh are due to stricture of the rectum and can be cured by a daily introduction of the rectal bougie! The London physicians, finding that all their patients were leaving them in order to go to Bath to see the new celebrity, held a meeting, and elected the most serious-minded, stolid, and matter-of-fact gentleman of their number to set forth for the express purpose of studying and exposing the methods of the irregular practitioner who was threatening to rob them of all their patients.

The delegate departed, and in a week wrote back to the committee, praising Providence that had so willed it that he should have been selected for the mission, for, said he, "I have found the doctor to be a most honest and learned gentleman, and I have discovered that I myself have stricture of the rectum, and I am now daily having a bougie passed for its relief—to my great betterment!"

This pleasantry, of course, is not detailed to condemn the practice of vesicular massage, because there is most positive merit in it, but to put the young practitioner upon his guard. I have had a man come to my office and appeal to me almost tearfully to relieve the dreadful pain in his back by milking his vesicles. I tested him by simply introducing my finger through the sphincter, without touching his vesicles, and the pain disappeared at once. This man had been having his vesicles stripped for a year and liked it, but, naturally, such treatment could not be expected to cure him—at least so I thought.

Yet there are cases in which the vesicle is manifestly distended and sensitive; the patient cannot sit squarely upon a cushioned seat for the discomfort it occasions; there is positive pain across the back low down, and perhaps also radiate neuralgia in the sciatic or anterior crural nerves; and disgorgement of the distended vesicle by pressure surely gives relief to all of these symptoms at once.

If vesicular massage be practised the intervals ought to be about five days. The douche may be tried first in all cases. If it succeeds, well and good; if not, massage may be tested; but sometimes both are ineffective.

Yet neither douche nor massage can be expected to effect a rapid cure. If the symptoms are moderately acute rather prompt relief may be looked for—perhaps in a month or six weeks. In chronic cases a longer period must be allowed for improvement to manifest itself, and it may take six months or a year to effect a cure.

While the success of the treatment of chronic spermato-cystitis, as of so many other maladies of these regions, often depends more upon a comprehension of the patient's nervous calibre and sexual hygienic irregularities than upon the technic of local treatment, correction of diatheses and of dietetics, with tonics—medical, moral, and hygienic—is of the utmost value.

Perivesicular Abscess.—Chronic abscess and infiltration of the perivesicular tissues occur now and again, causing retention of urine, impotence, local pains, etc.

Fuller[1] suggests that these abscesses be attacked by the Kraske sacral incision. I consider the perineal route preferable (p. 789). He reports 2 cases—1 cured, the other disappeared. This example has not been followed.

---

[1] J. of Cut. and Gen.-Urin. Dis., 1896, xiv, 330.

CHAPTER IX

EXTRA-GENITAL AND METASTATIC GONORRHEA

The gonorrheal maladies so far considered all affect the genital apparatus. Acute gonorrheal cystitis, confined as it is to the neck of the bladder, is in reality only a part of the picture of acute gonococcal posterior urethritis. But there are numerous other morbid conditions directly due to the specific germ, involving the urinary tract, the other mucous membranes, and many other structures of the body. Indeed, modern laboratorial research has achieved for gonorrhea the distinction of ranking as a general systemic malady, since the gonococcus has proved its ability to establish a habitat outside the urethra.

A mass of literature upon this subject is collated in the classical work of Marcel Sée.[1] It covers the subject entirely up to its date (1896). Since then there has been no stint of workers in the field, both in the clinic and the laboratory, and the extent of the *rôle* of the gonococcus is doubtless now fairly well understood. It is impossible to follow all these modern investigations minutely in a work of this character, but it is interesting to append Young's [2] list setting forth the chronological advance of our knowledge and the names attached to each new step.[3]

---

[1] Le gonocoque. Paris, 1896. [2] J. of Cut. and Gen.-Urin. Dis., 1900, xviii, 240.

[3] Neisser in 1879 demonstrated that the gonococcus is the cause of ophthalmia neonatorum.

Bumm in 1887 successfully cultivated the gonococcus.

Arthritis—Gonococcus demonstrated in Pure Culture. Lindemann, 1892.

Salpingitis and Circumscribed Pelvic Peritonitis. Wertheim, 1892.

Abscess, Subcutaneous. Lang and Paltauf, 1893.

Teno-synovitis. Tollemer and Macaigne, 1893.

Pleurisy. Mazza, 1894.

Perichondritis. Finger, Gohn, Schlagenhaufer, 1894.

Abscess, Intramuscular. Bujevid, 1895.

Acute Cystitis. Wertheim, 1895.

Endocarditis and Septicemia. Thayer and Blumer, 1895.

Adenitis—Glands of the Neck. Petit and Pichevin, 1896.

Chronic Cystitis, Pyonephrosis, Diffuse Peritonitis. Young, 1898.

Abscesses, cutaneous, subcutaneous, and muscular [1] (the inoculation being through the sheath of a tendon or direct, as after incising an infected joint), have yielded pure cultures. So also general diffuse peritonitis in the female (Cushing, Young). In animals diffuse peritonitis has been induced by inoculation, but diffuse pure gonococcal peritonitis has not yet been found in the human male. Peritonitis in the male, due to rupture of seminal vesicular abscess, has always bacteriologically proved to be a mixed infection.

GONOCOCCAL CYSTITIS

Wertheim in 1895, Lindholm in 1896, demonstrated a pure gonococcal cystitis without mixed infection. By aseptic suprapubic aspiration Young obtained gonococci in the urine thrice, and a pure culture once. In this instance the urine was full of blood, and Young attributes his failure to obtain pure cultures in the other cases to the fact announced by Colombini that the gonococcus does not develop in non-albuminous urine. This is due not to the acidity of the urine, but to the fact that it contains no albumin. Young states that out of many hundreds of cases of urine in gonorrheal cystitis examined bacteriologically in only 3 (Wertheim, Lindholm, and Young) has a pure culture been obtainable, and in only 6 has the diagnosis been made by cover-slip staining,[2] a failure explained by Colombini's discovery. Young has one case, however, in which the urine did contain gonococci, although there was no cystitis, an absence which he ascribes to lack of co-operating cause for cystitis and variability of gonococcal virulence. He also obtained a pure culture from a severe chronic gonorrheal cystitis of five years' duration. The urine was foul and alkaline.

Treatment.—For the acute stage the treatment has been given (p. 139). When chronic it is that of other forms of chronic cystitis (p. 393) with a special leaning towards rather strong local irrigations with the nitrate of silver. But in *very* old cases there is always, I believe, contracture of the vesical neck, and in these I have never been able to effect a cure except by perineal cystotomy and thorough division of the vesical contracture. This has always been successful (p. 317).

---

[1] Their study commencing with Lang and Paltauf in 1893, through Jundell in 1897, and ending with Young in 1898.

[2] Melchior, 1; Barlow, 2; Bastianelli, 2; Young, 1.

GONOCOCCAL PYELITIS AND PYONEPHROSIS

Moderate and sometimes most intense pyelitis has been observed during the course of an acute gonorrhea. This pyelitis has always been considered, and doubtless justly, to be an acute ascending infection by way of the ureters, but the bacteriological demonstration of this fact has not yet been made. Nor, indeed, has a demonstration of the gonococcus often been made for pyelo-nephritis.[1] Many cases of pyelo-nephritis have been reported as gonorrheal. Young reviews them and casts doubt upon them. Sée also concludes that gonorrheal pyelo-nephritis has not been conclusively demonstrated. Young's own case, however, seems nearly to fill the required conditions. There was double pyelo-nephritis, and an aseptic aspiration of urine from the bladder gave a pure culture of the gonococcus.

Arpad Gerster,[2] of New York, reports an autopsy which showed staphylococci and gonococci in the kidney. Bransford Lewis,[3] of St. Louis, publishes a case of pyelo-nephritis; the patient had denied gonorrhea, and his lungs showed tubercular cavities; autopsy cultures from the pus of the cavities in the kidney showed pure colonies of gonococci decolourizing under the Gram solution.

ANO-RECTAL GONORRHEA

This malady undoubtedly exists, due to a continuation of the practice of the abomination of Sodom and to the trickling down of pus from the vagina upon the anus. Bumm [4] found the gonococcus in the rectum, and Neisser [5] in a discussion called attention to rectal gonorrhea as a cause of chronic ulceration in that region. Lang in the same discussion thought that rectal ulcer and stricture might be of gonorrheal origin. Neisser had already reported 2 cases, Frisch a case, Tuttle, of New York, 3, and so on. Neuberger and Borzecki [6] have 5 cases, and have collated a number of interesting facts and observations. Griffon is referred to by Sée as having demonstrated gonococci (intercellular) taken from the rectum of a man who acknowledged the etiological factor.

Symptoms.—The incubation period is not known, for the malady at best is very rare, but a smarting, burning, itching, swollen condition of the anus and rectum with more or less discharge, with or

[1] Univ. Med. Mag., 1899, xi, 504.
[2] N. Y. med. Monatsschr., 1897.
[3] J. of Cut. and Gen.-Urin. Dis., 1900, xviii, 395.
[4] Archiv f. Gyn., xxiii.
[5] Deuxième cong. de dermat. Vienna, 1892, p. 303.
[6] Ueber Analgonorrhea. Archiv f. Derm. u. Syph., 1894, S. 355.

without excoriation or ulceration and with a relaxed sphincter, suggests a suspicion which may be verified by discovery of the gonococcus in the pus.

There may or may not be swollen folds about the anus, and condylomata (pointed) may or may not abound; nor is the funnel shape of the anus and the disappearance of the ano-rectal folds, found in old pederasts, to be confidently expected in every case. The grade of inflammation has varied greatly in the reported cases from almost nothing up to an ulcerated condition with abundant purulent discharge, foul and putrid, flowing over excoriated fissures, amid fleshy tabs and rankly growing warts.

The subjective symptoms, of course, vary with the grade of local inflammation. Defecation may be normal or excruciatingly painful.

In the old chronic cases, when there is stricture and ulceration, the diagnosis may lie between gonorrhea and tubercle, a point that the laboratory will decide.

Treatment.—Cleanliness, hot sitz baths, laxatives to keep the rectum empty, suppositories of cocain and opium are indicated, and rest in bed is obligatory in bad cases. Injections should be given twice a day through a small soft tube, and should always be hot. Such injections should be soothing, bactericidal, not astringent. Boric acid, and very mild sulpho-carbolate-of-zinc solutions (1 : 2,000) are helpful. The permanganate of potash (1 : 5,000 or weaker) ought to be useful. I am not aware that it has been tried. Bichlorid is too irritating. Nitrate of silver, 1 : 20,000, and increased very materially towards the end of the trouble, is of undoubted value.

Light cases recover spontaneously with little or no care, and old chronic ones with ulceration, etc., which are rebellious, give rise to a suspicion of mixed infection, perhaps tubercular. No one has seen a sufficient number of these cases to formulate a satisfactory routine of treatment, which must be along general surgical lines, recognising the infective nature of the malady, with cleanliness, rest, drainage, and antisepsis as the objective points.

BUCCAL GONORRHEA

This alleged malady is as yet too obscure to require more than mention. The older cases of swelling of lips, gums, and tongue after bestial practices have no value, as gonococcal examinations were not made. The cases in which gonococci have been found, or diplococci, at least, are those of Cutler,[1] a woman confessing the cause,

[1] N. Y. Med. J., Nov. 10, 1888, p. 521.

but her mouth inflammation came on within less than twenty-four hours after exposure, and of Dohm,[1] several infants, one notably with purulent ophthalmia. The mucous membrane of the mouth became eroded on the eighth day after birth, and the false membrane showed gonococci from which cultures were made. The mother had putrid vaginal secretion and condylomata. Rossinski [2] records infants with coincident suppuration of the mouth and conjunctiva, and Leyden [3] has about the same testimony to adduce.

All this makes a pretty poor claim, but no harm comes of allowing it. These mouth lesions get well under a mild bichlorid lotion.

Still less definite is the gonorrhea of the nose, where, Heaven knows, it ought to be common if it occur at all, for the dirty fingers of dirty men approach the nostrils perhaps more often than any other mucous orifice. The nose may be dismissed in spite of specious claims, and finally, the testimony upon which umbilical gonorrhea rests is too trivial even for citation.

The same may be said of the alleged affections of the nervous centres, and of the undoubted involvement of the connective tissue, the skin, and the lymphatic system.

But two definite lines of gonococcal infection remain for serious consideration, the one mostly by direct contamination, the eye, the other by metastasis, gonorrheal rheumatism.

GONORRHEAL RHEUMATISM—SYSTEMIC GONORRHEA

Systemic gonorrheal infections, especially their more acute and malignant forms, have, within the past few years, claimed a greater share of the attention of the profession than their frequency warrants, a claim which is due to their activity and their severity.

Gonorrheal rheumatism has long been recognised. We have learned that it is caused by the presence in the circulation of the gonococci or of their toxins and the deposition of the germs or of their products in the affected joints. Gonorrheal rheumatism, then, is a form of systemic gonorrheal infection. This fact is attested by the febrile manifestations associated with the acute forms of the disease; but the more striking condition—which has been recently described by many authors—is a virulent septicemia or a pyemia arising from some focus of gonorrheal suppuration (usually from a prostatic abscess). This follows a course similar to that of a like condition produced by the ordinary pyogenic cocci, terminating usu-

[1] Revue des maladies de l'enfance, 1891, p. 282.
[2] *Ibid.* (citation from Zeitschr. f. Geburtsh. u. Gyn., 1891), S. 282.
[3] Centralbl. f. Gyn., 1894, S. 185.

ally in recovery if a septicemia, and in death if a pyemia. It is often associated with a malignant endocarditis.

Though rare, some 70 cases of the disease have been reported. The gonococci have several times been found in the blood and many times amid ulcerations upon the valves of the heart. Thayer and Lazear[1] and Prohaska[2] have reviewed this phase of the subject.

In spite of all these varieties of systemic gonorrheal infection, I must protest against the belief that gonorrhea is habitually a systemic, and not a local disease. In the innumerable majority of cases the local symptoms of gonorrhea constitute the whole malady, and these cases, in which the germ or its toxin escapes into the system, are altogether exceptional. It is entirely misleading to class gonorrhea with such diseases as diphtheria, in which, although a serious local lesion exists, the systemic condition is always paramount.

Systemic gonorrhea, or gonorrheal rheumatism, as it is usually called, affects a number of structures, fibrous and serous—the joints, the sheaths of tendons, the bursæ, the fasciæ, the eye, the nerves, the pleura, the valves and lining membrane of the heart, the veins, the periosteum, and the perichondrium. As to the cause: it would be idle now to cite the formidable array of names favouring toxins, gonococcus, nerve influence, mixed infection, etc. There is no end to it, but an ounce of positive proof is worth more than a ton of negative evidence, and it is now clear that the gonococcus has been found in and cultivated from all these tissues—and that puts an end to the question of theory.

The method of metastasis indeed may be said to have been detected by Wertheim, who announced it at the sixth general congress of gynecology in Vienna on June 6, 1895. Wertheim excised a small bit of mucous membrane from the posterior wall of the bladder of a young girl having gonorrheal cystitis, and found gonococci not only in the submucous tissue, but also in the venous capillaries, although the arterial capillaries showed none.

Gonorrheal rheumatism was first known when, at about the same time in the year 1781, Salle and Swediaur described an inflammatory articular affection dependent upon gonorrhea. Since then the identity of the causes of the two maladies, the gonococcus, has been amply demonstrated.[3]

---

[1] J. of Exper. Med., 1899, iv, 81. [2] Virchow's Archiv, 1901, clxiv, 492.

[3] Among the best names connected with the advance of knowledge along this line may be mentioned Hunter, Cooper, B. Brodie, Brandes, Bonnet, Diday, Rollet, Fournier, whose bibliography of older authors may be found in the Art médical, 1857, vol. vi; Observations et matériaux pour servir à l'histoire de l'arthropathie

But a personal idiosyncrasy also pervades the issue, since certain individuals, not ordinarily subject to rheumatic attacks, suffer from a peculiar form of rheumatism when they get a gonorrhea. They will remain well between the gonorrheal attacks, but have a new rheumatism whenever a new urethral inflammation is acquired. Brandes gives the history of such a case where a fresh attack of rheumatism attended six successive gonorrheas, and Fournier mentions a quadruple relapse. I have often seen double, once quadruple relapse. Königer [1] chronicles a patient, never rheumatic except during three successive gonorrheas at two and a half years' interval, once complicated with iritis, once with iridochoroiditis.

None of the ordinary causes of articular rheumatism seem to have any power to produce the gonorrheal variety. Gonorrheal rheumatism does not need for its production any co-operation of cold, of moisture, or of fatigue, nor, indeed, is its immediate cause any modification in the discharge, or any medicine taken, or any injection used. The only efficient cause is the gonococcus, and why the gonococcus is efficiently active in some individuals and not in others is unknown. Doubtless it always exists in the inflamed locality in the earlier stages of the rheumatic malady. Later other pyogenic microbes may coexist with it, and may even dominate and ultimately extinguish it, as in an old, suppurating, disorganized joint.

When this complaint has once complicated a gonorrhea, the chances are that every succeeding urethral inflammation will be attended by rheumatism in spite of all efforts to prevent it. Fortunately only a small minority of gonorrheal patients are liable to the rheumatic complication. An ordinary patient with gonorrhea, even though he have a pronounced rheumatic diathesis, may expose himself to cold, moisture, and fatigue without getting rheumatism; or, if he does get an attack, its course is not varied nor its symptoms modified by the coexistence of urethral discharge.

Women possess a strange immunity. They do have the malady, but only exceptionally. It is supposed that an explanation of this is the fact that the vagina and not the urethra is the usual seat of gonorrhea in the female, but this is the statement of a fact, not a reason.

---

blennorrhagique. Ch. Ravel and Fournier, Dict. de méd. et de chir. prat., and Sée, Le gonocoque, Paris, 1896, furnish valuable information for modern investigators. Among these are Finger, Gohn, Schlagenhaufer, Kammerer, Respighi and Burci, Horteloup and Bosquet, Bergmann and Bumm, Hartley, Deutschmann, Lindemann, Stern, Jacquet, Hoeck, Young, McCaskey (Ulcerative Endocarditis in which Gonococci were Found. N. Y. Med. Record, 1900, lviii, 1005), etc.

[1] Ueber die sogenannten metastatischen Complicationen der Gonorrhea. Inaug. Dissert., Berlin, 1873.

Gonorrheal rheumatism resembles rheumatic gout more than rheumatism. The local inflammatory character of the symptoms is often inconsiderable, and the constitutional sympathy is not of a severity proportionate to the trouble in the joints. But, on the other hand, desperate conditions of hydrarthrosis and of suppurative destruction of joints may also owe their origin solely to the gonococcus as a first cause.

The date of the appearance of the rheumatic complication is variable. It may be noticed as early as the fifth day after the beginning of the urethral discharge, but usually does not come on until later, the fifth to the sixteenth day (Fournier), more rarely during the second or the third month or at any later period. The gonococcal infection does not occur until the microbe has reached the deep urethra, and as long as the malady lingers there rheumatism is a possibility.

The discharge is not generally modified, although it sometimes diminishes a few days after the rheumatic symptoms have set in, which may be explained either by the fact that the rheumatism keeps the patient more at rest, or by the revulsive action that any intervening inflammatory affection may exert over a purulent discharge. When it comes on late in a gonorrhea its advent is often preceded by an exacerbation of the discharge for a few days.

The seat of the disease is variable. Joints take the first rank, the synovial sheaths of tendons and muscles next, then come the synovial bursæ and the nerves. The eye not infrequently suffers. The pericardium, pleura, meninges of the brain and cord suffer occasionally. Fournier tabulates 120 joint cases. In these the knee was involved most often—in over two-thirds of all the cases—the ankle in about one-fourth. Bornemann's statistics [1]—278 collated cases—record the knee as involved in seven-eighths of the cases; while Finger's more extensive collection, added to his own experience, gives the knee the preference in only about one-third of the observations—136 times in 375 cases.[2] These variations, while notable, always leave the knee the first place, so that the conclusion is justified that the large joints, particularly the knee, are by far the most often involved. The affection is not absolutely confined to a single joint, but shows a tendency to be mono-articular. Fournier's division into three prominent varieties is convenient and practical.

Varieties.—*The first form, hydrarthrosis*, is common, usually attacks the knee, sometimes the ankle or the elbow, and is habitually

[1] Studier over den Gonorrhoiske Rheumatismus. Copenhagen. Cited by Taylor, Venereal Diseases, p. 262.

[2] Archiv f. Derm. u. Syph., 1894, xxviii, 2, S. 296.

mono-articular. It comes on insidiously, but the effusion, which is often considerable, may also take place rapidly. Pain is moderate, increased by moving the joint, but the discomfort may be so moderate as to be ignored. The skin over the joint is not reddened, there may be no constitutional disturbance. The affection remains indolent, usually lasting for months.

The second form is more like ordinary rheumatism. Some local and general febrile reaction is the rule, more than one joint is usually implicated, and there is often trouble in the tendons, the eyes, etc. The symptoms are those of ordinary rheumatism, only less acute. The pain, at first severe, is commonly much modified by rest, far more so than is the case in ordinary rheumatism. Constitutional symptoms occur, but fever is slight, and subsides after a few days while the local disturbance continues. This relative lack of proportion between the constitutional and local symptoms is one of the diagnostic features. In moderate cases, when only one joint is involved, there may be no constitutional symptoms whatsoever. When several joints are implicated they are implicated consecutively. The malady, however, never becomes so general as inflammatory rheumatism sometimes does. It is more stationary, less mobile, and does not jump from one joint to another. When a new joint is involved those previously implicated continue to suffer, with, of course, occasional exceptions. Resolution is even more tardy than in ordinary rheumatism. A secondary hydrarthrosis, rare in simple rheumatism, is not uncommon in the gonorrheal variety. The sweating, so constant in simple rheumatism, is unusual and of short duration. The acid, concentrated urine seen in simple rheumatism does not occur, nor does the blood show the same excess of fibrin. Finally, inflammations of the pericardium, the pleura, etc., are rarely encountered,[1] and do not differ in symptoms or treatment from the same conditions due to other causes. The same is true of the occasional pyemic and spinal-cord gonorrheal affections, which are occasionally recorded.

Slow resolution is the usual termination of polyarticular gonorrheal rheumatism; but pains in the joints and very persistent stiffness may be left behind, more rarely chronic hydrarthrosis, chiefly

[1] Baudin, Recueil de mém. de méd. de chir. et de pharm. mil., septembre et octobre, 1875; Marty, Archiv. gén. de méd., 1876; Desnos, Gaz. hebd., 16 novembre, 1877; Morel, Thèse de Paris, 1878; Fleury, J. de méd. de Bordeaux, 9 septembre, 1883; Schedler, Zur Casuistik der Herz Affectionen nach Tripper, Inaug. Dissert., Berlin, 1880; Young, *loc. cit.*; McCaskey, *loc. cit.*, the bibliography of Sée and Lartogau, deal with recent literature; a study of a case of gonorrheal ulcerative endocarditis with cultivation of the gonococcus, Am. J. of the Med. Sci., Jan., 1901, p. 52.

of the smaller articulations (Brandes), ankylosis, or even suppuration and disintegration of the joint, more especially in lymphatic, tuberculous, and debilitated subjects. Acute secondary suppuration is rare.

The third form which the affection may assume is that of vague ambulatory—sometimes very persistent—pains in joints, which do not appear to have suffered any structural alteration, and of which the function is undisturbed—the knee, wrist, shoulder, foot, and jaw. This pain, which may be the only symptom, is rebellious to treatment, and, after it has gradually subsided, is likely to return if from any cause the amount of urethral discharge increases.

The synovial sheaths of the tendons of the extremities may be affected, either alone, or, more commonly, in connection with whatever joints are involved. There are tumefaction along the course of the tendon, redness of the integument, occasionally very intense if the tendon be superficial, severe pain on pressure, and partial or entire abolition of the movement of the muscle belonging to the involved tendon. This affection, like the others, undergoes gradual resolution. Hot local anodyne fomentations are indicated, blisters, or, best of all, the Paquelin cautery.

The bursæ also may suffer. In this case we have an acute or a subacute hygroma, which is peculiarly painful and sensitive to pressure for a long time. Two bursæ seem most vulnerable, the one lying between the tendo achillis and the os calcis, the other beneath the inferior tuberosity of the same bone. This explains the pain in the heel so often complained of by these patients. Other bursæ suffer, but more rarely.

The acute symptoms accompanying inflammation of the bursæ usually yield rapidly to local depletion and sedatives—later to a blister. Fournier mentions a case of gonorrheal hygroma of a bursa over the ischium. The attending symptoms were so severe as to lead to a diagnosis of deep suppuration. After preparations to incise the swelling had been made a sharp pain suddenly appeared in the knee, and the operation was postponed. In a few days the hygroma disappeared "with surprising rapidity," while the knee-joint became acutely inflamed.

Diagnosis.—Gonorrheal rheumatism may attack the muscles as well as the joints. The nerves do not always escape. Fournier observed sciatica 5 times among his 39 cases. Diplopia (Fournier), deafness (Swediaur, Fournier), and small superficial collections of serum near the affected joints (Fournier, Ricord, Féréol) have been mentioned as rare occasional complications, to which may be added perichondritis and periostitis. The following excellent table, arranged by Fournier, gives at a glance the characteristics distinguishing gonorrheal from ordinary rheumatism:

Gonorrheal Rheumatism	*Simple Rheumatism*
1. Cause: Gonorrhea. No influence of cold in the production of the rheumatism.	1. No etiological relation with the state of the urethra. Habitual causes: Cold, inheritance, rheumatic diathesis, etc.
2. Very rarely observed in women.	2. Common in the female, although less frequent than in the male.
3. Non-febrile, or much less so than simple rheumatism. Even in acute cases reaction never attains the habitual intensity of rheumatic fever.	3. Reactional phenomena much more intense and prolonged than in gonorrheal rheumatism.
4. Symptoms habitually limited to a small number of joints. The affection never becomes general to the same extent as does simple rheumatism.	4. Symptoms usually involve a number of the articulations; sometimes nearly all of them.
5. Less movable than simple rheumatism, going from one joint to another less quickly. No delitescence; no real jumping from one joint to another.	5. Symptoms: Movable, ambulatory fluxions; rapid delitescence, jumping from one joint to another.
6. Local pains generally moderate, always less than in simple rheumatism; sometimes remarkably indolent.	6. Pains always rather intense, sometimes excessive, disappearing less rapidly than those of gonorrheal rheumatism.
7. Frequently a tendency to hydrarthrosis following the acute fluxion.	7. Little or no tendency to consecutive hydrarthrosis.
8. No sweating.	8. Abundant sweats, constituting a symptom almost essential to the malady.
9. Urine not modified.	9. Urine specially modified.
10. Blood not furnishing a marked buffy coat.	10. Blood forming a firm, concave clot with buffy coat.
11. Cardiac complications very exceptional.	11. Cardiac complications frequent.
12. Frequent coincidence with a special ophthalmia, inflammation of the synovial sheaths of the tendons, inflammation of the bursæ, etc. The latter localities may be exclusively implicated.	12. Acute rheumatism does not affect the eye; the bursæ escape, as do usually the sheaths of the tendons.
13. Relapse in the course of successive gonorrheas very frequent.	13. Relapse frequent, but always independent of the state of the urethra.

Treatment.—Ordinary treatment for acute or for chronic rheumatic or gouty maladies does not benefit patients with gonorrheal rheumatism. Neither salicylic acid, iodid of potassium, colchicum nor quinin modifies the symptoms in a specific or a notable manner. Although in special cases any of these remedies may sometimes seem to do much good, they are not to be relied upon. Local measures are of the first importance. The treatment internally is tonic, dietetic, hygienic—in short, rational—with an alkali if the urine is overacid. The sooner the urethral discharge is controlled the more quickly will the rheumatic symptoms cease, although the latter may outlast the former many months. Rest is most important, the joint being splinted in the acute stage. Leeches, hot fomentations, or a blister will soon bring on the subacute stage, if indeed the inflammatory phenomena have not been subacute from the first. The diet should be low while the patient is confined to bed. Probably the best early treatment in acute and subacute cases is absolute rest with hot fomentations, the joint being first lightly rubbed with pure salicylate of methyl, then wrapped up in moist hot flannel and covered with gutta-percha tissue, while large doses of the oil of wintergreen are administered internally, and energetic local treatment is employed to cure the urethral discharge. Sometimes pure ichthyol spread over the joint seems to work fairly well in the earlier stages, but nothing can be surely counted upon as helpful unless the urethral discharge is controlled.

In the later stages, when hydrarthrosis is established and threatens to become chronic, the surgeon must face a serious responsibility, for the integrity of the joint is involved in the ultimate issue.

In my opinion, no treatment for this condition can be compared to the irrigation of the joint with hot bichlorid-of-mercury solution at a strength of 1: 5,000 to 1: 1,000. I used this many years ago upon the knee-joint, making two punctures with rather large trocars, one on each side of the joint (for the fluid is not always limpid, but may contain viscid and clotted fibrinous material), and first thoroughly washing the joint cavity with prolonged hot-salt irrigation, and then with two quarts of a bichlorid solution, and putting it up under moderate pressure, later using blisters or the Paquelin cautery, and finally elastic pressure.

That these cases are serious is shown by Halstead's statistics given in Young's[1] paper. Halstead opens the joint, irrigates with bichlorid, and then closes the joint with sutures. He reports 11 cases with the result—cured 3, improved 2, ankylosed 1, not improved 1, not stated 4.

In acute bursitis I know nothing so good as the Paquelin cautery or a blister generously applied.

In chronic cases, wherever situated, the choice in local treatment lies between tincture of iodin, ichthyol, Paquelin cautery, and repeated small blisters, followed by rubber bandage, massage, hot and cold douches, Russian and Turkish baths.

---

[1] *Loc. cit.*

Finally, in very chronic cases a mercurial course sometimes assists, and the iodid of potassium as well, although there be no suspicion of syphilis attaching to the history; and ultimately in very old cases, in broken-down subjects, nothing excels iron, strychnin, mineral acids, hypophosphites, and cod-liver oil judiciously alternated, unless it be a course of treatment at suitable hot springs.

A suppurating disorganized joint calls for the knife, drainage, or excision, as the case may be, along general surgical lines.

But be it remembered first, last, and always, that the urethral discharge must be controlled by local measures in order to obtain the best and quickest results, and the patient must not feel discouraged if his recovery is slow. It is the nature of the malady to be obstinate.

AFFECTIONS OF THE EYE DUE TO GONORRHEA

All gonorrheal affections of the eye are directly due to the gonococcus, the lighter varieties to metastatic infection, the virulent conjunctivitis only to direct contamination by gonorrheal pus.

The eye has been an excellent field for the study of the gonococcus, both clinically and laboratorially, and all investigators who have there sought the gonococcus intelligently have found it in the pus and in the tissues. It is a waste of time to cite the legion of authorities on this point. Sée [1] may be profitably consulted for all earlier bibliography up to his date. The clinical side has been amply established long ago by the inoculations made purposely in the effort to cure pannus.

The concomitance of arthritic infantile maladies with gonorrheal ophthalmia has been noted by Vignaudon (cited by Sée), who in a study of 20 cases of arthritis in children found that 10 had coincident vulvitis and 12 ophthalmia; and the very frequent concomitance of latent gonorrhea in the mother with ophthalmia neonatorum in the child has long since been established, notably since the researches by Kraus,[2] Zweifel,[3] and Kroner.[4]

But yet not every case of this last-named malady is of gonorrheal origin, as proved by the repeated instances in which the gonococcus is not found in the conjunctival pus of ophthalmia neonatorum. Yet even in the metastatic sero-vascular ophthalmia the gonococcus has been detected in the secretions, surely much attenuated in virulence or a specific conjunctivitis would have ensued.

[1] Le gonocoque, 1896.
[2] Centralb. f. prakt. Augenheilk., 1882, S. 134.
[3] Archiv f. Gyn., xxii, S. 318.
[4] *Ibid.*, xxv, S. 109.

This is established by the case of Morax,[1] in which the gonococcus was found in the secretions of both eyes, simultaneously involved in the course of a rheumatic attack. The conjunctiva had the peculiar injection of the rheumatic malady, not the vivid inflammation of virulent conjunctivitis. It is especially notable that a relapse occurred six weeks later, coinciding with renewed articular pains. In this second attack no gonococci could be detected in the ocular secretion.

There are two distinct forms of ocular trouble caused by gonorrhea. The first is rheumatic in character and nearly always, but not invariably, accompanied by other signs of gonorrheal rheumatism. It has no connection with local contagion, and affects the membrane of Descemet, the iris, or the conjunctiva.

The second form is conjunctivitis, depending always upon contagion. The distinction between these two affections should be kept constantly in view.

Rheumatic Gonorrheal Ophthalmia

To Abernethy, to Mackenzie, and particularly to Ricord, is due the credit of having first accurately described this affection. It is generally associated with the polyarticular variety of gonorrheal rheumatism. It may precede or follow the development of the disease elsewhere. Contagion will not produce it. Its essential cause is the urethral gonorrhea. According to Fournier it is 14 times more frequent than gonorrheal conjunctivitis. Knapp (personal communication) thinks this ratio inaccurate, believing that in their fright the virulent cases of conjunctivitis habitually seek relief from the oculist, and are not seen by the genito-urinary specialist. Cold, fatigue of the eye, etc., have no power to produce it. An individual idiosyncrasy seems to preside over its appearance. Should it occur with one urethral inflammation, the chances are that it will reappear with the next. It is far more common in the male than in the female. Sometimes it seems to exercise a revulsive action upon the joint trouble, and *vice versa*, the one disappearing to be replaced by the other, but this is exceptional. In brief, rheumatic gonorrheal ophthalmia is a localization of gonorrheal rheumatism upon the eye, the remainder of the body perhaps escaping.

Symptoms.—*Inflammation of the membrane of Descemet* (aquocapsulitis) is the most common form of attack. Here the conjunctiva is only moderately injected. The cornea is transparent. A cloudy, smoky appearance of the fluid of the anterior chamber is

---

[1] Thesis cited by Sée, p. 73.

the most characteristic objective symptom. Sight is slightly troubled, objects looking misty. There is no pain, but sometimes a sensation of uneasiness about the eye. Photophobia is absent or very mild. Sometimes there is a slight flocculent deposit on the posterior face of the cornea, with escape of a little blood into the aqueous humor (Cullerier). The iris is unaffected, perhaps a little slow in its movements. There is no deformity of the pupil, no change in colour of the iris, no other sign of iritis—points strongly insisted on by Cullerier.[1]

When the iris is attacked the symptoms do not differ from those of simple iritis: there are redness of the cornea, radiate pericorneal injection, contracted deformed pupil, sluggishness or abolition of the movements of the iris, change of colour, effusion of lymph into the pupil, plastic deposits in the anterior chamber, gelatinous or spongy iritis (Knapp), more abundant in gonorrheal than in ordinary iritis (Mackenzie), obscurity of vision, photophobia, lachrymation, and periorbital and ocular pains.

Fournier has described a rare *conjunctival form*. There is simple conjunctivitis, injection of the conjunctiva, uniform or marked at certain points, the secretion scanty and muco-purulent. Lachrymation is slight, the eyes are but little irritated. There is sometimes absolutely no pain, no photophobia, no alteration of vision, no symptom of iritis or of aquocapsulitis.

These varieties of ophthalmia, unlike the contagious conjunctivitis, are not often monocular; when so, the form is usually iritis. Both eyes are rarely attacked simultaneously. After one has recovered, inflammation may attack the other, run its course, and then return to the eye first involved. To get the disease the patient himself must have gonorrhea, whereas the conjunctivitis of contagion may be produced in any healthy individual by the mere contact of gonorrheal pus.

This malady runs a rapid course, declining with unusual speed. It may last several weeks or only a few days. Relapse is not infrequent. Of the three forms, conjunctivitis is the least harmful, aquocapsulitis is not grave, the iritis alone may leave trouble behind in the shape of adhesions, but even its (seemingly) fiercest form, spongy iritis, gets well, the exudate being absorbed from the centre towards the periphery, and leaving a sound eye (Knapp). This same spongy appearance occurs in the vitreous, but also clears up spontaneously (Knapp).

---

[1] Des affections blennorrhagiques. Leçons cliniques publiées par Eugène Royet, Paris, 1861, p. 165.

Treatment.—Treatment is mainly expectant. The eye must be kept at rest in all cases. The best local applications are emollient lotions of boric acid frequently used, with atropin, in case of iritis. Astringent collyria are useless, even harmful. Irritating pediluvia, the judicious use of revulsive cathartics, and a low diet constitute the general treatment. In iritis blood-letting by leeches is often of great value, as is sometimes moderate purgation. In mild cases patients do better if not confined to the house. They may even attend to business, if the eye be kept covered. When the symptoms run high housing is necessary. When in iritis the periorbital and frontal pains are severe recourse must be had to morphin, purgatives, atropin instillations, and to the salicylate of soda—from 2 to 4 grammes a day.

Virulent Gonorrheal Ophthalmia—Conjunctivitis

The sole and only cause of this terrible malady is contact of gonorrheal pus with the conjunctiva. It has no other relation to gonorrhea, and may affect the surgeon or the nurse as well as the patient, provided only a drop of contagious pus touch the conjunctiva. Hence the necessity of forewarning patients of the danger they run in neglecting the most scrupulous cleanliness of the hands after dressing the penis, using injections, or passing water. For the surgeon this precaution is equally necessary, together with the other one of burning all pieces of sponge, cotton, linen, lint, etc., that are brought into contact with gonorrheal pus whether derived from the urethra or from the eye. Neglect of this precaution may jeopardize some healthy eye.

Gonorrheal conjunctivitis fortunately is rare. Bumstead, who was an expert ophthalmologist as well as the best-known venereal specialist in New York in his day, found that out of 37,034 cases of disease of the eye treated at the New York Eye Infirmary, it occurred but 59 times, 1 in 628 cases. It is much more frequent in the male than in the female for obvious reasons. The right eye suffers oftener than the left, since most people are right-handed, and that more of both sexes do not become afflicted is due to the fact that dried pus loses its virulence. The gonococcus is not a very hardy parasite.

Symptoms.—The symptoms are those of purulent conjunctivitis intensified. The rapidity of their march is often appalling. The slight dry, sandy feeling attending the first congestion of the eye is of the shortest duration, as is the secretion of tears and of mucopus. Within a few hours after contagion the discharge is frankly purulent and the inflammatory symptoms go on, increasing rapidly in severity until, in three or four days, often sooner, destruction of sight is threatened. Sometimes the safety of the eye is compromised in a few hours (ten to twelve). The vessels of the conjunctiva rapidly fill with blood, and its tissues become distended with serum (chemosis). The border of the infiltrated conjunctiva overlaps and partly conceals the cornea, the latter lying, as it were, at the bottom of a cup filled with pus. The eyelids have an erysipelatous redness and are very edematous and swollen. The upper overrides the lower. Pus is retained in large quantities. Pain, ocular and periorbital, is often intense. The cornea soon falls into ulceration if the chemosis continue. There is, first, a purulent infiltration between its lamellæ, then softening and ulceration, superficial to begin with, and usually situated near the circumference, perhaps obscured from casual inspection by the overhanging chemosed conjunctiva. This ulceration rapidly progresses to perforation, the aqueous humor escapes, and hernia of the iris usually occurs. The cornea may be pressed out into an anterior staphyloma, or be destroyed by the ulcerative process, or fall out whole, like a watch-glass, permitting the contents of the eye to escape. The general symptoms are moderate. Fever is usually mild, except in rare cases of suppuration of the globe, and soon gives place to a nervous, depressed, irritable condition, attended by insomnia, agitation, restlessness, more rarely by stupor.

Diagnosis.—The following table, prepared by Fournier, but slightly modified, sets forth the distinguishing characteristics of the two ocular affections found in a patient with a urethral discharge. These distinctions cannot be too strongly insisted upon on account of the liability to confusion of two conditions, one of which is so harmless and so little benefited by remedies, the other so destructive and so urgently in need of intelligent and careful treatment. The specific gonococcus always abounds in the pus of gonorrheal conjunctivitis, is usually absent or very difficult to find in rheumatic gonorrheal ophthalmia:

Virulent Gonorrheal Conjunctivitis	*Rheumatic Gonorrheal Ophthalmia*
1. Essential cause: Inoculation of the conjunctiva with gonorrheal pus.	1. Contagion plays no part in the production of the malady, which is developed under the influence of an internal cause the nature of which is unknown. (Now known to be metastatic.—KEYES.)
2. A rare affection.	2. An infrequent complication of gonorrhea, but still much more common than the contagious ophthalmia (14 : 1). (Knapp thinks that the specific form is undercredited.)

3. May affect subjects not suffering from gonorrhea.	3. Only attacks patients already suffering from gonorrhea.
4. Usually only one eye involved.	4. Commonly both eyes.
5. The symptoms are those of the gravest kind of purulent ophthalmia. They affect the conjunctiva primarily.	5. The symptoms are those of an inflammation of the membrane of Descemet, of an iritis, or of an oculo-palpebral conjunctivitis.
6. Symptoms fixed, not going from one eye to the other.	6. Sometimes the inflammatory phenomena are mobile, passing from one eye to the other.
7. No tendency to relapse in subsequent gonorrheas.	7. Frequent relapse in the course of subsequent gonorrheas.
8. No coincidence with rheumatic manifestations.	8. Coincidence with gonorrheal rheumatism very habitual, almost constant.
9. Prognosis excessively grave, often loss of the eye.	9. Prognosis without gravity.
10. The eye is saved only by a most energetic and careful treatment.	10. Expectation, or the simplest treatment sufficient for a cure.

Prognosis.—In severe virulent gonorrheal conjunctivitis the prognosis, under the best of conditions, is most grave. Unless treatment be started early and carried out faithfully the eye is lost, or at least its efficiency is impaired. A clouded cornea, anterior staphyloma, or trachoma may be left behind.

The real danger in gonorrheal virulent conjunctivitis is due to the dense episcleral or subconjunctival ridge of tissue which by strangulation tends to produce ulceration and sloughing of the cornea. This it is that produces chemosis—an edema of the superficial subconjunctival tissues. Scarifying the chemosis or even cutting through the tense ridge of episcleral tissue does not mend matters much. The aim of treatment is to prevent or to moderate the formation of this ridge by keeping down inflammation.

The prognosis also varies with the intensity of the case, which intensity is apparently regulated by the grade of virulence of the infecting pus.

That the gonococcus varies greatly in virulence is not to be doubted. When attenuated in the urethra by vigorous bactericidal treatment ophthalmic infection is certainly modified. Dr. Chetwood had recently a case in point under my observation. A patient gave himself double gonorrheal conjunctivitis while under most active permanganate-of-potash-irrigation treatment for a recent virulent gonorrhea. Dr. Knapp treated his eyes, finding the gonococcus in the secretion of both, and cured him in a couple of weeks with little else than ice compresses and protargol. The symptoms never ran high.

The prognosis in ophthalmia neonatorum of gonococcal origin is very much better than in the adult malady, and the reason clearly is attenuation of the virus which exists in a mild form (latent gonorrhea) in the passages of the mother, for surely the tissues of the child lend themselves most freely to the suppurative process.

Treatment.—For the line of treatment here laid down I am indebted to my friend Dr. Knapp, whose authority on these matters few will contest, none will deny. He totally condemns the old-fashioned strong nitrate-of-silver treatment in the early stages of the malady, believing that this always does harm, and never aborts the disease, but by adding a new irritative element only kindles the flame and adds to the danger of producing the hard episcleral ring already alluded to. This new theory I accept most readily, as it accords with my own experience about the urethra. Formerly nitrate of silver was used in the urethra early in gonorrhea. I myself advocated and practised this abomination. I have now totally discarded it. The nitrate is a coagulating agent. It does not penetrate. It does irritate the surface traumatically, preparing the soil for invasion by the fresh seed from beneath—seed protected by the tissues from the germicidal effect of the nitrate.

The only instance in which it is perfectly proper to apply nitrate of silver early in this malady is immediately after known infection, before any redness is seen or any irritation felt, as, for instance, when a little pus from an infected eye is accidentally spattered and gets into the eye of the surgeon or the nurse. In such a contingency a 2% solution of the nitrate may be once freely instilled into the contaminated eye with fair hope of aborting the malady. Two per cent of the nitrate of silver does no harm to the normal eye, and if the gonococcus is still upon the surface and has not penetrated beneath the epithelium, it may be fairly hoped that one thorough application will destroy it. After three hours it is hopeless.

Cocain should never be used upon the eye in virulent conjunctivitis. Its own primary contractile action, its capacity to produce anemia locally, as a first action, cause a sucking in of all the tissue juices, and with this a deeper penetration of the gonococcus. It also weakens the nervous vital tone of the tissues and makes them more susceptible.[1] In making local examinations of and applications to the inflamed eye the utmost care and caution should be exercised lest the fingers or the retractors touch the cornea, thus detaching the

---

[1] Dr. R. H. Derby praises without reserve the constant free use of a 1% solution of holocain during the entire course of this malady, believing that while it possesses certain analgesic qualities it is free from the evils of cocain, and is at the same time antiseptic. Dr. R. O. Born thinks highly of $\frac{1}{2}$% to 1% eserin ointment, or 1% pilocarpin, to relieve tension in impending or actual corneal ulcer.

soaked epithelium, and causing surface corneal excoriation. The pavement epithelium protects the deeper tissues and an excoriation lets in the microbes, changing it at once into a corneal ulcer.

In making manual and instrumental exploration this fact must be kept constantly in mind. The greatest danger in virulent gonorrheal ophthalmia is corneal ulcer with prolapse of the iris and its consequences. If this prolapse should occur, its removal with scissors or any cutting instrument is to be deprecated. The plug of iris is a sort of bar to deep microbic invasion. With its removal the door to the interior is opened, and panophthalmitis is imminent. Therefore it should be let alone until the patient gets well.

For the same reason, if the anterior chamber becomes tense and distended by fluid it should by no means be tapped, as formerly advised, because the puncture is an easy road for microbic invasion, a thing of all others to be dreaded.

If an eye is destroyed by gonorrheal or other purulent inflammation the danger of sympathetic inflammation of the opposite eye is very slight, if it ever occurs (Knapp). It is not therefore proper to remove the stump for fear of this dreaded complication, a fact well to bear in mind, because a shrivelled stump of an eye furnishes a better base of support for an artificial eye than does enucleation or its substitutes.

In treating virulent gonorrheal conjunctivitis not a moment is to be lost. Delay may jeopardize the eye. The essentials of treatment are three:

1. Antiphlogosis: Cold.
2. Cleanliness: Irrigation.
3. Antiseptics: Bactericides.

The greatest possible care is necessary in handling the tender swollen eye. No pressure is allowable. Two skilled nurses are essential—one for day and one for night work.

All dressings should be the lightest possible, and tenderly placed by a delicate hand. The swollen upper lid is already weight enough. The utmost care should be used in protecting the sound eye from contagion. Buller's shield, a watch-glass set into perforated squares of rubber plaster, is not so good as Knapp's suggestion, a mica spectacle plate (to be obtained from any optician) fastened on with rubber plaster strips. This is transparent, very light, and does not steam.

The moist absorbent cotton used for wiping the pus from the inflamed borders of the lids should be at once destroyed. Mild purgatives and a light diet are of advantage at first. Perfect rest of body, and, if possible, of mind, should be secured. The sick-room should be obscurely lighted. If the patient is not robust no depleting measures are allowable, and the laxative, if any be given, must be light, while the diet must be supportive, even stimulating when the condition is low.

Under no circumstances is a mercurial course advisable or a continued depressing treatment harmless. Under all diet rules lies the general principle that the strength must be kept up, for there are on record cases of children who in the period of recovery acquired summer diarrhea, and at once suffered an aggravation of inflammation of the cornea which, by regulation of diet and arrest of diarrhea, immediately improved.

Local treatment is the same for all cases. Cold applications are of the utmost importance, but their application must be unremitting night and day, and for this reason two or even three trained nurses are necessary. Thin compresses should be kept laid out flat upon a cake of ice, and these should be placed upon the closed lid, being renewed about every five minutes night and day, and the applications continued as long as they feel grateful to the patient, yet not too long, and the cold must not be too intense, especially during the decreasing stage, as it may interfere with the nutrition of the cornea—an interference which manifests itself by a misty appearance commencing at the centre of the cornea. Should this be noticed, the cold applications must be stopped at once.

Cleanliness and drainage must be constantly assured by gently separating the lids and freely instilling with a dropper or an irrigator (not a syringe for fear of sputtering the pus into the eye of the attendant), either chlorin water, or 4% boric-acid solution, or weak permanganate-of-potash solution.[1] These applications are made freely to the entire conjunctival sac about every two hours—or even oftener if the pus be very abundant—and a solution of protargol (5% to 15%) is to be painted over the entire ocular and palpebral conjunctiva with a soft camel's-hair brush (everting the lids) three or four times a day.

These applications are continued as long as the irritative symptoms and the swelling of the conjunctiva continue to increase, probably one or two weeks. The pus meantime is getting thicker, and must be scrupulously removed from within the conjunctival sac by antiseptic irrigation and from without by the aid of moist absorbent cotton.

---

[1] Constant permanganate weak irrigation has been used, and much stronger applications of the same drug, at longer intervals, but the treatment has not found general favour or adoption in New York, strangely enough, since this remedy has earned for itself such a notable reputation in the urethra.

Cerate or vaselin should be smeared along the edges of the lids to facilitate the escape of the pus which the swollen lids tend to keep inside the conjunctival sac, though the constant irrigation meets this difficulty pretty well. Cantholysis—slitting the outer commissure to the bone—formerly much insisted upon, is much more rarely called for since the introduction of modern methods. It is very rarely, if ever, required.

This treatment is to be kept up unremittingly with irrigations every two or three hours until the symptoms begin to decline—one or two weeks—and then, as the swelling abates and the mucous membrane assumes a velvety appearance, the nitrate of silver in a 2% solution may be applied with a brush once a day, the other means being continued with diminishing intensity.

Chemosis is no longer treated by scarification. This does no real good, as it only removes the symptom (the edema) and not the cause (the episcleral indurated ridge). The best testimony as to its inefficiency is furnished by the fact that the numerous scarificators formerly in evidence have disappeared from the shops.

The indication furnished by chemosis is to persist in antiphlogosis—cold.

If the cornea becomes opaque, or even before this, atropin should be used, in order to prevent congestion and implication of the iris.

Preorbital pains are treated like those of rheumatic gonorrheal ophthalmia (p. 160).

Finally, in the last period, after the gonococci have disappeared and the stage of catarrhal conjunctivitis has arrived and all acute symptoms have subsided, then astringent collyria are in order, such as—

℞ Alum.. 0.5% to 1%
℞ Zinci sulph................................ 0.5% to 1%

used with a dropper 2 or even 3 times a day—more or less often and more or less strong, according to the effect.

CHAPTER X

SPASMODIC AND CONGENITAL STRICTURE

An abnormal narrowness of any portion of the canal of the urethra constitutes stricture, or, since the urethra is naturally a closed canal, Sir Charles Bell's definition may be more accurate and loss of dilatability may be termed stricture. This contraction of the canal, according to the first definition, to constitute stricture must be unnatural, for the urethra has certain points of normal contraction—namely, the meatus, the middle of the pendulous, and the beginning of the membranous urethra, and these are not strictures. They became so, however, if unduly small. Thus, an individual with an average-sized penis and urethra, whose meatus will only take No. 10 French, has stricture (congenital) of the meatus, although he may never suffer any inconvenience therefrom. Again, any inflammatory condition of the walls of the canal, or spasmodic contraction of the same, constitutes stricture in a certain sense, as does also any growth upon or beneath the mucous membrane—cancerous, tubercular, syphilitic, or membranous. In the same way a collection of fluid outside the canal may constitute stricture—abscess, serous or hydatid cyst, etc.—anything, in short, which lessens the size of the canal when distended by the stream of urine, foreign bodies, of course, excepted. In all the last-named conditions, however, stricture is only an epiphenomenon, and not the disease itself.

True stricture is of two kinds: 1. Muscular or spasmodic. 2. Permanent or organic—the latter congenital or acquired. Inflammatory stricture does not exist as a disease of the urethra. Any inflammation will lessen the calibre of the canal, just in proportion to the turgescence of the mucous membrane; but this is unimportant. No amount of simple inflammation of the urethral mucous membrane constricts the canal enough to occasion serious inconvenience (retention), unless occurring in connection with organic stricture, assisted by muscular spasm or complicated by congestion. A croupous membrane may exist within the urethra, and more or less obstruct the flow of urine; but this is exceedingly uncommon. Roki tansky speaks of "very rare cases" where "we find primary croup occurring on the urethral mucous membrane"—this chiefly in children. Membranous deposits may occur upon the surface of organic stricture, or behind it, and may there form the nucleus of stone. But obstruction of the urethra by stone, membrane, foreign body, abscess, or tumour, whether within or without the canal, is in no sense a constriction. It is therefore inaccurate as well as confusing to term such conditions stricture.

MUSCULAR OR SPASMODIC STRICTURE

Spasmodic stricture is a symptom, not a disease. It always depends upon some separate and distinct condition. It varies with the variations of this etiological factor and disappears with its cure. Of all reflexes, spasm of the urethra is the most reflex.

Spasmodic stricture is an involuntary contraction of the compressor urethræ muscle of sufficient force to impede or to prevent, temporarily or permanently, the passage of urine from the bladder. I have encountered no case of spasm of the pendulous urethra, though De Bovis[1] records 2 cases. The so-called spasm of an organic stricture is elastic or congestive, except when it occurs in the compressor muscle, at the membranous urethra (see below).

An active predisposing cause is a sensitive, high-strung nervous organization, often in connection with an irritable, a gouty, or a rheumatic constitution, and particularly in those who are sexually astray. Such a one is unable to urinate in the presence of his fellows, and the more anxious he is to pass his water, and the more water there is to pass, the more difficult does he find it to satisfy his desire. Certain mental suggestions contribute to increase or to diminish the spasm. The sound of running water often breaks the spell, while derision or absolute silence has the opposite effect. I have known a commercial traveller who, during twenty years of life spent mostly on the road, could not urinate in a railroad car except by means of a catheter. Yet such a man may well go through life with no great inconvenience from his urethral idiosyncrasy, his *urethrismus*, as Otis termed it. But let him acquire an organic stricture or a vesical calculus, let him be operated upon for hemorrhoids, or suffer any local or constitutional strain or shock, and his urination immediately becomes difficult or impossible to accomplish for a greater or less space of time. I have known an operation for hemorrhoids to occasion complete retention lasting ten days, long after the patient was up and

---

[1] Gaz. des hôp., 1897, lxx, 583.

about. Such a spasm, if unrelieved by catheterization, may even cause rupture of the bladder. Thus there is this much in the theory of Otis that an abnormally small meatus may cause urethrismus, that if the meatus is small enough to irritate the urethra by impeding urination, it may excite a spasmodic stricture, though I have never known it to do so.[1]

Symptoms and Diagnosis.—The one symptom of spasmodic stricture is inability to urinate. Hence it is sometimes confounded with organic stricture. Indeed, not a few cases of stricture deemed impassable when put upon the operating table have been found to admit a full-sized sound, being cases of spasm with little or no organic contracture. The following differentiating points are therefore memorable:

1. Spasmodic stricture occurs only in the membranous urethra.
2. Unless there is some organic lesion of the urinary tract the urine is bright and sparkling, which it very rarely is if there is organic stricture sufficiently marked to seriously arrest urination.
3. Although it may be impossible to introduce a filiform bougie or a small sound, a full-sized sound, if allowed to rest for a few moments against the face of the stricture, will usually tire the muscle, and finally slip into the bladder. If it slips in by its own weight its course will often be jerky and irregular, as the muscle gives way by succeeding spasms of lessening intensity.
4. When the instrument is once introduced the obstacle is wiped out, and the withdrawal of the instrument is not opposed by any such grasping as is felt when there is tight organic stricture.
5. Even though a spasmodic stricture be absolutely impassable, general anesthesia will entirely relax it and permit the passage of any instrument that the normal canal will take.
6. Organic and spasmodic stricture often coexist. Indeed, organic stricture is the most common cause of spasm, and spasm may be the notable symptom of an organic stricture of large calibre.

Treatment.—The retention may be relieved by a hot sitz bath, by an opiate, by ice in the rectum, or by catheterization, with a metal instrument, if necessary.

The tendency to spasm is overcome by removing the cause and improving the general hygiene, special attention being paid to sexual irregularities, concentrated urine, and organic stricture.

To prevent recurrence of the spasm I know nothing better than the passage of a full-sized steel sound to overstretch the muscle, and nitrate-of-silver instillations to blunt the sensibility of the deep urethra.

---

[1] J. of Cut. and Gen.-Urin. Dis., 1887, v, 2.

CONGENITAL STRICTURE

Congenital stricture or occlusion of the urethra may occur at 3 places in the urethra:

1. At the meatus.
2. At the outer limit of the fossa navicularis, and
3. At the membranous urethra.

Such strictures are caused by inaccurate apposition in the embryo of separately developed sections of the urethra. Stricture in the deep urethra is most unusual. Guibé [1] relates an interesting fatal case in which the stricture only admitted a needle. On the other hand, congenital stricture at the meatus, or at the outer end of the fossa navicularis (aptly termed the second meatus) is very common. Indeed, the size of the meatus is no more fixed than the size of the mouth or the nose, though, in general, a small penis is far more likely to have a contracted meatus than is a large one. Moreover, the second meatus is very rarely smaller than the first, hence congenital stricture need not be looked for here unless congenital stricture of the meatus externus is seen to exist.

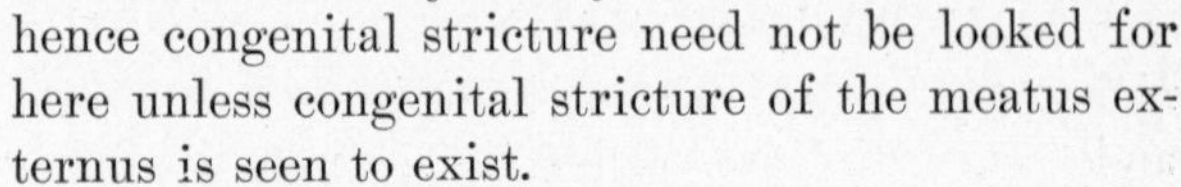

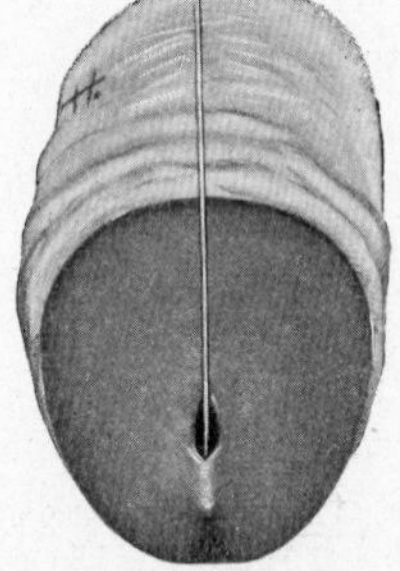

FIG. 35. — CONGENITAL STRICTURE OF THE MEATUS.
A probe is inserted into the pocket behind the stricture.

The solution of the question, how much contraction constitutes stricture of the meatus, depends upon one's point of view. Strictly speaking, a meatus is strictured if a probe, introduced into the fossa navicularis and rotated so as to sweep the point outward along the floor of the urethra, encounters a thin membrane which it must surmount in coming out through the meatus. This obstruction always occurs on the floor of the canal, and is never anything more than a fold of mucous membrane that may be pushed out by the probe (Fig. 35). The second meatus is strictured if it is not so large as the normal true meatus.

Strictly speaking, the above rule holds good. Practically, however, stricture of the meatus—to which so many reflex ills were once attributed—rarely produces any symptoms. If actually so small as to interfere with urination it may, perhaps, like a tight prepuce, cause hernia or even epilepsy in a child, and spasmodic stricture in later life (see above), and the urethra may become considerably dilated behind it. But such cases are exceptional. Most men can go through life in blissful ignorance of the size of their meati unless

[1] Bull. de la soc. anat. de Paris.

they fall foul of the genito-urinary surgeon, who, to permit the passage of his sounds, may justly claim the right to enlarge an orifice that had otherwise been sufficient for all Nature's claims.

Treatment.—The only way to cure a stricture of the meatus is to cut it. As above remarked, this is, as a rule, quite unnecessary, except for the surgeon's purposes.

The operation of *meatotomy* has occasioned the invention of various more or less ingenious *meatotomes,* of which the best is a blunt-pointed straight bistoury. This is the only instrument required, and the operation may be very elegantly performed as follows: A small cocain tablet is inserted within the meatus and pressed into the little pocket below it. This is allowed to remain in place for five minutes. If the urethra is very dry, instillation of a single drop of water upon the tablet will hasten its solution. Then the undissolved cocain, if any remain, is extracted and immediately replaced by a pinch of desiccated suprarenal extract. In a few moments the tip of the meatus is seen to blanch. The bistoury is then inserted and the membrane deliberately divided upon a finger placed beneath the frenum, which appreciates the fibrous ring about the meatus and at the second meatus, and by feeling the blade of the bistoury beneath the skin recognises when they have been effectually divided. The passage of a bulbous bougie proves that the obstructions have been sufficiently cut. If this technic is observed there will be no pain and little bleeding. The meatus is flushed clean and packed with cotton upon which glutol has been thickly dusted. This substance combines hemostatic and antiseptic properties. The glutol cotton is removed and replaced at each act of urination, and the wound is kept open by inserting the curve of a clean hairpin into the urethra once a day. The hemorrhage may be profuse if no hemostatic applications are made, but there are no other complications, and in the most extreme case pressure will check the flow of blood. Infection need not be feared, even if the patient is suffering from an acute attack of gonorrhea.

CHAPTER XI

ORGANIC STRICTURE OF THE URETHRA—ETIOLOGY, MORBID ANATOMY, SYMPTOMS, RESULTS, DIAGNOSIS

ALTHOUGH two conditions commonly known as stricture have been described in the preceding chapter, the one, spasmodic stricture, is a mere symptom, and the other, congenital stricture, a condition which, except in extreme cases, is absolutely innocuous. True stricture, the stricture that is never innocuous and always active in its work of undermining its possessor's health, except when kept at bay by the surgeon's efforts, has yet to be considered.

True organic stricture of the urethra is a cicatrix of the urethral wall left there by some injury or inflammation, and manifesting a constant tendency to contract, and thus to diminish the lumen of the urethra. This tendency to contraction, which is always manifested in a greater or less degree, is doubtless caused by the irritation incident to micturition, the impact of the stream against the barrier; for the deepest stricture, the one that most obstructs the flow of urine, is always the tightest, and if the stricture is kept dilated so as to afford little or no obstruction, the tendency to recontraction is very slight.

Varieties.—Strictures may be classified from several points of view: thus, for prognostic purposes, strictures are considered as anterior (at or in front of the peno-scrotal angle) and posterior (behind this point); therapeutically considered, strictures are of large calibre (admitting a 15 French bulbous bougie) or of small calibre; while from a pathological and etiological point of view strictures are classified as gonorrheal and traumatic. The old descriptive division into linear, annular, and tortuous or irregular stricture is clinically convenient to describe the nature of the obstruction to the exploring instrument, and the terms soft, fibrous, and inodular (or indurated) are descriptive of important features.

ETIOLOGY

All true strictures are either inflammatory or traumatic, and almost all inflammatory strictures are gonorrheal. An excessively severe or prolonged simple urethritis may cause stricture, and so may urethral chancres, ulcers, neoplasms, and loss of substance following periurethritis. But these causes appear so rarely as to be quite negligible.[1]

By far the greater number of strictures are gonorrheal. Thus out of 220 cases studied by Thompson, 164 (75%) owed their origin to gonorrhea; while Martin found among 219 cases 187 gonorrheal strictures (85%).

The *causes of gonorrheal stricture* are, however, many. The inflammation itself may cause the stricture, and doubtless this is usually the case; but it is difficult to estimate what proportion of strictures is due to breaking a chordee, to a false motion in coitus causing a tear in the inflamed mucous membrane, to the ill-advised use of caustic injections for the purpose of aborting the attack, or to the injudicious use of instruments in the urethra before the attack has subsided. Such strictures are properly traumatic, since trauma of the same kind, but greater in degree, may cause stricture when the mucous membrane is not inflamed and the gonorrhea thus only plays the *rôle* of a predisposing cause.

There is a small class of *intermediate cases* in which the stricture is neither absolutely inflammatory nor traumatic. To this class belong strictures caused by urethral chancres and ulcerations, or loss of substance from periurethritis, etc.

The *causes of traumatic stricture* vary widely. The *penile* portion of the urethra may be divided by knife or bullet, or torn by bending the erect penis, by a false motion in coitus, or by breaking a chordee. The *bulb* is the portion usually affected by trauma from within, by ulceration from stone, foreign body, or retained catheter, or by the sharp point of a blundering instrument. The *prostatic* urethra is said to become strictured when torn by disruption of the pelvis.

But of all traumatic strictures, recognisable as such, stricture of the *membranous urethra* or at the bulbo-membranous junction is the most frequent. The stricture is caused by a crushing force applied to the perineum, which brings the urethra sharply into contact with the subpubic ligament, crushing it beneath the sharp edge of this structure or tearing away from it in front.

The injuries which have caused traumatic stricture in the perineum, with or without a penetrating wound, are innumerable. Among the most classical may be mentioned falls from a height

---

[1] Ten cases of diffuse urethral syphiloma have been reported. Guyon's Annales, 1898, xvi, 892.

astraddle a beam, a chair, a stump, a manger, the limb of a tree, the corner of any blunt object, such as a trunk, a box, etc.; falls astraddle a fence while walking upon it, of a wheel while mounting an omnibus, of the tongue of a wagon; falls upon a sharp object, as a chisel, the breakage of a chamber-pot upon which the patient is sitting; falls with one leg through a hole in the ice, or down a coal-hole in the sidewalk; being thrown forward upon the pommel of a saddle, while riding; fracture of the pelvis, kicks in the perineum from man or beast, etc., *ad infinitum.* This perhaps unnecessarily minute detail of injuries capable of causing stricture is given because they are all occurring constantly. The authors have seen cases from each cause, and very many from some. They may be overlooked by the patient if they do not give rise to immediate hemorrhage or retention. The injury is then slight, not causing much immediate disturbance, and the patient forgets it; he never has a gonorrhea, perhaps, and yet in after years symptoms of stricture come on, and the canal is found highly contracted at its membranous portion; or, in trying to relieve retention in fever, the physician finds his catheter unexpectedly arrested.

Pathogenesis.—The most notable modern theories upon the formation of stricture are the theory of Finger and the Guyon school, Harrison's theory and the theory of Guiard.

The Finger-Guyon theory [1] makes stricture the result of chronic urethritis. According to these authors, chronic urethritis is essentially a sclerotic process, characterized by deposits of cicatricial tissue in the submucosa and even in the corpus spongiosum. This fact is illustrated by numerous pathological findings that would prove its truth were it not flatly contradicted by two notorious clinical facts. First, that stricture not infrequently occurs when there has been no chronic urethritis. Second, that chronic urethritis is habitually a posterior urethritis confined, that is, to a region where inflammatory stricture does not occur; while a chronic anterior urethritis is usually associated with a stricture, but as a result not as a cause, and chronic urethritis may exist for years without ever causing stricture.

Harrison's theory [2] is that the mucous membrane of the urethra, when inflamed by gonorrhea, becomes slightly permeable to the urine, which thus infiltrates the urethral wall at some place or other. To oppose this infiltration a circumscribed inflammation is set up which results in a local deposit of scar tissue, and ultimately in stricture.

[1] Finger. Internat. klin. Rundschau, Februar 12, 1893. Wassermann and Hallé. Guyon's Annales, 1891, ix, 143 *et passim.* Wassermann and Hallé, *ibid.*, 1894, xii, 244, 321.

[2] Mettsonian Lectures, 1888.

Guiard's theory[1] is that stricture depends upon the virulence of the urethral inflammation; the more severe the initial attack the more intense the chordee; the more frequent and violent the relapses, and the longer the gonococcus can be found in the discharge, the greater is the probability of stricture. He believes that in a mild or a chronic stage the urethral inflammation is simply catarrhal and neither deep-seated nor productive of any permanent lesion; while the acute inflammation, with its involvement of the lacunæ and glands, its circumscribed or diffused areas of periurethritis, is the inflammation calculated to leave behind permanent scars in and beneath the mucous membrane.

Of these three theories the latter two may be accepted. Indeed, a single stricture may owe its origin to a periurethritis, and then, after the first band of exudate has been thrown out, the impact of urine against the congested and ulcerated mucous membrane may be enough to permit a microscopic infiltration, followed by the reaction, which will pile up a new barrier of inflammatory tissue that will in turn cause renewed infiltration, and so on; or the infiltration may result from a trauma, the breaking of a chordee, or some such accident. But in cases of simple inflammatory stricture to assume that the primary accident is an infiltration seems hardly warranted. In short, the essential primary cause of simple inflammatory stricture would seem to be a periurethritis occurring during the acute stage of gonorrhea. The secondary cause, the factor that encourages the development of stricture and its constant contraction, is doubtless the impact of the stream of urine, whether this impact causes an excessive deposit of cicatricial tissue by setting up a minute infiltration or simply by a surface irritation. Long-continued chronic inflammation in the anterior urethra may, however, cause stricture. Thus in prostatic cases a slight linear stricture is often met with in the bulb. Its presence is denoted by the spasm it evokes in the cut-off muscle. This stricture is due, I believe, to a simple urethritis secondary to the prostatic catarrh.

In the etiology of traumatic stricture urinary infiltration must always play some part. It is true a severe contusion and laceration of the urethral wall are ample causes for stricture; but it is incredible that the muscular disturbance of urination and the distention of the wound with a fluid containing urinary salts and urethral bacteria should cause no increase in the inflammatory reaction. (See Infiltration of Urine.) Indeed, the admirable results obtained by simple perineal section and diversion of the stream of urine from

[1] Les uréthrites chroniques chez l'homme. Paris, 1898, p. 90 *et seq.*

the wound, confirm the belief that here again urinary infiltration is important as a secondary cause of stricture.

In this connection *the time of occurrence of stricture after gonorrhea and injury* is of interest. Of the 164 cases of stricture following gonorrhea, tabulated by Thompson, in 10 symptoms appeared immediately after or during the attack; 71 within one year; 41 between three and four years; 22 between seven and eight years; 20 between eight and twenty-five years. J. D. Hill,[1] from a discussion of 140 cases of stricture from all causes, makes the length of the period between the cause and the first symptoms of stricture noticed: after gonorrhea, shortest period two years, longest thirteen years; after urethral chancre, shortest period ten months, longest three years; after injury, shortest period four months, longest eighteen months. Guyon, among 142 cases of gonorrheal stricture, found only 4 cases within the first year, 10 during the second year, 79 distributed between the second and tenth years, and 49 after the tenth year. On the other hand, I have seen an impassable stricture in the perineum six weeks after a severe injury, and Guyon [2] has met a stricture which only admitted a 16 French sound two weeks after injury, and another which would not admit a 12 French after six weeks.

The deductions from the above statistics, confirmed by daily observation, are that the symptoms of stricture appear earlier after traumatism than after gonorrhea, the date of their appearance being measurably proportionate to the extent of the injury, and that the greatest divergence is noticeable after gonorrhea. It is totally exceptional, however, for symptoms of organic stricture to come on immediately after or during the attack of gonorrhea—as Thompson states occurred in 10 of his cases—unless stricture existed previous to the attack, unnoticed by the patient.

Morbid Anatomy

Number of Strictures.—While Thompson,[3] in examining 270 pathological specimens, found only 44 cases of multiple stricture, Guyon [4] lays down the clinical rule that gonorrheal strictures are multiple, while traumatic strictures are single. These statements, properly interpreted, conform perfectly with each other and with the facts. Concerning traumatic strictures there is no doubt; they are almost always single. But gonorrheal strictures, while fre-

---

[1] An Analysis of 140 Cases of Stricture of the Urethra. London, 1871.
[2] Leçons cliniques, 1894, vol. i, p. 239.
[3] Stricture of the Urethra. 2d Ed., 1858, p. 76. [4] *Op. cit.*, i, 139.

quently single from the pathologist's point of view, do present with equal frequency a number of ridges to the examining sound. Clinically, therefore, gonorrheal strictures are multiple, pathologically they are single.

Seat of Stricture.—Upon this subject the laborious investigations of Thompson, upon the 270 specimens above referred to, must be considered final, especially as daily experience with patients bears out the truth of his conclusions. He divides the urethra into three regions:

1. The bulbo-membranous, including 1 inch in front of and $\frac{3}{4}$ inch behind the junction of the spongy with the membranous urethra.
2. From the anterior limit of region 1, to within $2\frac{1}{2}$ inches of the meatus, embracing from $2\frac{1}{2}$ to 3 inches of the spongy urethra.
3. The first $2\frac{1}{2}$ inches of the canal from the meatus.

The 270 preparations showed 320 strictures.

Region 1 contained	215 strictures—	67 per cent.	
" 2 "	51 "	16 "	
" 3 "	54 "	17 "	

There were 185 cases of one stricture only, situated in region 1.
" " 17 " " " " " 2.
" " 24 " " " " " 3.

Otis places a majority of all strictures within the first $1\frac{1}{4}$ inches from the meatus—the next most common position being somewhere in the middle portion of the pendulous urethra. He believes deep urethral stricture to be far less common; but these views, which Dr. Otis has for years laboured earnestly to advance, are largely influenced by his theory that the urethra is a tube evenly calibrated throughout, and therefore what most other authors believe to be points of physiological narrowing (perhaps exaggerated in many individual instances) of the normal healthy urethra, he denominates stricture.

It is convenient to associate the region in which the stricture occurs with its cause. Thus, strictures at or near the meatus, if not congenital, are usually caused by chancrous or chancroidal ulceration, less frequently by caustic injections and by gonorrhea. Strictures of the pendulous urethra are commonly gonorrheal. Strictures in the bulb and at the bulbo-membranous urethra are also commonly gonorrheal. Strictures of the membranous urethra are never gonorrheal, always traumatic. Stricture in the prostatic urethra is very rare, to say the least. Thompson has not seen it, and French authors believe it only occurs as a complication of fracture of the pelvis. On the other hand, Walsh[1] describes a stricture in the museum of the Royal College of Surgeons, Dublin, as commencing in the posterior part of the membranous and extending into the prostatic urethra. Leroy d'Etiolle[2] says that he has in his collection one specimen showing prostatic stricture. Ricord[3] and Civiale[4] have encountered it, and Mastin[5] makes the same assertion.

Form of Stricture.—As has been said above, the descriptive distinction of strictures into linear, annular, and irregular or tortuous is merely a matter of clinical convenience, indicating that the amount of scar tissue in a stricture varies from a slight band or membrane to a broad and irregular mass, extending, perhaps, over the greater part of the anterior urethra. There are two points of much greater importance in this connection.

In the first place, the stricture is usually chiefly built up from the floor of the canal. This is most notable in the bulb, and commonly results in an eccentric position of the orifice of the stricture, close to the upper wall of the canal. The cause is not far to seek. It is in the loose floor of the canal, especially in the pocket of the bulb, that the gonococci commit their greatest ravages. It is the floor of the canal that is most often torn or crushed. It is the floor of the canal that is damaged by overdistention, when urination is obstructed (Bazy[6]).

In the second place, it is a matter of clinical experience that in broad, irregular strictures, strictures that are clinically multiple, the constrictions become progressively narrower as they approach the bladder. Beginning, perhaps, at the penoscrotal angle, there is a constriction which admits a 20 French sound. A short distance farther on this, too, is obstructed, and only a 15 French will pass, and finally the stricture in the bulb admits only a filiform instrument. In other words, the deeper extremity of the stricture, which receives the strongest impact of urine, is more irritated than the rest and contracts more rapidly.

Gross Pathological Changes (Figs. 36, 37, 38).—When the strictured urethra is slit longitudinally, the mucous membrane may be found only slightly thickened and congested. The surface may be quite normal in recent cases, though it has usually lost its polish, and may be cicatricial in character or covered with granulations. If

---

[1] Dublin Medical Press, January 26, 1856.

[2] Des rétrécissements de l'urèthre. Paris, 1845, p. 83.

[3] Notes to Hunter on the Venereal. 2d Ed. Philadelphia, 1859, p. 168.

[4] Maladies des organes génito-urinaires. 2de éd. Paris, 1850, i, 158.

[5] Boston Med. and Surg. J., 1879, p. 878.

[6] La semaine méd., 1891, xi.

the stricture is more advanced, a band or a mass of cicatrix may be found to replace the mucous membrane throughout its thickness, and it may even penetrate the corpus spongiosum, the meshes of which will be found obliterated. This tissue may be slight in extent, cicatricial in character, tightly contracted; or it may be exuberant, knobbed, and excessive in amount, so as to be readily felt from the outside of the canal, having a cartilaginous or even woody hardness. In this callous, fibrous mass there may be irregular areas of recent inflammation, soft congested patches, minute abscesses, and small cavities with ulcerated walls. Behind the stricture the canal is distended and more or less extensively ulcerated, and immediately in

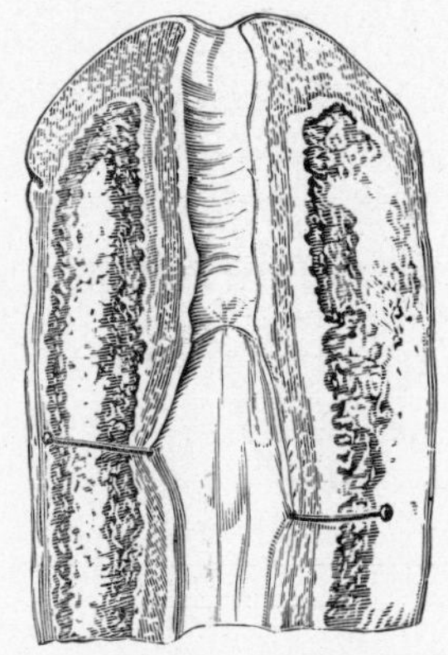

Fig. 36.—Voillemier.

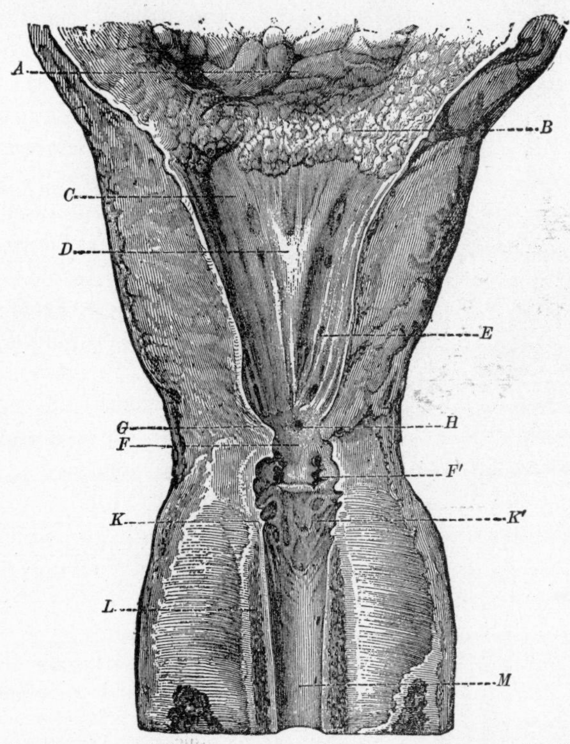

Fig. 37.—Traumatic Stricture of the Membranous Urethra (Voillemier).

A, bladder; *B*, bladder neck (ecchymotic); *C*, dilated prostatic urethra; *D*, verumontanum; *E*, one of the prostatic ducts; *F*, *G*, *K*, the stricture; *F′*, dilatations in front of the tightest part of the stricture; *H*, orifice of small abscess cavity; *K′*, mucous membrane in front of the stricture, thin and ulcerated; *L*, corpus spongiosum; *M*, anterior urethra.

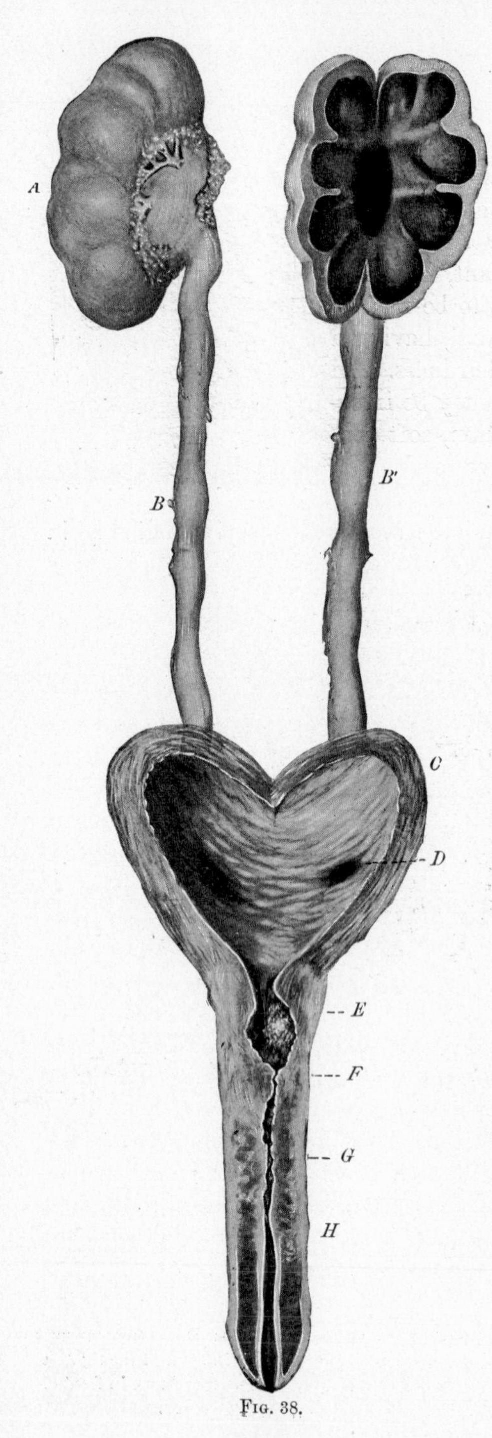

FIG. 38.

front of the stricture, or between two constricting bands, there are other lesser dilatations and ulcerations.

Microscopical Appearance.—The mucous membrane over the stricture is at first congested, and its epithelium thickened. When the congestion has become chronic the deeper layers of epithelium are increased in number and made up of cuboidal cells, while the more superficial layers are pavimentous or mere scales. In the dilated regions behind, and to a less degree in front of the stricture, the epithelium is thinned and flattened. Ulceration may destroy a part or the whole of the epithelium on and about the stricture, and if the ulceration heals the epithelium is in great part permanently replaced by scar tissue.

Beneath the epithelium appear the essential lesions of the stricture. Irregular areas of inflammatory tissue surround the canal and invade the corpus spongiosum.

FIG. 38.—RESULTS OF STRICTURE.

A, *A'*, Kidneys dilated, sclerosed, pyonephrotic; *B*, *B'*, ureters irregularly dilated; *C*, bladder contracted and thickened (concentric hypertrophy); *D*, dilated ureteral orifice; *E*, prostatic urethra dilated (prostatic abscess); *F–H*, the stricture; *F*, its tightest point; *G*, corpora cavernosa involved in the scar.

The glands are chronically inflamed, cystic, or obliterated, and they are seen to be the centres from which the inflammation spreads (Finger, Oberländer, Hallé, and Wassermann). When minute abscesses are present they, too, may often be found to originate in some inflamed gland, the duct of which has been obliterated. Areas of normal tissue are interspersed among the masses of pathological tissue.

Associated Lesions.—The chronic urethritis, cystitis, vesical hypertrophy, pyelitis, nephritis, etc., so often resulting from stricture will be considered under the title Results of Stricture, while abscess, fistula, extravasation, etc., will meet detailed treatment elsewhere. (See Index.)

Subjective Symptoms

Organic stricture may exist in a man for years, producing no symptoms and unsuspected. On the other hand, the usual symptoms of stricture, gleet, the irregular stream of urine, and the final dribble, are of daily occurrence among men who have not, and never had, stricture.

Gleet.—The initial symptom is the presence of shreds (*Tripperfäden*) and more or less free pus in the urine. If the stricture follows immediately after a gonorrhea the urethral discharge is perpetuated, but more often there is a lull while the shreds, and perhaps the general cloudiness of urine, persist, but, in the absence of a notable gleet, do not attract the patient's attention. These shreds and pus are evidence of the local inflammation on and about the stricture, which is adding fuel to the flame, and encouraging extension and contraction of the fibrous tissue.

As the stricture contracts the urethral catarrh grows worse and, sooner or later, produces a moderate chronic discharge, perhaps only visible in the morning when the urethra has not been scoured by the urinary stream for eight hours, perhaps persisting throughout the day. This is *gleet.* It is usually the first symptom noted by the patient. The gleet of stricture gets better or worse according to the general condition of the patient, the degree of acidity of the urine, and the amount of sexual indulgence or of venereal excitement. Exacerbations of gleet from slight causes, or repeated attacks of gonorrhea, as the patient usually considers them, often constitute the most marked feature of the case. In fact, it is the rule in mild cases for the patient to be wholly unconscious that his urethra is at all narrowed. He applies for treatment, on account of his gleet, for an attack of gonorrhea, as he calls it (bastard gonorrhea), and often refuses to believe that he has stricture, or that, if stricture does exist, it is of sufficient importance to occasion his symptoms; and he repeatedly asserts that he makes as large a stream of urine as ever. Nothing so well as the bulbous bougie will convince such a patient of his condition. The evidence of this instrument he must admit. The gleety discharge, once commenced behind the stricture, rarely ceases entirely until the constriction is relieved.

Changes in the Stream.—As the stricture tightens, fresh symptoms are added. A cartilaginous hardness may often be felt from the outside of the urethra at the constricted point. The meatus urinarius looks blue and congested, as does sometimes the whole glans penis, from obstructed circulation. The gleet continues, *the stream of urine is small and irregular*, often forked or curving up in a curious manner just after leaving the meatus, or there may be several streams running in different directions, or often one stream is projected for a certain distance, while another drops down perpendicularly from the end of the penis.[1] *The last few drops of urine are retained in the canal*, both mechanically by the obstruction of the stricture, and because the wave of blood, impelled by the contraction of the accelerator urinæ upon the bulb in the final effort at clearing the canal, cannot pass along the corpus spongiosum, on account of the obliteration of its meshes at the point of stricture, and thus fails in its function of expelling the last few drops of urine from the canal. By this same obliteration of spongy tissue, erection is sometimes rendered imperfect and painful.

Frequent Micturition.—In time the surface congestion of the stretched urethra behind the stricture extends backward to the bladder, and brings on irritability (so called) of that organ. The intervals between the acts of micturition grow shorter and shorter, and somewhat painful. Next to gleety discharge this frequency of micturition is the symptom of stricture which is least often absent. A slight narrowing of the canal may occasion it. It is undoubtedly attended by congestion about the neck of the bladder, but not necessarily by any true cystitis.

Retention.—The congestion of the urethra behind a stricture easily becomes greater, is kindled into acute inflammation by a heavy dinner, a little excess in drink, or a chilling of the legs; the mucous membrane swells up, the stricture closes, and the patient has retention of urine. If this retention is unrelieved, the bladder becomes overstretched; after many hours a few drops of urine will escape

---

[1] It is to be noted that while an impediment anywhere in a water-pipe (such as the urethra) modifies the *force* of the stream, the *shape* of the stream depends chiefly upon the shape of the nozzle (the meatus). Thus the shape of the stream, upon which so much stress is commonly laid, has no bearing on the diagnosis of stricture. It is modified by the meatus itself more often than by any other cause.

from the meatus (overflow), and the patient thinks he is getting better. If this condition of overdistention is allowed to continue unrelieved, the contractile power of the bladder may be permanently injured (atony).

Retention may be the only disagreeably prominent symptom connected with a case of stricture. The gleet may not have been noticed, the gradual decrease in the size of the stream may have been ignored, when, after exposure, excess, or a carouse of beer, retention suddenly comes on. Some patients will have had several attacks of retention before they apply for relief. The spasm and inflammation which cause the narrow canal to become obliterated in these cases cease after a few hours, and then the patient goes on perhaps for a year or more without another retention, not suffering noticeably in the meantime.

If retention does not come on, the inflammation, once aroused behind a stricture, gradually, sometimes rapidly, travels back to the prostatic urethra, and there is posterior urethritis. Now commences what before was absent, or present only to a mild degree, a *frequent desire to urinate*, at first every three or four hours, once at night, and gradually at shorter and shorter intervals, until, when the patient seeks relief, he may be passing water in a fine stream every half hour or fifteen minutes, with great pain and straining.

Hematuria.—Blood sometimes flows with the urine at the beginning or end of the act. Exceptionally *hematuria* may be the most prominent symptom of stricture, indeed the only one noticed by the patient for a long time. I have had several such cases, and have seen the hematuria cease upon relief of the stricture.

Pain.—Along with symptoms of vesical irritation, often before any actual inflammation of the bladder has occurred, are found pains various in character and situation: pain in the urethra, aching of the glans penis, in the testicle, along the cord, or running up into the back or hip; pains across the lumbar region, in the perineum, around the anus, in the rectum, over the pubis, etc., and other obscure pains of a neuralgic sort, in the thighs, the legs, or the sole of the foot [1] (Brodie), all of which pains are cured by dilating the stricture. Urination is often painful (sometimes excessively so), the pain being at the neck of the bladder, in the perineum, at the point of stricture, or near the glans penis.

Sexual Symptoms.—Erections may be painful, the venereal orgasm attended by pain, the semen not being discharged during the

[1] Or in the great toe. The pain is sometimes compared to intense heat, sometimes to icy cold, sometimes it is actual pain over a small area.

sexual act, but often dribbling away afterward, perhaps stained with blood, or running back into the bladder, to be discharged at the next flow of urine. Impotence sometimes accompanies this condition. The sexual appetite is often impaired, sometimes nearly obliterated, in old severe cases. But, in mild cases, the congestion kept up behind the stricture may be just enough to excite and irritate the patient, causing frequent erections, erotic fancies, and nocturnal emissions.

Results of Stricture

Hemorrhoids and Hernia.—The constant straining in urination keeps the hemorrhoidal vessels congested. This not infrequently results in an attack of piles or of rectal prolapse; occasionally, hernia occurs from the same cause. The straining may be so violent that the bowel protrudes at every effort to empty the bladder, making it unsafe for the patient to attempt to urinate except upon a close-stool, for fear of the passage of feces at the same time as the flow of urine.

Cystitis.—The inflammation of the bladder caused by stricture is usually superficial, but it may become parenchymatous, perhaps accompanied by abscess in the walls of the bladder, or in the connective tissue around it. In cases of stricture the bladder-walls, as a rule, thicken, while their dilatability diminishes. The muscle, constantly called upon to force the urine through a narrow orifice, becomes thickened and hypertrophied. Trabeculæ of muscular tissue project upon the mucous surface of the bladder, and between these trabeculæ the mucous membrane may protrude, forming pouches or sacculi. The bladder may contract to such an extent as to be almost totally obliterated, its muscular walls having undergone fibrous degeneration, which has rendered them non-distensible. In this condition (concentric hypertrophy) there may be a constant flow of urine from the urethra, which the patient cannot control (incontinence), to be carefully distinguished from atony, with overflow (in the one case the bladder is constantly empty, in the other constantly full).

Stone.—Instead of incontinence the patient may be obliged to empty his bladder every few minutes, after a few drams of urine have accumulated, which seem to be bursting the organ. The urinary salts sometimes deposit in vesical sacculi, or a small renal calculus lodges there, forming a nucleus for stone. The greater the urethral obstruction the more pressure is brought to bear upon the sacculi, and the larger they become, so that sometimes they equal or exceed the size of the cavity of the bladder. As the sacculus enlarges, its neck remains unchanged, and, if stone form in it, the stagnant urine (for there is no surrounding muscular tissue to empty it) constantly furnishes fresh supplies of urinary salts to increase the size of the stone, so that finally the latter may fill up the sacculus, constituting what is known as encysted calculus.

Atony.—Instead of contracting, the bladder may (rarely) dilate. In these cases there has not been so much irritability, and the bladder has not been called into such constant use; or overstretching may have been followed by atony, in which case overflow occurs, not to be mistaken for incontinence. Inflammation of the mucous membrane is also found in these cases of eccentric hypertrophy, together with the trabeculæ of hypertrophied muscular tissue and the sacculi.

Reflex Urinary Paralysis.—These conditions of vesical and urethral irritation, or others, such as stone, are sometimes, but very rarely, attended by partial paralysis of some groups of muscles of the lower extremities, or indeed by paraplegia. These various conditions, commonly known as reflex urinary paralysis, seem to depend upon the morbid condition of the urinary organs, and to be relievable, sometimes even curable, by treatment of the urinary difficulty.[1] Not very infrequently locomotor ataxia is mistaken for urinary reflex paralysis, especially if the urethra or the bladder happens to show any trifling lesion.

The Urine.—The urine in cases of stricture always contains shreds or free pus. As long as there is little or no posterior urethritis the second flow (p. 83) is clear. But as the inflammation extends backward the urine becomes clouded throughout. When cystitis supervenes the urine may become foul and ammoniacal.

Pyelo-nephritis.—Ultimately the back pressure makes itself felt upon the ureters and kidneys. The ureters sometimes enlarge to the size of the thumb. Their walls are thinned and contain areas of thickening from chronic inflammation. The pelves of the kidneys undergo the same distention, the kidney tissue being forced outward and compressed by the retained urine. Simultaneously, the inflammation extends up the ureter to produce *surgical kidney* (p. 361).

Indirect Results.—The less direct results of stricture, such as infiltration, extravasation, abscess, gangrene, fistula, prostatitis, vesiculitis, epididymitis, and cowperitis, are discussed elsewhere. (See Index.)

Constitutional Disturbance.—The constitutional disturbance in stricture is very variable. The stricture itself produces no general

[1] Brown-Séquard. Lectures on the Diagnosis and Treatment of the Principal Forms of Paralysis of the Lower Extremities. Philadelphia, 1861. Lecture on Reflexed Paraplegia. Lancet, 1863.

reaction whatever. It is the retention and inflammation that affect the patient's health, and the consequent *urinary toxemia and septicemia* have no special features to distinguish them from similar conditions due to other causes. The toxemic symptoms usually come on insidiously (unless there is complete retention), while septicemia usually affects the type of urethral fever and is evolved by instrumentation. In the more severe or acute varieties of cystitis and pyelitis septic intoxication is always found.

Recapitulation of Subjective Symptoms and Results of Stricture.—The *symptoms of stricture* are, briefly, narrowing of the canal, with dilatation of the urethra behind, blueness of the meatus, irregularities in the stream of urine, shreds and pus in the urine, pain, neuralgia of the urethra, retention of urine, overflow, dribbling, imperfect erection, irritability of the bladder, hematuria, and impotence—from urethral obstruction to escape of semen. The *remoter results of stricture* are the various inflammatory, functional, and structural changes in the bladder, ureters, kidneys, and rectum, also stone, infiltration, abscess, fistula, rupture of bladder, epididymitis, and sterility—from obliteration of the canal of the epididymis, and the various forms of urinary toxemia and septicemia.

A word must be said here concerning the effect of the sexual element in aggravating the symptoms of stricture. This concerns especially the painful, neuralgic, and functional disturbances. An unmarried man frequently tortures himself with fancied ailments, which he ascribes to stricture; or declares himself strictured when the canal is sound, imploring sympathy and demanding energetic treatment. Fancied stricture, next to fancied spermatorrhea, is the most common hypochondriacal expression of perverted sexuality, such as is found among those who heedlessly allow the brain to stimulate their erotic fancies and sexual needs, without being able to set Nature at rest by satisfying her demands, or who, on the other hand, abuse themselves sexually by physical as well as by intellectual excess.

These patients require kind and gentle management. They must be instructed about the cause of their troubles, and their sexual hygiene must be regulated. This can be accomplished by marriage, or by purity of thought and absolute continence.

Objective Symptoms and Diagnosis

Few diseases are more easy of diagnosis than organic stricture of the urethra. Few, perhaps, are more often wrongly diagnosed. The glaring fault is not overlooking an existing stricture, but attributing to stricture all the ills to which the urinary or the genital tract is heir. Some are born with stricture (at the meatus); let us respect the design of their Creator. Some acquire stricture; we can help them much. Alas! many have stricture thrust upon them; their road to neurasthenia is hewn with the urethrotome.

Before entering upon the positive points of diagnosis, let the surgeon disabuse himself of three prevalent errors. Let him recognise that—

1. Every case of gleet is *not* due to stricture, even if it is improved or cured by the use of the sound.

2. Every irregularity in the calibre of the anterior urethra, every contracture of the meatus is *not* stricture, nor a cause of stricture.

3. Every spasm of the urethra, every acute retention, every obstruction to introducing an instrument, however absolute, is *not* organic stricture, nor caused by organic stricture.

Given these negative data, three facts must be positively determined before the diagnosis of stricture can be made:

1. Shreds or free pus in the urine.
2. An obstruction, slight or marked, to urethral instrumentation.
3. Evidence that this obstruction is caused by organic stricture.

These facts are elicited by exploration of the urethra.

Exploration of the Urethra.[1]—In exploring a given urethra for stricture for the first time, I prefer to use a blunt steel sound which will just pass the meatus—that is, when the latter is not itself abnormally small (p. 170). The blunt sound causes less pain than either the bulbous bougie or the urethrometer. It should be cleansed, warmed, lubricated, and introduced with the utmost gentleness. If obstructed anywhere, there is stricture, for normally the meatus is the smallest part of the canal. When an obstruction is encountered, a smaller blunt sound is tried, and then another, until some sound will enter the bladder. It is always well in searching for stricture to commence with a large size and work down. To begin with a small instrument leads to confusion. I have more than once in hospital and in my office had a case referred to me as one in which a filiform instrument could not be made to enter the bladder, and have at once easily passed a full-sized blunt steel sound into the bladder. The explanation of this is that spasm of the deep urethra frequently fails to permit a fine instrument, especially a pointed one, to pass, while spasm in that region, in my experience, at least, always yields to gentle pressure slowly and accurately applied with a blunt steel sound. Moreover, a false passage, or a pouched sinus of the bulb,

---

[1] The instruments and maneuvres are described in detail in the next chapter.

or a dilated follicle, will frequently catch the point of a fine instrument, while a blunt sound will escape the obstacle, and, presenting fairly at the bulbo-membranous junction, will presently pass, perhaps smoothly, perhaps with a little jump, as it rides out of the sinus of the bulb into the membranous urethra.

The stricture, once detected, may be located, calibrated, and measured with the blunt steel sound, with the bulbous bougie, or with the urethrometer. Obstructions beyond 6½ inches may be set down as due to prostatic enlargement, particularly in patients more than fifty-five years old. If the bulbous bougie or the urethrometer be used alone, there is danger of assuming that the point of physiological narrowing, at about the middle of the pendulous urethra, is a stricture requiring treatment by cutting when there is no real occasion for the operation. If this point is covered by granulations, however, and bleeds as the bulb passes it, it is in a diseased condition, and may require sounding, although no true stricture exists—only a granular condition due to prolonged chronic inflammation. These are among the so-called strictures of large calibre so popular at the present day, so common in occurrence, so rich a field for the young surgeon, and sometimes the occasion of unnecessary cutting, as it appears to me, since the gleet they occasion may be permanently removed by a few passages of a large sound without recourse to the knife, and in most instances, when the gleet has been cured by the sound, although the physiological narrowing continues, the patient becomes and remains well without the necessity for further use of instruments in his urethra.

Just within the meatus—at ⅛ to ¼ inch—there is very often a point of congenital narrowing (meatus secundus) which may be cut if there is any occasion for using an instrument larger than it will admit—otherwise it may be disregarded. It is always wise to divide it if stricture exists beyond, because a free meatus greatly facilitates the use of large sounds (p. 170).

Differential Diagnosis.—So much for the method of examination. The presence of an obstruction having been determined, the differential diagnosis lies between organic stricture, spasm, and chronic inflammation. The position of the obstruction and the various points dwelt upon in the preceding paragraphs, and in the chapter on Spasm, are elements in the diagnosis. But the most distinguishing characteristic of all is resiliency. Organic stricture is always elastic and resilient, the others are not. To test this resiliency a sound—the largest that will pass—is gently introduced through the supposed stricture. It is allowed to rest in place for a moment, and then an attempt is made to withdraw it. *If there be* *organic stricture the withdrawal of the instrument will be opposed by a firm grasping* as long as the instrument remains engaged in the stricture. If there be no grasping there is no organic stricture.

To tabulate these features briefly—

	Organic Stricture.	Spasm.	Urethritis.
Shreds or pus..	Always present.	Not present unless there is an inflammation.	Always present.
Obstruction....	" "	Only in membranous urethra.	Sometimes.
Grasping......	" "	No.	No.

On the other hand, when the stricture is impassable and situated at the bulbo-membranous junction it may be impossible to distinguish it from spasm without the aid of general anesthesia. Yet in most cases the two may be differentiated by patient pressure with a blunt sound.

CHAPTER XII

STRICTURE OF THE URETHRA—INSTRUMENTS AND MANEUVRES EMPLOYED IN TREATMENT

Before passing to the treatment of stricture, it is better to describe at once the instruments used, the methods of manipulating them, and the operations in which they are employed, in order to avoid endless repetition.

Great mechanical ingenuity has been displayed in the construction of instruments for the detection and treatment of stricture. Such of them will be mentioned as are considered best suited for these objects. Space will not allow a description of more than the type instruments of each class.

The instruments which it is necessary for the surgeon to possess in order to meet the requirements of all cases of stricture are: different varieties of bougies, sounds or dilators, and catheters with a scale; instruments for internal and external urethrotomy, and an aspirator.

BOUGIES

Filiform Bougies.—Filiform or hair-like bougies are such as measure 1 mm. or less in diameter—size No. 3 (1 mm. diameter) being the smallest size that can be accurately measured on a scale-plate. There are three varieties of filiform bougies: the French, the English, and the whalebone. They are all made conical, narrowing down to a fine point, and gradually increasing for an inch or two until the full size of the shaft is reached. The whalebones are olive-tipped.

Woven French filiforms are used as guides to certain urethrotomes (Maisonneuve), being joined to them by metallic screw ends (Fig. 39). They are also employed at Necker as guides for sounds. The Maisonneuve urethrotome, or any other, can be guided into the bladder as well upon a whalebone guide as following a soft one. I have not found that sounds needed any guide. The English filiform instruments have no especial value; they are a little stiffer than the French, but not so good as the whalebone.

Whalebone filiform bougies are thin, hair-like strips of whalebone, very smooth and conical, with slightly bulbous points. By dipping them into hot water the ends may be variously shaped (an expedient employed in difficult catheterism since the last century)—twisted into spiral, bent into zigzag (Fig. 40), a modification which is of vast assistance in threading tortuous strictures and escaping false routes and lacunæ. The instrument may be rotated during its passage, and its point thus presented at different parts of the circumference of the canal, so as finally to engage in the orifice of the stricture. These bougies, about 2 feet long, are also used as guides for larger instruments, not by being screwed upon them, but by being threaded through a metallic loop made for the purpose upon the under side of the instrument which they are to guide—an adaptation of Desault's principle. Such instruments are called tunnelled (Fig. 46). Prof. William H. Van Buren[1] originated this device. These guides render splendid service as conductors, but three cautions are necessary:

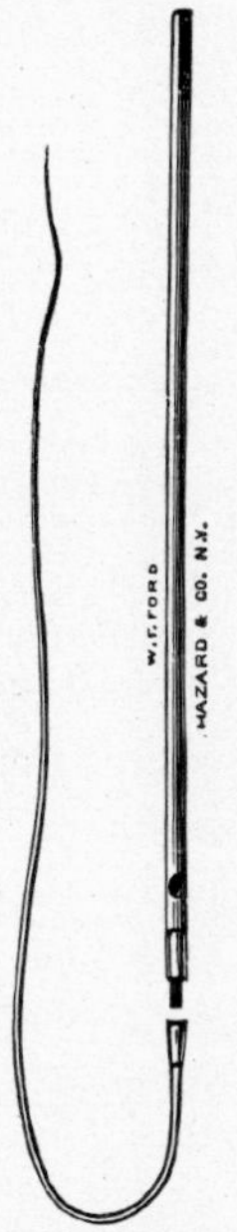

W.F.FORD HAZARD & CO. N.Y.

Fig. 39.

1. The guide should be 18 inches long. No cracked, bent, fissured, or frayed-out instrument should ever be used.

2. In employing a whalebone as a guide, it should first be introduced into the bladder, then threaded into the instrument to be guided, and the latter pushed gently down to the strictured point, while the whalebone is held stationary at the meatus. If force be used here, the slender guide may double up and a false passage may be made; but this may always be avoided by gently and continuously retracting the guide as the conducted instrument is passing the dangerous point, and until it reaches the bladder. The length of the guide permits this to be done.

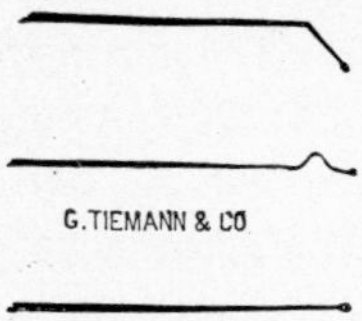

G.TIEMANN & CO

Fig. 40.

3. The loop of the instrument to be conducted should always be amply large, and be smoothed off in front so as to have a rounded and not a cutting edge; and, if the movement of extracting the guide, as the tunnelled instrument is being introduced, cannot be performed as above described, both instruments should be withdrawn; for, if the one be forced forward or the other pulled back, there is danger of cutting off a portion of the whalebone and leaving it in the canal—an accident which has occurred in very competent hands.

[1] Refer to note, p. 127, first edition of this treatise, Van Buren and Keyes.

Large whalebone bougies, having several inches of filiform tip and then suddenly growing larger in the shaft, have been devised by E. A. Banks, of New York. They are equivalent to a filiform bougie and a tunnelled sound (Fig. 41).

Manipulation.—Regarding the method of introducing filiform bougies, a few words will suffice. Their fine points are likely to catch, chiefly in the lacuna magna, but also in any of the numerous sinuses of Morgagni, in any false passage, or against membranous

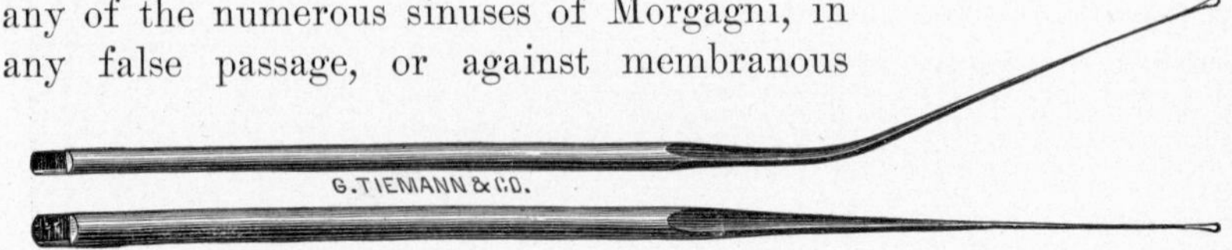

Fig. 41.

bands and folds of the urethra, in the tortuous turnings of a stricture, or in the softened, reticulated membrane behind it. With the whalebone bougie—perhaps with any filiform instrument—these obstacles may generally be surmounted. There are two special maneuvres for accomplishing this:

1. When an instrument catches, partially withdraw and slightly rotate it, pushing it forward while making the rotatory movement. This device rarely fails in finally engaging the instrument in the orifice of the stricture, especially if the filiform point be bent or twisted in any direction (spiral or zigzag), so that its extremity may lie outside of the axis of the shaft of the instrument.

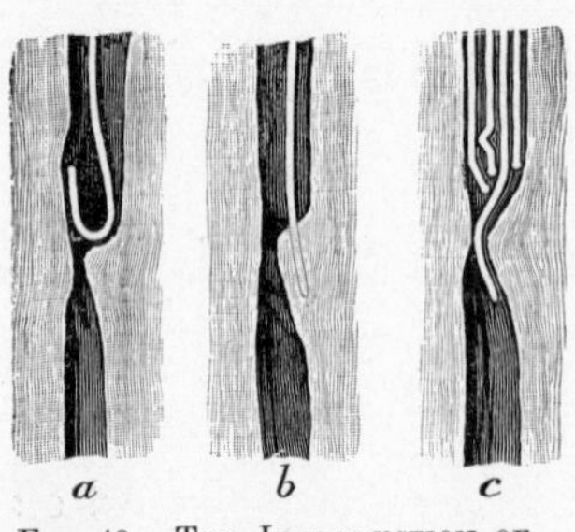

Fig. 42.—The Introduction of Whalebone Guides (Bryant).

a, guide bent upward; *b*, guide in lacuna; *c*, numerous guides in urethra, one passing stricture.

2. An excellent method of finding the orifice of a stricture, especially where false passage exists, consists in cramming the urethra full of filiform bougies, engaging their points in all the lacunæ and false passages, and then trying them, one after another, until that one is pushed forward which is presenting at the orifice of the stricture, when it will at once engage (Fig. 42).

The use of filiform bougies in threading tight strictures is greatly facilitated by first injecting the urethra with warm oil. Filiform bougies, intelligently used, make impassable strictures the greatest rarities in a surgeon's practice.

Woven Bougies.—Of other bougies (not filiform) only the French and English conical need be described—the blunt are not useful. Bougies are woven instruments covered with gum or varnish. They come of all sizes, and are necessary in the treatment of stricture up to size 15 or 20 (French). The olive-tip is of advantage in

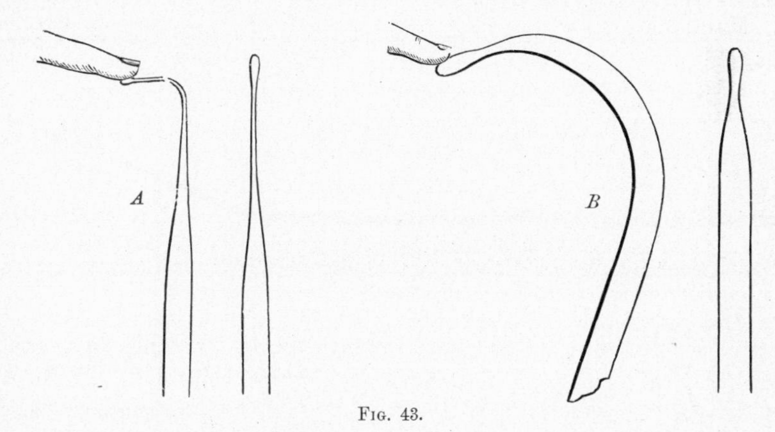

FIG. 43.

the large sizes, objectionable in the small. When choosing olive-tipped bougies, preference should be given to such instruments as are rather stiff, but have a long, slender, flexible neck supporting the bulb. When held vertically, bulb uppermost, and touched upon the olivary tip, the neck should yield at once (Fig. 43, *A*). Such an instrument will guide itself safely and override obstructions. The English olivary bougies lack this quality (Fig. 43, *B*).

Of late years the French have far surpassed the English in the manufacture of woven instruments, and I know of no American instruments that equal the French in durability, flexibility, and polish. The best French bougies may be boiled without injury.

Bulbous Bougies.—The bulbous bougies (*bougies-à-boule*) are useful instruments for the accurate diagnosis of stricture. They are either woven or metallic. They consist of a flexible, woven shaft headed by an acorn extremity of a diameter much greater than that of the shaft, and are sized according to the diameter of the head. A set of them, running from 5 to 30, is required. Anything too tight for 5 (5 mm. in circumference) may be said, practically, only to admit a filiform instrument (size 3). A bulbous bougie should have a short conical head and an abrupt shoulder (Fig. 44). Instrument makers have them of all varieties, with very pointed, even oval heads and no shoulders—occasionally with two or three bulbs. These are not useful. The metallic silver bougies are more durable and more easily sterilized than the woven, but, being stiff, they are more irritating and less accurate.

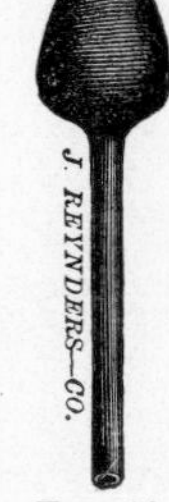

FIG. 44.

The Urethrometer.—The urethrometer (Otis's) is a very ingenious little instrument, which is designed to take the place of a whole set of bulbous bougies, from size 20 to 40 (Fig. 45). By turning the handle the bulb is expanded to a size indicated upon the register at the handle. A rubber cap prevents its bars from scratching the mucous membrane. It is especially useful in calibrating the pendulous urethra. It is to be introduced beyond the deepest point of stricture, screwed up, and then drawn forward. The shaft is marked in inches and half inches, and, as it is drawn out, the location and size of the various narrow points of the urethra may be read off and located at once. The objection to the instrument is that it is more irritating than ordinary bulbous bougies, while the findings of these simpler instruments will satisfy the most fastidious. Other urethrographs and urethrometers are objectionable for the same reason—viz., that they encourage a fanciful accuracy at the patient's expense.

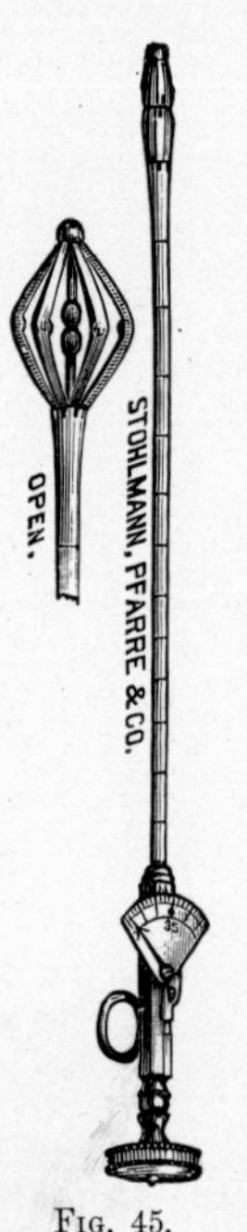

Fig. 45.

CATHETERS

Silver Catheters.—Silver catheters do not wear out, and it is well to have a case of them on hand, of short curve, from size 9 to 22 French. They should be made blunt, not conical. No one not accustomed to manage difficult cases can safely use a silver catheter of a less size than No. 9 without a guide. Fine silver catheters may be used with safety and advantage only when guided—that is, with a soft filiform guide screwed upon the tip, as in the instrument of Bumstead, or tunnelled for a whalebone guide, after the manner of ordinary tunnelled instruments (Fig. 46).

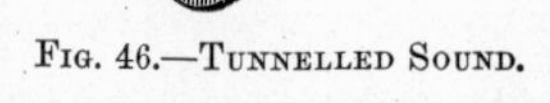
Fig. 46.—Tunnelled Sound.

Soft Catheters.—Three varieties of French flexible catheters may be mentioned: the flexible olivary, particular attention being given, in choosing the instrument, to the flexibility of the neck (Fig. 43, *A*); the flexible catheter, open at both ends; and a flexible instrument armed with a metallic tip, to be screwed upon a filiform guide. Only the first variety is in general use. In ordinary cases all soft catheters should be introduced without a stylet.

Soft-rubber (Nélaton) and elbowed woven catheters belong rather to the prostatic armamentarium, where they are described, together with the woven and metal catheters employed in cases of hypertrophied prostate.

SOUNDS

The most essential instrument for the treatment of stricture is the steel sound. It is the best instrument with which to obtain a cure, the only instrument to maintain one.

The sound should be made of the best steel and nickel-plated. Its proper curve has been described (p. 6). Straight sounds are used in the anterior urethra. Steel sounds are blunt and conical.

Blunt.—Blunt sounds, used in diagnosing a stricture, have a spherical extremity and the same calibre throughout. A complete set of them runs from 10 to 30 French. Alternate sizes suffice, for strict accuracy is unessential.

Conical.—Conical sounds increase from 7 to 14 sizes in the first 2 or 3 inches of their length. For a number of years I have employed a *double taper sound* (Fig. 47). This instrument spares the meatus while it is distending the deeper parts of the canal. A set of conical instruments runs from 13 to 35 French. Yet below 20 French I prefer the woven bougie, and it is scarcely ever necessary to use an instrument larger than 31, except for overstretching immediately after urethrotomy. The double taper is unnecessary below 24 French.

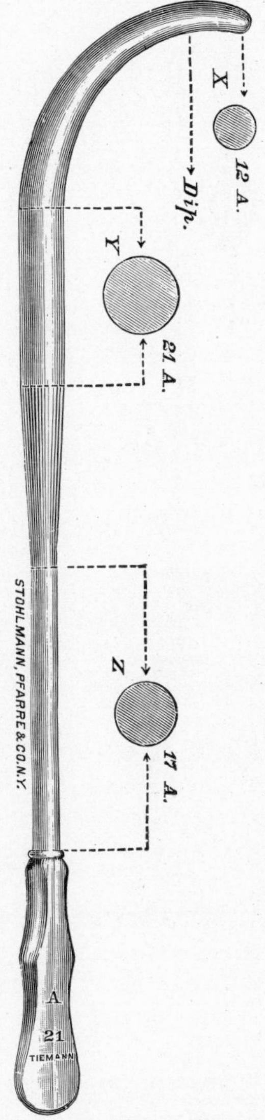

FIG. 47.—DOUBLE TAPER SOUND.

In employing conical instruments of steel it should be remembered that the surgeon has the advantage of using a wedge as well as a lever, and, by carefully inserting any given conical steel instrument through a stricture, he practically does (with less violence) the same thing as if he passed a number of blunt instruments, since the conicity of the sound runs through many sizes.

Advantages of Steel Instruments for dilating Stricture.—Since Thompson, one of the most brilliant minds connected with the subject of genito-urinary surgery, decided at one time in favour of the use of soft instruments for dilating stricture, a word will be necessary to state the reasons why the authors of this treatise hold a contrary opinion. In regard to facility of manipulation, that depends upon practice, and he will use this, that, or the other instrument the best who has used it the most. Less harm can be done with flexible than with solid instruments, undoubtedly, and on this account they are to be recommended for the unskilled, and for all, however expert, in the low sizes—below No. 15 French. In trained hands, however, the steel sound is perfectly safe; it is smoother than any soft instrument, and certainly can be passed into the urethra with less pain than any other instrument, and is capable of effecting more dilatation, in the same length of time, with the employment of less force. Steel instruments, made with the curve and conicity already described, possess all the powers of the wedge, and of a lever of the first order. The surgeon holds the long arm, the fulcrum is a sliding one, situated at the junction of the shaft with the curve, perhaps steadied by the surgeon's finger. The immense power which the application of this compound mechanical principle, in the construction of the instrument, gives to it, is not appreciated by surgeons.

The ease with which harm may be done, in using force with conical sounds, is rarely realized until after an accident has occurred, and then the surgeon often ascribes the mischief to chance rather than to his own carelessness. Swelled testicle, congestion of the neck of the bladder, irritation of the stricture, even false passage, may be produced by a surgeon in too great a hurry, or using force. It is a rule, from which no departure should be made, either on account of solicitation by the patient, or of desire to push the case to a rapid termination, *never to use force with any instrument in the urethra—especially with conical steel sounds.* The character of the stricture may, occasionally, in the judgment of the operator, sometimes require force, but the motive for its use must never be haste, or desire to effect a rapid cure. The weight of the instrument, aided by a little coaxing, will usually exert all the power necessary. "*Festina lente*" is the golden rule. Patience and gentleness will effect more in the long run than force.

The method of preparing and introducing a sound has already been described (p. 26).

DILATORS

From time to time various instruments termed dilators have been devised for the purpose of replacing a set of sounds by a single instrument. Thompson's dilator (Fig. 48) and Kollmann's dilators are the best known. The former is a dangerous instrument, and should never be employed except to remove foreign bodies from the urethra (p. 40). Kollmann's instruments (Figs. 49, 50) have, however, the advantage of an irrigation attachment, by means of which the urethra may be thoroughly washed out while distended. Great virtues are attributed to the instrument on this account. Moreover, with it the urethra may be stretched to any size, regardless of the calibre of the meatus. This is a distinct advantage in that it may spare the patient a meatotomy. But, on the other hand, the dilator is not and cannot be a smooth instrument, and it is even more likely to be used roughly than the steel sound. These two facts overbalance its virtues and lead me to reject it.

The operation of *divulsion*, as practised with these instruments, is never warranted.

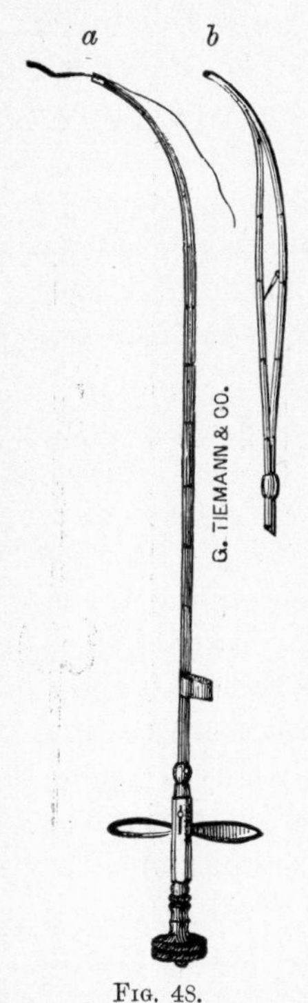

Fig. 48.

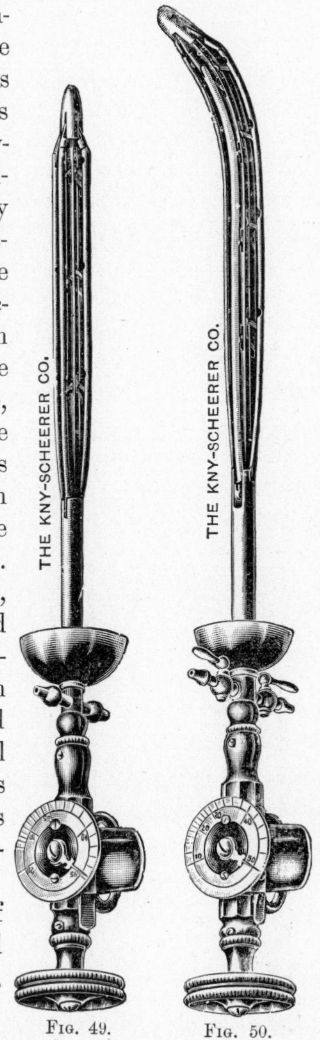

Fig. 49. Fig. 50.

URETHROTOMES

Only four cutting instruments, suitable for dividing strictures in different portions of the urethra, need be described.

Bistoury.—The straight, blunt-pointed bistoury is the best instrument for dividing strictures at and quite near the external meatus. These should always be cut upon the floor of the urethra to an extent sufficient to cut through *all* the morbid fibrous thickening which constitutes the stricture. (See Meatotomy.)

Civiale's Urethrotome.—This instrument (Fig. 51), of which there are many modifications, is used almost exclusively by Thompson and others for cutting permeable strictures of the anterior urethra.

It has a small, straight shaft terminated by a flattened bulb which conceals a rounded blade. By means of a mechanism in the handle this blade may be protruded to an extent indicated upon a register in the handle. The bulb is to be passed through a given stricture, withdrawn until it encounters the stricture, when the blade is to be protruded, and the stricture is cut by withdrawing the instrument. It is a very safe urethrotome. It is most serviceable for cutting a single linear, well-defined stricture of the pendulous urethra.

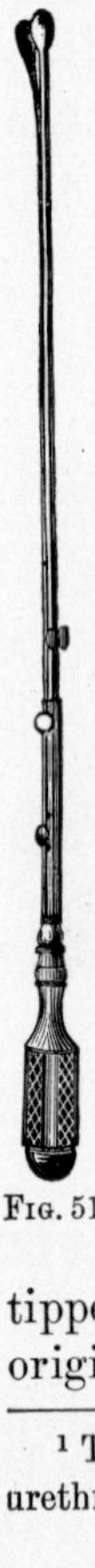

Fig. 51.

Maisonneuve's Urethrotome.—This instrument (Fig. 52), or one of its modifications, is used by those who perform internal urethrotomy on strictures of the bulbo-membranous urethra.[1] It is, moreover, the only urethrotome that will cut a stricture which only admits a filiform bougie. It consists of a hollow wire with a linear opening on the side corresponding to the roof of the urethra. The knife (of different sizes), cutting from before backward, and from behind forward, with its exposed obtuse angle always blunted, is attached to the end of a long stylet which fits into the groove of the instrument. The blade is prevented from slipping out by a projecting shoulder on each side which runs inside the hollow wire. It is used with a screw-tipped filiform bougie. Bumstead has advantageously modified the original instrument by making the knife run only to the beginning

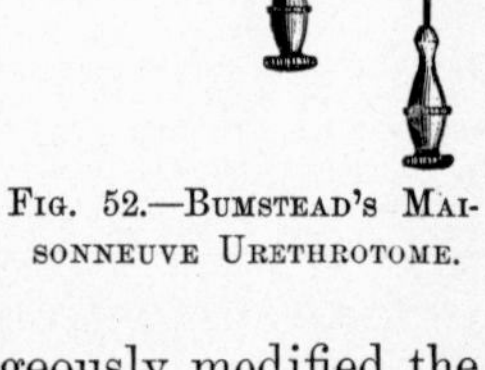

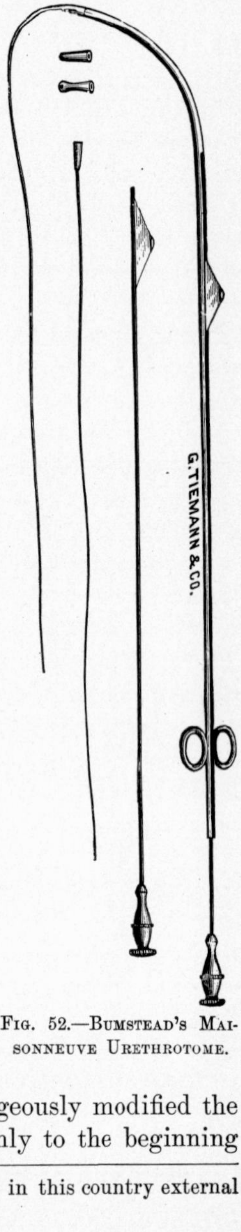

Fig. 52.—Bumstead's Maisonneuve Urethrotome.

[1] This is the practice of most continental surgeons, but in this country external urethrotomy is preferred for these cases.

of the curve, instead of up to the point, and by making the tube a little more solid. Bumstead's instrument has the blade on the lower side, and therefore is not appropriate for strictures of the pendulous urethra, since these should always be cut on the roof. Other varieties of the Maisonneuve instrument do this.

The instrument is introduced, following its guide, and depressed until the straight portion of the tube has passed the stricture. Then the blade is entered, pushed rapidly down as far as it will go, and immediately retracted. The objection to the instrument is that it incises the urethra blindly and throughout its length if a large blade is used, while it may fail to divide the whole thickness of the stricture if a smaller blade is selected. Another objection—that the soft woven filiform is liable to curl up in front of the stricture instead of engaging—is overcome by the use of a stiff woven filiform or of a whalebone bougie threaded as for the tunnelled sound.

Otis's Dilating Urethrotome.—This powerful instrument (Fig. 53) is a very valuable one for cutting strictures in the pendulous urethra. It has a straight, oval shaft, about size 20 (a smaller and correspondingly lighter instrument is made, but the stiffer one is the better). The end of the shaft is tunnelled for the passage of a whalebone guide. The two segments of the shaft are separated by turning the screw in the handle, the extent of separation being registered upon a plate on the handle. The limit of this separation is 45 French. The knife is narrow, concealed in the shaft at a point near the end of the instrument. It is disclosed by withdrawal, when it rides upon a ridge which is continuous up to the handle. The instrument is introduced until the point of emergence of the knife is about $\frac{1}{2}$ inch behind the deepest stricture to be cut. The blades are then separated until the stricture is well upon the stretch. The knife is withdrawn, cutting the tense tissues. The instrument may then be still further screwed up if desired, and the cutting continued to any extent upon the roof of the urethra. The whole roof or a part of it may be cut. The knife is then returned, the instrument unscrewed and withdrawn.

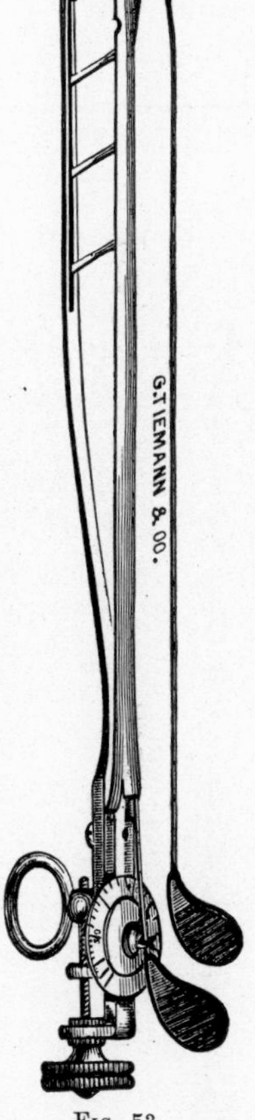

FIG. 53.

The Choice of Instruments.—The Otis urethrotome is the instrument generally used in this country, and the preference is justified by the facts in all cases of stricture of the pendulous urethra. At and beyond the bulb external perineal urethrotomy is called for. The Otis instrument has the advantage over the Maisonneuve of cutting the stricture from behind forward intelligently, and cutting nothing but the stricture. It has the advantage over the Civiale of cutting the whole stricture in a single stroke, or at most in two strokes, whereas with the bulbous instrument this is not always possible.

INTERNAL URETHROTOMY

Preparation.—As preparation the patient should take $\frac{1}{2}$ to 1 gramme of urotropin 3 times a day for two days beforehand. If cocain is used, the urethra should be distended with a 2% solution of the drug for five minutes before the operation. If general anesthesia is employed, the customary catharsis is appropriate. For local preparation the urethra and bladder should be thoroughly irrigated immediately before the operation (a small catheter will usually pass), while if there is any marked inflammation, it should be reduced as far as possible as a preliminary measure.

The Operation.—The operation should be conducted according to certain rules—viz.:

1. All incisions, except those at or near the meatus, should be made upon the roof of the urethra. The reason for this is that there is usually less scar to cut through in the roof than elsewhere, and there is also less tendency to inflammation and infiltration, since the incision, after dividing the corpus spongiosum, enters the intercavernous septum and not the subcutaneous tissue.

2. The operation should be completed by one cut, if possible, or at most by two, and the stricture should be cut at least three sizes (French) larger than the normal (p. 170) meatus.

3. No instrument should be introduced into the posterior urethra either during or for two weeks after the operation. If this rule is observed no urethral chill or other infectious complication need be feared after section of any stricture in the penile urethra.

4. If the hemorrhage is alarming, and not to be checked by finger pressure, it may be controlled by the injection of a saturated solution of desiccated suprarenal capsule (after which secondary hemorrhage may occur), or by bandaging the penis after introducing a medium-sized woven catheter into the anterior urethra, or by binding the penile urethra tightly between two narrow strips of wood laid like splints along the dorsum and the venter of the penis.

After-treatment.—The patient should usually remain in bed until the third day. The urotropin is continued, and on the second day a full-sized sound is passed through the stricture, but not into the posterior urethra. This operation is quite painful and may excite as much hemorrhage as the operation itself. The next day, if all is well, the patient gets up, unless a cystitis, a fever, or any other complication makes his stay in bed advisable. The same sound, or one a size or two smaller (if there is much congestion), is introduced on the fourth, sixth, tenth, and fourteenth days. After this the full-sized sound is introduced twice a week as long as there is any tendency to contraction or bleeding. Sometimes two or three sizes are lost at first, but, in the end, the urethra should take a sound one size smaller than that to which it was cut. If the stricture continues to contract in spite of sounds, it must be cut again and to a larger size than before.

After the stricture is conquered the sound should be passed twice at intervals of ten days, twice at intervals of a month, and twice at intervals of six months. Any recontraction is appropriately treated by sounds (p. 220), and if at the end of this period there is no sign of recontraction, and the stricture was at or anterior to the peno-scrotal angle, the patient may be pronounced cured. If the stricture is deeper, the permanence of the relief must be proved by annual soundings for five years before the cure is assured (and this it very rarely is).

EXTERNAL URETHROTOMY

The Instruments.—1. A staff, tunnelled (Fig. 54), a tunnelled catheter or a Wheelhouse staff (Fig. 55).

2. A blunt probe-pointed bistoury, or a Blizard knife (Fig. 56).

3. A female catheter.

4. A gorget or grooved director (Fig. 57).

5. A soft-rubber perineal tube with terminal and lateral eyes (size 32 to 40 French) (Fig. 58).

6. A large syringe or an irrigator.

7. Several sounds.

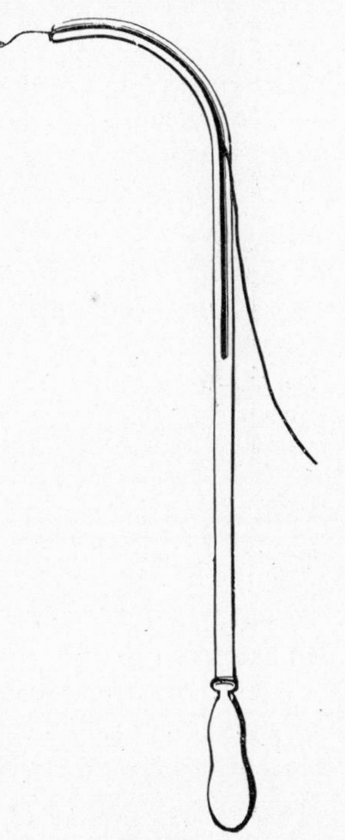

Fig. 54.

8. Clover's crutch (Fig. 59) or Pritchett's anklets and wristlets.

9. Scalpels, clamps, retractors, catgut and silk, probes, etc.

The Choice of Instruments is, to a great extent, a matter of taste. Some surgeons insist upon a Blizard knife, but an ordinary straight blunt-pointed bistoury serves as well. Again, a tunnelled staff will do for all purposes, although a blunt instrument or a Wheelhouse

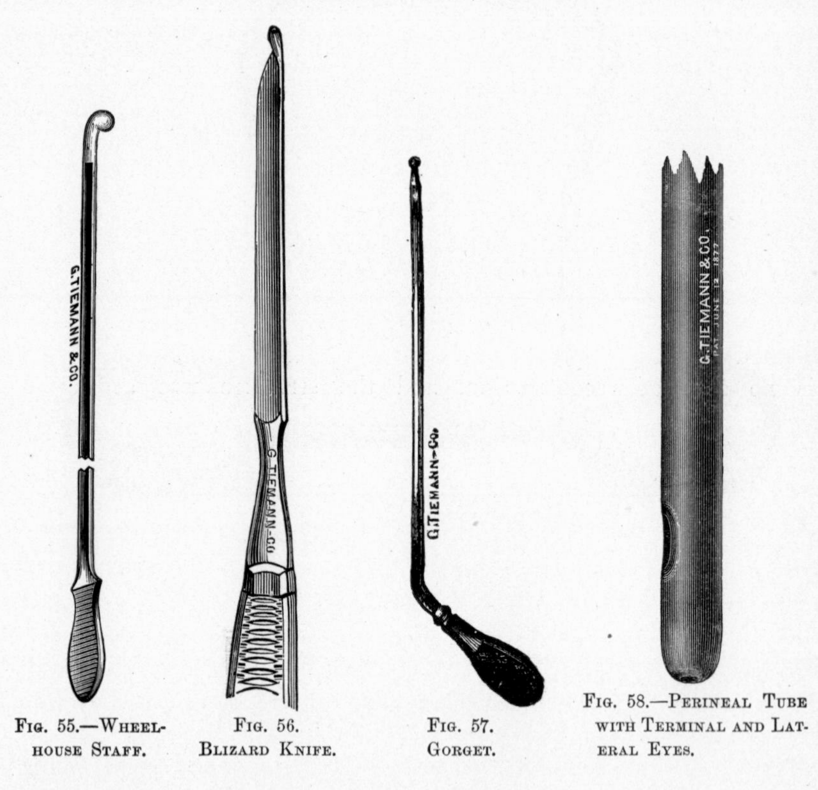

FIG. 55.—WHEELHOUSE STAFF.

FIG. 56. BLIZARD KNIFE.

FIG. 57. GORGET.

FIG. 58.—PERINEAL TUBE WITH TERMINAL AND LATERAL EYES.

staff is rather more convenient for urethrotomy without a guide. Some surgeons prefer to terminate the operation by inserting a urethral catheter *à demeure;* but the large perineal tube is far safer.

Preparation.—The patient is prepared as for any major surgical operation. Unless there is an immediate emergency, it is well to put him on urotropin, 1 to 2 grammes a day, for two days. The perineum is to be shaved and prepared antiseptically.

Anesthesia.—Local anesthesia may be employed by injecting a 5% solution of cocain into the urethra and infiltrating the tissues with a 1% solution. My personal preference is for general anesthesia, although, when the operation is done without a guide and the opening of the stricture is hard to find, the patient, if only anesthetized locally, may pass a few drops of urine, and so indicate the passage.

The Operation.—After the anesthetic has been administered every effort should be made to engage at least a filiform bougie in the stricture. If this succeeds, the operation, *external urethrotomy*

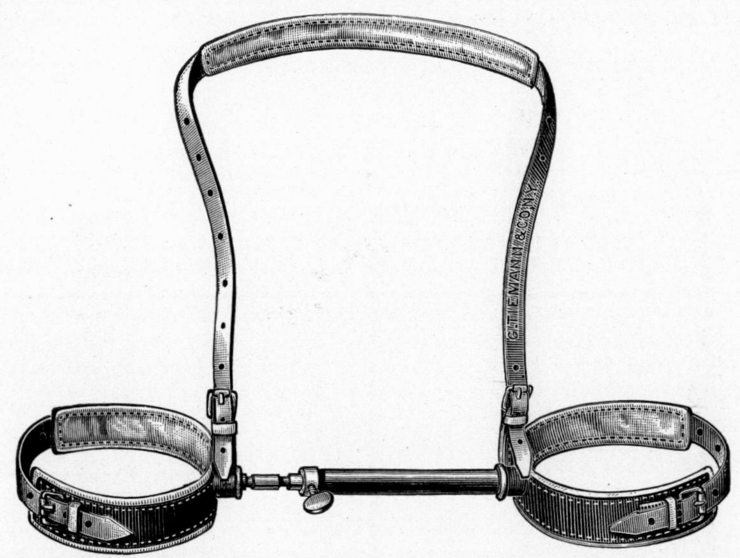

Fig. 59.—Clover's Crutch to hold the Legs, with Strap to go over the Shoulders.

with a guide, is perfectly simple. The bougie is carefully held in place, the patient put in the lithotomy position, and the tunnelled staff threaded over the filiform down to the face of the stricture.[1] One assistant occupies himself solely with holding the scrotum well up out of the way and keeping the staff directly in the median line and pushed outward in the perineum to form a resistance for the surgeon's knife. The surgeon seats himself on a low stool facing the perineum, and makes in it an incision 1 inch long down to the staff (*A–B*, Fig. 60). As soon as the tip of the staff is laid bare it is withdrawn a little, and the filiform is seen disappearing among the tissues. By following this a grooved director is readily introduced into the bladder, and, by running a blunt bistoury along it, the floor of the urethra may be freely incised without damaging the adjacent tissues. The director should not be removed until the index finger has been passed into the bladder. If there is contracture of the bladder neck this is to be broken, cut, or burned through (p. 317).

---

[1] The patient may be conveniently held in the lithotomy position by two assistants, or by the Clover's crutch (Fig. 59), or by a bandage tied at each end just below the patient's knees and slung around his neck, over one shoulder and under the other, or by Pritchett's anklets.

Having thus opened a way into the bladder, all instruments are withdrawn and all fibrous bands in the *roof of the urethra* must be cut with the knife, and any fibrous material detected in the floor of the canal, at either extremity of the incision, should be freely excised. Finally, a blunt steel sound, as large as the urethra will admit, should be passed through the meatus into the bladder, the meatus and any anterior strictures being cut if necessary. This sound should be introduced several times, to make certain that it glides easily and without obstruction. If the stricture is an old one, it is always well to search the bladder for stone after the operation, and to remove any that may be found.

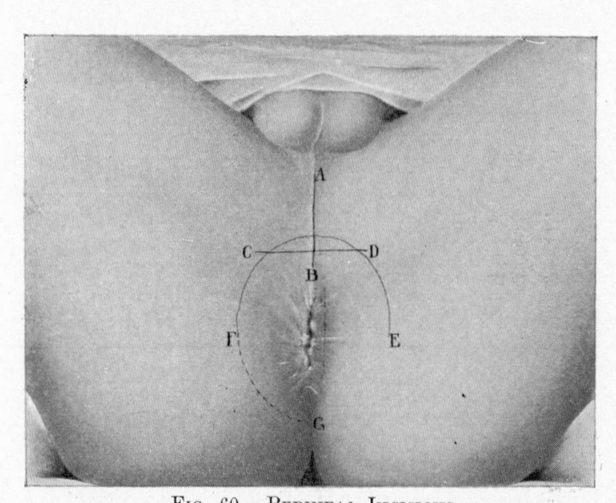

Fig. 60.—Perineal Incisions.

A–B, median incision; *C–D*, transverse incision; *E–F*, curved pre-rectal incision; *E–F–G*, incision for extirpation of the right seminal vesicle.

To close the operation the large perineal tube is inserted and the bladder washed free of clots with boric-acid solution. It is then filled once with nitrate of silver (1: 4,000) to check hemorrhage and prevent chill. The tube is so placed that its eye is just within the bladder, and is pierced by a silk suture to mark the point where it emerges through the incision. Hemorrhage is sometimes considerable, but is readily controlled by packing about the tube. The tube is secured by two tapes passing X-wise over each groin and gluteal fold to a bandage belt. Over these a few pads of gauze are slipped about the tube and held in place by a T-bandage, split to pass up on each side of the scrotum. It is not advisable to use any sutures, since the patient's safety may depend upon free drainage, and healing is not materially hastened by sutures. The scrotum should be slung up out of the way to prevent infiltration of its loose tissues by blood and urine.

Without a Guide.—The operation just described—external urethrotomy with a guide—is simple and straightforward; but the same operation without a guide may still be accounted one of the most difficult operations known to the surgeon. Hence no effort should be spared, either before or after anesthesia, to insinuate an instrument through the stricture. This failing, the operation without a guide must be undertaken. A large staff is passed into the urethra, and if any filiform is thought to have engaged ever so little it is left in place. The surgeon then cuts down upon the staff and lays the urethra freely open at this point. Much time may be saved if the surgeon—as soon as he has made this linear section of the urethral floor—inserts a stout silk suture into each side of the cut urethra and the adjacent tissues as near the stricture as possible. The ends of the ligatures are then knotted, and they make the best possible retractors and serve to identify the urethra, which otherwise may be hopelessly lost (Fig. 61).

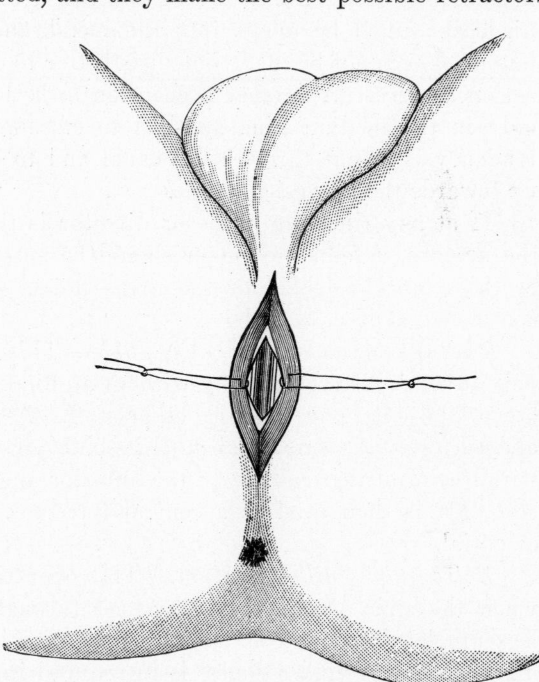

FIG. 61.—THE OPERATION OF EXTERNAL PERINEAL URETHROTOMY. Grooved staff seen between separated borders of incisions.

Now the tedious part of the operation—the hunt for the opening of the stricture—begins. *The only guide is the roof of the urethra*, which should never be cut until the stricture has been laid open. Patient methodical searching usually ends in the discovery of this point, but wild or hasty jabbing is almost sure to fail. The two sutures mark the lateral walls of the urethra. Between them is the roof. Follow it back to where it is lost in cicatricial tissue and there is the opening. It is not plainly visible, but gentle sponging and probing may be depended upon to find it. As long as these bearings are kept in mind fifteen minutes is not too long a time to spend in finding the orifice.

Failing in this, three courses are open to the surgeon:

1. To cut directly back through the scar tissue until the urethra is opened.

2. To search behind the scar tissue for the dilated portion of the urethra.

3. To perform retrograde catheterization.

The first course is usually selected, yet, although the chances of its success are great, it generally results in the destruction of an inch or two of the urethra. A safer plan is to feel for the membranous urethra by a finger in the rectum. This portion of the urethra lies in the median line between the prostate and the anus. Having identified it, the surgeon makes a clean incision from the last recognisable part of the urethral roof downward (as the patient lies upon his back) until he opens into the membranous urethra. If these landmarks cannot be made out, it is better to do retrograde catheterization at once. A further precaution to be borne in mind is to cut only in the median line, and not to cut too deeply. The natural tendency is to cut through the canal and to search for the opening up towards the prevesical space.

If at any time the probe or director is thought to have entered the urethra, a female catheter should be passed alongside of it, and as this enters the bladder the urine flows. The operation is then completed as described above.

The Wheelhouse Staff (Fig. 55).—This instrument is for use only in external urethrotomy without a guide. It is inserted, groove down, and cut upon like any other staff. As soon as the urethra is opened, the staff is revolved until its bulb presents in the wound, and withdrawn until it catches in the anterior angle of the urethral incision. It is then used as a central retractor. I have not found it essential.

Retrograde Catheterization.—This operation is the last resource when the stricture cannot be opened through the perineum. The legs are let down and suprapubic cystotomy is performed (p. 459). Through this wound a sound is introduced into the urethra down to the posterior face of the stricture. Upon this the urethra is readily opened. Most urinary surgeons in this country pride themselves never to have performed retrograde catheterization; but in Europe, where external urethrotomy is less often done, retrograde catheterization seems to be resorted to quite frequently.

After-treatment.—The patient is placed in bed with hot bottles about him and stimulated as much as necessary. To the perineal tube is attached a long rubber tube leading into a bottle containing a known quantity of 2% carbolic-acid solution. This is emptied from time to time, and the amount of urine accurately noted. The tube remains in place four days, during which time the bladder is injected through the tube once or twice daily with boric-acid solution.

If cystitis is severe 1 : 8,000 nitrate-of-silver solution serves better. The dressings are changed as often as necessary.

On the fourth day the tube is removed, a full-sized sound introduced, and a few drops of 1 : 1,500 nitrate-of-silver solution injected along the urethra. This is repeated twice a week until the wound is healed, and then at longer intervals (p. 218).

After the removal of the perineal tube the wound is kept clean and covered with a pad. For the first few days there is incontinence, and all or nearly all the urine is passed through the perineum. But the incontinence ceases, and the urine comes to pass entirely through the penis during the second or third week. Ten days later the wound is healed.

Complications.—Hemorrhage, spasm, and infection are the three complications to be feared.

Hemorrhage usually does no harm beyond blocking the tube or filling the bladder with clots, thus exciting spasm. But I have known a man to bleed persistently from a perineal wound until his death was imminent. Alum injections stopped the flow after other astringents and packing had failed. The bleeding is usually free for the first day, after which it decreases rapidly.

Spasm of the bladder is excited by distention of the organ with clots or by obstruction or slipping of the tube. The spasm may also be set up by the mere presence of the tube or of packing in the perineal wound. Clots may be removed by repeated gentle injections and aspirations of hot boric-acid solution, or by replacing the tube with a litholapaxy tube and aspirator. The injection of hydrogen peroxid may do more harm than good. On the other hand, if the spasm is due to the mere presence of the tube, the patient should be kept under the influence of narcotics for the first twenty-four hours, and if spasm persists at the end of that time the tube must be replaced with a smaller one or removed entirely. In the latter event the frequent use of the catheter may be required.

Infection is the great danger. It may assume any of the forms of urethral or urinary fever. Our great safeguards are diluent waters and urotropin by the mouth, nitrate of silver locally, and the perineal tube. If the integrity of the kidneys is assured no septic complications need be feared. Unfortunately, the kidneys are often congested, or even infected, and the mere cutting may suffice to excite a urethral chill, in spite of the most minute precautions; but this chill will not recur if there is efficient drainage and the patient is flooded with water by mouth or rectum (p. 46).

To recapitulate: The points in external urethrotomy that require special attention are:

1. Perfect familiarity with the operative field.
2. Methodical deliberation at every step.
3. Plenty of light and a wide dry wound.
4. Preservation and recognition of the urethral roof.
5. Division of all bands and excision of all masses of stricture tissue, especial care being taken to free the roof of all ridges and to pass a full-sized sound.
6. Proper use of the perineal tube.
7. Intelligent after-treatment.

Other Operations

Sir Reginald Harrison,[1] instead of cutting deep perineal strictures from without, has devised a rapid method which he calls *combined external and internal urethrotomy.* It consists of an internal urethrotomy done with a Maisonneuve instrument upon the roof of the canal, followed by the introduction of a staff and a puncture in the perineum large enough to admit a perineal tube. This operation commends itself by its simplicity and rapidity for use in all cases where excision of cicatricial tissue is unnecessary. I believe it essential to introduce a finger into the bladder to be sure that the way is clear.

Certain other operations have been devised to minimize the scar tissue which remains after any urethrotomy, and whose practical persistence in deep strictures, and especially in traumatic strictures, sooner or later causes recurrence, unless sounds are used indefinitely. Of these operations the simplest is the *immediate suture of a lacerated urethra* (p. 38). In a similar manner, if a great deal of scar tissue is excised in doing an external urethrotomy, the divided urethral roof may be brought together by buried catgut sutures. For traumatic stricture the scar is often wholly excised and the urethral ends approximated. Developing along these lines a number of surgeons have applied *Thiersch grafts* to urethræ from which considerable lengths of scar have been removed. The inner layer of the prepuce has usually been called upon to supply the graft, but any skin upon which no hair grows does as well. The graft should be sutured to the urethral roof at each end and kept in place by packing. I have thus succeeded in filling a gap 1 inch long to the patient's entire satisfaction.[2]

Time has judged the use of *caustics* and condemned them, while the same fate awaits *electrolysis.* My experience with it has been unfortunate and my verdict pronounced.[3]

[1] Brit. Med. J., 1885, July 18th. [2] J. of Cut. and Gen.-Urin. Dis., 1891, November.
[3] N. Y. Med. J., 1871, xiii, 569.

SUPRAPUBIC ASPIRATION

When there is complete retention, either from stricture or from hypertrophy of the prostate, and the urethral obstacle is insurmountable, it is often expedient to relieve the patient by aspiration. This operation is absolutely simple and may be repeated a number of times. Not infrequently an impassable stricture will admit a filiform bougie after aspiration.

Any form of aspirator may be used. I prefer Potain's (Fig. 62). The needle should be of fine calibre and 2 inches long. The

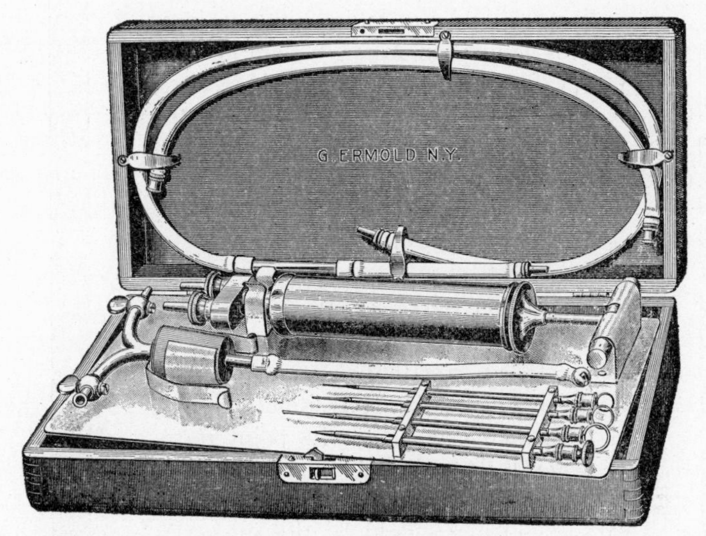

Fig. 62.—Potain Aspirator.

pubic region is shaved and scrubbed with green soap, then washed with alcohol and ether. The needle is boiled and the rest of the apparatus rendered as clean as possible. While it is not necessary that the surgeon's hands be surgically clean, they should at least be washed. Immediately before inserting the needle its permeability and the efficiency of the aspirator should be tested.

The suprapubic region should be percussed; a flat note indicates that the distended bladder lies beneath with no loops of intestine intervening. The needle is plunged through the abdominal wall in the median line at a point about ½ inch above the pubes. The aspirator is then attached and its piston withdrawn to form a vacuum. If no urine flows the needle is pushed in until some does. Then it is held stationary until the contents of the bladder have been drawn off. Only one other precaution need be observed—namely, to maintain suction while the needle is being withdrawn. Unless this is done a drop of infected urine may be left in the suprapubic space and cause a prevesical abscess.

Aspiration through the rectum or perineum, and simple puncture without aspiration are dangerous operations, and should not be practised.

THE RETAINED CATHETER

The retained catheter (*sonde à demeure*) is employed for dilatation or drainage. For the latter purpose it is far less popular in America than abroad. We prefer external section and perineal drainage to internal section and catheter drainage for reasons to be given in the next chapter.

The Instrument.—Filiform, rubber, or woven bougies or catheters may be selected, *but no metal instrument should be tied in the urethra.* Within twenty-four hours a metal instrument will cause severe ulceration at the peno-scrotal angle, at the bulbo-membranous junction, and in the bladder, wherever its point rests. In general, the softer the instrument the better for the canal. Hence a new stiff-rubber catheter should be the surgeon's choice. If this cannot be introduced, a smooth woven instrument should be employed.

Self-retaining catheters of various designs may be employed. Pezzer's catheters are the most satisfactory. They have a flange which rests against the neck of the bladder. One form (Fig. 63) is for introduction over a mandrin through the urethra. The other (Fig. 64) is intended for retrograde catheterization. A sound is introduced into the urethra and brought out through the suprapubic wound. The catheter is fitted over its point and so drawn into the urethra.

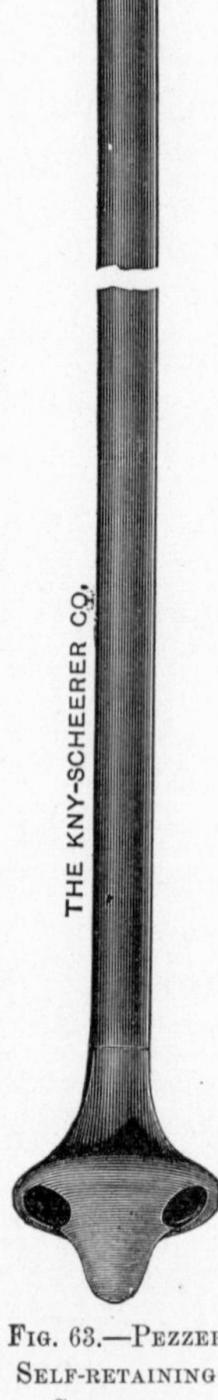

Fig. 63.—Pezzer Self-retaining Catheter.

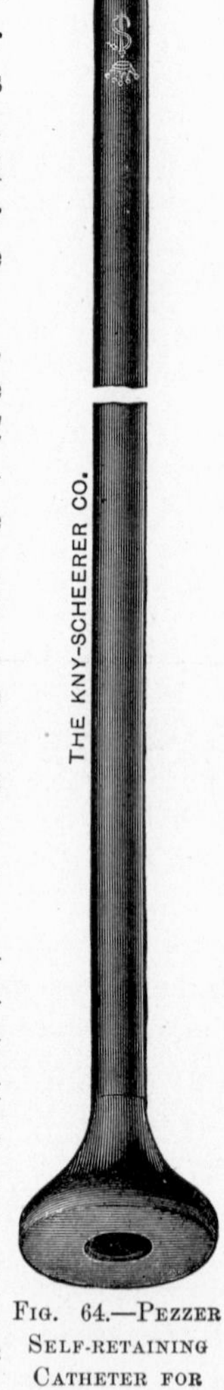

Fig. 64.—Pezzer Self-retaining Catheter for Retrograde Catheterization.

The instrument employed should fit loosely in the canal. Even when dilatation is aimed at, an instrument that fits rather loosely in the stricture will do more good than one that is introduced only with difficulty.

Introduction.—For dilatation the filiform instrument should only be introduced far enough to engage thoroughly in the stricture. It should be changed every twenty-four or forty-eight hours.

For drainage, if a self-retaining catheter is employed, it is placed with its collar resting lightly against the neck of the bladder. An ordinary catheter should be introduced until the urine flows through it, then withdrawn until the flow is cut off, then reintroduced ½ inch, and there fixed. With the catheter in this position the surgeon may feel sure that the outflow will not be interfered with, nor will the point of the instrument make any undue pressure upon the floor or the posterior wall of the bladder. The catheter should be removed and cleansed at least twice a week.

Fixation.—Even when a self-retaining catheter is employed, it should be further guyed at the meatus. Several varieties of apparatus have been devised for this purpose, but none is more efficient than the following: A large flat bone button, with its centre cut out to fit snugly over the catheter, is slipped over it close up to the meatus. A piece of tape or coarse silk thread is then tied tightly around the catheter just beyond the button. The two ends of the thread are tied together at about 1 inch from the catheter, then carried around the corona glandis and again knotted, thus forming a collar too tight to slip over the glans, but not tight enough to strangulate it. This maneuvre is repeated with another piece of silk or tape carried in the opposite direction. The four ends are then carried back along the penis and bound to it by several turns of adhesive plaster, or tied to the pubic hairs.

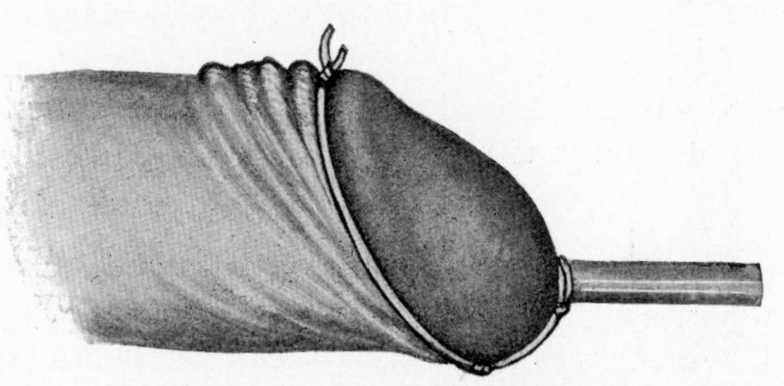

Fig. 65.—Filiform Bougie tied in.

To tie in a filiform no button is needed and only one strand of silk, the ends of which may be cut short after the corona has been snugly encircled (Fig. 65).

Dressings.—After the catheter has been tied in place a dressing of sterile gauze is wrapped about it and the penis, and the whole slung up over the groin by a T-bandage. If the instrument is used for drainage it is then inspected. If the urine flows drop by drop the catheter is properly placed. Its end is attached to a tube leading over the side of the bed into an antiseptic solution.

Complications and Precautions.—Some patients cannot endure a retained catheter. It sets up continuous vesical spasm. The selection and proper introduction of a small smooth instrument will go far to overcome this in some cases, and, if necessary, the patient should be kept under the influence of morphin for twenty-four hours before the attempt is abandoned.

A purulent urethritis almost invariably results from the use of a retained catheter. It is due to the presence of the catheter, but in a sense is bacterial as well, since it is associated with and in part caused by a pullulation of the urethral bacteria. This urethritis usually produces few symptoms beyond a free discharge of pus from the meatus, and it subsides when the catheter is withdrawn; but if neglected it may lead to ulceration of the canal, and so increase the stricture. To minimize the urethritis a smooth clean instrument should be chosen and the anterior urethra irrigated by the Janet method before the introduction of the catheter, as well as every time it is changed.

Urinary fever and urethral chill may be unavoidable. But if the antiseptic precautions just laid down are observed, if the catheter is working properly, so that no fluid is allowed to accumulate in the bladder, and if urotropin is administered, the danger of septic complications is minimized. A single chill may be disregarded, but if, in spite of all precautions, the patient's condition gets worse instead of better, the catheter must be withdrawn.

Cystitis and stone may be avoided by cleanliness and frequent changing of the instrument.

CHAPTER XIII

STRICTURE OF THE URETHRA—PROGNOSIS AND TREATMENT

PROGNOSIS

Although the prognosis of stricture depends upon the treatment more than upon any other one thing, the progress of the disease varies according to the nature and location of the scar. Traumatic strictures often contract rapidly, in spite of all the surgeon's efforts. Gonorrheal strictures, on the other hand, contract far less energetically. Strictures of the perineal urethra are far more difficult to cure than strictures of the pendulous urethra. The latter contract slowly and are commonly curable; the former contract more rapidly and are, in the majority of cases, incurable—that is, they may be relieved by sounding or urethrotomy, but they usually relapse after a time. Finally, the more extensive a stricture the more irregular its surface, and the denser the cicatricial tissue composing it the more difficult will be its treatment and the more dubious its cure.

In the matter of life or death, however, the prognosis of stricture is far less gloomy. Stricture is not often fatal, except in neglected cases, such as are sometimes encountered in hospitals. Death occurs in various ways. Not to mention the rare cases of sudden death following the simple introduction of an instrument, and only alluding to rupture of the bladder and death following surgical operations for the relief of stricture, the causes of fatal termination in cases of stricture are three:

1. Extravasation of urine, which, if extensive, kills at once by shock, or, later, by exhaustion, suppuration, abscess, gangrene, or pyemia.

2. Chronic uremia, usually associated with septicemia, from the involvement of the kidneys in the inflammatory process. The patient may die from such a cause even after the stricture has been dilated, or, as is more commonly the case, the treatment itself, whether by sound or knife, may induce a reflex congestion of the diseased kidneys, which closes the scene.

3. Cachexia and exhaustion, attended by pain, loss of rest, and inability to eat, due to the torment of constant unrelieved desire to urinate, and the agony and labour of the act. No more pitiable sight can be imagined than that of a man with pericystitis, trying to pass water every five minutes through an old tight stricture. Standing up, with his body bent forward, his head leaning against the wall, or on his knees, and half doubled up, his hands clutching at anything within reach, he writhes and groans in agony, the sweat starting from his face, his whole body quivering and convulsed with pain. After a minute of this torture, he finds he has passed, perhaps, a teaspoonful of bloody, purulent, putrid urine, perhaps nothing at all, and he sinks exhausted upon his bed, only to renew the effort after five or ten minutes. No man can long endure torture of this sort. If the surgeon does not soon bring him relief, death will be more kind.

TREATMENT

The principle governing the treatment of stricture is simplicity itself. *Enlarge the urethra by dilatation, aided, if necessary, by cutting. Then maintain its calibre by dilatation.* Or perhaps the negative view is more forcible. *Never cut if you can dilate; and recognise that the patient is not cured unless he stays cured.* Cutting is at best a substitute for dilatation, while divulsion and electricity are no substitutes.

Prophylaxis

Since most strictures are caused by gonorrhea, and the occurrence of gonorrheal stricture is favoured by the intensity and the duration of the inflammation, every effort made to control this inflammation is so much towards the prevention of a possible stricture. Yet this is but an indirect prophylaxis, since it is impossible to prophesy which case of gonorrhea will culminate in stricture and which will not. But when the disease becomes chronic *in the anterior urethra,* although there be no stricture present the inflammation is encouraged by and is in turn encouraging a periurethral sclerosis, which may soon develop from this chrysalid state into a veritable stricture. Therefore, the systematic treatment of chronic anterior urethritis is the surest preventive of stricture.

For traumatic stricture the proper prophylaxis is immediate perineal section at the time of injury (p. 38).

Curative Treatment

The Action of Sounds.—Since the sound is the instrument best adapted to the cure of stricture, and since, unfortunately, it is easier to use a sound wrongly than rightly, a few words on the use and effects of sounds are required.

The surgeon attacking a stricture of the urethra may fairly analyze the therapeutic problem thus: "Here is a scar with a congested surface; shall I cut or shall I massage it?" If he cuts through it the symptoms are relieved, the obstruction is apparently removed, but the scar is still there. In fact, there is rather more scar than ever, and if the former scar contracted and gave trouble, so much the more will this one. To prevent this he will keep the lips of the wound separated by sounds, so that it may heal with so broad an insertion band that the contraction will be of no moment. Such a course may well succeed in the pendulous urethra; but, if the stricture is in the perineal urethra and of such density as to give the shadow of an excuse for cutting, it will certainly relapse after the operation unless subjected to systematic massage by sounds. The knife only relieves the congestion plus a temporary relief of the contraction, while the sound actually causes the resorption of the scar tissue. The effect is quite comparable to the reabsorbing effect of massage applied to the outside of the body. The exact nature of the process is not known, but the practical conclusion of universal experience is that *the maximum of effect is produced by the minimum of effort*, or, as Guyon puts it, "the effect is due, not to the pressure of the sound, but to its mere contact."

It is a matter of every-day experience that the brutal passage of a sound, bruising and tearing the congested urethra, is followed by a sharp inflammatory reaction, which probably increases rather than diminishes the scar tissue. Such treatment is inexcusable. The stricture is already congested, the mucous membrane already inflamed. What more futile procedure than to add irritation to irritation! Such is not the object of the sound. On the contrary, the sound, if a metal one, should slip in as nearly as possible by its own weight; slowly indeed, but surely. Such a maneuvre has the treble effect of lessening congestion at the point of contact, straightening out irregularities in the canal, and stimulating the deeper tissues to a favourable reaction, which will result in softening the cicatrix. But to do this the sound must press without bruising. If a given sound will not pass, try a smaller one. The effect is readily judged. If a sound is properly introduced, it may usually be followed by sounds of the next larger sizes with less pain than the first. Larger sounds may be introduced at each sitting; the rapid amelioration of the symptoms shows that the congestion is relieved, the obstruction is disappearing, and the canal is resuming its normal condition. Yet, however gently a sound is introduced, it will be followed within forty-eight hours by a congestive reaction of more or less intensity. Hence, in treating stricture by dilatation it is bad surgery to introduce instruments—unless filiforms—before the lapse of seventy-two hours, and even longer intervals will often produce better results.

Lastly, and above all, gently, *gently*, GENTLY!

The Treatment of the Various Kinds of Stricture

The treatment of stricture at the meatus and of spasmodic stricture has been dealt with. The treatments of fistula, extravasation, etc., and of the remoter complications are considered under their respective titles. Apart from these, the treatment of stricture may be considered under the following captions:

1. Stricture of large calibre.
2. Stricture of small calibre.
3. Stricture admitting only a filiform.
4. Stricture complicated by retention.
5. Impassable stricture.
6. Traumatic and resilient stricture.
7. Inodular or indurated stricture.
8. Stricture complicated by prostatitis. (Irritable stricture.)

1. Treatment of Uncomplicated Stricture of Large Calibre.—The majority of strictures which the surgeon is called upon to treat are of large calibre. The symptom of which the patient complains is persistent gleet, following gonorrhea, with, possibly, some frequency in urination. These cases are of daily occurrence and often pass unrecognised, the gleet being treated, the stricture overlooked. Too much stress cannot be laid upon the importance of exploring the urethra with the bulbous bougie in such cases. One, two, or more strictures are found, the smallest, which is probably the deepest, allowing passage, perhaps, to a No. 15 bulb.

Treatment here is most simple. After the diagnosis has been made, no further instrumentation is advisable (if the patient can spare the time) until the effect of exploration has been observed. The chances of urethral chill after first examinations must be remembered. The patient's general condition and habits must be studied, and his urine tested for acidity or possible kidney disease. He must be instructed in urethral hygiene, the nature of his malady must be explained, and, to forestall future disappointment, he should be informed at the outset that, after his symptoms have been removed by treatment, the permanence of his cure, *if his stricture is in the deep urethra*, may depend upon his use of an instrument upon himself at proper intervals, in order to prevent recontraction.

Being instructed not to mind the smarting at his next urination, and given such alkali, balsam, or injection as the condition of the urine and amount of discharge seem to call for, the patient is dismissed to return in two days for treatment. I have recently adopted urotropin as a preventive of urinary chill from sounding, as well as in the other operations of the urinary tract. One gramme (15 grains) a day may be administered, either alone or in combination, beginning two or three days before the urethral exploration or operation. It has proved most efficacious.

Sounds.—The treatment best adapted to the majority of these cases is dilatation with a conical double taper steel sound. One of these instruments properly warmed and sterilized is introduced in the manner already detailed. Its size should correspond to that of the blunt sound that has passed the stricture, and the utmost delicacy, care, and gentleness should be used in its introduction. The wedge and lever should not be forgotten, nor should we abuse power because we possess it. To overcome resistance, patience is better than force. As soon as the instrument has entered the bladder it should be gently withdrawn at once. Nothing is gained by leaving it even for a moment. During withdrawal the stricture is usually felt to grasp the sound. After one sound has been withdrawn, a second and even a third may be introduced, if considered safe. No rule, nothing short of personal experience, can indicate how far the dilatation may be pushed at one sitting. The tendency is always to hurry and to use force, a course detrimental to rapid progress. It may be stated as a rule, subject to judicious exception, that *if a conical steel instrument of any size larger than No. 15, when held in proper position, will not enter a stricture by its own weight after a little delay, it should not be used.* Every urethra, however, has its own temper; some are aroused by the slightest disturbance, while others bear considerable violence without protest. A surgeon should acquaint himself by gradual experiment with the temper of a given urethra before he takes liberties with it.

The mischief to be feared from the employment of large sounds with force, besides false passages which are not likely to be produced by large instruments, is threefold:

1. Epididymitis, a common result of violence to the urethra, and a complication which suspends treatment and confines the patient to bed for several days, or, it may be, weeks.

2. Inflammation in the stricture, which aggravates its condition and defeats the end of the treatment.

3. Chill and urethral fever.

In rare instances epididymitis may come on in spite of care. This complication must be properly attended to, and all treatment of the urethra suspended until the pain in the testicle has subsided and the swelling of the epididymis has assumed an indolent character. It is not necessary to wait for the latter to disappear entirely, and, if extra care be employed in resuming the use of instruments, there is little danger of provoking relapse. While using instruments in the urethra, especially at the beginning of a course of dilatation, the patient may be advised to wear a suspensory bandage.

If the stricture is really uncomplicated—i. e., if there is no cystitis or prostatitis—it cannot be irritated except by overtreatment. The management of a stricture complicated by these inflammations deserves special mention (see below).

The third danger, the chill and fever, is very unusual after manipulation of the pendulous urethra—witness the impunity with which many young surgeons cut far and wide through that part of the long-suffering canal—and increases as we approach the bulbo-membranous junction. Some persons have a predisposition in this regard, and the presence of some catarrh of the prostate is almost essential as a predisposing cause of any real septic chill. Yet in no given case can the prognosis be definite, and the only safety lies in hedging the operation about with all possible precautions. The rule which I have found most efficacious is—

Urotropin before,
Gentleness during,
Nitrate of silver after.

The nitrate is best applied by instillation in the strength of 1:1,000 (p. 134). While not essential, it is safe to *end every séance with this instillation.*

At each subsequent visit of the patient, the surgeon commences with a sound from one to two sizes smaller than the last instrument introduced at the previous visit, and carries the dilatation as far as possible without the employment of force—this till the full size is reached.

The most important feature in the treatment of stricture by dilatation is a proper regulation of the intervals to be allowed between the visits. The intervals usually recommended are too short. Occasionally we see patients who attempt to treat themselves, introducing a bougie into the urethra daily, or twice daily, perhaps at every act of urination, aggravating every symptom, worrying the urethra and bladder into a state of inflammation, and wondering why the stricture does not get well. Some surgeons, unfortunately, are guilty of the same error. We can only repeat that *it is bad surgery, in treating stricture by dilatation, to reintroduce instruments—unless fili-*

form—before the lapse of at least seventy-two hours, and even longer intervals will often produce better results.

As to the degree of dilatation which is to be aimed at, every urethra has its own gauge in the size of its meatus—provided that meatus be not congenitally small, nor contracted by disease. If there is any cicatricial tissue in the circle of the meatus, or if a probe can make out any pouching below the lower commissure (Fig. 35), the meatus is too small.

The normal meatus, however, is the smallest part of the healthy canal, and the object in view is to bring all available pressure to bear upon a morbid narrowing of some other portion of the tube. To do this the meatus must be lightly put upon the stretch. When this is done, the feeling is one of discomfort, which subsides after the instrument has been in place for a moment. If the meatus is overstretched, a distinctly marked, narrow white line will be seen encircling the instrument upon the lips of the urethral orifice, indicating that the latter have been deprived of blood by pressure. The use of double taper sounds makes this stretching transitory, and therefore much more bearable.

In the majority of cases this physiological gauge—the normal meatus—is absolutely satisfactory. A stricture once dilated to this size—which will vary from 27 to 32 French—will stand the test of a cure—that is, the inflammation about it (not necessarily the prostatitis) will rapidly disappear, and the stricture will not recontract during the lengthened intervals of sounding that constitute the after-treatment. But occasionally the meatus is too small a gauge. The outer fibres of the scar lie so deep and are so elastic that they are unaffected by the pressure and tend to recontract as soon as the lengthened intervals of sounding permit them to do so. Such strictures must be cut or stretched until a point is reached where they do not recontract. To do this the integrity of the meatus must often be sacrificed.

Otis's Theory.—Such was the basis of Dr. Otis's famous theory. Meeting many strictures incurable by the half-hearted methods of dilatation then in vogue, and finding that a generous incision cured stricture of the anterior urethra, he evolved the theory that the urethra is an evenly calibrated tube whose size bears a direct relation to that of the flaccid penis. This ratio he fixed at 10 mm. of urethral circumference to every inch of penile circumference. Thus, a 3-inch penis should take a 30 French; a $3\frac{1}{2}$-inch penis a 34 French. The objection to Dr. Otis's theory is that it is incorrect. The urethra is no more an evenly calibrated tube than the ureter, the esophagus, or the bowel. Its size no more varies with that of the penis than does the size of the esophagus with that of the neck. The objection to Dr. Otis's practice is that it involves an unnecessary and harmful amount of cutting, since, as a rule, the patient can get well without it, and the operation leaves the canal defective in expulsive power. The last drops of urine dribble away drop by drop, to the great inconvenience of the patient. Moreover, though this wide cutting cures strictures of the pendulous urethra, it does not cure deep strictures. The latter get well sometimes under all varieties of treatment—in most instances they require the occasional use of sounds for an indefinite period.

Yet Dr. Otis's work deserves the highest praise, in that he has shown us what great sizes may be attained with safety. And although he has not proved that his treatment is always essential, he has proved it most desirable in strictures of the anterior urethra incurable by a moderate course of sounds. Only recently Albarran and Guiard in France have insisted that some strictures must be dilated above 23 French!

Urethrotomy.—If at any stage of dilatation the stricture rebels and will not be dilated any further, the urethrotome must be resorted to.

Choice of Urethrotomy.—As was mentioned in describing the operations, external section is best suited to deep strictures, internal section to strictures of the pendulous urethra. There still remains a choice of instruments for internal urethrotomy, which choice is simply a matter of taste. For my part, I like Civiale's urethrotome for strictures near the meatus, Otis's dilating urethrotome for any other stricture large enough to admit the instrument, and Maisonneuve's urethrotome only for those strictures through which an Otis instrument will not pass.

After-treatment.—The after-treatment depends upon the location of the stricture.

If the stricture is in the pendulous urethra, the surgeon may feel confident that a cure persisting three months will prove permanent. When the stricture has been dilated fully, so that there are no longer any large shreds in the urine (unless from the posterior urethra), the patient may be dismissed to report in two weeks. If at that time there is no recontraction, he may be dismissed for a month, and again for two months, when his cure may be pronounced permanent. If, however, there is a relapse on any of these occasions, biweekly visits must be renewed, and the patient's cure insured by higher dilatation or a further cutting.

If the stricture is in the bulb the matter is different. In all such strictures, except those soft bands that yield to one or two passages of a sound, recontraction will almost inevitably take place, unless the cure be maintained by the patient. This is easily done, and no intelligent patient objects to it. In a few lessons he acquires the art of gently passing a sound upon himself, and he should be seriously cautioned to perform this trifling but important operation at first weekly, then fortnightly, then monthly, studying his own case to determine how long an interval he may allow without sensible recontraction of his stricture. In this way, in some cases, the use of instruments may be gradually abandoned; in the majority, it will have to be continued indefinitely, at intervals varying from a week to a year. Thus the cure becomes radical. The surgeon is responsible for the cure only on condition that the patient carries out this plan; or, rather, the patient is responsible for the permanence of his own cure, and this he must be made distinctly to understand.

2. **Stricture of Small Calibre.**—To this class belong strictures admitting any instrument less than No. 15 French. They are considered separately, not because they require different treatment, but in order to emphasize the fact that they are better treated with soft than with steel instruments. The danger of making a false passage in an obstructed urethra with a small metallic instrument cannot be overrated. No one can appreciate the ease with which a false passage is made until he has himself made one. Indeed, it is not very uncommon for a patient or a surgeon, not well acquainted with the urethra, to make a false passage, and to go on dilating it instead of the stricture, wondering meantime that the size of the stream is not increased nor the symptoms alleviated. A surgeon who knows every line of the urethra may occasionally assume the risk of using a small metallic instrument in the canal without a guide, but only in exceptional cases. Below No. 15, soft instruments only should be employed, unless there be a guide through the stricture.

Dilatation is carried on as already directed, steel instruments being used as soon as the stricture will admit No. 15. Progress is slower with soft than with steel instruments.

Cutting (internal or external urethrotomy) operations are daily growing in favour in the treatment of strictures of small calibre; yet, in a case of uncomplicated stricture in the deep urethra, no matter how tight, if not resilient, and not of traumatic origin, if any instrument at all can be passed, dilatation is still the best method of treatment. Scarification and divulsion are mentioned only to be condemned. If you cannot dilate, cut; never divulse. Cutting may be resorted to:

a. If the stricture will not dilate.

b. If the patient has not the time to go through a long course of dilatation.

c. If urethral fever follows all attempts at dilatation.

3. **Stricture admitting only a Filiform, but not complicated by Retention.**—In commencing the treatment it may be impossible to enter the bladder with any instrument, either on account of the tightness of the stricture, or because the point of the instrument does not engage in the latter, or is arrested by some fold or lacuna beyond. In these cases gentle perseverance and skill will rarely fail of success. The different varieties of filiform bougies, with the maneuvres and expedients of introduction already detailed, will rarely fail to triumph over all difficulties. Sooner or later the bladder is reached,[1] and the case is under control. On the third or the fourth day the same filiform instrument will pass with greater facility, and a larger one will usually follow; the treatment by dilatation is fairly under way.

In those exceptional cases just alluded to, where a filiform bougie can be introduced only after long and persevering effort, it becomes a serious question whether it is not better either to tie it in, thus obtaining a more rapid and certain dilatation, or to perform urethrotomy at once rather than to incur the risk of having to operate without a guide later. The temptation to operate on such a case is great, but the necessity for operation is more apparent than real. The selection of treatment depends upon the requirements of the case. Urethrotomy is certain, and is usually the speediest cure, but it puts the patient in bed for a week, perhaps longer. Continuous dilatation, with the filiform tied in, is somewhat dangerous if the patient is up and about, but is a very satisfactory way of commencing treatment if he is willing to go to bed for a few days. Intermittent dilatation may result in retention, leaving him worse off than at first; yet, as a rule, on the third day the filiform may be reintroduced and followed by larger instruments, and the cure is under way. The alternative so frequently employed of introducing a tunnelled sound forcibly over the filiform usually amounts to divulsion, and as such is a dangerous practice; but, if the tunnelled sound can be insinuated gently this is an excellent measure.

If continued dilatation is selected, the filiform should be replaced on the second or the third day by a slightly larger instrument, and this removed one or two days later, after which intermittent

---

[1] In one (personal) case it required ten sittings, most of them over one hour long, before any instrument could be made to enter the bladder. At the tenth effort, the instrument passed.

dilatation may be taken up, or dilatation may be begun when the filiform is removed.

4. **Retention.**—A patient with stricture may be enjoying good health, when suddenly, after exposure to cold, after a dinner or a carouse, or after the passage of a small instrument through his stricture, he finds that he cannot pass water. If he does not get relief, his bladder fills up, and after twenty-four to thirty-six hours, most of which time is passed in acute suffering, a little urine forces its way through the stricture, and he has overflow (often inaccurately styled incontinence). Such an overdistention of the bladder ultimately causes atony; hence every means should be employed to avert it, and to preserve the bladder from an injury the effects of which are sometimes permanent.

The most frequent cause of retention is sudden acute inflammation of the stricture, by which the already narrow canal becomes occluded. In this condition, as a rule, a fine catheter, or filiform bougie, can be introduced by the exercise of patient gentleness and skill. If the bladder is reached, a flow of urine will follow the withdrawal of the instrument. If the bladder cannot be reached, the patient should be placed in a hot bath, more hot water being added after he has become accustomed to the first heat, and this carried as high as bearable. He should remain in the bath from fifteen to twenty minutes, and will often be able to empty his bladder while in the water. A sitz bath, at a temperature of 100° to 104° F., is sometimes more effective than a full bath, but it should only be continued for about three minutes, and may be repeated after an interval of fifteen minutes. If the heat is sufficient to induce nausea or faintness, it is more likely to produce the desired effect of relaxing the stricture.[1] A piece of ice in the rectum every few minutes may be tried (Cazenave).

If these expedients fail and percussion reveals a bladder only slightly distended, reaching not more than half-way up to the umbilicus, 5 centigrammes of opium may be given every hour. The nervous excitability attending retention is thus relieved. The pain soon ceases, the patient's fears become quieted, and after the fourth or fifth dose urine will generally flow. Twenty-drop doses of the sesquichlorid of iron, administered every fifteen minutes, for two hours, at the same time with the opium, seem to facilitate relaxation of the stricture. Finally, an instrument can often be introduced under the entire relaxation of anesthesia.

---

[1] In a robust and full-blooded subject, blood may be drawn from the perineum by leeches.

In a case of retention, if a filiform bougie can be passed into the bladder, the advantage so gained should not be lost, but the instrument should be tied in and treatment by continuous dilatation (see above) or urethrotomy instituted. If no instrument can be passed and all other means fail, the bladder may be aspirated every eight hours for one day. Then the patient is put into a hot bath for twenty minutes, a 2% solution of cocain is injected into the urethra and held there for five minutes, and a final attempt made to introduce a filiform. This failing, the stricture may be fairly considered impassable.

In drawing the urine from a distended bladder it is well not to remove more than 25 c. c. (℥viij) at a time. If there is more than this draw off the remainder after twenty minutes. Too quick emptying of an acutely distended bladder has been followed by hemorrhage, collapse, and sudden death.

5. **Impassable Stricture.**—No stricture (congenital atresia excepted) is impervious unless the urethra has been cut across and united anteriorly, all the urine escaping behind the cut, or unless stricture has gone on contracting for an indefinite period, the urine escaping through large fistulæ. If a drop of urine can pass, the stricture is pervious, but nevertheless it may be impassable to any instrument, or to any skill and patience we may bring to bear upon it, and that, too, although the urine flows in a considerable stream. The absence of retention relieves the surgeon of the immediate necessity of emptying the patient's bladder and gives him time to coax the stricture into admitting an instrument. When there is retention time may be gained by aspiration.

How far the surgeon shall continue coaxing the urethra before resorting to external urethrotomy without a guide is a matter to be decided on the merits of each individual case. If the patient has had retention before, his experience then will aid in forming a judgment. If the surgeon is acquainted with the temper of the urethra and the character of the stricture (resiliency, traumatic origin), he may found his opinion on such previous knowledge. If the patient is difficult to manage, and there is fear that, once relieved from his present necessity, he may not submit to treatment, it would be only a kindness to take advantage of his misfortune by insisting upon perineal section at once, thus putting him in the way of keeping off further trouble by the passage of a large instrument.

But external perineal urethrotomy without a guide is an exceedingly difficult operation, and is not to be undertaken unadvisedly. If it is the patient's first retention, if he was previously passing a fair-sized stream, and if the bladder is not already too full, it is always well to try palliative measures. But, on the other hand, it is not wise to fritter away time to the permanent detriment of the patient's bladder and kidneys when a single stroke of the knife would solve the difficulty.

6. **Traumatic and other Resilient Strictures.**—As has been observed (p. 37) traumatic strictures close down with great rapidity and are very rebellious to treatment. They are resilient. When dilated ever so little they recontract and often are made worse, rather than better, by sounds. Under such conditions dilatation is a losing game. The knife must be used. When the scar is linear, simple perineal section will suffice to render it amenable to the sound. When, as is often the case, the scar is annular and fibrous, all the scar tissue, both on roof and floor, must be cut away. The urethral wound may need to be closed by suture or graft, but that does not signify: the scar must be removed at all costs, since it never loses its retractile quality, and simple section will be followed by a recontraction almost as rapid as after the original injury.

Other resilient strictures must be dealt with similarly.

7. **Inodular or Indurated Stricture.**—Strictures which involve a considerable length of the urethra, masses of scar whose irregularities can be felt externally, and strictures complicated by fistula often do ill under dilatation. When they come to operation they may perhaps be improved by simple section, but the only way to do them justice is to excise the urethral roof and floor and if necessary to fill in the gap by suture or graft.

8. **Stricture complicated by Prostatitis** (*Irritable Stricture*).—Many strictures classed as irritable in reality present no peculiar irritability in themselves, but, situated in the bulb, they are complicated by a catarrhal prostatitis. As soon as the point of the sound or the bougie passes well through the stricture it glides over the prostatic urethra—the really irritable point—though, be it understood, only the minority of strictures complicated by prostatitis are irritable—and provokes an exacerbation of the prostatic inflammation, and very likely a sharp chill. When such a complication presents itself the simplest solution is perineal section; but this is not always essential. By bracing the patient's general health, by treating the prostatic inflammation, by using the utmost gentleness in sounding, by preferring bougies which are less violent to the prostatic urethra than sounds, or else blunt sounds whose points need not enter the prostate at all, and by treating the stricture only sufficiently to permit local treatment of the prostatitis until the latter is materially

improved—by such means the operation may often be avoided. Yet I know no condition which may more tax the surgeon's experience and ingenuity.

Summary of Treatment of Stricture

1. Alkalies, diluents, and rest are serviceable in most cases of stricture—sometimes indispensable if there be any serious complication.

2. All uncomplicated strictures, not highly irritable or resilient, should be treated by dilatation with soft instruments up to No. 15 French, and with conical steel sounds afterward; reintroductions being made every third or fourth day.

3. Until well acquainted with the temper of a given stricture every sounding should be preceded by urotropin, followed by nitrate of silver.

4. Dilatation need rarely be carried beyond the calibre of the normal meatus.

5. Any stricture resisting dilatation must be cut.

6. For the pendulous urethra, internal urethrotomy. For the perineal urethra, external urethrotomy or the combined operation.

7. In general, anterior stricture of the urethra is curable, deep stricture of the urethra incurable.

8. Impassable stricture without retention may usually be overcome with whalebone bougies by time, patience, and skill. If finally proved impassable, the treatment is external perineal urethrotomy.

9. Retention is treated by hot baths, ether, opium, tincture of the sesquichlorid of iron; failing these, by aspiration, or by external urethrotomy without a guide.

10. Traumatic stricture may be prevented by section at the time of injury. Once having shown itself, it usually requires excision for a cure.

11. Resilient and inodular strictures are best treated by excision.

12. Irritable strictures may often be cured without cutting.

Case of Urethral Instruments

The subjoined list includes the instruments required by the general practitioner for the treatment of stricture:

Gauge.

Conical steel sounds, Nos. 15 to 33, preferably double taper from 24 up.

Several whalebone filiform guides.

Conical woven French bougies, sizes 5 to 18.

Set of bulbous bougies, or blunt sounds, or a urethrometer.

1. The more the bladder is distended the less able is it to exert any great force or to produce more than a dribbling stream, even after the urethral right of way has been re-established.

2. When a urinary pocket is opened, and its urethral orifice found, the urine never gushes out, but flows drop by drop.

In short, although the mechanical theory of urinary extravasation explains with charming simplicity the type cases of extravasation—a large invasion of the tissues behind a tight stricture—it does not explain all the phenomena, nor even all the cases of extravasation, and is not compatible with certain clinical facts. Indeed, Escat[1] and Cottet[2] go so far as to deny that the clinical picture of mechanical extravasation exists. The terrible straining and agony suddenly relieved with a feeling of something giving way in the perineum, and soon followed by extravasation, is, it would seem, a description devised to fit a theory.

But if a purely mechanical theory fails to explain the facts, they are fully elucidated on the basis of infection. Without discussing the details, which may be found in the essays of Escat and Cottet, the theory may be set down thus: Although many patients go through all the other complications of stricture, and even come to their deaths thereby, they may never develop any marked urethral dilatation, nor any urinary pouch, abscess, or extravasation. Yet others—even some with stricture of large calibre—especially if enfeebled by alcoholic or other excess or by a long continuance of the disease, may suffer any or all of these local complications. The underlying lesion, therefore, in all (or nearly all) these cases is a stricture, commonly an old stricture. Hallé and Wassermann[3] make the following remarks:

"The most striking feature of a stricture resulting from a chronic urethritis" (read, "an old stricture") "is the extent of the lesion; the whole canal is involved from the meatus to the neck of the bladder. Though constriction has only occurred at a few points, the sclerotic urethritis has implicated the greater part of the canal. . . . To these long-established sclerotic lesions recent inflammatory changes are often added at certain points. Underneath the epithelium confluent areas of small-celled infiltration appear. These usually occur at points of flexure and about irregular areas on the surface of the canal. Perhaps this area of round-cell infiltration extends and invades the spongy tissue. Such a focus has manifestly a suppurative tendency."

---

[1] Guyon's Annales, 1898, xvi, 897 and 1026.

[2] Thèse de Paris, 1899, and Guyon's Annales, 1899, xviii, 590.

[3] Guyon's Annales, 1894, xii, 244, 321.

Such is the soil. Upon its surface there is chronic catarrh; in its substance areas of tissue tending to suppuration in the midst of a dense sclerotic mass—fit nest for any inflammation. Grant any determining factor—deterioration of health, local trauma, acute retention, exposure or excess—and inflammation ensues. Hence any of the following types:

1. Suppuration within the stricture causes *periurethral abscess*, which—

   a. Remains localized and quiescent.

   b. Is absorbed.

   c. Extends into the perineum and scrotum.

   d. Opens into the urethra and—

      α. Discharges and heals.

      β. Remains as a fibrous sac filled continuously or intermittently with urine, and communicating with or shut off from the urethra. (*Urinary pouch.*)

      γ. Fills with urine and bacteria, whose ravages rapidly spread the infection, causing *infiltration*, *extravasation*, *phlegmon*, *abscess*, *or gangrene.*

2. Suppuration on the surface of the sclerotic tissue, usually behind, sometimes at, and rarely in front of the stricture, may cause *dilatation of the urethra*, *periurethritis*, *periurethral abscess* (with the associated lesions just noted), or, if the physical and bacterial conditions are appropriate,[1] *gangrene of the urethra* alone or of the surrounding tissues as well.

3. To fill out and complete the theory that these accidents depend solely upon the combination of individual predisposition and bacterial virulence, two other conditions may be explained by it: the one, *malignant gangrene of the genitals*, a spontaneous gangrene extending over the genitals, sparing the deeper tissues, terminating in recovery, occurring in young subjects with genito-urinary history or disease, and quite comparable to noma, though not fatal; the other, *genital gangrene of old prostatics* long habituated to catheter life, a similar condition, not diabetic in origin, terminating in death (Guyon and Albarran, quoted by Escat). These rare conditions can arise from no source other than a fortuitous combination of soil and seed, comparable to that presented by gangrenous extravasation.

---

[1] Cottet quotes Veillon and Zuber's law, "No gangrene or putrefaction without anaërobic bacteria," and finds in all the cases examined by him that when anaërobic bacteria were present there was gangrene, and when they were absent, even with extensive infiltration, there was no gangrene. He confesses that the suggestion requires further clinical confirmation.

Clinical Types

Periurethritis.—In almost any long-strictured urethra there can be felt, by introducing a sound and palpating the canal against it, irregular masses of cicatricial tissue occupying more or less of the whole length of the canal. A sensitive nodule in this mass indicates an area of periurethral inflammation that may, at any time, develop into an abscess.

Periurethral Abscess.—With the onset of suppuration in this tissue there is a sharp, septic febrile reaction—one of the many septic fevers classed by patients as dumb ague. The lump grows rapidly larger, more painful, and tender, and it may encroach upon the urethra sufficiently to cause retention. Ultimately, as indicated above, it opens into the urethra, or passes into a chronic stage, or more commonly extends into the perineum, burrowing thence throughout the subcutaneous tissue of the external genitals, the thighs, the groins, and even to the lower belly, discharging at many points, and leaving the whole region a mass of fistulæ, through which the urine escapes, perhaps not one drop passing by the natural channel. In these cases the patient makes water sitting, the urine escaping as though through the sprinkler of a watering-pot. Civiale reports a case of urinary fistula with fifty-two external openings.

Urinary Infiltration (*Periurethral Phlegmon, or Urethral and Periurethral Gangrene with or without Urinary Infiltration*).—Beginning as an acute or a chronic periurethral abscess, or as a gangrene of the urethral wall, the acute infective process rapidly spreads over the perineum and the genitals. The first sign is a tender edematous swelling in the median line of the perineum which rapidly increases in size and spreads superficially in every direction. If there is gangrene this reaches the surface within twenty-four or forty-eight hours, and spreads with frightful rapidity. If there is not gangrene the enormous edematous swelling, which may reach the size of a child's head, breaks up into innumerable foci of suppuration, from which pus, and, later, pus and urine pour out. Accompanying all this are shock, severe septic symptoms, and usually retention of urine.

It is usual in these cases for the tumour to be extensively infiltrated with urine, and to contain one or more irregular central cavities filled with urine, necrotic tissue, and pus; but there may be no appreciable infiltration nor any communication with the urethra, and urethrotomy without a guide may be required to relieve the retention.

The bladder never becomes gangrenous, though the urethra slough to its very neck. The suppuration and gangrene may leave a urethro-rectal fistula, but the cavity of the pelvis is never invaded. In practice it is always found that infiltration starting from the membranous urethra at first extends forward to the perineum and only secondarily passes backward to the rectum.

Inasmuch as urinary infiltration usually occurs in debilitated persons, and is itself a very virulent septic process, it usually terminates fatally.

Treatment.—*Prophylaxis.*—No serious disorder is more entirely preventable than urinary infiltration. Intelligent treatment of the stricture and early incision of all foci of suppuration about the perineal urethra would suffice to obliterate the condition. But even passing over these precautions, there is a very fair proportion of cases that have their dumb ague for days with but slight local symptoms until, finally, they burst into full infiltration, and it is too late. A careful physical examination would disclose the tender perineal mass, the proper incision of which might save a life.

Radical Treatment.—There is no sane palliative treatment of periurethritis and its complications. The *simple inflammatory areas* should be treated by methodical soundings, perhaps aided by hot sitz baths and leeches to the perineum. Under such a course they rapidly suppurate or disappear.

Periurethral abscess (p. 129) requires prompt evacuation and drainage by median perineal incision. The urethra should be opened and the stricture cut. In dealing with small abscesses this is a simple matter. Large ones should be cut and drained like infiltrations.

Infiltration of urine demands immediate and radical incision. The patient's life is entirely in the surgeon's hands. Timorous incision is the patient's death-warrant. The infiltrated area must be slit open from end to end. Necrotic tissue must be sacrificed with no thought of ultimate disfiguration. Every boggy pocket must be opened up and drained. Although each case presents its own special features, all may be made subject to certain general operative rules:

1. Operate immediately and fearlessly, with the knife, not the thermo-cautery.

2. With the patient in the lithotomy position, let the first incision be from end to end of the infiltrated area in the median line. Below it may reach to within ½ inch of the rectum. Above it may split the scrotum to the root of the penis, thence up one or both groins. (Escat reports a cure after an incision 16 inches long.) Carry the incision down to the perineal urethra, and then with the fingers break into all urinary necrotic and suppurating foci, and destroy the partitions between them. Next, with scissors and knife,

clip away all masses of necrotic tissue and make the way clear for drainage of all parts of the wound. Parallel lateral incisions are rarely required.

3. The bladder must be opened and drained, either through the perineum or above the bone, before the patient leaves the table.

4. The stricture must be cut, but occasionally this may be deferred until a later date.

5. The after-treatment must be supporting and cleansing; stimulants, irrigations, and drainage.

URETHRO-PERINEAL FISTULA

Varieties.—Urethral fistulæ are congenital (p. 13) or acquired. Acquired fistulæ are penile (p. 129), perineal, or urethro-recto-perineal. Perineal fistulæ are blind internal (urinary pouch), blind external (perineal sinus), or complete. Fistulæ may originate in the pendulous (p. 129), the prostatic (p. 247), or the bulbo-membranous urethra. Only the last concern us here.

A fistula from the bulbo-membranous urethra, though commonly spoken of as perineal or perineo-scrotal, may extend to any point that infiltration can reach—rectum, groin, thighs, abdomen. Desnos mentions one extending to the lower angle of the scapula.

Rectal fistula will be considered in another place (p. 247).

The fistula usually follows abscess or infiltration, rarely trauma, or cancerous, calculous, or tubercular ulceration. Its internal orifice is usually single, however many the outward openings. The fistula, if long and tortuous or branched, contains diverticula which repeatedly close, form abscesses, and discharge; or, again, they contain foreign bodies or calculi, or the entire tract may be encrusted with calculus.

Complete urethro-perineal fistulæ have been classified by Thompson [1] as simple fistulæ, fistulæ with induration, and fistulæ with loss of substance.

Simple fistula is a direct tract without indurated walls.

Indurated fistula is embedded in a mass of sclerotic tissue. It may be branched, and is often tubercular or epitheliomatous. Fibromata (Monod) and fibromyomata (Cocteau) are found in the walls.

Prognosis.—Blind internal fistulæ tend to close unless there is stricture. If they persist, there is danger that they may suppurate and form the starting-point for abscess or infiltration.

---

[1] Stricture of the Urethra, 2d Edit., Lond., 1858, p. 357.

Blind external fistulæ close spontaneously, or after cauterization or curettage.

Complete fistulæ will close when the impediment to urination (stricture, calculus, foreign body) is removed, unless there is considerable loss of substance, or the fistula is tuberculous or cancerous.

Treatment.—The chief point in the treatment of fistula is to remove the impediment to urination—in most cases to *dilate the stricture.* This done, every simple fistula will close itself; but as long as the urethra is obstructed the urine will seek the freest outlet —viz., the fistula.

Indurated fistula is usually associated with resilient or impassable stricture. To cure it all the scar tissue about the fistula and the urethra must be excised and external urethrotomy performed.

Fistula with loss of substance may sometimes be cured by a median section connected by radiating incisions with all the branches of the fistula and the insertion of a graft between the separated ends of the urethra. Too often, however, such an operation simply leaves the fistula larger than ever.

Sir Astley Cooper [1] records the closure of a fistula "the size of a pea" by injections of nitric acid after two operations with hairlip pins and suture had failed. Such a result encourages the hope that the injection of a concentrated solution of hydrogen peroxid, which has proved so eminently curative of the baffling penile fistula (p. 129), may also prove serviceable for the cure of perineal fistula with loss of substance.

Tubercular fistula closes only when thoroughly curetted or excised.

Cancerous fistula is a minor complication of a mortal disease.

The catheter *à demeure* and epicystotomy have been employed in the cure of fistula.

Symanowsky's operation may also be applied to fistula with loss of substance in the perineum. Sabine first adopted it for the perineum, and McBurney,[2] in an admirable paper, clearly detailed his experience with it in 6 perineal cases, 5 of which were successful. The operation apposes two large, raw, flat surfaces to each other, and covers the fistula with a double thickness of flap. I have found this very easy of execution.

A straight incision in the skin is made through the centre of the fistula in the pendulous urethra, at its right edge in the perineum— always in the long axis of the urethra. The parts must be clean, washed, and shaven, and it is better, if hairs grow on the flap to be turned in, that they should be removed by electrolysis as a first step

---

[1] Surgical Essays, Lond., 1819, p. 205.

[2] New York Med. J., 1886, v, 513.

in the operation. The edges of the fistula must be curetted and cleaned of all suppurating granulations. The length of incision in the anterior urethra varies with the size of the fistula. In the perineum the incision commences $\frac{3}{4}$ inch in front of, and terminates at the same distance behind, the fistula. The incision goes through the superficial fascia. On the right of this incision, the skin and superficial fascia are dissected up to form a half-oval pocket, sufficiently deep to take in a flap turned over from the other side. On the left of the first incision, another half-oval flap is made of skin and superficial fascia. Its greatest width in the perineum is $\frac{3}{4}$ inch. This flap is dissected up towards the median line until it can be turned over as on a hinge. Enough tissue is left at the hinged line to insure the vitality of the flap. The cutaneous surface of this flap is freely rawed with curved scissors, except that part which, when the flap is turned over into its place, covers the fistula.

Catgut sutures, passed from the right edge of the undermined flap into the pocket, take in the free edge of the flap to be inverted, and are again passed through the pocket and out upon the surface near the point of entrance. In this way a number of loops are formed, with which the inverted flap is pocketed and drawn snugly into place. A few more catgut sutures are passed from the surface of the undermined flap through the raw surface of the inverted flap, and serve to bind together the raw surfaces. Finally, the edge of the undermined flap at the line of the first incision is united by many points of suture to the curved edge on the other side, from which the inverted flap has been cut away. Bichlorid irrigation, iodoform, cotton, and a T-bandage with pressure, complete the dressing. An opiate confines the bowels at first, and a catheter is used for many days every time the patient urinates, the bladder being washed with a solution of boric acid each time. One of McBurney's cases took over three months to get well. The other 4 were healed in thirteen, seventeen, nineteen, and thirty-four days respectively. Of course the entire urethra must be freed from stricture before the plastic operation is attempted.

CHAPTER XV

THE PROSTATE: ANATOMY, PHYSIOLOGY, EXAMINATION, TUBERCULOSIS, CONCRETIONS, FISTULA

ANATOMY

THE prostate (*προστατα*, *standing before*) is a sexual organ, partly glandular, partly muscular, lying in front of the bladder about the prostatic urethra (Fig. 67).

In shape the prostate is an irregular truncated cone. It has been aptly compared to a horse-chestnut. Its apex rests against the posterior layer of the triangular ligament. Its base, towards the bladder, is pierced above by the urethra, below by the ejaculatory ducts. Its upper (anterior) and lateral surfaces are rounded, its lower (posterior) surface presents a boss on each side of the median line. It is to this lower surface particularly that the title heart-shaped or chestnut-shaped applies.

The *diameters* of the prostate, as given by von Frisch[1] (and Thompson[2]) are: length, 33 to 45 mm. (25 to 30 mm.); width at the base, 34 to 51 mm. (32 to 40 mm.); thickness, 13 to 24 mm. (20 to 25 mm.). Its *weight* is 16 to 20 grammes. In *position* it is 8 to 12 mm. below the symphysis, and its apex is 30 to 40 mm. from the anus. Its long axis makes an angle of 20 to 25 degrees with the perpendicular.

The prostate is supported by the pubo-prostatic ligaments and the levator prostatæ (anterior fibres of the levator ani).

It is fixed in its relations to the urinary organs by the urethra, which pierces it from base to apex, as well as by the decussation of its muscular fibres with those of the bladder and the urethra. It is separated from the pubic arch above and in front and from the rectum behind by a loose fascia containing the large prostatic plexus of veins.

The prostate is composed of two *lateral lobes* that develop inde-

[1] Nothnagel's Specielle Path. u. Therap., 1899, xix, ii, iii, 4.

[2] The Diseases of the Prostate, 1883, p. 5.

pendently during the first half of intra-uterine life, and then become united behind the urethra by the so-called *posterior commissure* (isthmus, pars intermedia), at the same time covering over the urethra by a thin layer, the *anterior commissure*. In the adult prostate the lateral lobes are felt as bosses on the under surface of the organ, the posterior commissure as the groove between them. The so-called *third or middle lobe* and the prostatic *bar* are products of senile and inflammatory changes, and are not found in the normal prostate (p. 256).

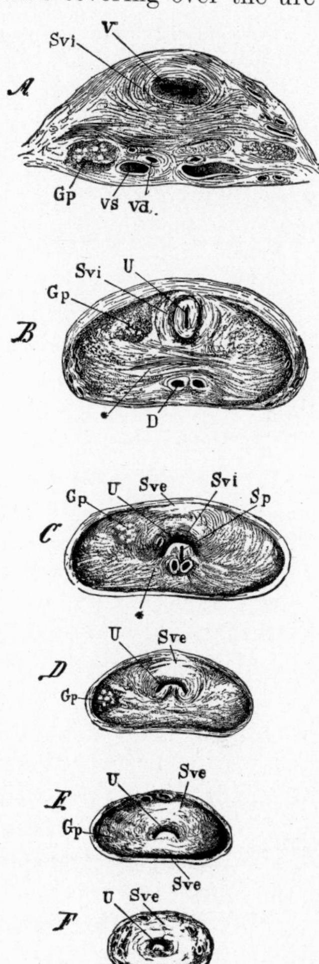

FIG. 67.—CROSS-SECTIONS OF THE PROSTATE IN A SERIES FROM BASE TO APEX.

V, urethral orifice of bladder; *U*, urethra; *Vd*, vas deferens; *Vs*, vesiculæ seminales; *D*, ejaculatory duct; *Sp*, utricle; *Svi* and *Sve*, sphincter vesicæ internus and sphincter prostatæ externus; *, muscular septa.

Structure.—On section the prostate is found surrounded by a dense fibrous capsule that sends thin septa inward between the glands and among the muscle fibres. The organ itself is composed mainly of unstriped muscle and glandular elements. There is a framework of connective tissue, which contains many elastic fibres. Authorities are curiously at variance as to the relative amount of muscular and glandular tissue in the organ. Thus Kölliker (von Frisch) states that from two thirds to three fourths of the organ is muscular; Rüdinger (*ibid.*) says that the glands occupy from one third to four fifths of the whole; finally, Walker insists that the glandular substance forms five sixths of the organ.[1] However this may be, it is acknowledged that the glands are densest in the lateral masses and the posterior commissure (especially its upper part), while in the anterior commissure the glands are few or wanting altogether.

The *muscular tissue* is arranged in so irregular a manner that no two observers are agreed as to its exact distribution. Walker believes that the

[1] Johns Hopkins Bull., 1900, xi, 242.

prostatic muscle is so arranged as to compress the gland as a whole, and each individual lobule of it in particular, but is not calculated to compress the urethra. This view is in accord with the fact that women — who possess no prostate — have complete control of the bladder without any additional muscle to take the place of this gland.

The *glands* are of the compound racemose type with columnar epithelium, which may be flattened by pressure. They are collected into lobules, each lobule surrounded by a layer of muscle and emptying by a duct into the lateral portions of the floor of the prostatic urethra, some behind and some in front of the verumontanum. Walker has shown that in dogs all these ducts point towards the orifices of the ejaculatory ducts, so that the prostatic secretion is mingled with the semen at the moment of ejaculation. The lobules of glandular tissue are chiefly contained in the lateral lobes and the posterior commissure. In later life both glands and ducts commonly contain concretions (p. 246).

The Prostatic Urethra.—The urethra extends from the bladder downward and forward through the prostate, so that, although the major part of the gland lies below and behind it, the urethra emerges quite at the centre of the apex of the prostate. The prostatic urethra is fusiform in shape when dilated with fluid, crescentic when empty (Figs. 5 and 67). Its roof and lateral walls are smooth, pierced by but a few ducts. The floor consists of two lateral portions pierced by the prostatic ducts, and a central irregular part. This central portion rises slowly from behind forward to form a little mound, the *verumontanum* (colliculus seminalis, caput gallinaginis). The anterior slope of the verumontanum is hollowed out by a little cavity, the *sinus pocularis* (utricle), the analogue of the uterus. The ejaculatory ducts open upon the edges of the sinus.

Structure.—The epithelium of the prostatic urethra is squamous, like that of the bladder. Its muscle consists of a thin internal longitudinal and an external circular coat. From this latter is developed the internal (involuntary) sphincter of the bladder. Most authors place this muscle as an annular mass of fibres at the bladder orifice, the so-called neck of the bladder, and consider it an integral part of the prostate rather than of the urethra. In a recent publication, however, Kalischer[1] has brought to light several new and interesting facts. After a searching investigation of the literature and a series of observations on sections made from both the infant and the adult cadaver of each sex, he concludes (1) that the internal

[1] Die Urogenital Musculatur des Dammes, Berlin, 1900.

vesical sphincter is part of the urethra and quite distinct from both bladder and prostate, and (2) this muscle is made up of fibres that encircle the canal obliquely, so that (3) this sphincter muscle forms what is commonly known as the trigone of the bladder below, whence passing upward and obliquely around the urethra, (4) it is, on the roof of the canal, separated from the cavity of the bladder by the transverse layers of the bladder muscle. According to this theory the trigone of the bladder is in reality the lower part of the sphincter, and the neck of the bladder is constituted by bladder wall above and urethral sphincter below.

The *verumontanum* is analogous in structure to the prostate. It is a mass of glandular tissue surrounded by unstriped muscle.

PHYSIOLOGY

The prostate is the sexual heart. It has nothing to do with urination, and is quite passive during this act.[1] But towards the sexual function it acts as a muscle, a sensory organ, and a gland.

As a *muscle* it acts to open the ejaculatory ducts, thus permitting the escape of the semen into the prostatic urethra, to express its own secretion into the prostatic urethra, and probably to expel it into the anterior urethra. The accepted function of the verumontanum —viz., to close the vesical orifice and prevent regurgitation of semen into the bladder—has recently been denied (Walker).

The seat of *sensation* in the prostatic urethra is, perhaps, throughout its mucous membrane, but more probably it is confined to the verumontanum. When erection has been stimulated by friction of the glans penis the verumontanum becomes congested and irritated, perhaps by a spinal reflex, perhaps by the gradual influx of semen into the prostatic urethra, and ejaculation results. Thus it is quite logical that pollutions and premature ejaculations should be caused by hypersensitiveness in the prostatic urethra, and should be curable by treatment directed towards blunting the sensitiveness of that region.

The *glandular function* of the prostate is no less interesting. Many investigators confirm the observation that the spermatozoa are immobile in the testicle and the seminal vesicle. This immobility is in part due to the density of the semen, for dilution with any fluid provokes evidence of life in these micro-organisms. The prostatic

---

[1] For the various aspects of this disputed question consult, besides the authors already quoted, Rehfisch, Virchow's Archiv, 1897, cl, 111; Finger, Allg. Wien. med. Zeitung, 1893, xxxviii, 427, 439, 452.

secretion performs this function. But besides acting as a simple diluent it adds something to the semen that keeps the spermatozoa alive some twenty-four hours, whereas other diluting fluids keep them alive only three or four hours.

The *secretion* of the prostate is a thin, turbid fluid of watery consistency (not ropy or sticky), of slight acid reaction, and of seminal odour. Under the microscope it is seen to contain epithelia from the prostatic glands and phosphatic crystals. Concretions are occasionally met with. *Böttcher's crystals*, very rarely seen in normal prostatic juice, are said to be common in azoöspermatous semen. They can be produced in any semen by mixing it with a 1% solution of ammonium phosphate. These crystals are dagger- or cuttle-fish-shaped, large, colourless, and transparent, and are found in sheaf-like clusters. Lubarsch [1] claims to have found them in the testicle, but Fürbringer [2] denies their existence there.

EXAMINATION OF THE PROSTATE

The examination of the prostate includes—

1. Rectal palpation.
2. Determination of the urethral length.
3. Cystoscopy, and
4. Combined examination.

1. **Rectal Palpation.**—Rectal palpation is of all these the most important. To examine the patient to the best advantage his bladder should be moderately full. He should stand facing a table or desk, with his left knee on the seat of a chair (to relax the buttocks and separate the thighs). He is instructed to lean well over the table, and he is then ready for examination. (Dorsal decubitus is also employed.) It is convenient to cover the examining index finger with a cot. The cot or the finger should then be anointed with vaselin and slowly introduced into the rectum. As soon as the finger has passed the internal sphincter it enters a pouch upon the anterior wall of which is felt the membranous urethra for perhaps half an inch, then the prostate.

The normal prostate is but faintly perceptible as a heart-shaped body 1½ inches long, with its apex downward. It should be investigated for evidence of tenderness, hard nodules, enlargement, pulsation, and fluctuation. Above each lobe of the prostate lie the seminal vesicles; if healthy, these cannot be felt.

---

[1] Virchow's Archiv, 1896, cxlv, 316.

[2] Deutsch. med. Woch., 1896, xxii, 603, and Virchow's Archiv, 1896, cxlv, 644.

The so-called stripping or massage of the prostate is a maneuvre executed by rectal touch. The finger, pressing firmly but forcibly against the extreme upper point of one of the lobes, is carried slowly towards the apex with a to-and-fro sinuous course, all the while making firm pressure on the gland. This is repeated several times on each side. To reach the seminal vesicle for a similar procedure it may be necessary to make counterpressure on the abdomen.

2. **The Urethral Length.**—The urethral length or urinary distance is, clinically, the distance a catheter must travel from the meatus before drawing any water from the bladder. While the length of the urethra varies in the healthy individual between 16 and 22 cm. ($6\frac{1}{2}$ and 9 inches),[1] this variation is due to the length of the penis, and, in the great majority of cases, the length of the urethra, estimated by the distance at which the urine begins and ceases to flow when a catheter is pushed in and out, is between 19 and 21 cm. ($7\frac{1}{2}$ and $8\frac{1}{4}$ inches). Any increase in this distance indicates that the prostate is enlarged (p. 257).

3. **Cystoscopy.**—Cystoscopy is of no great value in the diagnosis of diseases of the prostate, although it is sometimes employed on the ground that certain peculiarities of the urethro-vesical fold are characteristic of prostatic hypertrophy.

4. **Combined Examination.**—If a stone-searcher is introduced into the bladder, inverted, and drawn tightly up against the neck of that organ, the prostate may be mapped out between the instrument and the finger in the rectum. This procedure is sometimes quite painful and may usually be dispensed with.

DEFORMITIES OF THE PROSTATE

Deformities of the prostate are exceedingly rare. Its roof is open in exstrophy of the bladder, but its floor seems never to fail. It is never wanting except in connection with extensive lack of development of the whole genital system.

INJURIES OF THE PROSTATE

The prostate by its position is well protected from ordinary casualties, and rarely suffers unless the general injury is very extensive, in which case its implication may be considered unimportant.

The *wounds* of the prostate are incised wounds made in the operation for stone, lacerated wounds in the same operation from the in-

---

[1] Am. J. Med. Sci., 1898, cxvi, 125.

troduction of dilating instruments or the extraction of a large, rough stone, and penetrating wounds (false passage) made by accident or design in trying to pass a metallic instrument of an improper curve through an obstructed urethra (p. 286). The prostate is a patient organ, and bears all these injuries well. Healing after stone operations is exceptionally rapid, and the prostate may even be punctured by a catheter without any evil consequence, unless it be the seat of chronic disease. Injuries to the prostate usually get well if let alone, even if abscess forms in the organ, and abscess is not frequent even after extensive laceration, although the parts be constantly bathed in purulent urine. Injuries of the prostate do not excite much constitutional derangement. Very different, however, is the case if the injury extends beyond the limit of the fibrous capsule of the gland. In such cases the worst complications (pelvic infiltration, abscess, peritonitis) are to be feared, and if the patient escape with his life he is fortunate. These consequences are more likely to occur in the operation for extraction of very large stone (p. 444). Large incisions and thorough drainage constitute the treatment of such injuries.

INFLAMMATIONS OF THE PROSTATE

For obvious reasons the inflammations of the prostate have been considered as complicating gonorrhea (p. 72).

TUBERCULOSIS OF THE PROSTATE

Tuberculosis of the prostate is the central point, as it were, of genito-urinary tuberculosis. The point of origin of genital and urinary tuberculosis is much discussed (pp. 398, 735). Suffice it to say that I believe the prostate is usually primarily involved in the former, sometimes in the latter. But, however this may be, it is through the prostate that tuberculosis of the urinary tract reaches the genitals, and *vice versa*, and it is through tuberculosis of the prostate that the inflammation crosses from one testicle to the other.

Etiology.—Those who consider tuberculosis of the prostate a primary lesion find its chief cause in chronic gonorrheal prostatitis. Sexual excess, calculus, etc., have been incriminated, and in some cases the disease has evidently nothing to do with previous inflammation. Like other tubercular manifestations, it is commonest in the young adult of a tubercular predisposition. I cannot accept infection *in coitu*.

Morbid Anatomy.—Tuberculization seems always to begin just beneath the glandular epithelium. It goes through the ordinary stages of caseation, abscess formation, and fistulization, or it may terminate by cicatrization.

At the beginning the disease is usually confined to one half of the gland, and to the genital apparatus of one side, viz., half the prostate, the vesicle, the vas, and the epididymis. These may all be involved for years before the disease crosses to the opposite half of the prostate. The usual course is thus typically unilateral for a long time, and finally bilateral. Direct extension to the bladder wall is not rare. The anterior urethra is not often invaded. When abscess forms, it may extend to the periprostatic tissue and may burst into the urethra, rectum, bladder, or perineum.

Symptoms.—The disease begins in one of four ways:

1. It is secondary to a chronic posterior urethritis, assuming its specific characteristics imperceptibly, and patient and surgeon are often unaware of the change until rudely aroused by some of the typical manifestations of tubercle.

2. It is apparently spontaneous. The patient comes complaining of gleet or dysuria for which he fails to account.

3. It is a minor feature of an epididymal infection. The patient complains of the enlarged testicle, and is not aware of the shreds or pus in his urine that testify to the prostatic inflammation.

4. Less frequently a spontaneous hematuria or a urethrorrhagia is the first sign of the disease.

Diagnosis.—The course of the malady is peculiarly slow, and it may for a long time simulate simple posterior urethritis. The features that serve to distinguish it from ordinary chronic urethritis are: 1. Tubercular antecedents. 2. Tubercular lesions elsewhere in the body. 3. The discovery of tubercle bacilli in the urine. 4. The discovery by rectal touch of several small hard nodules of tuberculization in the affected half of the gland. 5. A spontaneous tendency to hemorrhages. 6. A peculiar irritability, often so intense that any instrumentation may excite swelled testicle, simple or tubercular, abscess of the prostate, or at least a violent attack of dysuria. 7. The occurrence of tubercular abscess and fistula.

Prognosis.—The prognosis is bad. Death may ultimately occur from gradual deterioration of the patient, or from tubercular disease elsewhere; the latter, perhaps, being of the true miliary type. Recoveries are entirely possible under the continued efficient action of hygienic conditions and proper food. The course of the malady is always exceedingly slow.

Treatment.—Curative treatment is general rather than local. For local treatment the rules laid down for tubercular cystitis (p. 406) apply. The general measures are hygiene, fatty food, tonics, proper clothing, life out of doors, travelling, change of climate, antistrumous medication. These means, intelligently combined, sometimes effect a cure. The climatic cure is the best. If an abscess is found before it has burst into the bladder or the rectum, it should be opened from the perineum, drained and scraped. Curetting the prostatic urethra is likely to do more harm than good. Prostatectomy should not be thought of.

PROSTATIC STONES AND CONCRETIONS

Prostatic stones or calculi are, properly speaking, urinary calculi which have become lodged in the prostatic urethra or in the prostate itself. Prostatic concretions [1] are the result of a concentration of the prostatic secretion, and originate in the gland itself. These are very commonly met with in the prostates of middle-aged men. They are formed of phosphatic salts and epithelial detritus. They rarely attain the size of a pea, and, unless they exceed this size, have no clinical significance. The larger concretions become coated with phosphates, and when they give trouble they are quite indistinguishable from prostatic calculi of vesical origin.

These prostatic calculi are met with of all sizes and shapes. Several may be found separated from one another, perhaps embedded in cysts, which are dilated follicles, or, if many are present, they cause atrophy of the prostatic substance, until the prostate resembles a sack full of small stones, which may be felt rubbing against one another on pressure per rectum, giving an emphysematous-like crackling (Adams). In bad cases prostatic calculi tend to unite, projecting into the urethra, and forming curiously distorted, branched masses, dipping down into the substance of the prostate, and extending forward into the canal of the urethra, and backward perhaps into the bladder. Such masses have been found 4 or 5 inches long. One, removed by T. Herbert Barker, is referred to by Thompson as composed of 9 portions, weighing, collectively, 3 ounces, 4 drams, and 1 grain—about 110 grammes.

Symptoms.—The stones may simply give rise to a rebellious prostatitis, to abscess of the prostate, or to symptoms closely resembling vesical stone. They are often the unrecognised cause of long-standing trouble. Unless they can be felt from the rectum or by a urethral

[1] *Cf.* Siegert, Virchow's Archiv, 1892, cxxix, 513; Pasteau, Guyon's Annales, 1901, xix, 417; Spencer, Phil. Med. J., 1900, vi, 457.

instrument, their existence remains unsuspected until disclosed by perineal section.

Treatment.—The stones should be removed by median perineal section.

URETHRO-RECTAL FISTULÆ

Urethro-rectal fistulæ are very rare. They commonly involve the prostatic urethra. They are caused by trauma (catheterization, lithotomy), abscess of the prostate, tuberculosis, or malignant disease. Tubercular and cancerous fistulæ are quite incurable and need not concern us. Traumatic and inflammatory fistulæ, on the other hand, commonly recover. I once opened a prostatic abscess into the rectum only to find that it had just burst into the bladder. The resultant fistula healed in four weeks. Thompson's [1] case, cured by urinating while on his hands and knees, would, perhaps, have recovered spontaneously.

Treatment.—A large proportion of the cases do not recover spontaneously. They require operative interference. Preliminary cauterization of the fistula may be tried, but success need not be anticipated from such treatment. As a preliminary measure all strictures of the urethra must be cured. Whatever operation is performed should include division of the sphincter ani, preferably by posterior proctotomy. By these means the urethral and rectal channels are freed from all impediments. Continuous drainage of the bladder through the perineum or the urethra is advisable.

Among the many operations suggested to cure this condition the one advanced by White and Martin [2] may be selected. The fistula is exposed through a curved prerectal incision, and thoroughly scraped or excised. Rectal and urethral orifices are then freshened and sutured with catgut. The wound is lightly packed. The authors omit any mention of draining the bladder by a retained catheter or a perineal tube, or of dividing the rectal sphincter by posterior proctotomy, both of which procedures would seem essential to success. An operation successfully carried out by Zembieski and by Fuller may be borne in mind. The feature was dissecting loose the end of the rectum like a cuff, and rotating it so that the two fistulous openings were not opposite each other. In this and all similar attempts it is wise to drain the bladder by perineal tube. (*Cf.* Orville Horwitz [3] and J. P. Tuttle.[4])

---

[1] Diseases of the Urinary Organs, 8th Ed., 1888, p. 175.

[2] Genito-Urinary and Venereal Diseases, 1898, p. 259.

[3] Phil. Med. J., 1901, vii, 70.

[4] Matthews's Quarterly J., 1898, v, 103.

ATROPHY OF THE PROSTATE

Atrophy of the prostate is uncommon. It may occur after the substance of the organ has been materially injured by abscess within or by pressure of a stone outside. Physiological atrophy of the prostate occurs in a certain proportion of old men. This atrophy Thompson observed 11 times among 164 persons over sixty years of age. Messer met with it 20 times in 100 cases (von Frisch), and others give still higher estimates.

The prostate fails to develop in eunuchs, and many authors believe that it atrophies after castration in later life. Idiopathic failure of development has also been observed.

In the atrophied prostate the glandular tissue is shrunken and wasted, and the stroma is but little affected.

Symptoms.—The symptoms of atrophy of the prostate are somewhat obscure. Both enuresis and retention have been attributed to it. Although I have met with it a number of times in old men I have never seen any symptoms referable to it. On the contrary, I have seen retention with atrophy of the prostate relieved by the removal of its cause—contracture of the neck of the bladder.

CHAPTER XVI

HYPERTROPHY OF THE PROSTATE

THE true nature and pathogenesis of hypertrophy of the prostate are not known. We can only describe it as a disease of the latter years of life, a chronic, non-inflammatory hyperplasia of all the tissues of the gland, but especially of the epithelial elements, diffuse in its character, and subject to inflammatory attacks and secondary fibrous metamorphosis.

ETIOLOGY

Age.—The one thing known about the etiology of prostatic hypertrophy is that it occurs at middle age, never giving any trouble before the forty-fifth year, and rarely appearing after the seventieth. Although individual cases have been reported at the ages of nineteen (Stretton), twenty-five (Englisch), thirty-seven (Thompson), etc., the disease cannot be looked for before forty-five. Lydiston and others believe that the prostate begins to hypertrophy in the third decade of life, yet there is no clinical evidence of any such change until twenty years later. In fact, the patients begin to suffer, for the most part, between the ages of fifty and sixty.

To explain the relative infrequency of hypertrophy of the prostate after the seventy-fifth year, Thompson has advanced the theory that the physiological atrophy of old age makes itself felt at this time of life, so that if a man escape until then he is all the more likely to escape thereafter. This senile atrophy does not, however, promise any relief to the sufferer, for when once the urinary mechanism has been upset by the hypertrophy the secondary phenomena cannot be alleviated by any slight atrophy of old age.

Frequency.—According to Thompson's figures, 34% of men reaching the age of sixty have enlarged prostates, and less than half of these (15% to 16% of the whole) suffer from the disease. Many authors give far higher estimates. Thus Johnson,[1] in examining the prostates of 360 men, found hypertrophy present in 79%, yet only 16%

[1] Internat. J. of Surgery, 1899, xii, 98.

—Thompson's own estimate—suffered from the disease. This is only one example of the wide discrepancy in all the statistics relative to hypertrophy of the prostate, a discrepancy founded on confusion of prostatic hypertrophy with contracture of the neck of the bladder, more than on any other one thing (p. 317).

The size of the hypertrophy bears no relation to the age of the patient, nor, as we shall see, to the symptoms.

Pathogenesis.—The popular conception of the nature of prostatic hypertrophy has long been, and still remains, that it is a neoplastic change, fibroma, myoma, or adenoma, according to different theories; while these theories, all proving insufficient to explain the conditions found, have encouraged still other suppositions, such as Guyon's [1] of *arterio-sclerosis*, White's [2] of *sexual senility*, and the theory maintained by many in various phases, that a chronic congestion of the gland is the predisposing cause of prostatic hypertrophy. The theory of arterio-sclerosis has been amply disproven by Casper [3] and Motz,[4] that of sexual senility by the failure of castration to achieve changes in the prostate demanding the support of the theory.[5]

The *neoplastic theory* of prostatic hypertrophy is so immediately suggested by the very appearance of the enlarged gland—which seems to be full of tumours—that it has not been seriously questioned until recent years. Since the time of Griffith, indeed, we have known that the so-called myoma of the prostate was, in fact, fibroma, or adenofibroma, and strict thinkers have always recognized that the prostate was not the analogue of the uterus, and, therefore, the adenofibromatous gland not comparable to the fibromatous uterus.

But these small differences sink into insignificance in the light thrown upon the subject by Ciechanowski's observations. This Polish pathologist has proven that the so-called hypertrophy of the prostate gland is not due to a neoplastic formation; that the senile changes in the prostate—whether they be atrophy or hypertrophy—are essentially the same; that these are due to obscure, inflammatory processes originating in the stroma of the gland; and that the so-called adenomata and fibromata are secondary changes due to the dilatation of gland ducts and acini whose mouths are obstructed.

These revolutionary doctrines have been confirmed by Greene and Brooks [6] and Crandon,[7] and indirectly by Rothschild,[8] and have not been controverted.

---

[1] Guyon's Annales, 1885, iii, 148. [2] Annals of Surgery, 1893, xviii, 152.

[3] Virchow's Archiv, 1891, cxxvi, 139.

[4] Structure histologique de l'hypertrophie de la prostate, Paris, 1896.

[5] So-called Prostatic Hypertrophy, translation edited by Dr. R. H. Greene, 1903.

[6] J. Am. Med. Ass'n., 1902. [7] Annals of Surgery, 1902.

[8] Centralblatt f. d. Krankheiten d. Harn- u. Sexual-organe, 1904.

It is impracticable here to go into the details of the theory, since this is a very complex matter. It need only be observed that the great majority of prostates of men at middle age show evidences of chronic inflammation in the stroma. If these areas of chronic inflammation are situated chiefly in the periphery of the gland, their tendency is to compress it and to cause prostatic atrophy. If located near the urethra, such areas of inflammation may surround and obstruct any or all of the efferent ducts of the prostate. When this occurs the ducts behind the obstruction dilate, and, inasmuch as these ducts run in a crescentic manner and their tendency to dilate is restricted by the dense, fibrous capsule of the prostate, they become somewhat distended by the products of secretion, forming the small cysts (Fig. 69) that are seen throughout the hypertrophied prostate, but they tend more particularly to flatten out and to curve around islands of glandular and muscular tissue. These islands, varying in size, may thus become almost completely encapsulated by the dilated duct.

Such are the pseudo-adenomata which secondary fibrous changes resulting from further inflammation may transmute into fibromata.

The Effect of Gonorrhea.—Ciechanowski notes the fact that the underlying stroma changes found by him in the prostates of old men are the same as those found by Casper in the prostates of young men who had suffered from gonorrheal prostatitis. Hence the inevitable corollary that perhaps the hypertrophy of old age is due to the gonorrhea of youth. This suggestion, tentatively set forth by Ciechanowski, has been seized upon by several writers as an unavoidable inference, and is by them flaunted to the great shame of a large and respectable army of prostatics.

In order to test this theory from the clinical side, I have collected [1] the histories of a great number of men who have reached the age of fifty after having suffered prolonged attacks of chronic gonorrhea, and cannot find that they show any special tendency to suffer from prostatic hypertrophy. This, taken in connection with the fact that every established genito-urinary practitioner can call to mind many prostatics who—he may be morally certain—never had gonorrhea, seems to establish the fact that this underlying prostatic sclerosis is not necessarily gonorrheal, but may be due to the congestion of sexual excess or of continence, to gonorrhea, or simply to advancing years. Where chiefly to lay the blame we do not know; in the meanwhile let charity temper our provisional conclusions.

It seems probable that whatever conclusion is ever reached in this obscure matter will be based upon the fact that the prostate tends to undergo retrograde changes with cessation of its sexual function, as

[1] J. Am. Med. Ass'n, 1904, xliii.

do the uterus and the female breast. How far prostatic hypertrophy will be found attributable to this normal involution, and how far to the congestion of sedentary life, to the inflammations of youth, and to the congestion of sexual excess, the future must determine.

Morbid Anatomy

Microscopic Changes.—There are three general types of hypertrophied prostates—a diffuse, soft "adenomatous" type, a diffuse, hard, fibrous type, and a type characterized by the growth of encapsulated tumours within the gland. No given example of hypertrophy adheres strictly to any one type; indeed, it is the rule to find all three types existing in different parts of the specimen: in one place a diffuse, soft enlargement, in another dense masses of fibrous tissue, and scattered everywhere enucleable tumours, large and small, the larger ones (Figs. 68, 69) complex in structure and composed, like the whole organ, of soft and hard tissue and of enucleable "adenoma."

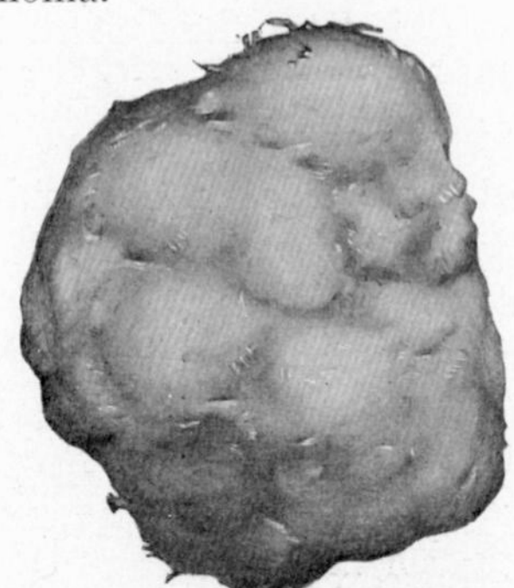

Fig. 68.—Adenoma enucleated from a Hypertrophied Prostate.

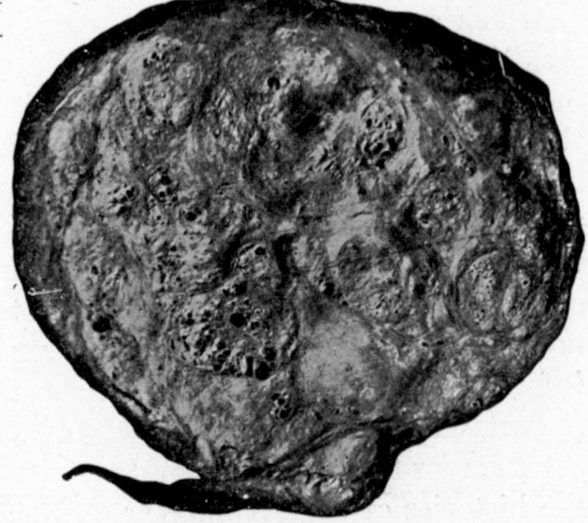

Fig. 69.—Section of a Large Prostatic Adenoma, showing its Composite Character.

These changes are due, as we have seen in the preceding paragraphs, to chronic interstitial fibrosis of the prostate; and however descriptive the terms adenoma and fibroma may be in this connection, we must remember that in using them we do not refer to true neoplasms, but to the pseudo-neoplasms resulting from inflammation of the gland and obstruction of its ducts.

To describe the various changes encountered in the tissues of the hypertrophied prostate would require pages of pathologic detail, interesting only to the special student and already accessible in the works of Ciechanowski, Greene and Brooks, and Crandon.

Diffuse Soft Hypertrophy.—This represents a general distribution of obstructed ducts and of dilated ducts and acini. The cut surface is soft and bulging, dotted with cyst-like spots filled with hard, yellow concretions, or softer, inspissated prostatic secretion. The microscope shows ducts and alveoli widely dilated, their epithelium flattened, their lumen filled with desquamated epithelial cells and detritus, sometimes with pus. Careful examination of serial sections often reveals the point of constriction where a duct is strictured by interstitial infiltration about it and dilated beyond.

Fibrous Hypertrophy.—Here the cut section is hard and fibrous, though scattered traces of soft hypertrophy may be seen. The microscope shows masses of scar tissue, into which the soft " adenomatous " tissue has been transformed by inflammation. Clinically, therefore, fibrous hypertrophy may be regarded as " adenomatous " hypertrophy scarred by prostatitis.

Pseudo-adenoma.—The pseudo-adenomata so constantly found in the aged prostate, whether hypertrophied or not, are due to the excessive dilatation of a large duct which, running normally in a curve and forced to increase this curve as it enlarges, finally almost completely encircles a portion of gland tissue which has undergone soft, hard, or, as in Fig. 69, pseudo-adenomatous hypertrophy.

Macroscopic Changes.—Inasmuch as the hypertrophy may concern any or every part of the organ, a number of varieties of hypertrophy exist and may be tabulated as follows:

		Thompson.[1]	Prédal.[2]	Desnos.[2]	Motz.[3]	Watson.[4]	Total.
Total hypertrophy.	General	74	7	17	8	14	120
	Notably median	19	23	..	1	..	43
	Notably lateral	..	..	..	5	..	5
	Notably unilateral	19	..	5	2	..	26
							194
Partial hypertrophy.	Lateral only	5	15	12	10	4	46
	Anterior commissure only	3	..	..	..	..	3
	All but the median lobe	3	..	..	..	..	3
	Median only	..	19	14	..	9	42
	Median and unilateral	..	..	..	1	2	3
	Pedunculated tumour	..	..	..	..	1	1
							98
		123	64	48	27	30	292

This table shows that all parts of the gland were involved in 65% of the cases, while at least one lateral lobe was enlarged in 84%, both

[1] *Op. cit.*, p. 39.
[2] Desnos, Maladies des voies urinaires, 1898, p. 386.
[3] *Op. cit.*
[4] Operative Treatment of the Hypertrophied Prostate, 1888.

in 83%. Hence, in 84 out of every 100 cases the prostatic enlargement may be diagnosed by rectal touch. My own clinical observation would lead me to put the percentage even higher. Desnos's cases of hypertrophy ranged in weight from 23 to 85 grammes (the normal prostate weighs 20 grammes). Much larger tumours are occasionally met with, but in the usual run of cases the prostate is smaller than an orange.

The most notable changes associated with hypertrophy of the prostate are (1) bulging of the posterior surface of the gland, (2) elevation of the urethral orifice, (3) production of a middle lobe, and (4) lengthening and distortion of the prostatic urethra.

1. **Posterior Enlargement.**—We have seen that in a large proportion of cases the lateral lobes of the prostate are enlarged. Such

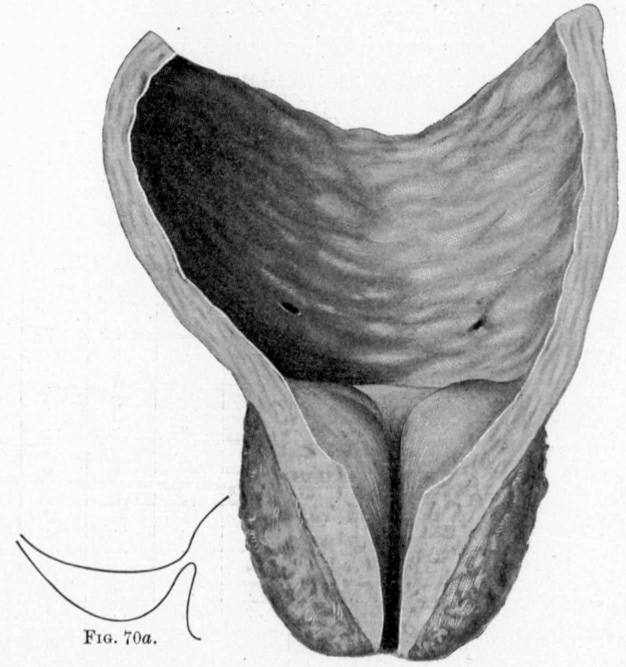

Fig. 70.—Bilateral Hypertrophy of the Prostate without Median Enlargement. The sagittal section (70*a*) shows the elevation of a fold of mucous membrane between the lateral lobes.

an enlargement may always be felt by rectal touch. The examining finger, instead of impinging upon a scarcely perceptible organ, encounters a large mass, perhaps the size of a plum or a mandarin orange, perhaps so much enlarged that its upper border cannot be reached. To estimate the size of the growth the finger is swept over it from side to side, into the sulci between it and the lateral wall of the rectum, and, if possible, over the top of the tumour. Its pro-

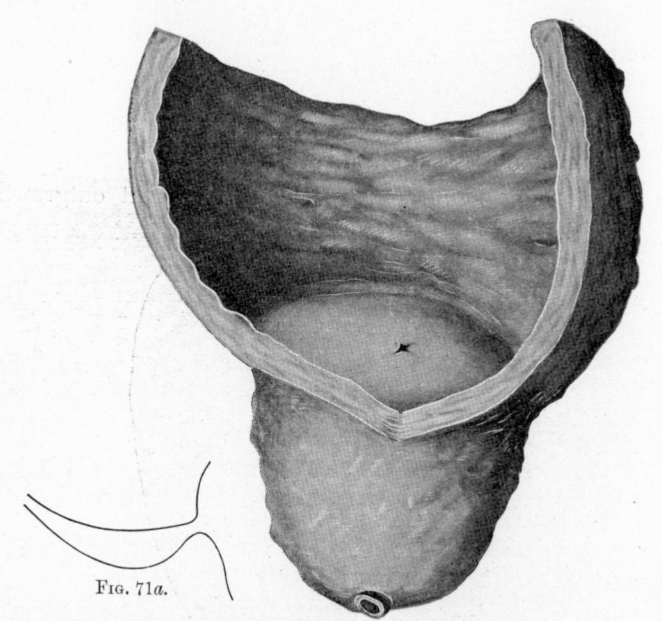

FIG. 71.—GENERAL HYPERTROPHY OF THE PROSTATE, THE MEDIAN AND LATERAL LOBES FORMING A SINGLE MASS.

The sagittal section (71*a*) shows the elevation of the urethral orifice.

jection may thus be fairly estimated and its general character of elasticity or hardness determined. In shape the mass is usually quite globular. It may be furrowed down the centre, showing that the overgrowth has chiefly affected the two lateral lobes, but has spared the posterior commissure. One lobe may be more hypertrophied than the other. Small phleboliths may be felt upon the gland, or hard nodules within it.

2. **Elevation of the Urethral Orifice.**—When bladder and prostate are normal, the urethral orifice practically lies on the same level as the trigone and the floor of the bladder. But every form of prostatic hypertrophy disturbs this relation. If the growth is purely lateral, whether on one or both sides, the tumour lifts a fold of mucous membrane at the urethral orifice (Fig. 70). If there is general hypertrophy, the posterior commissure projects upward into the bladder, pushing the urethra before it and forming the so-called *bar at the neck of the bladder* (Figs. 71, 72). The *third lobe* (Fig. 73) acts in the same way. Finally, the chronic posterior urethritis, so often met with in this disease, may cause a true *contracture of the*

neck of the bladder (p. 317) with increased elevation of the urethral orifice.[1]

In order of clinical frequency the causes of elevation of the urethral orifice are: (1) Bar and contracture with about equal frequency, (2) the third lobe, and (3) rarely, the lifting of the orifice between lateral projections.

3. **The Third or Middle Lobe.**—This term is loosely used to indicate any projection into the bladder, be it bar or tumour. Properly speaking, the middle lobe of the prostate is a distinct outgrowth

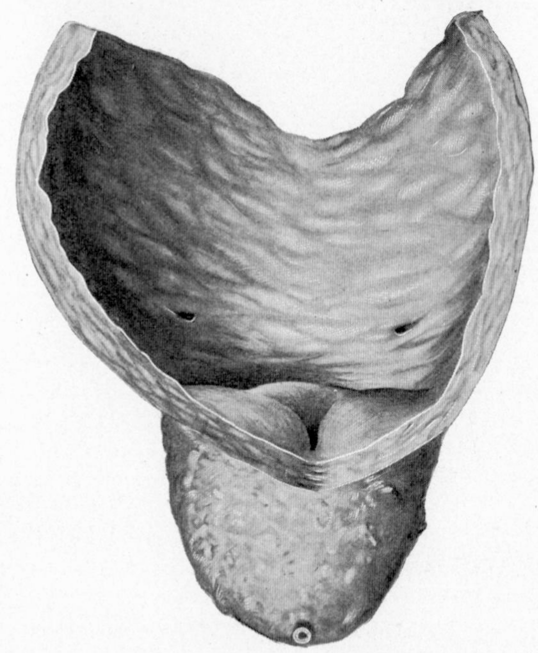

Fig. 72.—General Hypertrophy of the Prostate, with relatively Slight Median Enlargement in the Form of a Bar.

The sagittal section is similar to 71*a*.

from the neck of the bladder or from the floor of the prostatic urethra (Fig. 73). This tumour springs from the posterior commissure of the gland, and was supposed to originate within it. But Jores[2] showed that "its first beginning occurs in the accessory prostatic glands which lie just under the mucous membrane, and the projec-

[1] Rochet (Traité de la dysurie sénile, Paris, 1899) gives some space to the consideration of those unusual forms of hypertrophy in which the upper lobe is chiefly affected, and there is no elevation of the urethral orifice. Such a case was also illustrated in the previous edition of this treatise.

[2] Virchow's Archiv, 1894, cxxix, 224.

tion into the bladder is due at first to the hypertrophy of these alone." Later, the hypertrophy of the pars intermedia usually forms

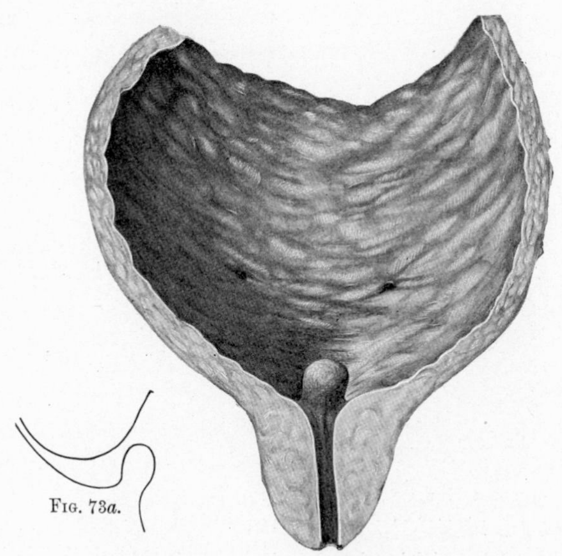

FIG. 73.—PEDUNCULATED MEDIAN ENLARGEMENT.

The sagittal section (73*a*) shows an obstruction quite as pronounced as in 70*a* and 71*a*, but less lengthening, and distortion of the prostatic urethra.

the base of the tumour with the third lobe as its apex. These outlying glands are usually situated at the urethral orifice "directly beneath the mucous membrane and between the circular fibres of the bladder and the middle isthmus of the prostate" (Alexander[1]). There are a few similar glands lying along the floor of the urethra, and occasionally these become hypertrophied and form projections in the floor of the urethra itself. The middle lobe is rarely more than 2 cm. in diameter. It will be observed that some median enlargement is noted in 81% of the tabulated cases (p. 253).

4. **Lengthening and Distortion of the Prostatic Urethra.**—The prostatic urethra is altered in length, size, and curve (Figs. 70*a*, 71*a*, 73*a*, 74, 75). *The urethra is always lengthened* by the increased size of the prostate, whether the hypertrophy be general or circumscribed. But the lengthening of the canal is not very great, unless there is a middle lobe or a prostatic bar to be surmounted before the bladder is reached. This is an important point in relation to prostatectomy, since a long urethra means that a great deal of tissue must be removed to enable the bladder to empty itself, while, if the urethra

---

[1] Med. Record, 1899, lvi, 982.

does not exceed 21 cm. ($8\frac{1}{2}$ inches) in length, a mere incision will set things right in most cases (p. 299).

The urethra is dilated chiefly by the growth of the lateral lobes which enlarge on each side of it and spread it out on a vertical plane, so that, from being a transverse slit, it is altered to a vertical one, with perhaps a curve to one side or the other, where a projection in one lobe fits into a depression in its fellow of the opposite side. The dilatation may be so great that an ordinary sound can be rotated quite freely within the canal, thus giving the false impression that the bladder has been reached. *The curve of the urethra is lengthened.* That is, its internal orifice is carried upward and backward, and the canal, instead of having the short normal curve, sweeps in a curve of much longer radius, a curve that will not transmit the ordinary steel sound, but requires special instruments with the long prostatic curve (Fig. 78). The urethra is further deformed by the presence of the bar, behind which the canal forms a distinct pouch, or by the projection into it of tumours from the various lobes, notably the middle lobe, which sometimes blocks the way completely after the fashion of a ball valve, or may allow the urethral current to flow in one or two streams at either side of its base.

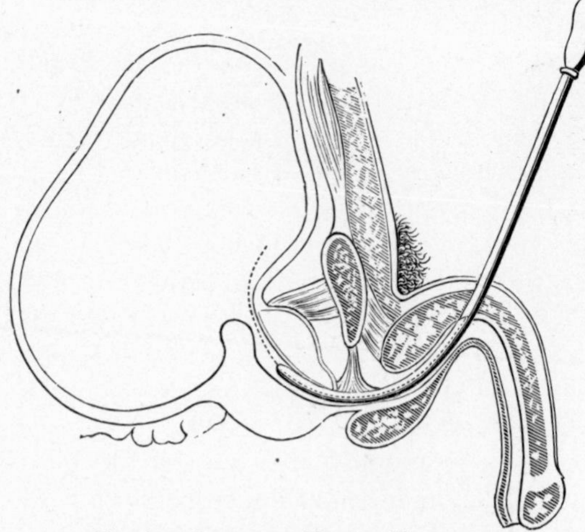

FIG. 74.—POSTERIOR MEDIAN HYPERTROPHY.
Compare the urethral curves in Figs. 74 and 75.

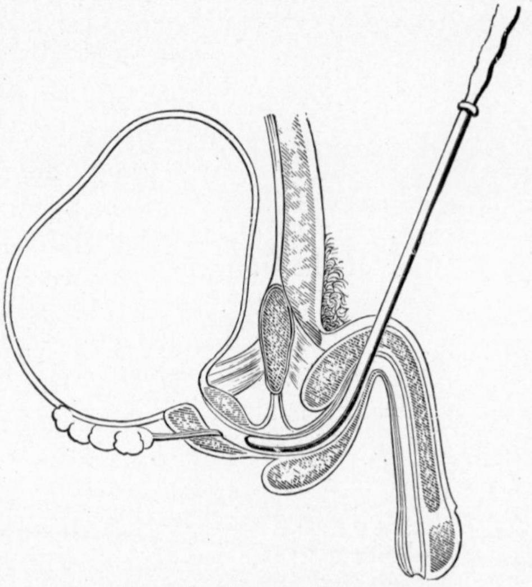

FIG. 75.—HEALTHY PROSTATE.

Pathological Physiology and Secondary Morbid Changes

Retention, Congestion, Inflammation—these are the Fates of the prostatic.

Retention.—The causes of retention of urine are to be found both in the prostate and in the bladder. The prostate is primarily at fault. I do not remember to have seen retention of urine, whether complete or incomplete, in any prostatic who had not some obstruction at the neck of his bladder, some elevation of the urethral orifice (whether such elevation was absolute or merely relative to the bladder), by bar, middle lobe, or contracture of the neck of the bladder. These changes about the urethral orifice disturb its physiological relation to the bladder. When in the act of urination the bladder contracts, it forces the urine over the prostatic bar with great difficulty, and thus it is overstrained. To estimate the effects of this strain, the condition of the bladder at this time of life must be borne in mind. In the child the organ is ovoidal with the sharper end at its neck: it has no floor. But as adult life is reached it settles down into the pelvis. Its trigone becomes more and more horizontal. It acquires a floor. As age advances it tends to sag more and more. In the female it bulges down until it forms a cystocele. But in the male the bladder neck is supported by the urethral and prostatic attachments to the pubes, and, as the bladder sags, it thus tends to pouch behind the prostate, the trigone swings around until it forms the anterior incline of this pouch—the *bas fond,* as the French call it. While there may be some *bas fond* without prostatic hypertrophy, without obstruction of the urethra, such a *bas fond* has no clinical significance. But when there is urethral obstruction, with an extra strain upon the bladder, and heightened vesical tension at a time of life when the muscles are becoming fibrotic and losing their energy, the result is a relatively rapid pouching of the floor of the bladder, a general weakening of its muscle, and an inability of the organ to empty itself completely. The *bas fond* is never dry; there is always some urine left in the bladder; in short, there is *partial retention* of urine. It is as though the bladder were a tank with the outlet upon one side instead of at the bottom. However often the water is allowed to drain off from the tank none of its contents below the level of the outlet pipe can escape and the tank cannot be completely emptied.

As a result of this vesical derangement, and because of the low vitality of its adenomatous structure, the prostate, perhaps still bearing the scars of ancient battles with the gonococcus, is very subject to attacks of *acute congestion.* A Christmas dinner, an exposure to cold, particularly of the legs, a slight alcoholic excess, may bring on acute congestion in a prostate that has given no previous trouble. The patient may have had a little retention of urine quite unconsciously, until some day his acute congestion comes and he cannot pass water. Perhaps he succeeds in relieving himself by dint of hot baths and straining; perhaps his urine has to be drawn from him. The attack may be lasting, or transitory, it may or may not terminate in inflammation; in any case, it causes a temporary *complete retention of urine,* increases the chronic partial retention, and enhances the effects of this retention upon the upper urinary organs. And the constant pressure of the retained urine produces in turn a *chronic congestion* of the prostate.

The Bladder.—The bladder is far from healthy. Its walls, instead of being smooth on the surface and of even thickness, are thickened in some places, thinned in others, and the mucous membrane is thrown into irregular ridges by isolated bundles of hypertrophied muscle, while between these ridges it is bellied out into pouches or diverticula. In general, the cavity of the bladder is dilated or contracted, its wall thickened or thinned, but in all cases, even when the thickened muscular wall bears every sign of great strength, an examination of the muscle tissue reveals that, although there be some real hypertrophy, the bundles of muscle fibres are surrounded and infiltrated by a notable amount of fibrous tissue, sufficient evidence that the bladder is fighting a losing battle (p. 341). Clinical evidence of this soon appears in the guise of a veritable atony of the bladder (p. 344). Many French authors, following Guyon and Lannois, consider this sclerosis of the vesical muscle a feature of the *sclérose urinaire,* natural in old age; but English and American writers attribute the sclerosis, as well as the macroscopic changes in the urinary organs, entirely to the triad of retention, congestion, and inflammation. According to this more plausible view no special *sclérose urinaire* need be invoked.

The Ureters and Kidneys.—After the bladder has begun to feel the effects of its futile struggle, and is undergoing the changes just noted, the upper urinary organs feel the distention. The ureters begin to dilate, first at their vesical orifices, then higher and higher up. In places they attain 2 and 3 times their normal size. Next, the renal pelvis, with the surrounding kidney substance, gives way before the ever-increasing pressure. A hydronephrosis—usually small—is established, and the renal parenchyma slowly and silently atrophies (p. 544).

Congestion.—The prostate is surrounded by a plexus of veins so large and so closely interwoven as to suggest the cavernous spaces of an erectile tissue. (*Cf.* Guépin.[1]) A similar, but smaller, plexus gives erectile power to the verumontanum and the floor of the prostatic urethra, and the gland itself is pierced by numerous branches connecting those plexuses. These groups of veins form one of the connecting links between the portal and the inferior caval systems. Such is the basis of prostatic congestion. An organ so bathed in venous blood falls an easy prey to active, *acute congestion*, the result of exposure to cold, overeating, overdrinking, overexertion, sexual irritation; or to passive, *chronic congestion*, from pressure of residual urine, from overdistention of the bladder, or from the torpidity of intestine so common with advancing age—in fact, due, fundamentally, to that general sluggishness of the pelvic venous circulation that shows itself under the form of varicose veins of the leg, hemorrhoids, and chronic constipation. The congestion is always more marked at night. Whether this is due to spinal or to local congestion is not clear; clinically, however, the congested prostate is always more irritable by night than by day. Hence the characteristic nocturnal frequency of urination of the prostatic.

Inflammation.—We have seen how easily retention leads to congestion. Congestion and inflammation are even more closely allied. It would be to no purpose to recite here the whole tale of inflammations spreading from the prostate and the prostatic urethra to the surrounding tissues and to the remotest corners of the genital and urinary tracts. Suffice it to say that the prostate may become inflamed spontaneously, or as the result of instrumentation, and that any and all of the genito-urinary organs may be infected from it, while the bladder and kidney are necessarily involved soon after the prostatic inflammation is established. This train of *ascending urinary inflammation* once it has become chronic does not disappear so long as the obstacle to urination remains; and in the great majority of cases it is to this that the patient ultimately succumbs, unless relieved by the surgeon.

Phosphatic vesical *calculus* is a common result of the combined retention and inflammation.

In the more advanced stages of prostatic disease the patient gradually fails under his *urinary toxemia* and *septicemia* (p. 561).

---

[1] Guyon's Annales, 1897, xv, 305.

CHAPTER XVII

SYMPTOMS AND DIAGNOSIS OF PROSTATIC HYPERTROPHY

Symptoms

The cardinal symptoms of prostatic hypertrophy are *frequency of urination*, chiefly by night, *difficulty in urination*, and *dribbling* from overflow, irritation, or incontinence.

Frequency of Urination (*Pollakiuria*).—Nocturnal frequency of urination is almost pathognomonic of hypertrophy of the prostate. That the urine is passed too often is due to the congestion of bladder and prostate, which, as a rule, makes them sensitive to a less distention than when in their normal state. We shall see later that increase in local irritability plays the chief part in causing this pollakiuria.

Nocturnal polyuria is, in my opinion, in no way related to the question of residuum. The nocturnal polyuria, which these cases also often manifest, is more an evidence of failing vital force than of dilatation or congestion of the kidney. Indeed, congestion of the kidney is more likely to produce diminution than increase of urinary flow. Surely there is no evidence that hysteria produces kidney congestion, or that anxiety induces it—both of which agencies occasion intense polyuria. If the patient is nervous he may, perhaps, urinate as often by day as by night, but, as a rule, this is not the case. The nocturnal frequency still predominates.

The polyuria—increase in quantity—seems to be uniformly distributed throughout the night; not so the pollakiuria, of which a distinct feature is its tendency to increase towards morning. The urinary intervals shorten as the night wanes, so that, while the early hours of the night may be passed in comparative comfort, the morning hours are constantly disturbed.

Difficulty in Urination (*Dysuria*).—When there is prostatic obstruction the act of urination is always a tedious, a difficult, and even a painful process. This prostatic dysuria has four striking features:

1. The stream is very slow to start. Sometimes the sufferer struggles several minutes before his water will come.

2. The flow lacks force and body. There is no gush of water. It comes in a thin stream, the jet is not great, perhaps it only dribbles forth drop by drop.

3. The greater the strain the less the result. It is curious to note how often patients themselves remark that the more anxious they are to hurry the less they succeed. Their predicament is almost that of the young neurotic subject, to whom any hurry in urinating is an absolute preventive.

4. At the end of the act there is no sharp piston-stroke finish. The urine dribbles away by irregular jets and drops, and the act might be said rather to fade away than to terminate.

The amount of *pain* on urination and general uneasiness in the intervals depends upon the amount of congestion and inflammation.

Dribbling.—Of all the symptoms of prostatic hypertrophy, a constant dribbling is the source of greatest discomfort. Many other symptoms disturb the patient more acutely, but none is more constantly annoying. This dribbling may be due to three widely differing causes:

1. **Overflow.**—When there is complete retention the bladder fills until it can hold no more. Then, instead of bursting, it overflows. The mere elasticity of the bladder wall finally overcomes the obstruction, and urine drips away from the meatus at about the same rate at which it arrives in the bladder. The bladder remains full. There is no true incontinence. There is simply a continuous overflow.

2. **Irritability.**—In many cases, with but little residual urine, there is constant dribbling, not from overflow, nor yet from true incontinence, but due to unusual irritability of the neck of the bladder, whereby every few moments a drop or two of urine is expelled. This condition is rather an abnormal frequency of urination than an incontinence, since the urine does not drip away in spite of every muscular effort to control it, but is constantly expelled by a muscular spasm.

3. **True Incontinence.**—This is rare. Occasionally a patient is encountered whose persistent dribbling of urine suggests overflow. But his urethra readily admits a catheter and his bladder is found to be empty. This is true incontinence. It seems due to a distortion of the urethral orifice in such fashion that the sphincter cannot close, so that the urine is allowed to flow from the bladder as fast as it enters. In such a case the prostatic hypertrophy is confined to

the lateral or to the anterior lobes. There is no bar, middle lobe, or contracture of the neck of the bladder.

Course of the Disease

The patient may date the beginning of his troubles from an acute retention, from a tendency to dribble between the urinary acts, or, less frequently, from a hematuria. He may have simply noticed an increasing frequency and difficulty in urination; but close questioning will usually show that the malady has passed through three stages: 1. The stage of congestion without retention. 2. The stage of partial retention. 3. The stage of retention with overflow. The second and third stages may be introduced or interrupted by attacks of acute complete retention.

1. **Congestion.**—During a period of many months, perhaps years, ever since there began to be a little hyperemia around its neck, the bladder has been gradually becoming irritable. The patient does not readily notice this, and will never be able to fix a precise date for the commencement of his troubles. An old man does not sleep soundly nor pay the strictest attention to the performance of his habitual functions, and he so gradually acquires the habit of getting up a little earlier than usual in the morning to empty his bladder that he pays no attention to it. Soon he finds that he wakes up once at night, perhaps twice, with a feeling of fulness in his bladder. He passes water, and goes to sleep again. He is also troubled in the daytime a little more frequently than usual, but he looks upon this as a condition natural to advancing life. He has learned that the little ills of the flesh, if let alone, usually regulate themselves. He has passed water without trouble for fifty or sixty years, and he thinks that he ought still to be able to manage it without applying to the surgeon. He shrinks from acknowledging a weakness, which he must admit to be, if nothing more, a symptom of advancing age, and so he goes on lulled to security, making water at intervals which gradually, but steadily, become shorter, and constantly annoyed by a faint, obscure sense of weight and heaviness about the lower part of his belly, with, perhaps, a fulness in the rectum, and a dull pain behind the pubes. During this first period of the disease attacks of neuralgia of the neck of the bladder (p. 314) and surface prostatitis (p. 85) may occur from insignificant causes, and a sexual irritability almost amounting to priapism may prove very annoying.

2. **Partial Retention.**—The passage from the first to the second stage of the disease, unless marked by an acute retention, is quite insensible; but ultimately the time arrives when the *bas fond* is

formed and the bladder is no longer quite able to empty itself; only an excess above a certain residuum can be passed off, but the patient does not know it. He only notices that his urinary intervals are getting shorter and shorter; that he has to wait a little before the urine begins to flow; that the stream is small, and is not projected away from him with any force, and that, perhaps, a part of the urine dribbles down perpendicularly from the meatus, while the rest flows as a continuous stream. He cannot make the *coup de piston*, the final spasmodic clearing of the urethra, and finds that a few drops dribble away upon his clothes after each urinary act. He does not experience quite so much ease and relief as usual after micturition; but this has come on so gradually that he disregards it. He may notice the return of morning erections, which had long since ceased to trouble him.

At this juncture he dines out, and drinks a glass or two of wine, or he neglects a call to urinate, or gets a wetting, or his feet and legs get chilled (this is the commonest cause of trouble), and suddenly he finds that he cannot pass water at all. After vainly trying at intervals for a number of hours, if he does not seek surgical relief, at last the urine will begin to dribble away from him. The bladder has been distended to its utmost, the mouth of the urethra has been dragged slightly open, and the excess of urine trickles away involuntarily. This is overflow and not incontinence. Meantime the patient has been suffering the torments known only to those who have had retention, and he hails the overflow with delight, believing that his sufferings are about to cease. The hope is vain. The congestion of the bladder neck, brought on by the use of liquor, or by the chilling, and which, added to the already large prostate, has swollen it sufficiently to shut up the urethra entirely, may subside spontaneously, or be relieved by the catheter, leaving the patient little worse off than before, or it may continue, thus leading to the third stage of the disease.

During this stage of incomplete retention pressure begins to be exerted upon the kidneys; polyuria, especially by night, may ensue —nocturnal pollakiuria is certain.

3. **Complete Retention.**—Now the bladder is literally full all the time. During the day the patient may be able to prevent a continuous overflow by urinating a few drops every ten or fifteen minutes; but the bladder is now quite atonied, and, at night, at least, is quite unable to cope with the inflow of urine, which therefore dribbles away, disturbing the patient's rest and adding shame to his other sufferings.

By this time the ureters and their pelves have begun to dilate and the kidneys to atrophy. The polyuria becomes considerable. Two, 3, or 4 quarts of urine are passed, chiefly at night, of a specific gravity of from 1.005 to 1.010, containing casts and albumin, and a very low percentage of urea and salts. There is a general urinary toxemia. The tongue is dry, glazed, and red at the edges, brown or gray in the centre. The appetite is poor, the bowels constipated and full of gas. The patient loses flesh and becomes feeble and worn.

Variations in the Course of the Disease.—While the above description applies to many cases, the progress from one stage to the next may not be so systematic. Appropriate treatment may carry the patient back from the stage of partial retention to that of mere congestion, or from complete back to partial retention; or an isolated acute retention may be relieved and be followed by a long interval, even an interval of several years, during which the patient suffers not at all, and there is no retention whatever; or there may be true incontinence (see above).

The *inflammatory complications* are, however, the chief agencies in modifying the course of the disease. These complications occur sooner or later in almost every case, and once the inflammation has set in it is almost impossible to get rid of it. *The inflammation is usually due to catheterism.* Spontaneous infection does occur (p. 357), but, as a rule, the complication is due to the surgeon's misfortune or fault.

Inflammation of the Prostate.—*Catarrhal prostatitis* is always present in every case of cystitis, and indeed the posterior urethra and the neck of the bladder are the places from which it is least possible to dislodge the inflammation. *Abscess and periprostatitis* (pp. 88, 90) are relatively uncommon. *Seminal vesiculitis* is common and usually unimportant.

Epididymitis.—Epididymitis may occur in acute attacks, spontaneous or following instrumentation, or it may appear as a sluggish, chronic induration at one end of the epididymis, with occasional subacute or acute attacks of recurrent inflammation.

Cystitis.—Inflammation of the bladder is the most common and important complication of prostatic hypertrophy. The cystitis is usually due to catheterism, less frequently it is spontaneous (p. 383). When due to the catheter, it usually begins acutely, often with a chill, while spontaneous cystitis is commonly chronic from the outset. Although the type of the inflammation may be severe throughout, the cystitis of prostatics is often of a mild and superficial type for many months, not causing any great pain or frequency of urination, or, at any rate, easily controlled by local treatment. The urine is usually alkaline, or, even if faintly acid, it has an ammoniacal odour, and often a fetid, sickening smell, which occasionally disappears. When the urine is acid, and yet ammoniacal, it is so because it comes down strongly acid from the kidneys, and its acidity has not been neutralized by mingling with the ammoniacal residuum. Whatever urine has been alkalinized, deposits crystalline and amorphous phosphates, so that, even in those cases where the urine is still acid, it is murky, cloudy, filled with little strings and clots and clouds of pus, and with gouts of ropy muco-pus (pus agglutinated and made translucent by ammonia). A few blood-corpuscles will nearly always be found, and more or less amorphous urates or phosphates (perhaps both), with crystals of triple phosphate entrapped in the stringy mucus. This is the so-called catarrh of the bladder.

On the other hand, the cystitis may be intense and uncontrollable, with interstitial cystitis, pericystitis, etc. (For further description, see Cystitis.)

Pyelo-nephritis.—No prostatic can have cystitis for any length of time without extension of the inflammation up the ureters to the kidneys. The urinary stasis permits the bacteria to work up against the current, and the kidneys—already partly disabled—fall an easy prey to the bacterial invasion. The pyelo-nephritis often remains for years a mild catarrhal inflammation, recognisable only by a careful urinary examination; but, mild as it is, this inflammation is an aid to the urinary pressure in its work of debilitating the kidneys and slowly leading to the patient's death. (See Pyelo-nephritis.)

Stone.—Phosphatic stone is the natural result of a protracted ammoniacal cystitis.

One stone, or several, may exist under these circumstances without giving rise to any symptom. They are usually smooth, and do not greatly irritate the floor of the bladder, nor add much to the already existing pain. The fibres of the weakened detrusor cannot, during micturition, force a stone thus formed against the sensitive tissues at the neck of the bladder and produce the striking symptoms which characterize vesical calculus when found in a healthy subject (p. 435).

Diagnosis

When a patient of over fifty comes to seek relief for frequent micturition, suspicion falls at once upon the prostate. It is rare that stricture causes trouble for the first time so late in life; moreover, with enlarged prostate, the inconvenience will, as a rule, have been first noticed at night—the reverse of what is observed in stricture. As the first step in the examination, a digital exploration should be made through the rectum (p. 242). By this means alone general prostatic hypertrophy can always be demonstrated. In place of the soft, chestnut-like body, hardly recognisable except by the skilled touch, the finger will encounter a rounded, dense mass, smooth and symmetrical, or variously distorted and nodulated. The median fissure between the lobes may be more than usually perceptible, or may be wholly obliterated; while the finger passed up on each side, between the prostate and the walls of the pelvis, recognises a deepening of the sulcus, and any undue prominence in size of one or the other lobe. By forcing the finger well up the rectum, it may be possible to hook the last phalanx above the posterior margin of the enlarged prostate, where the seminal vesicles can sometimes be made out on each side, partly embedded in the general hypertrophy.

Perhaps rectal examination may reveal no positive evidences of enlargement, median hypertrophy existing none the less. In such a case the finger readily detects the bladder, if it be distended, beyond the prostate; the latter apparently not at all or but little larger than normal. Pressure through the rectum upon an enlarged prostate does not cause pain, unless there be some inflammation about the neck of the bladder, but it often provokes a desire to urinate.

The next step in the examination is to make out the condition of the bladder by palpating and percussing the hypogastrium. Usually this gives no hint of the condition of the prostate, unless it is exceedingly large, when pressure upon it through the rectum may be recognised by the hand upon the hypogastrium. This same resistance may be felt in severe cases of concentric hypertrophy of the bladder with excessive hypertrophy of the walls and contraction of the cavity. As a rule, hypogastric palpation only excites a desire to urinate from transmission of the force to the sensitive neck of the bladder. Sometimes, however, an oval tumour is found, as large as a child's head, filling up the lower part of the belly, perhaps as high as the umbilicus, flat on percussion, and causing a desire to urinate when pressure is made upon it. This tumour, formed by the overdistended bladder, may often be plainly seen, but the patient is usually unconscious of its existence. If the finger in the rectum can reach beyond the posterior border of the prostate, fluctuation can be felt between it and the other hand pressed upon the hypogastrium.

The patient is now asked to stand up and to pass water into a glass vessel. A little gleety discharge may often be found at the meatus, originating from the congested surface of the prostatic urethra. Occasionally, if questioned, the patient will confess that he is troubled with frequent erections, the cause of which lies in this same congestion. Sometimes, on the other hand, erections are absent.

As the urine is flowing off, it will be noticed that it commences tardily, and in a small stream, which gradually enlarges. There is very little force to the flow. There may be two streams, the one projected, the other dribbling perpendicularly from the meatus, indicating an obstacle to the escape of urine at the outlet of the bladder. If there is retention, the urine will not flow at all, or comes away only by drops. While the stream is flowing, if the patient be requested to strain, instead of becoming larger or flowing with greater force, it may be diminished in size and power. If the bladder be inflamed, there may be severe tenesmus and pain during the attempt to urinate, and the rectum may protrude or feces be passed during the act. Hernia may be occasioned by the violent straining. At the end of urination the stream gradually dribbles away in drops, and often the final jet is wanting, although this may be perfect or even exaggerated.

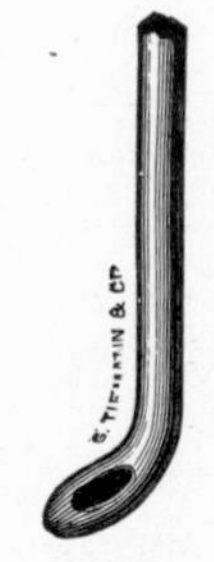

Fig. 76. Elbowed Catheter.

If the urine which has been voided be now held up to the light, it will be found cloudy, perhaps bloody, often ammoniacal, and containing white flocculi of pus, or perhaps stringy muco-pus, or again, it may be perfectly clear. The condition of the urine indicates the amount of cystitis present, while its quantity (in residuum) and the force of its flow, after the catheter has been introduced, measure the degree of atony. Yet there may be considerable irritability, with little or no cystitis, and in such cases the urine is nearly or quite clear, generally strongly acid, and of high specific gravity.

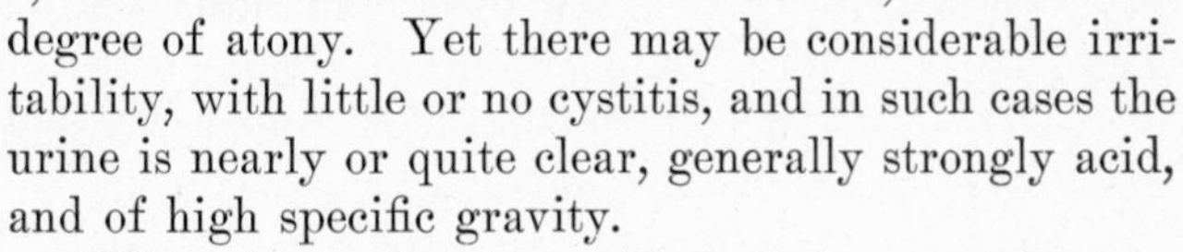

When the patient has voided all the water he can, he is again placed upon his back, and a soft-rubber catheter (18 French), previously sterilized, is gently introduced into the bladder. If it will not enter, a woven catheter, of the elbowed (Fig. 76) or double-elbowed pattern (Fig. 77), is sterilized and introduced. No force should be employed in introducing these instruments. Dexterity and patience will succeed where brute force will only light up inflammation or open a false passage. The elbowed catheter is especially designed to ride over the prostatic obstacle, and can almost always be introduced, if properly and patiently manipulated, and aided by a finger on the perineum or in the rectum, unless there is a stricture of the urethra, which arrests the catheter before it reaches the prostate, or unless the hypertrophied organ has been damaged by previous rough attempts at catheterization.

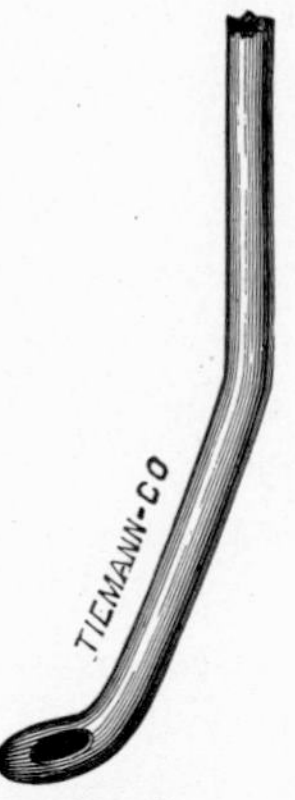

Fig. 77.—Double-elbowed Catheter.

When the elbowed catheter fails to pass, the olivary woven instrument (Fig. 43) may succeed; but, as a rule, it, too, will fail. In this event, two courses are open to the surgeon: he may send the patient home, with directions to employ such measures as may tend to diminish the prostatic congestion, or he may persist in his manipulations. In examining a patient for the first time it should never be lost sight of that he is an old man whose urinary passages are in a more or less irritable condition, and probably unused to local disturbance. Any examination at all rough or too prolonged is pretty sure to be followed by some aggravation of the symptoms, and, unless the condition be urgent (retention), it is often advisable to make only a partial exploration at the first sitting, leaving the rest for another day. If made worse by his first examination, the old man becomes far less docile for future management. If, however, there is retention with or without overflow, it becomes the surgeon's duty to make judicious use of all available means to enter the bladder with a catheter. But such persistence is justifiable only for the purpose of relieving the patient's retention, not for diagnosis. (See Treatment.) A large silver instrument with a very long curve will sometimes find its way when nothing else will enter.

When the catheter reaches the bladder the urine will jet from it. The *atony* of the bladder may be estimated by the force of the stream. If atony is complete, and the patient recumbent, no urine may issue from the catheter, even though the bladder be quite full. Pressure on the hypogastrium, or catheterization in the erect position, will start a sluggish stream. *The amount of residual urine* measures, in a general way, the depth of the *bas fond*, though a strong bladder will almost empty a fairly deep *bas fond*, while an atonied organ can only spill off the upper layers of fluid. Finally, a third point is estimated by the catheter—viz., the urethral length (urinary distance). The catheter having been introduced until water is drawn, is immediately withdrawn until the flow stops, then introduced until it comes again and the eye thus placed accurately at the orifice of the bladder. The catheter is then grasped at the point where it issues from the meatus, and the distance from this point to the eye of the instrument measures the length of the urethra. This measurement is simplified by having the catheter marked in centimetres with nitrate of silver beforehand.

In thus emptying the patient's bladder two rules must ever be borne in mind:

1. *Close the operation by a mild antiseptic irrigation*, with hot boric-acid solution if the bladder is clean; with nitrate of silver, 1:8,000, if it is infected.

2. *If the bladder contains a pint or more of fluid the patient must lie down while his urine is being drawn, and the bladder must be immediately refilled to one half its former capacity with boric-acid solution.* Neglect of this precaution has caused syncope and instant death. A more common result from the sudden relief of pressure is an acute congestion, which may terminate in profuse hemorrhage (*hematuria ex vacuo*) or in cystitis.

After the first passage of the catheter the patient should remain warm and quiet, but not necessarily in bed, for some hours—preferably for an entire day. After a few days the process may be repeated, and presently the bladder may be entirely emptied and left empty.

Further discussion of this subject, notably of the dangers of urinary fever and cystitis after catheterization, is deferred to the chapter on Treatment.

Diagnosis of the Shape and Size of the Prostate.—The size of the lateral lobes having been estimated by *rectal touch* and the intravesical projection by the *urinary distance*, no more accurate diagnosis need be attempted until the surgeon has familiarized himself with the temper of the patient's organs and put him in the best possible condition to undergo a more thorough investigation. The best implement for this purpose is the Thompson *stone-searcher* (Fig. 105). With it all irregularities in the urethra, the presence of bar or of middle lobe, and the existence of *stone* may be at once determined. But its use involves some damage to the neck of the bladder, for which reason it is rarely to be employed, unless there is distinct evidence pointing to the presence of stone.

The bladder should contain about 100 c. c. of urine or boric-acid solution. The instrument is sterilized, lubricated, and introduced gently into the urethra. It will sink into the canal by its own weight, guided only by a light touch of the finger, which is thus able to appreciate the obstacles to its progress. At the bulb some difficulty may be experienced in entering the membranous urethra; but a little patience will overcome this obstacle. The instrument now slips easily into the prostatic urethra, where its beak may be thrown to one side or the other by some projecting lobe. But it has not yet reached the bladder. It may be turned a little from side to side, but until it has definitely met and overcome the obstruction at the neck of the bladder it is not within that organ. The instrument, which up to this point has entered by its own weight, now meets a very definite obstacle. To overcome this the handle must be still further depressed. Perhaps all that is required is a firm crowding down of the suprapubic fat and a light touch upon the handle of the searcher; perhaps the shaft of the instrument will have to be carried well back of the median plane of the body before it will enter; perhaps it will not pass at all. No attempt must be made to push the instrument in. It is pocketed in the prostatic sinus behind an organic obstruction. Force may overcome the obstacle, but it may tear a tissue already diseased and most resentful. The result may well be a complete retention, a sharp chill, or a violent cystitis. *The only force allowable*—and that should not be violent—*should be directed to depressing the handle of the instrument.* The shaft pivots at the membranous urethra, and, as the handle is depressed, the beak rises, the point of the instrument enters the bladder, and, as soon as the heel reaches the height of the orifice, it slips in easily enough with a slight jerk. If this maneuvre fails, the attempt must be given up, with the consolatory thought that if the bar is so high the *bas fond* is, undoubtedly, too deep to be thoroughly explored for stone.

If the instrument slips in, the bladder is to be quickly searched for stone (p. 436). The projection of muscular trabeculæ into the bladder may often be appreciated, and, finally, in withdrawing the instrument, it will hook into the *bas fond* if its beak is turned downward. With the instrument held in this position, a finger in the rectum will appreciate the thickness of gland tissue intervening between it and the urethral instrument. If the *bas fond* is deep a small stone readily escapes the searcher.

Cystoscopy is rarely necessary, and often injurious.

Differential Diagnosis

The distinguishing features of inflammation, abscess, and tuberculosis, are too characteristic to require rehearsal here. When there is a diffuse, non-inflammatory enlargement of one or both lobes of the prostate, as felt by the rectum, the diagnosis rests between hypertrophy and cancer. When there is little or no lateral enlargement, but considerable urethral obstruction, the diagnosis rests between hypertrophy of the prostate and contracture of the neck of the bladder. In neither case is the differential diagnosis always possible.

Malignant Disease.—When a large, hard, ill-defined tumour is felt through the anterior rectal wall, the surgeon attempts to delineate the prostate. If that organ can be made out below and distinct from the mass, it is a cancer of the bladder or a pericystitis, not a tumour of the prostate. If the prostate is involved in the disease, and the mass is apparently fast to each side of the pelvis, and extends upward indefinitely, there is a question of cancer of the prostate or of periprostatitis; there is no question of hypertrophy. But if the finger can be swept across the tumour and into a deep sulcus on each side of it, and the enlargement is evidently confined to the gland itself, there may still be malignant degeneration. A single hard tumour the size of the ball of the thumb is extremely suggestive of carcinoma, whether the remainder of the prostate be hypertrophied or not. But in some cases all the signs and symptoms are those of hypertrophy of the prostate until the rapid advance of the disease betokens its malignant nature.

Contracture of the Neck of the Bladder.—If cancer and hypertrophy of the prostate are sometimes confounded, contracture of the neck of the bladder and hypertrophy of the prostate are, one might say, always confounded. Among the innumerable tomes, monographs, and pamphlets that appear month after month, torturing every aspect of the "old man's disease," I have not found one that makes the clear clinical distinction between retention due to contracture of the internal sphincter and retention due to hypertrophy of the prostate gland. This distinction is vital as regards prognosis and treatment, and the key to the situation is this: *When there are symptoms of prostatic retention without any hypertrophy of the prostate, the essential lesion is a contracture of the neck of the bladder.* The anomaly of prostatism without hypertrophy of the prostate, of inveterate cystitis cured by perineal section, of hypertrophied prostate cured by Bottini's operation—all these have been commented upon again and again; but since the days of Mercier and Civiale only faint glimmers of the truth have penetrated the writings on this subject. Suffice it to say here that, while contracture of the neck of the bladder complicates disease of the prostate, from the gonorrheal inflammation of youth to the hypertrophy of old age, and is present in many cases of long-standing hypertrophy, the diagnosis of contracture without hypertrophy may be passed upon all those who, with the symptoms of prostatism, have no increase in the urethral length and no hypertrophy appreciable by rectal touch (p. 317).

Prognosis

Hypertrophy of the prostate is not of itself a mortal malady. The tumour is benign and rarely undergoes malignant degeneration. (*Cf.* Albarran and Hallé.[1]) Yet it does not get well spontaneously although sufferers from it may have long intervals between exacerbations of the disease—and it is mortal by the retention and the inflammation that it causes.

The prognosis of the disease is bad. Its progress is slow; it may be controlled for many years (the prostate itself ceases to en-

---

[1] Guyon's Annales, 1900, xviii, 113, 225.

large at or about the age of sixty-five), but it slowly progresses. After the bladder has once become chronically inflamed it does not recover unless the obstruction is removed. After the kidneys have become inflamed or sclerosed they never return to their normal state. With each year sapping the sick man's powers of resistance his prostate gets the better of him in the end.

The surest criterion of prognosis is the patient's amenability to palliative treatment. He is safe so long as his symptoms can be controlled by palliative means. Systematic catheterism and irrigation of the bladder may hold the disease in check for years; but when they fail there is nothing left but operation or death. The post-operative prognosis will concern us later.

The common cause of death is urinary toxemia or septicemia through kidney insufficiency. In certain cases, acute retention, violent cystitis, or local inflammations have much to do in wearing out the patient.

CHAPTER XVIII

PALLIATIVE TREATMENT OF PROSTATIC HYPERTROPHY

The treatment of hypertrophy of the prostate is palliative and radical. Palliative treatment will be described first, while the detail of prostatic hygiene, which should be the background of every other treatment, demands preliminary consideration.

PROSTATIC HYGIENE

The prostatic man resembles the menstruating woman in that any exposure or overdoing reacts promptly upon his pelvic organs. "Beware of congestion" must be his motto, and upon this he must mould his life. He must avoid all exposure to cold: draughts are dangerous, wet feet fatal. His clothing, especially his underwear and footgear, must be regulated by the thermometer. Light exercise and fresh air are beneficial; but any excess, physical, mental, sexual, or alcoholic, must be avoided. Of alcoholic beverages, he may drink whisky, gin, and white wine in moderation; but no beer nor champagne. The stomach must not be overloaded. "*C'est souvent en lui souhaitant bonne fête,*" says Guyon, "*qu'on détermine chez un vieillard prostatique sa première rétention.*" The diet must be both light and laxative, for a torpid bowel threatens infection as well as congestion. Meats should be largely replaced by vegetables and cereals, milk by buttermilk, tea by coffee or cocoa, red wine by white. Fruits should be employed circumspectly, as their acidity may do more harm than their laxative qualities do good. Finally, the patient must keep his urine bland by drinking plenty of water, using alcohol little or not at all, eschewing all beer, ale, and champagne, and cutting off all rich and fried foods and such special articles as strawberries, asparagus, and grapefruit. If he has been a high liver these dietary changes will have to be worked out gradually, since too great insistence on them all at once will only make him disobey instructions.

GENERAL TREATMENT

During the active stages of the disease, local applications to the bladder and the prostate are of the greatest service in allaying symptoms; but they must always be seconded by attention to the rules of hygiene suggested above, and internal medication may be most efficacious in some cases, while in others it seems absolutely ineffectual.

If the prostate is simply *congested*, the urine clear, the residuum negligible, there may be marked irritability of the bladder with frequent and painful urination. To conquer this, astringents and irritants are often useful. Tr. ferri chlorid, 0.5 gramme, *t. i. d.*, and urotropin, 0.5 to 1 gramme, *t. i. d.*, often act like a charm, and, similarly, a desperate pint of beer or small cold bottle (of champagne) may drive away the symptoms which the surgeon has struggled to master in vain.

When there is sharp *inflammation* of the bladder, with torturing dysuria, the local treatment may sometimes be materially assisted by the following alkalin sedative combination:

℞	Liq. potassæ....................	5.00–15.00	grammes
	Extr. hyoscyami fl................	10.00–25.00	"
	Syr. aurant, cort..................	100.00	"
	Aq. cinnamon..................ad	200.00	"
M.	S.: Tablespoonful in water, *t. i. d.*		

Yet this medicine is somewhat hard to digest, and is therefore not suitable for prolonged use. In the endeavour to control a chronically inflamed organ, the routine internal medication may be antiseptic or sedative. In either case, the first essential is that the patient drink enough water to keep his urine at or below a specific gravity of 1.015. The medicine to be used depends upon the quality and intensity of the cystitis and the individual peculiarities of the patient; but it is a general rule that no medicine which is not easily digested will materially help the patient for any length of time. (For further details of the General Treatment of Cystitis, see page 367.)

The treatment of renal infections is fully detailed in its appropriate place.

The bowels and stomach often require special attention by cathartics, vegetable and saline, enemata, gastric lavage, etc. When the local conditions have been righted the general health may be improved by tonics.

Opiates.—A final word on the subject of opiates. Hypertrophy of the prostate is a chronic disease, and pursues a most uncertain course. The sufferer, writhing in agony to-day, may be entirely relieved to-morrow. The patient whose last sun seems to have risen may be relieved by operation, and survive for many a year. Under these circumstances, it is scarcely necessary to insist that opiates should be administered with extreme caution. The patient, a constant sufferer from a tormenting disease, is in an ideal condition to become addicted to narcotics. I have seen few sadder cases than those of old men whose prostatic disease was still apparently curable while their subjection to narcotics could not be overcome.

LOCAL TREATMENT

First Stage.—During the first stage of the disease the bladder empties itself completely. Catheterization is therefore quite unnecessary; indeed, it may be harmful. But there may exist, even during this stage, a considerable neuralgia of the neck of the bladder, which must be treated appropriately (p. 314). Or again, there may be prostatitis or cystitis, due to other causes (pp. 266, 383). Finally, an acute retention may be the chief feature of the disease, and this requires especial notice.

Acute Retention.—The therapeutic indication is perfectly clear. The urine must be withdrawn. Half-hearted measures are inefficient. The hot sitz bath may be employed with a hypodermic injection of morphin as a temporizer; but the patient, once thoroughly obstructed, is quite beyond emptying his own bladder. The surgeon must do that for him.

If the rubber or woven catheter passes easily there are only two requirements: (1) Absolute cleanliness, and (2) evacuation of the bladder, as already indicated (p. 271) by easy degrees. Under the head of absolute cleanliness must be included irrigation of the anterior urethra with salt solution before catheterization, and instillation of silver nitrate afterward (p. 218).

If flexible instruments will not pass, and there is no false passage (p. 286), the surgeon may employ Guyon's device.[1] This consists in mounting an elbowed woven catheter on an elbowed steel mandrin, and introducing this instrument until its beak is within the prostatic sinus, but *not touching the obstruction.* The catheter is then advanced and the mandrin held stationary, or withdrawn a little. The beak of the instrument is thus sharply elevated and will override a most abrupt obstacle. If this maneuvre fails, recourse must be had to a metal instrument. The ordinary silver catheter is

[1] Leçons cliniques, Paris, 1897, iii, 211.

useless, its curve is entirely too short. The long-curved prostatic catheter is required. Three or four such catheters of different sizes and curves constitute an outfit (Fig. 78).

In introducing such an instrument the surgeon must be gentler than gentleness itself. He must proceed slowly, guide his instrument by a finger in the rectum, and make its point hug the roof of the prostatic canal. Above all he must remember that there is no stricture in the prostatic urethra, no spasm (Rochet and von Frisch to the contrary, notwithstanding), no obstruction to be broken through. The dilated prostatic urethra is a cellar in which the instrument loses itself. The prostatic obstacle is a wall. At the top of that wall is a window, the vesical orifice. The difficulty is to find that window. When once found it is large enough to admit the instrument. It is to be searched for not along the obstructing bar but along the roof.[1]

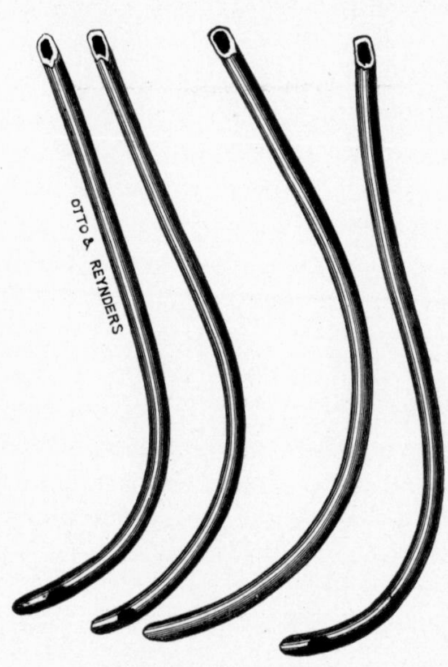

FIG. 78.—(THOMPSON.)

After the bladder has been reached, the case is treated according to the routine methods laid down below.

If all instruments fail to pass, the bladder may be aspirated (p. 209) every eight hours for a day or two. If the catheter still fails to enter, admission must be obtained by operation.

Second Stage.—The catheter is the instrument for treatment of the retention that characterizes the second stage of prostatic hypertrophy. But to be effective the use of the catheter must be intelligent, and the hygienic and medicinal treatment must not be lost sight of for a moment. For therapeutic purposes four classes of cases may be considered:

1. Simple, uninfected cases.
2. Infected cases.
3. Irritable cases.
4. Obstructive cases.

---

[1] Von Frisch employs an instillation of 2 c. c. of 5% cocain solution, followed by 5 c. c. of sterilized oil, as a preliminary to difficult catheterization. This diminishes pain, spasm, and congestion.

1. **Simple, Uninfected Cases.**—We have seen the precautions with which the first diagnostic catheterization must be surrounded. These are to be kept in view at all times, but especially when breaking in to catheter life a man with a large, soft prostate and a considerable amount of clear residual urine. Such a subject is especially liable to infection, with sharp chills and extreme systemic disturbance (p. 43). Gentleness and cleanliness will avert this, if carried sufficiently far, and in such cases they must be carried to the extreme limit. The cleanliness must be threefold: cleanliness of the instrument, the cleansing irrigation both before and after using the instrument, and urotropin administered internally (p. 373).

After the first diagnostic evacuation of the bladder the catheter is passed, with the same precautions, as often as required. While the irritability and infection of each case present special indications that must be respected, the ideal to be aimed at is removal of the congestive and infective dangers of residual urine by means of the least possible number of catheterizations. Every introduction of the catheter is one more trauma, be it ever so slight, one more possibility of infection for the prostate to contend with. Hence the catheter should never be introduced except for a definite purpose. The prostatic with clear urine is the worst possible subject to experiment upon.

In general, the number of catheterizations is regulated by the amount of residual urine. *If the residuum is less than 75 c. c. (2 ounces) no catheterization is required.* The patient's symptoms of nocturnal pollakiuria may still be alleviated by the sounds and the astringent injections employed during the first stage. But *with a residuum running from 75 to 125 c. c. (2 to 4 ounces) the bladder must be emptied by catheter every evening.* Without this the nocturnal symptoms cannot be controlled. The congestion kept up by the retained urine more than counteracts the influence of sounds and astringents alone. *A residuum running from 125 to 200 c. c. (4 to 6 ounces) provokes diurnal symptoms and requires the catheter twice a day, morning and evening.* Finally, *for larger quantities, three or more catheterizations are required daily to control the symptoms.* Although it is often possible by the methodical use of the catheter to reduce the amount of the residuum—and even to do away with it entirely—this end is not to be attained by frequent catheterization. On the contrary, the less frequent the catheterization, within reason, the better the result. Thus the use of the catheter should be *cleanly, gentle, infrequent, and systematic.* The first three points require no further insistence. The last is quite as cardinal as any of the others. To use the catheter systematically is to use it intelligently.

Irregular catheterization is valueless. When the instrument is required but once in the twenty-four hours, it must be used immediately before retiring. When it is required twice, before retiring and on rising. When it is required three or more times—this part of the rule is the least observed—it must be introduced at regular intervals. As the dyspeptic stomach must be fed regularly, so must the overburdened bladder be emptied regularly. The intervals should be made mathematically even, if possible. Six in the morning, two in the afternoon, and ten at night are favourite hours, or, if the patient retires late, seven, three, and eleven. The evening catheterization must be at bedtime. The morning one seems early, but the patient's bladder will awaken him betimes.

Thus far *catheter life* has been considered as though entirely conducted by the surgeon. This is far from being the case. The surgeon must initiate catheter life. He must perform the catheterizations for the first few days; but, at the same time, he must instruct the patient, by both precept and example, how to perform the operation himself in a cleanly, gentle, systematic manner. The gentleness and system are the same for patient as for surgeon. The details of cleanliness differ somewhat. The patient should be instructed as follows:

1. Urotropin (0.5 to 1 gramme a day) must be taken throughout the institution of catheter life and indefinitely as long as the bladder remains clean, to avert the ever-present danger of infection.

2. The hands must be washed with soap and water before each catheterization. Most surgeons advise that the glans penis be washed also. This the patient will very rarely do; he will give it up, and, finding no harm results, he will perhaps give up washing his hands as well. I am therefore contented with the hand-washing.

3. The catheter is to be flushed inside and out with running water after using. It is then boiled for ten minutes, dried with a clean towel, and placed in a metallic box or between the folds of a towel, where it remains until again needed. Before using, the catheter is again flushed out. The metallic box must be kept scrupulously clean. The catheter is flushed out by holding it in a faucet of running water, so that the water runs down it outside and in. If a woven catheter is used, and a boilable one cannot be obtained, the catheter must be washed carefully with soap and water and then flushed with running water before and after each catheterization.

4. The lubricant used must be aseptic and kept in collapsible tubes.

5. The bladder must be washed daily with a hot solution of boric acid for from three to six months. After this time it will have

acquired a toleration to the instrument, and the wash may be discontinued on the condition that urotropin is still taken.

6. Special attention must be paid to combating constipation.

The *technic of auto-irrigation* must be described in detail to the patient, and he must be made to perform the operation in the surgeon's presence. I shall describe only the method which I have employed for twenty-five years, having found it universally acceptable to my patients with no modification of the apparatus. I have used various solutions, but now employ, in clean cases, only a boric-acid solution, for the reason that this is easily made, and it is impossible for the patient to make the solution strong enough to irritate. Its antiseptic properties, though not great, are sufficient for the present purpose.

The patient is supplied with a pint measure, a glass rod, a pound tin of granular boric acid,[1] a fountain-syringe, a two-way stop-cock (Fig. 79), and two or three catheters. He proceeds as follows: First washing his hands and obtaining some water so hot that he can only just keep his finger in it (*circa* 115° F.), he fills the pint measure with this, adds a heaping teaspoonful of the granular boric acid, and stirs with the glass rod until the crystals are dissolved. This solution he pours into the fountain-syringe, to which the two-way metallic stop-cock is attached, and hangs it just above his head. He then attaches the hard-rubber nozzle to the clean catheter, lubricates the latter, and introduces it gently into his bladder. He introduces the catheter only far enough to strike water—the natural tendency is to push it in too far, and then to pull it out and in until the right spot is reached—and drains the bladder dry. Then he opens the stop-cock, allows the water to escape from the bag until it runs warm, turns off cock, couples cock and nozzle, turns on the stream

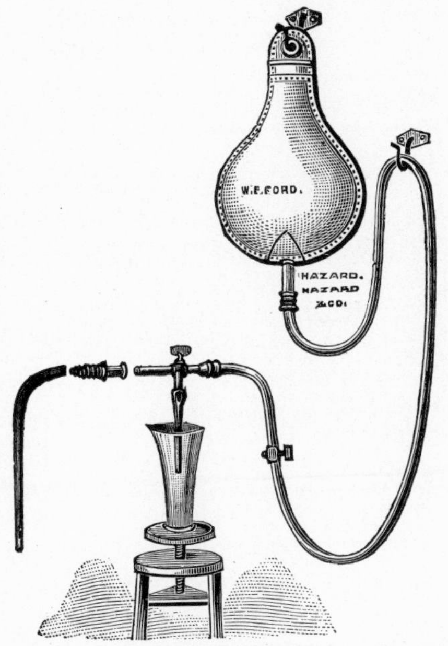

Fig. 79.—Apparatus for Auto-irrigation of the Bladder.

[1] Pulverized boric acid dissolves very slowly.

again, and allows the bladder to fill. As soon as he feels any intravesical tension he turns the cock off and the fluid escapes into the vessel. By turning the cock on and off the bladder may be filled and emptied several times; for the present purpose one filling suffices.

The *results* of catheter life may be the reduction or the abolition of symptoms and residuum, or both may continue, or the bladder may, in spite of the best care, become infected.

2. **Infected Cases.**—Infection introduces several new features in treatment. The same cleanly, gentle, and systematic catheterization is required,[1] but beyond this the infection itself must be treated along the same lines as a posterior urethritis or a cystitis, independent of hypertrophied prostate (pp. 131, 393). If recent it should be attacked vigorously with the hope of conquering it. The stronger remedies—nitrate of silver, protargol, permanganate of potash, mercurol—should be injected instead of the mild boric acid, and the surgeon should apply them himself; while internally, balsamics and alkalies are usually more efficient than antiseptics. If the infection is acute, rest in bed and anodynes may be required; instillations are preferable to irrigations, and in some cases even these do more harm than good, and all local treatment, except catheterization, must be suspended. Urethral fever may occur and require appropriate treatment (p. 46). In these acute cases the danger of administering opium freely, whether by mouth or by rectum, should not be forgotten; the patient's future must not be unduly imperiled to assure his present comfort.

Chronic inflammation assumes one of two forms: (*a*) The urine is bacterial, acid or neutral in reaction, and contains little pus; (*b*) the urine is ammoniacal and loaded with stringy muco-pus. Either form, if long continued, leads to pyelitis. For each the best general remedy is usually urotropin, or, if this is not tolerated, salol, or boric or benzoic acid. The mild form of inflammation is, in a sense, a boon to its possessor. It toughens his organs, as it were, and lessens the danger of serious inflammatory complications. Though not readily overcome, it is very easily controlled, and, if the patient is faithful to his urinary toilet with urotropin, catheter, and daily irrigation, he may indulge in the little irregularities of aseptic technic, which all patients allow themselves in the long run, without any harm coming to him. Severe ammoniacal cystitis, on the other hand, is always a menace. Phosphatic stone, abscess of prostate, bladder,

[1] It is sometimes advantageous to modify the system of catheterization to suit the irritability of the bladder. Thus, I have at present under my care a gentleman who has 125 c. c. residuum, and gets more comfort by using his catheter at 5 A. M. and 5 and 10 P. M. than under any other *régime*.

or kidney, and urinary fever, either acute or chronic, result from it. Urotropin and energetic local treatment are required to control it. On the Continent, the retained catheter is often employed for this purpose with advantage when the prostate is not irritable, yet I have rarely used it. Stone should be suspected and searched for, and, if the ammoniacal cystitis, whether due to stone or not, cannot be controlled, operation is required.

3. **Irritable Cases.**—Irritable cases are very rebellious to treatment. An irritable case is one whose symptoms are made worse by all local measures, whether simple catheterization or irrigation. If the residuum is small, internal remedies, whether antiseptics, balsamics, or alkalies, may conquer the irritability; the rectal douche (p. 131) may be of assistance. But if these means fail, if the case does badly without local treatment and equally badly with it, there is no alternative but the knife.

4. **Obstructive Cases.**—Obstruction to catheterization is often an important feature. It may be impossible to introduce soft-rubber or even woven instruments into the bladder on account of spasm of the cut-off muscle or of some crookedness in the deep urethra. Spasm of the cut-off is oftenest caused by a soft linear stricture at the bulbo-membranous junction, and the passage of a few sounds then solves the difficulty; and even if there is no stricture, the gentle passage of a sound is often the best treatment to relieve spasm or to iron out a tortuous prostatic canal.

The retained catheter is especially useful here. By fastening a rubber or woven catheter into the urethra (after introducing it upon a mandrin) for a few days, the rough canal can be smoothed down. By this means the urine is also drawn off continuously, and the lessened congestion thus obtained often results in a notable diminution in the size of the prostate and the amount of residual urine.

The *technic of the retained catheter* has been minutely explained by Guyon.[1] His rules may be summed up as follows (see also p. 210):

1. The instrument employed should be large enough to permit a free outflow of urine, and small enough not to make any pressure along the canal. Its eye must be near the end. Metal and olivary instruments are useless. The simple rubber catheter, the blunt woven catheter, or the Guyon-Pezzer catheter (Fig. 63) may be employed.

2. The instrument must be introduced only so far as to have its eye just within the bladder. When the catheter is properly placed

---

[1] Leçons cliniques, 1897, iii, 328.

the urine flows continuously from it, drop by drop. When the retained catheter proves irritating this is usually because it has been introduced too far or not far enough, and is not draining the bladder properly.

3. The method of fixation has been described (p. 211).

4. While the catheter is in place the penis should be laid up over the groin, or else an ulcer will form at the peno-scrotal angle.

5. Cleanliness is insured by using a clean catheter in the first place, by changing the catheter and cleansing it and the urethra every few days, by using daily irrigations of the bladder if there is cystitis, by wrapping the penis in a wet dressing of bichlorid (1:10,000), and by using an aseptic urinal. An ordinary glass bed urinal will suffice. A rubber tube is led into it from the catheter, and a little (1:40) carbolic solution kept in the vessel. The urinal is to be scoured and boiled daily.

When the retained catheter acts efficiently it reduces urinary fever and septicemia. When it acts inefficiently it produces them. Inefficient action may be due to plugging of the catheter by pus or blood, or to an idiosyncrasy of the patient. If his local irritability is such that the retained catheter stirs him up, there's an end to it; it must be withdrawn. A certain amount of local irritation is quite common during the first twenty-four to forty-eight hours; but, as a rule, this is controllable by anodynes.

If sounds and the retained catheter fail to diminish the obstruction, it must be endured or removed by operation.

Third Stage.—When there is complete retention with overflow the treatment is much the same as when the retention is incomplete. The first catheterizations must be conducted according to the rules laid down for acute retention (p. 277). The catheter should be passed not more than 3 or 4 times in the twenty-four hours, if possible, even though a pint is drained off each time, for the distended and atonied bladder endures this retention better than the more frequent passage of a catheter. If the complete retention is of short standing it may, perhaps, be relieved by the retained catheter. If there is much irritability or inflammation, the patient may have to pass the catheter 6, 8, 10, or more times a day to alleviate his sufferings. Such a condition is unbearable and demands operation if not speedily relieved by palliative measures, notably the retained catheter.

Overflow.—Overflow is the most disagreeable symptom of complete retention. If systematic catheter life can be instituted, the overflow is usually controlled; but if the bladder is contracted or irritable, the overflow may continue, to the great annoyance of the patient. If this symptom is not relieved by the catheter, irrigations, the retained catheter, etc., and the patient will not submit to operation, he must wear a urinal.

Of the many varieties of this instrument found in the shops, I know of only one that accomplishes the two necessary objects of being safe as well as comfortable. This urinal (Fig. 80) was devised by a gentleman suffering from true incontinence. It is made of soft rubber, in the form of a large pouch, capable of receiving the whole scrotum as well as the penis, and large enough to allow a free circulation of air around the parts, thus preventing sweating or excoriation. From this pouch two broad bands of rubber extend up flatwise, one over the belly, the other over the nates to the waist, where they are attached by buttons to the suspenders. Below, the pouch terminates in a long, flat bag, attached by tapes to the thigh and leg, and reaching nearly to the ankle, so that no urine can possibly spill out during any ordinary motion. A metallic cap at the bottom unscrews to drain off the urine and clean the instrument, which should be daily washed out with soap and water and occasionally boiled.

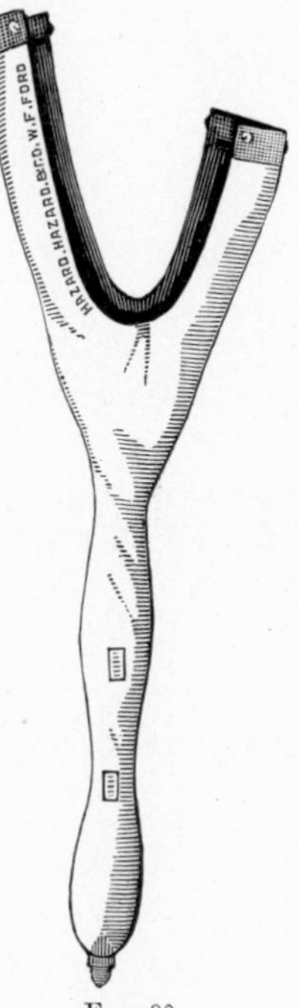

Fig. 80.

This urinal is useful only by day. During the night, when the patient's symptoms are at their worst, he must be satisfied to relieve himself as much as possible with the catheter and—wet the bed. A large rubber penis bag may afford some relief at night, if the patient can accustom himself to lie on one side and not to roll over in his sleep.

TREATMENT OF COMPLICATIONS

The treatments of *prostatitis*, *cystitis*, *irritability*, *obstruction to the catheter*, and *retention* have already been dealt with. True *incontinence* like overflow must be treated by the urinal. It may sometimes be relieved by stimulating instillations (nitrate of silver, 1 : 1,000) into the posterior urethra. If such measures fail, perineal section offers the hope of a cure, and can certainly do no harm.

Stricture.—Soft stricture in the bulb sometimes results from hypertrophy of the prostate and causes annoying spasm of the cut-off muscle. It is easily cured by the passage of a few sounds. Organic stricture requires dilatation in order that the prostate may be properly dealt with and this extra cause of retention removed. If there is much retention, and the kidneys are damaged, there is notable danger of chill and septicemia, to avoid which every precaution must be taken (p. 565). If dilatation is impracticable, external urethrotomy and perineal prostatectomy should be performed.

Stone.—It is often impossible to identify a small stone behind a large prostate. The X-rays and the cystoscope may be employed, but by neither means can stone be excluded with certainty if the bladder is sacculated or the *bas fond* deep. I have recently in my own practice had a striking example of this fact. I touched a stone in the bladder of a man suffering intensely with a large prostate and severe cystitis. I performed litholapaxy, and his symptoms were, if anything, aggravated. A month later—no stone being found—he submitted to epicystotomy. A stone the size of a lima bean was found in the *bas fond*, entirely out of reach of the searcher. It was removed, together with a prostatic middle lobe, and the patient became, and has remained, entirely well. This case exemplifies the general rule that if a stone complicates a hypertrophied prostate, it is futile to attempt litholapaxy. Perineal prostatectomy and litholapaxy or suprapubic section should be performed. If the stone is not found by the searcher or the cystoscope, the issue is only delayed. In the long run the patient will submit to operation as a happy relief to his symptoms, and the stone will be found and removed.

False Passage.—The clinical history of false passage is characteristic enough. A prostatic obstruction is encountered by the surgeon. He cannot surmount it; he uses force; something gives way, and the instrument (always a metallic one) is twisted out of its median course, and the patient cries out with pain. It may be forced into the bladder and the urine withdrawn, or the bladder may not be reached. In either event the withdrawal of the instrument is followed by free hemorrhage, and its reintroduction is usually more difficult and painful than ever.

With such a condition of affairs it is usually best to drain the bladder several times by suprapubic aspiration before attempting any urethral instrumentation. In the meanwhile hot sitz baths, enemas, etc., should be employed to relieve prostatic congestion (p. 131). After twenty-four or forty-eight hours of such treatment a double-elbowed catheter or Guyon's elbowed catheter (p. 277) is introduced with the greatest gentleness. These instruments, following the roof, will often escape the mouth of the false passage, which is on the floor. Where they fail the prostatic silver catheter may succeed. Special instruments, of which one part enters the passage while another avoids it, should never be used, since they keep the false passage open, whereas the surgeon's chief endeavour should be to encourage it to close.

If a woven instrument can be introduced into the bladder, it had better be tied in for two or three days. The false passage will thus be encouraged to close, and subsequent catheterizations will be comparatively easy. If, on the other hand, catheterism is impossible, or if an abscess of the prostate forms, the knife must be resorted to.

Epididymitis.—This is one of the most annoying complications of this disease. The epididymis may be stirred up by every passage of the catheter, and yet the passage of the catheter may be imperative. The treatment for such a case is that of recurrent epididymitis (p. 728), with vasectomy as a last resort. During an acute epididymitis the passage of the catheter should be dispensed with, if possible (p. 728).

Renal Complications.—*Nephritic retention* (p. 544), *pyelonephritis* (p. 553), and *urinary septicemia* (p. 563) require the treatment appropriate to them. There is no need to repeat the special features here, although these often take a prominent place in the treatment of prostatic hypertrophy.

CHAPTER XIX

THE OPERATIVE TREATMENT OF PROSTATIC HYPERTROPHY—THE CHOICE OF TREATMENT

TWENTY years ago no one operated upon the hypertrophied prostate. To-day every surgeon approaches this organ with a knife or a cautery in his mind if not in his hand. The mass of literature upon the subject is appalling. Every one operates; every one writes; every one defends his own views in his own way, and the result is that the variety of operations almost equals the number of operators. Some would operate always; a few would operate never. On one point only do they all agree implicitly, if not explicitly—viz., the prostatic may not be operated upon with impunity. The mortality of prostatectomy varies from 10% to 25% at the hands of different surgeons, while that of castration is, according to the latest statistics (Wood), 8.18%, and of vasectomy 6.7%. Even Bottini's operation has its 4½% to 5½% mortality (Freudenberg). In face of this single accepted fact I have not until now felt justified in urging early operation for this malady. We have been seeking many false gods. We have been diverted first to this side, then to that, in the hope of finding the safe and sure cure; from this diversity of effort has arisen a more correct understanding of what a hypertrophied prostate is and what must be done to cure it, and at last we are approaching the surgical ideal: an operation that removes the obstruction and does not kill the patient.

The Indication for Operation.—There is but one condition calling for operation, and that is *the failure of palliative treatment.* If the patient is failing in spite of the most minute care, if he cannot be got out of a precarious condition, or even if it is foreseen that palliative measures are about to fail—in any such case an operation should be strongly urged upon him. The presence of stone, unconquerable irritability of the bladder, persistent ammoniacal cystitis, progressive urinary toxemia or septicemia, increasing renal dilatation or suppuration—all these are indications for operation.[1] On the other hand, an old man with a patient bladder and an acid cystitis, with some pyelo-nephritis, is no candidate for the knife. He endures the catheter well, and, even though he depend entirely upon the instrument, he only has to use it 4 or 5 times in the twenty-four hours. He has no notable pain. His bladder gives him no more trouble than the rest of his organs. He can live out the full term of his life—ten, twenty years—in this condition. It is not fair, indeed it is not often possible, to persuade such a man to submit to considerable discomfort, with a very appreciable risk to his life, for the single purpose of ridding him of the catheter, to which he has become thoroughly accustomed.

But there are many cases in which the operative indications cannot be thus summarily decided. As for the patient, he will usually not acquiesce unless his symptoms force him to it. The agony of an acute retention or of a ceaseless strangury will quickly bring him to terms; yet either of these may often be entirely relieved by palliative means; while the slow progression of the disease, the persistent ammoniuria, the decreasing renal output, the failing appetite, the thinning, weakening limbs, the quickening pulse, the chalky white face, the hectic fever—these signs, so patent to the surgeon, make no impression upon the patient. He accepts them as the discomforts of old age, and will not hear of operation until too late.

As for the surgeon, let him beware of too earnestly advocating operation. Any operation upon an old man has some mortality which cannot be overcome, and though the most desperate case may

---

[1] The conditions that demand operative treatment for prostatic enlargement are summarized as follows by Alexander:

1st. When there is complete, or almost complete, retention of urine, due to prostatic outgrowths about the internal urethral orifice or projecting into the prostatic urethra, making the patient entirely dependent at all times upon the use of his catheter. The consequences cannot be doubtful in such cases, and operation affords the only means of averting fatal disaster.

2d. When there is marked and continuous vesical irritability, due to intravesical outgrowths, which cannot be allayed by the most careful catheterism and washing of the bladder. These patients usually suffer from frequent attacks of hematuria, and cystitis, when it develops, is usually severe.

3d. When, in spite of careful catheterism, the amount of residual urine is steadily and surely increasing, showing a gradual failure of expulsive force in the bladder.

4th. When catheterism is becoming more and more difficult, in spite of every precaution, and when it is frequently followed by hemorrhages.

5th. When catheterism, in spite of every precaution, is frequently followed by attacks of cystitis.

6th. In cases of long-continued vesical inflammation which do not yield to treatment.

7th. In cases in which the patients cannot or will not use a catheter and take the necessary aseptic precautions to make its use of value.

rally splendidly, no health, strength, or vigour is proof against an embolus or an apoplexy, nor are any old man's kidneys, however apparently sound, to be entirely trusted. One of the healthiest men I ever performed prostatectomy upon died on the fourth day by cardiac embolism. Therefore I urge that the surgeon expend every effort, every artifice at his command, before he says finally to his patient, "You are failing, you are losing ground, you are wasting time. You have now every chance of being saved by operation; the longer you delay the less your chances." Then the responsibility of choice is off the surgeon's shoulders. If the patient refuses operation, so be it. If he accepts, he does so knowing that he has come to his last stand, and his elation at the victory which, in all human probability, awaits him will only be heightened by the appreciation of the dangers he has avoided.

At the other end of the line, when kidneys, heart, head, and stomach all are failing, operation is still indicated. The mortality here is high, but the cures are little short of the miraculous.

PALLIATIVE OPERATIONS

Aspiration of the bladder { suprapubic, perineal, rectal.

Cystostomy {
- suprapubic { puncture, incision,
- perineal incision,
- prostatic puncture.

Aspiration

Aspiration we may dismiss briefly. Rectal and perineal aspiration are never to be employed. Suprapubic aspiration (p. 209) is of the most ephemeral value. By it we gain time—that is all. For acute retention it is an appropriate treatment (p. 277); for anything else it is futile.

Cystostomy

Cystostomy is the formation of a fistula in the bladder wall. A simple cystostomy does not interfere with the prostatic obstruction, but carries the stream of urine around it, and, although in some few cases the prostate, thus relieved of irritation, may shrink sufficiently to re-establish the urethral right of way, this outcome is not to be expected, and a cystostomy is always performed with the intention of establishing permanent drainage, often for the cure of chronic cystitis. The inconveniences of such treatment are obvious. No surgeon who has had to deal with a permanent vesical drainage, whether suprapubic or perineal, can delude himself into the belief that it affords the patient any very great comfort. It may well relieve pain and spasm, though sometimes it fails even to do this, but it does not necessarily cure cystitis, and it leaves the patient more or less incontinent, bound to an ungainly and stinking apparatus, chafed and wet in spite of infinite washings and powderings, and by no means a well man. Hence the field for this operation is daily becoming restricted by the extension of radical operations to more and more desperate cases, and when cystostomy is performed in these days, it is often only for the purpose of alleviating the patient's symptoms until he shall have gained sufficient strength to withstand a more radical procedure.

Of the varieties of cystostomy enumerated above the suprapubic operation is the best. Prostatic puncture is not employed because it does not afford satisfactory drainage. Perineal section is sometimes the source of unbearable irritation at the neck of the bladder. Suprapubic puncture is uncertain in its results and may allow urinary infiltration. On the other hand, suprapubic cystostomy allows free inspection of the field, thorough drainage, and the removal of stone, if one is found. The technic of the operation is described in another place (p. 459). I confess that I have not employed cystostomy for hypertrophy of the prostate for fully eight years. I have always felt justified in preferring a radical operation.

RADICAL OPERATIONS

Before discussing the merits of the numerous operations employed for the cure of hypertrophy of the prostate, it is necessary to have a perfectly clear idea on two points, viz.: (1) What constitutes a cure of a hypertrophied prostate, and (2) How much of a cure may be expected in any given case.

1. **What constitutes a Cure?**—We have seen that less than half the hypertrophied prostates produce any symptoms. We have seen that the symptoms of the disease, excepting only true incontinence, are primarily due to obstruction of the urethra. We shall see that even when the prostate is atrophied a urethral obstruction of an entirely different nature may give rise to a similar train of symptoms (p. 319). It needs no great wit to derive from these facts two important conclusions, viz.:

1. *To cure this disease the urethral obstacle must be removed.*

2. *Even if the whole gland be cut away or become atrophied urethral obstruction from another cause may still remain.*

These truths are fundamental. They are not commonly appreciated, yet an appreciation of them seems essential to enable one to test the merits of the various alleged cures of prostatic hypertrophy and to foresee what their ultimate outcome is likely to be. To take a practical example: What of castration? Does it pretend to cure the disease by attacking the urethral obstruction? By no means. It pretends to cure by causing atrophy of the gland. Even allowing that it does cause atrophy, there is no guarantee that such atrophy will free the urethra of its obstruction. Take Dittel's prostatectomy. By this method almost the whole prostate may be extirpated. Yet the urethra is not so much as explored to prove that the obstruction has been relieved. Bottini's operation has the same fault in a less degree. An honest attempt is made to relieve the obstruction, but no possible means is afforded to show that it has been relieved. Let me not deny that each one of these operations has its virtues and can boast its cures. That I grant. But we should advance a step further than these chance procedures. It is but prudent not to promise a patient an entire cure before his operation, but it is pitiful not to know, after it is all over, how radical the cure is to be, or even whether it is to prove a cure at all. For such reasons as these (it is not possible to enter into the infinite detail of the matter here) *the immediate and direct object of every operation should be the removal of the prostatic obstacle, and the technic of the operation should be such as to allow the surgeon to verify the fact that the obstacle is removed.* No one will deny that such an operation approaches very close to the ideal. I hope to show that it has been approached even closer by the practical.

The nature of the prostatic obstacle has been already noted. In every case there is the *bas fond* with an *elevation*, relative, at least, *of the urethral orifice.* The canal may also be distorted by large projecting lateral or median lobes. The elevated orifice and the enlarged lobes are what the surgeon has to deal with. The removal of these constitutes a cure.

2. **How much of a Cure may be expected?**—Here is the capital practical point. Supposing the obstructions are entirely removed. Supposing there are no post-operative complications. Supposing the operation is an entire success from the surgeon's point of view. Will the patient be satisfied with the result? Not always. When the patient comes to operation both bladder and kidneys have usually felt the effect of the strain. The former is contracted and irritable or dilated and atonied; the latter are dilated or septic. The patient's general health is sure to improve after a successful operation, for however badly off the kidneys, if they are strong enough to stand the strain of operation they are sure to perform

their functions better after the pressure has been removed from them. As for the local conditions, the pollakiuria and dysuria that are the patient's chief distress, they, too, will be relieved. If the bladder is atonied it will gain sufficient strength to empty itself. Urination will not be unduly frequent; but if there is sacculation or long-standing inflammation the patient may be forced to wash the bladder in order to keep this under control. If, on the other hand, the organ is contracted and irritable, it will still have to empty itself frequently, perhaps almost as frequently as before; but the pain and straining will be relieved and the bladder need no longer be washed. Where atony, contraction, or renal involvement is not extreme the result will be perfect, and, in any case, the conditions will improve with time and care, instead of becoming worse, as they had been doing before operation. (The complications to operation will be considered later.) It is evident, therefore, that the ideal time for operation is as soon as the surgeon is convinced that he cannot control the disease by palliative measures. Operation at such a time will give the lowest mortality and the highest proportion of complete cures. Delay beyond this time simply serves to drag the patient down, to unfit him for operation, and to diminish his chances of entire relief by operation.

Bearing in mind these principles, the surgeon is in position to judge fairly between the various so-called radical cures of this disease. These may be grouped into three classes, viz.:

1. Operations designed to cause atrophy of the growth by interfering with its nutrition indirectly.
   a. Ligation of the internal iliac arteries.
   b. Castration (including vasectomy, angio-neurectomy, venesection, injections into the testis).
2. Operations upon the prostate other than excision—
   a. Injections.
   b. Puncture.
   c. Prostatotomy.
   d. Bottini's operation.
3. Chetwood's operation.
4. Prostatectomy—
   a. Suprapubic.
   b. Perineal. { *α* Extra-vesical. *β* Intra-vesical.

Indirect Operations

The object of all indirect operations is not to remove the urethral obstacle, but to cause atrophy of the prostate. Thus their results are limited to the advantages that may be gained by causing atrophy of the gland, without reference to the main point at issue.

Iliac Ligation.—Ligation of the internal iliac arteries (Bier) may be dismissed with a word. Bier has performed the operation 11 times, with 3 deaths, 1 case unimproved, and 7 improved or cured. Of these 7 cases, 6 were examples of acute retention. They all showed a diminution in the size of the prostate; there were no relapses, yet only 1 case was relieved of his residual urine, and he still suffered from nocturnal frequency. The operation has found favour in the eyes of none but its originator. Willy Meyer alone has taken it up in this country, only to abandon it in favour of Bottini's operation.

Castration.—Castration (White [1] and Ramm [2]) has been so stoutly defended, has championed so many kindred procedures, and is still received with favour by so many of the profession, that it deserves more extended notice. Vasectomy (Harrison [3]), angioneurectomy of the spermatic cord (Albarran [4]), injections into the testicle for the purpose of causing it to atrophy, etc., have not proved reliable, and are quite universally condemned, although Harrison [5] still employs his own operation, and Wood [6] speaks favourably of it.

According to White's statistics (1895), derived from 111 collected cases of castration, the mortality was 18%, the cures 46.4%, improved 28.3%, and unimproved 7.3%. The recent statistics of Wood show, among 159 cases, a mortality of 8%, improved (more than 90% of the survivors benefited) 83%, and unimproved 9%. Other observers have not been so happy. No one has yet brought forward a single proved example of atrophy of the prostate after castration, while pathologists have reported no atrophy in prostates examined six weeks, twelve months, and, in a personal case,[7] sixteen months after castration. But if the removal of the testicles does not cause atrophy of the prostate, it does, nevertheless, relieve the symptoms of the disease in some cases. This it does, as Albarran [8] suggests, by relieving the congestion of the gland. Why castration should relieve prostatic congestion more than vasectomy does (which gives, according to Wood, only 67% improved and 6.7% mortality), and how much of the improvement is due to the loss of

[1] Annals of Surgery, 1893, xviii, 152, and 1895, xxii, 1.
[2] Centralbl. f. Chir., 1893, xx, 759.
[3] Brit. Med. J., 1893, ii, 708.
[4] Guyon's Annales, 1898, xvi, 262.
[5] *Ibid.*, 1900, xviii, 836.
[6] Annals of Surgery, 1900, xxxii, 309.
[7] Med. Record, 1900, lviii, 81.
[8] Guyon's Annales, 1898, xvi, 1, 113, 225.

blood, the rest, and the careful local treatment after operation need not concern us here. The practical conclusion to which those who practise this operation have been driven is that it is applicable only to cases of acute retention or congestion, cases which may often be temporarily relieved by palliative measures, and which are not always permanently relieved by castration. The ephemeral effects of castration are beautifully exemplified by Cabot's experience.[1] Excluding 1 case of unilateral castration and 1 case of cancer of the prostate, there remain 8 castrations.

Each of these cases might be said to have been improved by the operation. Yet in only 5 of the 8 cases was the improvement material or lasting, and 3 of these relapsed at the end of six months, while in the other two (II and IV) the result was in no sense a cure; the obstacle was not removed, and neither patient was insured against further accidents. My own experience is even less happy: 1 death, 1 case unimproved. Hence I join those who see little good in the operation. *It may relieve congestion temporarily, but it is not a radical cure for prostatic hypertrophy.*

The technic of castration and vasectomy is described elsewhere (pp. 729, 752).

---

[1] Annals of Surgery, 1896, xxiv, 265. Boston Med. and Surg. J., 1899, cxl, 393.

Case I. Castration and litholapaxy. Post-operative mania lasting two months. Somewhat improved, but relapsed and died of the disease three months after operation.

Case II. Intense cystitis (contracted bladder). Residuum ℥ ij. Eighteen months later frequency and residuum undiminished; irritation much less; very comfortable.

Case III. Acute retention. Rapid improvement. One month after operation residuum was ℥ v. At the end of six months it was down to ℥ ss. Still urinating every two hours and twice at night. At the end of a year he began to relapse, and six months later retention was again practically complete. This time one week of palliative treatment relieved him.

Case IV. Complete retention. Threatened suppression. Retained catheter. Castration. At the end of three weeks residuum ℥ ss. Still urinating once an hour. Dysuria and pollakiuria persist; general condition improved. Wears a soft-rubber catheter for continuous drainage at night.

Case V. Stone and prostate. Castration did not prevent recurrence of stone, and after several litholapaxies a middle lobe ("about the size and shape of the last joint of the thumb") was removed two years later.

Case VI. Litholapaxy and castration relieved him of the catheter (which he had used three years) for six months. Relieved by litholapaxy and again relapsed. Was relieved by suprapubic section of a "band of tissue forming a bar at the neck of the bladder."

Case VII. Chronic complete retention three years. Castration. Relief slight. Six months later suprapubic section. Thirteen stones and a middle lobe removed. The patient died four days later.

Case VIII. Chronic complete retention two years. Much relieved for six months, then relapsed. Projecting masses of prostate removed by suprapubic section.

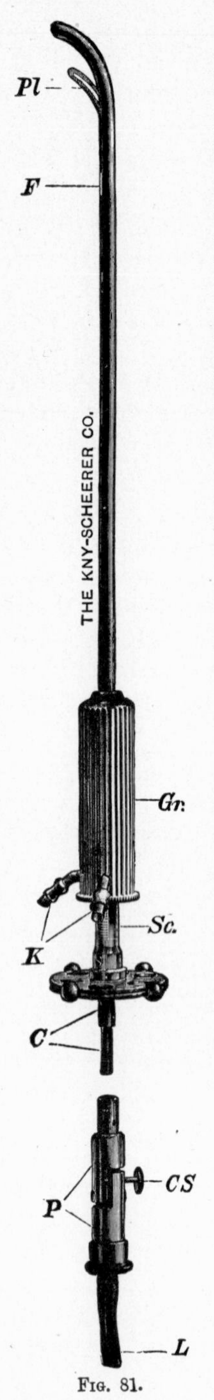

Fig. 81.

Prostatotomy.—Prostatotomy, in one form or another, has long been a favourite treatment for hypertrophy of the prostate. Mercier, with his prostatome, was among the first to agitate the question. Later, simple perineal section with incision of the offending lobe had some vogue. Harrison [1] suggested that a puncture be made through the prostate itself, and a tube left in for drainage and to cause atrophy of the gland. Electropuncture and injections of iodin, ergot, etc., have been employed with varying success at the hands of a few surgeons, but none of these procedures has appealed to the profession at large. Such cures as occurred were not permanent. It remained for Bottini to suggest how a prostate might be incised in such a manner that the incision would not heal and leave as much obstruction as ever.

Bottini's Operation.—Bottini's operation consists in burning a groove in the prostatic obstruction with a galvano-cautery introduced through the urethra. The instrument devised by Bottini has been advantageously modified by Freudenberg. This instrument (Fig. 81) resembles a lithotrite. The male blade is a strong, thin galvano-cautery knife. The female blade is provided with a cooling apparatus, a double-current tube through which cold water is allowed to run during the operation. The blades are connected by a screw handle similar to that of the lithotrite. The electrical apparatus attaches to the end of the handle. The electricity may be obtained from a portable battery or from any electric-lighting plant. The former is a heavy apparatus weighing some 80 pounds, and can never be employed unless freshly charged. To use the street current a transformer and motor must be interposed to reduce the strength of the current to about 4 volts.[2]

[1] Lithotomy, Lithotrity, etc., London, 1883, p. 65.

[2] Guitéras has given a detailed description of the apparatus. N. Y. Med. J., 1899, lxx, 588.

Fig. 81.—Freudenberg's Bottini Incisor.

Pl, cautery blade; *F*, shaft; *Gr.*, grip; *K*, irrigation tube; *Sc.*, screw; *C*, *P*, *L*, electrical connection.

Technic.—The operation is performed as follows: a preliminary cystoscopy determines as closely as possible the nature and shape of the prostatic obstacle. Unless general anesthesia is to be employed this cystoscopy is performed a day or two before the operation. The operation itself is often performed under cocain or eucain (see Cystoscopy), but the effects of these drugs is often illusory, and general anesthesia by chloroform or nitrous oxid is preferable. The patient is prepared by the administration of urotropin for forty-eight hours before the operation. Immediately before operation his bladder is washed as clean as possible with a solution of boric acid. One hundred and twenty-five c. c. (4 ounces) of this may be left in the bladder, or the organ may be inflated with air. The instrument is prepared by boiling. The surgeon's hands should be sterilized, the patient's penis scrubbed with soap and water, and the fossa navicularis washed out with bichlorid of mercury, 1:10,000.

Before introducing the instrument into the bladder all the connections are made. An irrigator full of cold water is attached, and the water from this is allowed to flow through the instrument for a moment. Then the electrical apparatus is turned on slowly until just sufficient current is obtained to heat the cautery to a bright glow. The ampèrage is noted, the electricity turned off, the male blade allowed a moment to cool, and then screwed home; now if all is well, the operation is begun.

With the patient lying on his back the instrument is introduced slowly and gently into the urethra, over the bar, and thus into the bladder. Its beak is then turned downward and hooked snugly against the prostate by traction on the handle. The position of the point of the instrument should be verified by a finger in the rectum, and throughout the operation the operator should keep the index finger of his left hand in the rectum, while steadying the instrument with his right. The water is then allowed to flow and the electricity turned on to the point previously ascertained (40 to 50 ampères). After a few seconds' interval the handle of the instrument is slowly turned by an assistant until the blade is extruded from 2½ to 3½ cm., as indicated by the scale on the shaft. The knife is then slowly returned and the current turned off. This maneuvre should take from one to two minutes. Other incisions may then be made (not over 2½ cm. long) in the lateral lobes or the roof of the prostate. The instrument is finally closed and withdrawn. Many surgeons prefer not to keep the finger in the rectum during the operation, but to employ both hands in manipulating the instrument. I believe, however, that the rectal finger is essential, for by it only is the surgeon able to judge how deeply he is cutting into the prostate.

After the operation there is almost always *retention* of urine, requiring a permanent catheter for three to seven days. There is commonly some *fever*, the temperature running to 101°, or even to 104° F. This fever lasts but a few days. There may also be severe *tenesmus* for several days. Towards the end of the second week after operation the sloughs begin to come away. They are cast off for four or five days, and the patient does not show the full benefit of the operation until the end of this time.

Results.—Freudenberg[1] has performed 86 operations upon 69 patients. Eight operations for inflammatory troubles may be thrown out, leaving 78 operations upon 61 patients. The operation was repeated 3 times on 2 patients, twice on 13 others (repetitions, 21.31%); 31 cases (50.82%) were cured—i. e., they abandoned the catheter, were no longer troubled with pollakiuria, and showed a residuum of not more than 50 c. c.—16 (26.23%) were much improved, 8 were unimproved, and 1 relapsed. There were 4 deaths (6.56%): 1 by pulmonary embolism, 1 by hypostatic pneumonia, and 2 on account of errors of technic. Willy Meyer[2] has performed the operation 30 times upon 24 cases, there being one double and four single repetitions (20.83%). According to Freudenberg's standard there were 7 cures (29.13%), 9 (37.5%) were much improved, 2 somewhat improved, 2 unimproved and died shortly after the operation. There were 4 deaths, 1 of acute sepsis (the case being already very septic), 1 of inflammation of the prevesical space, although the bladder had not been perforated, 1 of septic phlebitis and pneumonia, 1 suddenly after a secondary suprapubic cystotomy. (Mortality, 16.66%.) Finally, Freudenberg has collected 753 reported cases with a mortality of from 4½% to 5½%, and some 88% of satisfactory results.

The complications of the operation are numerous and frequent. Willy Meyer twice, Bangs[3] once, and Guitéras once have cut into the membranous urethra. In both of Meyer's cases there was urinary infiltration, and the patients were only saved by prompt perineal section. One patient required liberating incisions for a scrotal edema, another developed an abscess of the vas deferens. (Other surgeons have noted epididymitis and incontinence of urine as frequent complications.) Perusal of Meyer's detailed reports will give

[1] Wien. klin. Rundschau, 1900, xiv, 915.

[2] Deutsche med. Zeitung, 1900, xxi, 1, 13, 25, 37, 49, and 61. Med. Record, 1900, lvii, 705, 793. *Ibid.*, 1899, lv, 37, and *ibid.*, 1898, liii, 325.

[3] Med. Record, 1901, lix, 367.

an idea of the difficulties with which the operation is beset. Yet it gives satisfactory results in from 67% (Meyer) to 76% (Freudenberg), and a mortality varying from 6½% to 16⅔%. It is most attractive to patients, since it is not a cutting operation, and may be done under local anesthesia. But it has its disadvantages. The convalescence is often painful, tedious, and interrupted by complications, every fifth case requires a repetition of the operation, and there is a very appreciable mortality. Moreover, the operation presents grave fundamental defects from the surgeon's point of view. In the first place, even with the cystoscopic incisors lately devised, the surgeon cannot tell what he is cutting. If he cuts too much, urinary infiltration results; if too little, the operation has to be repeated. In the second place, it is against all the rules of surgery to make a hole in the wall of an infected cavity without supplying adequate drainage, and this is exactly what a Bottini operation, followed by retention, does. If these two difficulties could be removed, the good results would be many times multiplied and the mortality reduced almost to insignificance. This end can be obtained by performing the cauterization, not through the penis, but through the perineum.

Chetwood's Operation

Chetwood's operation[1] is a modification of Bottini's. A perineal cystotomy is performed, and through it the bladder is explored and the obstructing lobes cauterized to precisely the proper extent to lower the urethral orifice. This cauterization is supplemented, if necessary, by prostatectomy.

Technic.—With the patient in the lithotomy position, the bladder cleansed, and a staff in the urethra, perineal cystotomy is performed (p. 458). If there is no contracture of the neck of the bladder the finger enters readily and explores the prostatic obstacle (if there is a strictured vesical neck this should be cauterized forthwith, p. 320). An endeavour is made to outline the prostatic obstruction. The finger in the perineal wound, aided by pressure upon the hypogastrium, detects the projecting lobes, be they lateral or median, and may be hooked over the bar down into the *bas fond*, so as to appreciate its depth. The shape of the obstacle determines the method of attack. If there is a single lateral lobe this may be divided by a groove burned through its centre; or the cautery knife may be held at an angle and passed through the tissues where the lateral lobe holds up a bar of mucous membrane. A bilateral obstruction requires similar treatment—two lateral incisions or two oblique

[1] Med. Record, 1901, lix, 767; N. Y. Med. Jour., 1902, lxxv, 925.

ones. A bar or a projecting median lobe requires incision at one or both sides. If in any case the grooves burned by the prostatome do not seem to do away with the obstruction and fail to lower the floor of the urethra to the level of the floor of the bladder, a perineal prostatectomy may be performed forthwith. In this event it is convenient to perform the enucleation through the burned incision and to confine one's attention chiefly to removing the median bar, enucleating only those tumours in the lateral lobes that shell out easily.

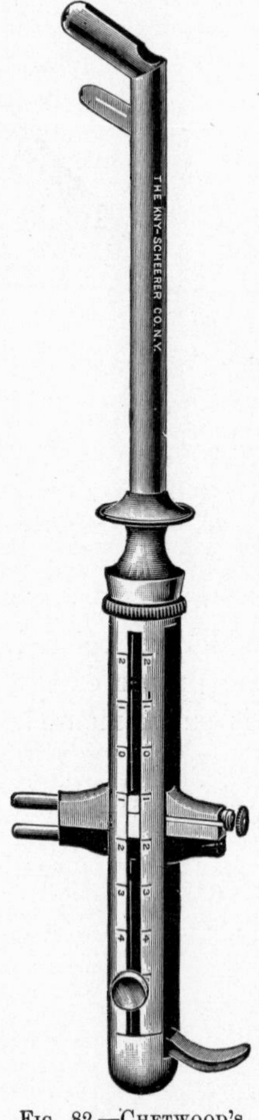

Fig. 82.—Chetwood's Galvano-prostatic Incisor.

The great advantage of this procedure is its simplicity. The surgeon's effort is not to remove the whole prostate, but simply to lower the level of the prostatic orifice. Lateral lobes are only attacked incidentally, and anterior outgrowths may be left to themselves. It is the median lobe and the bar that are chiefly assailed, so that even if prostatectomy be done it is only partial. It may be performed rapidly, and, on account of the cautery incisions made through the mucous membrane, it does not give rise to the hemorrhage that so often follows prostatectomy by other methods.

Technic of the Galvano Incision.—The accompanying figure shows the instrument employed (Fig. 82). It resembles a short, stout Bottini incisor, the knife of which is drawn out by the surgeon's direct pull instead of by a ratchet-wheel. The length of the incision is regulated by a small stop-pin, which may be set at any desired point. The battery is the same as that required for the Bottini operation, and it is customary to allow a stream of cold water to course from the meatus through the urethra and out of the perineal wound while the burning is being done. The instrument must be tested before using in order that the amount of electricity required to heat the knife to a white heat may be justly appreciated.

The surgeon introduces the instrument into the perineal wound, and turns it to hook over the prostate in the required direction. He then inserts the index finger of his left hand (protected by a rubber stall) into the rectum, and bears down on the point of the instrument until it can be distinctly felt on the front wall of the rectum above the prostate.

The cooling apparatus having then been adjusted and only a very small stream of water being allowed to flow, all is ready to begin. From this point it is best to proceed by the watch. The electricity is turned on, and five seconds are allowed for the knife to become heated. It is then very slowly withdrawn (Fig. 83), from sixty to ninety seconds being employed in drawing it out, and fifteen seconds for its return. The instrument is then extracted, the cold-water nozzle inserted into the perineum, so as rapidly to cool the incised tissues, and then a finger is introduced into the wound, and further

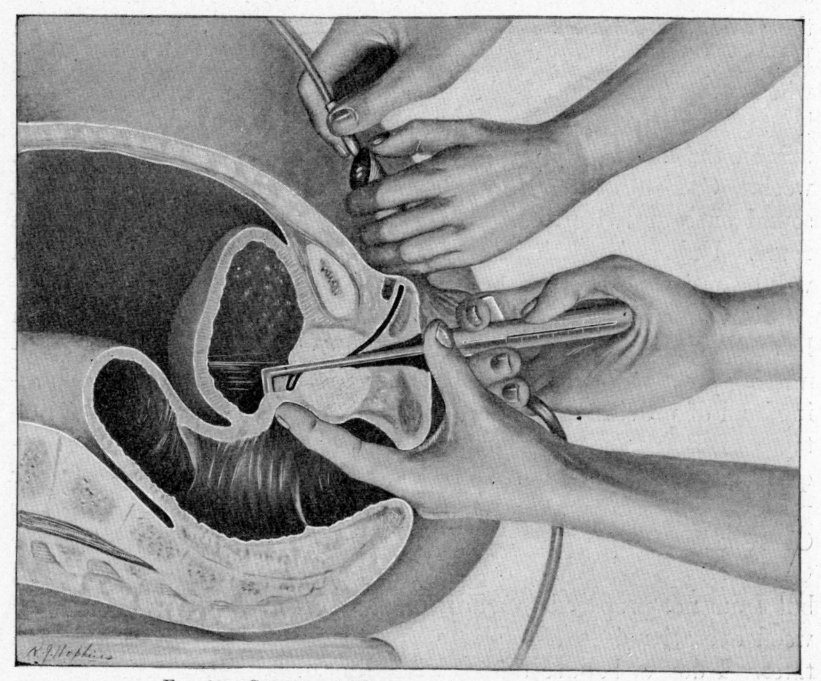

FIG. 83.—CHETWOOD'S PERINEAL GALVANO-PROSTATOTOMY.

incisions or excisions made according to the requirements of the case. The length of the incision varies from ½ to 3 cm., and can only be estimated according to the experience of the operator. Indeed, so much depends upon experience in this operation that, although one may expect good results from the start, the percentage of absolute cures will undoubtedly increase with the practice of the surgeon.

The instrument is fitted with knives of various sizes, but the largest knife is used almost exclusively. At the end of the operation a perineal tube is inserted and the bladder washed clean (p. 204).

After-treatment.—The convalescence from Chetwood's operation is notable for the absence of discomfort to the patient. Spasms may be expected to cease, even though there has been a great deal of irritation immediately before operation. It is customary to wash the bladder with a solution of boric acid once or twice a day; a mixture of iodoform, glycerin, and water may be substituted if the urine is foul. Alarming bleeding there never is. Spasms do not occur during the first four or five days if the cauterization has been adequate. On the fourth or fifth day the perineal tube is removed; it may be exchanged for a smaller tube at an earlier date. After its removal the patient is catheterized every six hours and washed twice a day. During this time there is likely to be a period of two or three days when every urination will be more or less painful and accompanied by a spasm; but this soon passes, and the patient is usually able to urinate through his penis—in part, at least—by the end of the second week. Catheterization through the urethra and the passage of a sound once or twice a week materially hasten the opening of this route. Unless the patient is greatly debilitated the perineal wound will be entirely closed by the end of the fourth week.

As compared with Bottini's operation, Chetwood's modification has the advantage of being accurate and certain in its action, of permitting prostatectomy if the obstruction is not removed by the burning, and of providing adequate drainage. It possesses all the advantages of Bottini's operation, and has the sole disadvantage of requiring perineal section and general anesthesia. I have never performed Bottini's operation, and doubtless never shall. I consider Chetwood's operation superior to it in every respect. It is true, the Chetwood operation has, as yet, been tried on no enormous prostate; but I am not prepared to admit that either the Bottini or the Chetwood operation is preferable to prostatectomy for very large prostates. I do not believe that any burning operation can be adequate to clear a way through a huge obstruction, but for the cure of the obstructions habitually encountered, be they prostatic or inflammatory, I consider the Chetwood operation ideal.

Prostatectomy

Prostatectomy—partial excision of the prostate—is the most difficult and dangerous operation employed for the relief of prostatic hypertrophy. Its mortality always has been and always will be relatively high. It is justified only in extreme cases, and yet my belief is that it will continue to hold its place and to give brilliant results in cases that without it are doomed to prolonged suffering and death.

The preparation for the operation should be of the strictest sort. Several days of milk diet, diluents, urotropin, or salol, and careful local treatment should precede prostatectomy whenever possible.

Suprapubic Prostatectomy (McGill [1]).—A suprapubic cystotomy is performed (p. 359), and the index finger is introduced into the bladder. Any stones that may be present are removed, and the position of the urethral orifice is then ascertained. It is usually found high up on the anterior wall of the bladder, surrounded by masses of hypertrophied prostate. Although no two prostates are exactly alike in shape, the obstructions may be grouped into four classes:

1. *Contracture of the Neck of the Bladder.*—There is little or no hypertrophy of the prostate. The urethral orifice does not admit the finger; it feels like the mouth of a sack with the string drawn tight (p. 317).

2. *Bar or Middle Lobe.*—The prostate juts boldly into the bladder below the urethral orifice. The shape and size of the tumour vary indefinitely. It may be a large mass entirely below the urethra; it may be a small tumour acting like a ball valve.

3. *Horse-collar.*—When the whole prostate is hypertrophied the urethral orifice is surrounded by a mass which may be roughly compared to a horse-collar. It is often asymmetrical, and contains projecting masses of larger or smaller size.

4. *Unilateral or Bilateral Overgrowth with no Median Lobe.*—A rapid search suffices to disclose the general outline of the tumour. The finger is then placed in the urethral orifice, and with the

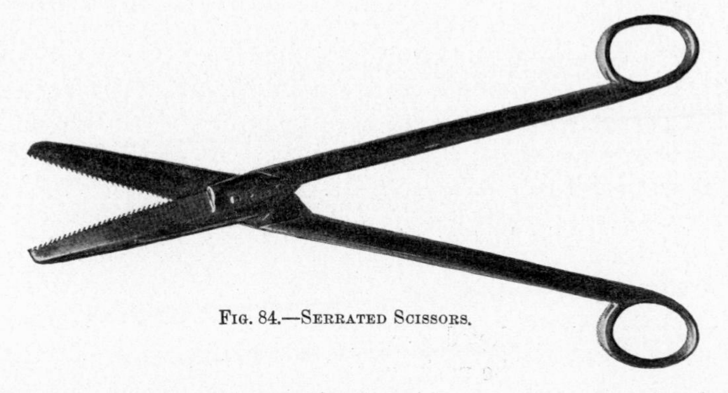

Fig. 84.—Serrated Scissors.

other hand the serrated scissors (Fig. 84) are inserted into the wound. With one blade of the scissors inserted into the urethra, and the other blade in the bladder, the isthmus or middle lobe is

[1] Brit. Med. J., 1889, ii, 863.

divided by one or two clips. Immediately the bladder fills with blood, but without stopping to try and control this hemorrhage the surgeon continues to cut down in the median line until he has completely divided the mass that separates the urethra from the bladder, until, in fact, the finger can be passed from the floor of the bladder to the floor of the urethra without riding over any prostatic obstacle. If there are any pedunculated growths, these are then caught and twisted off with the heavy rongeur forceps (Fig. 85). The finger

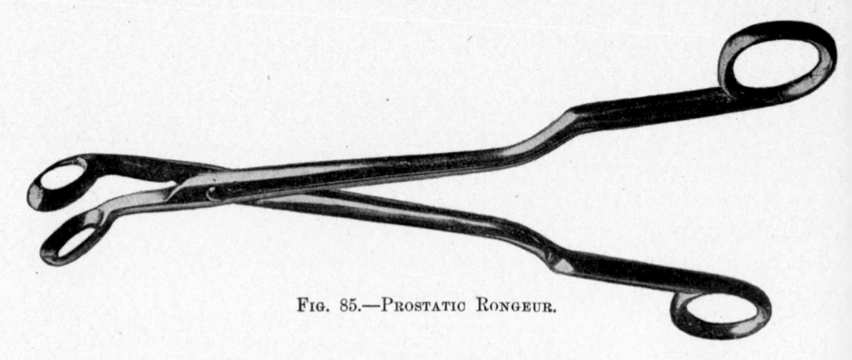

Fig. 85.—Prostatic Rongeur.

is then introduced into the median cut in the prostate, and, working on one side or the other, an endeavour is made to enucleate large encapsulated masses of glandular tissue (Fig. 68). If the prostate is large and glandular, these tumours are easily enucleated, and after their removal it will be found that the projecting masses have disappeared. This work is much facilitated by the firm counterpressure of a fist against the patient's perineum, or by a finger introduced into the prostatic urethra through a perineal cut (Belfield [1]). But if the prostate is fibrous the finger will make no impression upon the tumour. It will then be preferable to remove a wide groove of tissue from the bar with the rongeur, while leaving the lateral lobes untouched.

The hemorrhage all this while is profuse, so that the operation is performed at the bottom of a pool of blood. But a single irrigation with very hot saline solution, followed by an irrigation with nitrate of silver (1: 4,000), moderates the oozing. Some years ago I advocated and employed a graduated pad to be held in place by a loop passed through the perineum; but I no longer use this, nor have I lately had any great trouble with hemorrhage after this operation, although the bleeding commonly continues for several days, and clots may obstruct the drainage. By doing much of the work with

[1] Am. J. of Medical Sciences, 1890, c, 439.

in the prostatic capsule dangerous hemorrhage is avoided. Counter pressure from the rectum assists enucleation.

The double suprapubic tube (p. 465) provides for drainage. Urethral drainage is inadequate, perineal drainage unnecessary.

The operation attributed to Freyer appears to have been originated by Fuller. It purposes to remove the entire prostate including the prostatic urethra. So radical a procedure is scarcely necessary, though Freyer [1] reports singularly good results, and finds that excising the prostatic urethra does not cause vesical incontinence.

Perineal Prostatectomy.—Within the last few years perineal prostatectomy has become the operation of choice with the majority of surgeons. It requires more technical skill than does the suprapubic operation, and achieves, with the modern improvements in anesthesia, asepsis, and urinary antisepsis, end results little if any better and a mortality little if any less. Yet it is technically more promising, since it attacks the prostatic obstruction directly, and provides dependent drainage. Moreover, convalescence is far shorter and more comfortable after the perineal operation.

We may mention the pioneer names of Watson,[2] Thompson,[3] Dittel,[4] Nicoll,[5] and Alexander,[6] and proceed to discuss the two operations at present employed. These may be called respectively the intra-urethral and the extra-urethral methods.

Intra-urethral perineal prostatectomy is the operation I prefer for almost all cases. It is rapid, simple, and efficient.

With the patient in the lithotomy position, median perineal urethrotomy (p. 201) is performed and the finger introduced through the deep urethra into the bladder to palpate the obstruction, noting also the presence or absence of a contractured bladder neck (p. 317). Then withdraw the finger to the apex of the prostate, and break into the prostatic lobe to be enucleated. The finger should be gouged directly toward the centre of the offending mass until it feels the lobular convolutions of prostatic substance. Otherwise the mistake may be made of getting outside the prostatic capsule, and causing grave hemorrhage from the peri-prostatic veins.

Having thus entered the proper plane the finger sweeps around the lower and outer surfaces of the hypertrophied lobe (always within the capsule). When these are entirely freed so that the lobe adheres only to the bladder above and the urethra within, it is seized by a long, thin volsella and freed from above downward very gently.

This last step is the most difficult to accomplish. To simplify

[1] Lancet, 1904, ii, 197.
[2] Operative Treatment of the Hypertrophied Prostate, 1888.
[3] *Op. cit.*, p. 114.
[4] Wien. klin. Wochenschr., 1890, iii, 364.
[5] Lancet, 1894, i, 926.
[6] Med. Record, 1894, l, 841.

it, Alexander's suprapubic cystotomy and Parker Syms's [1] rubber bulb have been suggested. But most surgeons find that the finger alone, or aided by a long, narrow volsella, is able to do the work.

The enlarged lobes are thus attacked in turn. If fibrous, they may be so adherent as to require a rongeur to remove them; if very large, they may have to be broken up and extracted piecemeal. In fact, for very large lobes either suprapubic prostatectomy or extra-urethral perineal prostatectomy is the operation of choice.

Extra-urethral perineal prostatectomy is the only one of these operations by which the prostatic enucleation is done actually under the eye of the observer. It therefore appeals to the imagination as a simple, straightforward procedure. Yet it is actually more difficult, tedious, and dangerous (to judge by actual results) than any other accepted method of attacking the prostate. The experienced operator does well with it, but the beginner often tears bladder and rectum, and even the expert may lacerate the urethra.

The incision employed is the curved (or angular) pre-rectal incision (E F, Fig. 60, p. 204), enlarged if need be by a median incision. This opens up a wide space between urethra and rectum. With a sound in the former and a finger in the latter the bulb is exposed, and will be found attached to the rectum by a fibrous band, the central tendon of the perineum. Divide this, and immediately beneath appears the recto-urethralis muscle which holds the anterior wall of the rectum against the membranous urethra. Divide this, push the rectum back and expose the prostate by blunt dissection. A flat retractor in the lower angle of the wound depresses the rectum and leaves the prostate in full view.

Now enter the urethra by snipping it longitudinally just in front of the apex of the prostate; insert a finger into the urethra, outline the obstruction, and depress the lobe to be excised by hooking the finger over it. Incise the prostatic capsule in a line parallel to the urethra, and where it bulges most prominently into the wound. Enucleate the lobe within the capsule (see above) and, in order to spare the urethra, dissect on the urethral side with scissors, all the while keeping a finger in the urethra. All the enlarged lobes may thus be removed by one or two incisions in the prostatic capsule.

This is the operation done by Albarran. Exceptionally, the perineum is so deep as to require a hook in the bladder to pull it down. The best instrument for this purpose is Young's retractor.[2] Young pleads against using a median incision into the prostatic capsule in any case, lest damage be done to the median isthmus in

---

[1] J. Am. Med. Ass'n, 1901, xxxvii, 1154. [2] *Ibid.*, 1903, xvi, 999.

which run the ejaculatory ducts; for he believes the preservation of these ducts essential to potency and preventive of epididymitis.

Termination of the Operation.—At the close of perineal prostatectomy one must control hemorrhage and establish drainage.

Extra-urethral prostatectomy requires systematic, but not tight, packing of the cavities left by removal of the prostatic lobes. If the gauze is well dusted with glutol the control of bleeding will be more immediate. This gauze may be removed between the second and fourth days. Drainage is by a small perineal tube. Young uses a double tube and continual irrigation.

Intra-urethral prostatectomy requires drainage by a rather large tube (30–35 F), and gauze impregnated with glutol should be packed about this to control the bleeding both within the prostatic urethra and at the incision in the bulb.

After-treatment of Prostatectomy.—The after-treatment of prostatectomy differs little from that of cystotomy (p. 206). But the drainage tube should be removed and the patient got out of bed before the fourth day. Urotropin (p. 376) and Suwannee water (p. 378) and daily irrigations complete the routine treatment.

Causes of Death.—The special dangers of prostatectomy and the usual causes of death are shock, suppression, heart failure, sepsis, embolism, and hemorrhage. If the temperature rises, and there seems to be a progressive *infection* it must be combated by stimulants and frequent irrigations with antiseptics (I prefer nitrate of silver) as strong as the patient can bear. This failing, the wound is reopened, under primary anesthesia, if necessary, in the hope of finding some pocket or centre of suppuration. Unhappily, if infection gets a hold on an old prostatic he usually succumbs to it in spite of the surgeon's best efforts.

Embolism.[1]—Pulmonary or cardiac embolism is a still more desperate matter. This is one cause of death after operations upon the prostate that we cannot hope to eliminate. One of Freudenberg's and one of Meyer's deaths after Bottini's operation are attributed to this cause. One case of obvious embolism, and two others that might possibly be attributed to that cause, have occurred among my prostatectomies. But how great an importance to attach to this danger cannot yet be determined.

Hemorrhage.—Hemorrhage has not brought me a death. I have always been able to control it by hot irrigations or by packing. The packing may be placed around the perineal tube in a sac (the so-called shirted catheter), somewhat after the fashion of the abdominal Mikulicz drain, or the wound may be opened and a graduated pad

[1] N. Y. Med. J., 1902, lxxv, 577.

inserted into the neck of the bladder. This latter expedient I have never had to employ. Hemorrhage is, in fact, more often inconvenient than dangerous. The clots that accumulate in the bladder occlude the tubes and distend the viscus, causing a great deal of tenesmus. Repeated irrigations with salt solution at 120° F. will usually break up and carry off these clots. If this device fails the clots may be removed by aspiration through the litholapaxy apparatus. Serious hemorrhage does not occur after Chetwood's operation.

Early Complications.—Two other early complications, besides those already noticed, require special mention. Sloughing of the wound may occur as the result of overdosing with urotropin. I have met with only one such case.[1] The perineal tube may cause intense spasm and straining which can only be relieved by its removal.

Late Complications.—The four chief late complications of the operation are incontinence of urine, recurrence of the disease, post-operative insanity, and carcinoma. *Incontinence of urine* is often complete for three or four weeks after prostatectomy; but after the wound is healed and the patient up and about the incontinence rapidly diminishes. In many cases it disappears immediately. In some it persists for several months in the form of a dribbling after urination and slight overflow after the bladder has filled to a certain point, so that the patient is obliged to urinate every two or three hours to anticipate this overflow. Among some thirty odd operations for contracted neck of the bladder, I have produced permanent incontinence once or twice. Among my prostatectomies I know of one patient who, five years after the operation, still dribbles a few drops after urinating. The cause of this incontinence of urine is, apparently, the failure of the fibres of the divided internal sphincter to reunite. *Recurrence* of the obstruction is, I believe, always due to inadequate operation. I have never known a prostatic obstruction to recur, though it may well persist. The one such case that I have noted among my prostatectomies was caused by my neglect to attack a contracture of the neck of the bladder when removing a pedunculated middle lobe, and was cured by simple incision. *Post-operative insanity*, apart from uremic dementia, has occurred once in my practice. The patient, sixty-eight years of age, submitted to suprapubic prostatectomy. Three stones and a middle lobe were removed. He made an uninterrupted recovery, but a few weeks later his mind became deranged, and he died, two months after operation, of acute mania. *Cancerous degeneration* may declare itself after operation (p. 321).

---

[1] Phila. Med. J., 1900, vi, 606.

POST-OPERATIVE PROGNOSIS

From what has been said in the preceding paragraphs it is clear that the post-operative prognosis depends upon several factors, many of which cannot be expressed by statistics. Thus there are some persons whose bladders are so contracted before the operation that their urinary functions cannot be perfectly restored by any mechanical procedure. Others come to operation in such desperate straits of urinary septicemia that their deaths are almost foregone conclusions. Then, again, those operations which I consider quite unjustifiable, such as castration, vasectomy, Bottini's operation, certainly have a low mortality, and, in certain cases, do benefit the patient. I have endeavoured to express the merits of these operations in the preceding pages, and shall not therefore concern myself with them here; but, from a personal experience extending over many years, I can speak with some authority upon the subjects of suprapubic prostatectomy, perineal prostatectomy, and Chetwood's operation. In the appended table are classified my prostatectomies and the Chetwood operations thus far performed by Dr. Chetwood and by Dr. Keyes, Jr.

I have included all the Chetwood operations in order to show, as well as figures can show, how admirably safe and successful the procedure has been. I have carefully excluded from the prostatic tables all reference to cases of contracture of the neck of the bladder, although such statistics are commonly included, to the great lessening of the operative mortality.

Suprapubic Prostatectomy

1890–1894—12 cases (6 calculous)—5 deaths (3 calculous).

1895–1900—10 cases (4 calculous)—2 deaths (0 calculous).

Mortality—1890–1894—41.66%.

(Eight perineal prostatectomies during this time reduce the total mortality to 25%.)

1895–1900—20%.

Total mortality—31.81%.

Improved—5 cases.

One (my first case) was relieved of his stone, but his partial retention persisted.

One exchanged total retention with stone for partial retention.

One was relieved of his retention, but still suffers from a urethral stricture and pyelo-nephritis.

One had a recurrence of stone and was permanently cured (for three years) by perineal lithotomy and prostatotomy.

One, who was nearly dead at the time of operation, has clear urine and no subjective symptoms, but still passes a catheter once a day.

Secondary Mortality—2 cases—both were entire operative successes.

One of mania at the end of two months.

One of prostatic cancer at the end of two years.

Cures—1890–1894—2 cases, 16.66%.

1895–1900—6 cases, 60%.

Total cures—8 cases, 36.36%.

Five of these have been followed for ten, seven, four, three, and two years respectively.

Perineal Prostatectomy

1874–1895—8 cases—no deaths.

4 improved.

4 cured.

Chetwood's Galvano-prostatotomy

1900–1902.

For Chronic Urethritis.—1 case—cure.

For Tubercular Contracture of the Neck of the Bladder.—3 cases—improved.[1]

For Contracture of the Neck of the Bladder.—11 cases. No deaths.

One patient is still under treatment.

One who had complete retention and stone now has 150 c. c. residuum.

One was lost sight of before his cure was complete.

One who had slight incontinence of urine and a suprapubic fistula still has slight incontinence, but the fistula is closed.

Seven are cured. Two of these have been followed more than one year.

For Prostatic Obstruction.—16 cases (18 operations).

One death not attributable to the operation.[2]

One has incontinence of urine.[3]

One passed into the hands of another surgeon, refusing nephroto-

---

[1] It is noteworthy that in these cases the perineal wound healed slowly, but permanently. In each case the frequency of urination was lessened.

[2] This patient died by renal insufficiency five weeks after operation. The drainage afforded allowed him to pass his remaining days in peace. (*Cf.* Chetwood, Med. Record, 1901, lix, 767.)

[3] This patient was overcut; a second operation failed to relieve him, and two attempts at paraffin injection have been equally unsuccessful.

my for a severe pyelo-nephritis. I understand that his bladder symptoms have entirely abated.

Two are still under treatment, promising well.

One was only partially relieved by a first operation, but was cured by a second.

Eleven are cured (78%[1]), and no relapse has occurred in the five that have been followed for more than a year.

In order to estimate these statistics at their proper value it must be understood that I have never performed prostatectomy except in quite desperate cases—cases upon which every form of medication and instrumentation had been tried, and which, with not more than one or two exceptions, were suffering from pyelo-nephritis at the time of operation. Given these circumstances, the operative mortality is not bad. Two patients died of shock and suppression within forty-eight hours of the operation; 4 died within two weeks of uremia and heart failure, and 1 died of embolism. In spite of the relatively low mortality of perineal prostatectomy, I have never felt willing to prefer this method to the suprapubic in attacking massive enlargement of the prostate, but have reserved it for cases of bar and third lobe.

In comparing these operations with Chetwood's procedure, allowance must be made for the fact that while the latter has usually been employed late in the disease, and often as a last resource, there have been a certain number of cases (and with each success their number should increase) who have been persuaded not to wait until their kidneys had failed and their bladders were so dilated or contracted as to deprive them of the hope of a radical cure by any method. Some three or four have been operated upon *in extremis;* of the remainder all but three were failing under the best available palliative measures and in urgent need of operation; but in the days of prostatectomy this need was rarely acceded to until the stage of desperation had been reached.

On the other hand, I have been astonished to find what a wide range of usefulness there is for this operation. I have seen patients with very considerable prostatic enlargement cured by it. I have known a bar to cease obstructing after being burned at each extremity. I have seen cases of bilateral hypertrophy cured by cutting loose the attachments of the floor of the urethra from these lateral lobes. And I have been more than ever deeply impressed with the fact—which I long ago insisted upon—that "the main object of the operation is to cut away the bar and to depress the bladder open-

[1] Excluding the cases still under treatment.

ing into the prostate, so that the *bas fond* may drain." [1] In order to do this it has seemed proper in 5 cases to remove some prostatic tissue—once an outstanding middle lobe, thrice some portions of the bar, once an adenoma, which was loosened from a lateral lobe by the cautery incision.

I cannot believe that the perineal operation, whether a simple prostatotomy or a prostatectomy, is as suitable for very large prostates as the suprapubic route. But I repeat, an experience with the operation has shown it to be applicable to every case encountered during the past two years and has proved its efficiency to an unexpected degree.

The advantages which I have found attached to the Chetwood operation are, first, the *absence of shock*. The operation can always be performed within fifteen or twenty minutes (in Dr. Chetwood's record case the patient was away from his bed only fifteen minutes in all). Thus even in the gravest cases the shock of the operation has seemed to add nothing to the patient's dangers.[2] In the second place, the *absence of post-operative hemorrhage and urethral spasm* removes one of the greatest sources of annoyance. Any surgeon who has had much experience in operations upon the prostate must recognise the great distress often aroused and the grave danger sometimes incurred by reason of post-operative spasm, hemorrhage, and the filling of the bladder with clots. When I say that none of these immediate complications has been encountered after the Chetwood operation, the striking advantage thus gained can be understood. The patients, instead of straining and having to be irrigated and narcotized, rest peacefully after the operation and know no spasms before the fourth or fifth day, when the lacerated sphincter begins to resume its work. A third advantage, I think, is to be found in the fact that the burned incision is likely to stay open without the retention of the perineal tube any longer than required for purposes of drainage. Yet this permanence of the incision is not without its dangers, as exemplified by the one case of complete incontinence and the one case of partial incontinence resulting from this operation. It is not justifiable to burn completely through the neck of the bladder as it is justifiable to cut completely through, for the cut partially heals in spite of any tube, whereas the burn remains more or less as it is made.

I believe, therefore, that Chetwood's galvano-prostatotomy is the simplest and safest operation yet devised for the cure of prostatic

---

[1] Med. Record, 1891, vol. xl.

[2] In several desperate cases nitrous oxid has been the anesthetic employed.

hypertrophy; but it may well be inapplicable to the larger hypertrophies. I consider perineal or suprapubic prostatectomy the operation of second choice.

CHOICE OF OPERATION

From what has been said of the various operations above, we may briefly conclude that—

1. Castration and the allied operations, while they commonly reduce the congestion of the prostate, afford no permanent relief and fail to justify their statistical mortality.

2. Bottini's operation often gives excellent and apparently permanent results, but its action is entirely uncertain. It has occasioned serious and fatal blunders at the hands of the most experienced operators, and is often followed by annoying complications owing to the lack of proper drainage.

3. Chetwood's operation, while retaining all the advantages of Bottini's operation, except the purely sentimental one of "no cutting," adds to it precision and safety, and is always the operation of choice unless the prostate is enormous.

4. Prostatectomy, in spite of its relatively high mortality, cures certain cases that could not otherwise be cured.

In short, having decided that a sufferer from hypertrophy of the prostate is doing badly under palliative treatment, he should be cut in the perineum in the hope that Chetwood's operation may suffice to cure him, and, if the obstacle is too large to be burned down, prostatectomy—suprapubic or perineal—should be performed forthwith.

CHAPTER XX

NEURALGIA OF THE PROSTATIC URETHRA—CONTRACTURE OF THE NECK OF THE BLADDER—MALIGNANT DISEASE OF THE PROSTATE

THE three disorders considered in this chapter—viz., neuralgia of the prostatic urethra, contracture of the neck of the bladder, and cancer of the prostate—have nothing in common from the scientific point of view, but they are bound in strong clinical kinship by the fact that all three are frequently encountered in connection with hypertrophy of the prostate, and a correct knowledge of their characteristics is essential chiefly for the purpose of distinguishing them from that disease.

NEURALGIA OF THE PROSTATIC URETHRA

This disorder rejoices in many titles. By the French it is termed *névralgie du col*; in this country it commonly passes as irritability (or weakness) of the bladder. I have selected the above title as best expressing the nature of the condition, which may be defined as a non-inflammatory hyperesthesia of the surface of the prostatic urethra.

There are two classes of cases, the one due to sexual excess and common in the young, the other a pure neurosis, frequently an expression of excess with tobacco, wine, or women, or of the nervous strain brought on by business cares or family feuds, and commonest in middle and later life. This latter class of cases may be associated with some hypertrophy of the prostate, and perhaps the congestion of that gland may prepare the soil as it were. I am more inclined to incriminate an overacid urine loaded with crystals; but whatever the predisposing cause, the striking feature of the disease is the manifest effect of the general nervous tone upon the prostatic sensibility. With every outbreak—and it is difficult to ward off recurrences—there is some new nervous cause—overwork, an unhappy speculation, a turbulent son—in short, some nervous strain or other.

On the other hand, the sexual cases are often part of a general sexual neuralgia due to excessive, irregular, or ungratified sexual desire. Here the picture of deep urethral irritability is obscured by frequent nocturnal emissions, paresthesia of the scrotum and testes, etc. The clean-cut cases are not of this type.

Symptoms.—The symptoms of a pure case are as follows: Frequent desire to urinate, the attack coming on sometimes suddenly, sometimes gradually, without appreciable cause, or perhaps commencing in an inflammatory condition of the parts (gonorrhea), but not subsiding with this. The desire to empty the bladder may or may not be attended by a slight burning pain in the act. The relief after urination is usually not perfect, and the desire soon returns. There is often a certain slowness in the act, the bladder contracting without force, and the stream being small, or, on the other hand, the bladder may contract spasmodically when the call comes, throwing out the urine with great force. Again, there may be spasmodic contraction of the cut-off muscle, causing inability to urinate, or hesitation in the act.

There are some prominent peculiarities about these calls to urinate. They rarely disturb the patient at night. Once asleep, he rests quietly, but, if restless and wakeful, from anxiety or other causes, he is obliged to empty his bladder frequently, by night as well as by day. When under the stimulation of liquor, the urine can sometimes be held for a number of hours. When pleasantly occupied, or deeply interested in anything, as at the theatre, in agreeable company, or engaged at some earnest work, the bladder is often but little if at all troublesome. On rainy, damp, or cold days, the calls to urinate are more frequent, perhaps once an hour. The same occurs during idleness, and especially during mental worry or disquietude. The spirits are usually depressed, the patient anxious, perhaps hypochondriacal. The urine is usually clear, unless it contains an excess of amorphous phosphates. This deposit sometimes alternates from week to week with a deposit of urates. Sometimes both ingredients exist in excess. Crystals of oxalate of lime are not uncommonly present. There is no soreness over the pubes, though pressure there will sometimes call forth a desire to urinate. In the rectum there is often a slight sensation of heat and uneasiness. There is frequently a dull, dragging, uncomfortable feeling in the perineum, but pressure there is not painful. Spasmodic stricture of the urethra may come on as an accompaniment of this condition, while great irritability of the cut-off muscle exists as a rule.

Diagnosis.—When a patient comes complaining of frequent urination of the type just described, and his urine contains no pus, the diagnosis is clear; he has an irritable deep urethra. The introduction of a moderately large (22 French) blunt steel sound confirms the diagnosis. The whole canal is found sensitive and irritable.

At the membranous urethra, the cut-off muscles contract spasmodically, often sufficiently to bar the progress of the sound entirely, and give the idea of organic stricture. As the instrument advances, the cut-off muscle may be felt to quiver in slight partial contractions, while the patient complains greatly of pain. When the beak of the sound enters the prostatic sinus, the patient is very apt to feel faint. He may indeed go into syncope, or have an attack of nausea; or perhaps a sexual orgasm may be induced, in which case the prostate and the cut-off muscle contract violently upon the sound, causing the patient considerable pain. As the sound passes the neck of the bladder, either the natural feeling of a desire to urinate will not be perceived or (usually) the sensation will be highly exaggerated and painful. Sometimes spasm of the bladder will be induced, and the instrument will be forced out, or a jet of urine may gush out along the urethra outside of the instrument. On withdrawing the sound, a little blood may be found upon the beak, but, as a rule, the patient feels relieved, and will often experience for hours thereafter an ease and local comfort such as he has been a stranger to for months, perhaps for years, his interval of urination being decidedly lengthened, although the smarting at the next urinary act will be greater than before.

Treatment.—While tonics, climate, sexual hygiene, etc., may play a part in the cure, no remedy can be depended upon that does not blunt the urethral sensibility, and for this purpose nothing is so potent as the very gentle introduction of a steel sound or a few astringent deep urethral instillations. The sound need not be large enough to put the canal on the stretch; the instillations need not be strong enough to produce anything more than a passing discomfort. I do not commonly carry the sound higher than 26 French; the instillations I begin at 3% or 6% thallin sulphate; run this to 12%; then turn to nitrate of silver, 1: 1,500, carry this to 1: 500, and by that time the patient is cured. Sometimes sounds, sometimes instillations are best used alone, sometimes it seems more profitable to follow each passage of a sound with an instillation. The time for reintroduction will depend upon the duration of the effect of a single use of the instrument. If there is prostatitis or cystitis, the instrument will aggravate the local conditions; if neuralgia, its gentle use will always be followed by comfort, and the relief will last a variable time. In old subjects it is sometimes necessary at first to reintroduce the instrument every day; in younger people every second, third, or fourth day, until a cure is effected. The patient must be warned that relapses are likely to occur; but he may be assured that if he comes immediately for treatment a few local applications will suffice to set him right again.

CONTRACTURE OF THE NECK OF THE BLADDER

I know no common malady of the urinary organs more elusive than contracture of the neck of the bladder. I am confident that it may exist without causing any symptoms whatever. In young men it keeps up a severe posterior urethritis. In older men it simulates, and is commonly mistaken for, hypertrophy of the prostate. It is curious that this disorder, so much discussed by Mercier, Civiale, and the men of their time under the names *valvule du col*, *contracture du col*, should in our days be entirely overlooked, or classed as a variety of prostatic hypertrophy instead of receiving the clinical recognition to which it is entitled.

Contracture of the neck of the bladder is a rigid, fibrous, contracted condition of the ring of muscle constituting the vesical neck. The orifice is often so small and the contractured tissue so dense that the tip of the little finger cannot be forced through it, but the occlusion is never complete.

Varieties.—The line must be sharply drawn between tubercular (p. 404) and simple contracture of the neck of the bladder. The former possesses all the features of vesical tuberculosis, and is, clinically, quite distinct from simple contracture, although, pathologically, they resemble each other closely. At present we are concerned only with simple contracture.

Etiology.—Contracture of the neck of the bladder occurs in young and old alike, but it is not met with before puberty. The chief and almost the only cause of the disease (tuberculosis excepted) is chronic posterior urethritis. In some cases it is perhaps caused by stone in the bladder. It is so common in later life that it might almost be ranked with the arcus senilis and the fibrotic arteries as one of the evidences of the crystallization of age; but, in the great majority of cases at least, protracted inflammation of the posterior urethra is its sole cause, and many cases can be traced directly to a persistent chronic gonorrhea.

Morbid Anatomy.—The essential morbid change seems to occur in the band of muscle surrounding the neck of the bladder, the internal vesical sphincter. The fibres of this muscle, or at least those nearest the surface, lose their resiliency and become fibrous and inelastic, so that they no longer dilate or contract, except very slightly. The superimposed mucous membrane is commonly, if not always, in a state of chronic inflammation. As a result of the contracted condition of this muscle the bladder ultimately becomes pouched behind it, forms a *bas fond*, and contains residual urine, quite as though the obstruction were prostatic.

Symptoms.—Contracture of the neck of the bladder has no one clinical type by which it may be constantly identified. While it doubtless often passes unrecognised, and may in its milder forms be quite curable, I have only been able to identify it clinically under one of three forms. In each case it is a stubborn and unmanageable condition.

1. *Posterior Urethritis.*—Contracture of the neck of the bladder commonly occurs, as we have seen, as the result of a protracted chronic urethritis. Indeed, the contracture itself often enough seems to prevent the cure of the posterior urethritis. The onset cannot be clearly defined, but, clinically, the diagnosis of contracture of the neck of the bladder is clearly established by a combination of certain symptoms—viz., a protracted posterior urethritis that does not respond to any local or general treatment, imperative urination, and some pain during and after urination, a pain which is the more notable since there is no acute inflammation to account for it. Imperative urination is a most distressing symptom. When the patient feels the call to urinate he must respond at once under penalty of losing a few drops of his urine, enough to saturate the tail of his shirt. There may be other symptoms, partial retention of urine, cystitis, even pyelitis, or neuralgic phenomena; but, in this class of cases, the three characteristic phenomena are (1) chronic, unconquerable, posterior urethritis, (2) imperative urination, (3) dysuria. The history of such a case is simply that of a chronic urethritis that will not get well, plus imperative and painful urination.

2. *Stone in the Bladder.*—A contracted neck of the bladder is often met with in long-standing cases of vesical calculus.[1] Whether the contracture is due to the stone or the stone is secondary to the contracture, I do not know. Suffice it to say that the condition is similar to the third variety (see below), plus stone. The contracture may be quite unsuspected until, after the stone has been crushed, the case takes on the aspect of the first or the third variety of the disease, or in the course of a lithotomy a rigid vesical neck may be encountered. Occasionally, the diagnosis is made during a litholapaxy by the obstruction to the admission of instruments. This

---

[1] Exceptionally a contracture gives the symptoms to stone, although the urine is clear and no stone present.

obstruction is usually met with in the shape of a bar at the neck of the bladder (when, as a matter of fact, no prostatic hypertrophy exists) over which the instruments jump. Very rarely a large-sized litholapaxy tube may be caught in the grip of the contractured muscle. On forcing the instrument a trifle it is then felt to tear through the obstruction.

3. *Bar at the Neck of the Bladder.*—This variety of contracture covers a multitude of misinterpreted cases. Those cases of atrophied prostate with the retention and other symptoms of hypertrophy; cases of "prostatic hypertrophy" occurring abnormally early in life; cases in which the retention and other symptoms are out of all proportion to the hypertrophy of the prostate; cases of "hypertrophied prostate" in which the introduction of the Bottini instrument serves to show that the prostate is not really enlarged—a discovery which is usually explained on the score of congestion—these obscure forms of retention, wrongly ascribed to hypertrophy of the prostate, are, in reality, due to contracture of the neck of the bladder. It is needless to add that the contracture may occur when there is hypertrophy of the prostate as well as when there is none. It is not always possible to identify it, yet there are some cases clearly due to contracture and not to hypertrophy of the prostate. These are:

1. All cases in which the prostate feels normal or atrophied to rectal touch and the urinary distance does not exceed 20 cm., while there is retention of urine.

2. Most cases in which there is moderate peripheral enlargement of the prostate, a urinary distance not exceeding 20 cm., with a residuum of 100 c. c. or more.

In both these classes of cases the peripheral enlargement of the prostate is quite inadequate to account for the residuum, the shortness of the urethra precludes the possibility of a middle lobe or bar, and the only remaining factor to which the residuum can be attributed is a contracture of the neck of the bladder, and perineal section will prove this the *corpus delicti*. The course of the disease here is that of hypertrophy of the prostate.

Diagnosis.—After what has been said there is little to be added on the score of diagnosis. When a chronic urethritis, whether gonorrheal or not, drags on indefinitely and is rebellious to treatment, contracture may be diagnosed if dysuria and imperative urination are present without any acute inflammation, and if there is residual urine without hypertrophy of the prostate, that clinches the diagnosis. In the second place, when there are all the symptoms and signs of prostatic hypertrophy, and yet the prostate is not hypertrophied sufficiently to account for the symptoms, the existence of contracture of the neck of the bladder may be affirmed.

Prognosis.—The outlook in these cases is not good. When there is retention of urine recovery may not be expected spontaneously nor from topical applications. When there is no retention the cases are often equally intractable, although, occasionally, one is cured by the treatment of the posterior urethritis, whether by curing the surface inflammation or by causing the resorption of the deeper inflammatory tissue, I cannot say.

Treatment.—The indications for treatment are perfectly clean-cut. If the case affects the chronic urethritis type, it should be treated locally, until the patient's endurance gives out, in the hope that it may perhaps be cured thus. But if these means fail, or if the disease is of the prostatic type, it should be submitted to the knife. The only exception to this rule occurs in the stone cases. If these are submitted to litholapaxy, the bruising of the neck of the bladder by the large tubes, though this will cause a pretty active post-operative reaction lasting some weeks, may so tear the contracted bladder neck that a cure will result in the long run; yet such an uncertain and brutal treatment could not be advocated.

Operative Treatment.—Although I have kept no records of operations for contracture of the neck of the bladder, I have found in my case books 15 operations for contracture without a death. Among 8 other operative cases in which the contracture complicated a tight stricture there were 2 deaths. Although I have operated for contracture much more frequently than these figures show, I have never had a post-operative death. Among urethrotomies for stricture the mortality is entirely attributable to the stricture, and does not concern the contracted neck of the bladder.

My method of operating has always been to perform perineal cystotomy (p. 457) and to tear through the neck of the bladder with the finger, or, if this proved inefficient or impossible, to cut down the rigid neck obliquely to one side, just deep enough to allow the finger free access to the bladder. I prefer a lateral to a median cut, believing it less likely than the median incision to cause incontinence or to divide both ejaculatory ducts. To make the cut I now use the Chetwood galvano-cautery instead of a blunt-pointed straight bistoury, for the knife sometimes causes alarming bleeding, the cautery practically none. The great danger after this operation is incontinence of urine. If every fibre of the muscle at the bladder neck is divided incontinence may be complete and permanent, and I have known this unfortunate result to occur in two cases. Yet it is necessary to divide the contracture sufficiently to overcome the symptoms, notably the retention. A solution of this difficulty will, I believe, be found in Chetwood's operation. The cautery must be applied very moderately. A single incision 1½ cm. long is ample to divide the tighter fibres and to relieve the residuum.

The after-treatment of this operation depends upon whether the knife or the cautery has been employed. If the former, a perineal tube must be inserted and retained for at least a week, preferably two weeks, in order to force the wound to heal by granulation. The use of the cautery obviates this necessity, however, and after employing it I believe the tube need only be left in place for four days. The bladder must be washed daily for a few weeks.

The complications of the operation are hemorrhage and incontinence of urine. After cutting down the neck of the bladder there is often incessant bleeding for two or three days. I have not known this hemorrhage to be fatal, but it is often alarming. After burning operations it does not occur, and this constitutes one of the notable advantages of burning over cutting. On the other hand, incontinence may occur after either operation. Even after the most skilful manipulation it is not uncommon for the patient to dribble a little for several months after the operation; but permanent incontinence may be avoided by conservative cutting. It is true that if the patient is cut too sparingly the operation may have to be repeated; but this is far preferable to an incontinence which neither time nor art will cure.

MALIGNANT DISEASE OF THE PROSTATE

Malignant disease of the prostate is almost always primary. Extension of a vesical cancer to the prostate is extremely rare, while extension of a prostatic growth to the bladder is very common. Sarcoma occurs in youth, carcinoma in old age. Either form is rare, although such statistics as Tauchon's, which show among 8,289 cases of cancer only 5 cases affecting the prostate, certainly underestimate the frequency of the disease. Engelbach in 1888 collected 96 reported cases of malignant disease of the prostate. Nine occurred before the tenth year. There were only 18 between the tenth and the fiftieth year; while between the fiftieth and the eightieth were 69 cases. Ten carcinomata occur for every one sarcoma.

Morbid Anatomy.—*Sarcoma* may be round or spindle-celled; rarely it is an adenosarcoma, lymphosarcoma, or myxosarcoma.

Carcinoma is usually medullary or adenocarcinoma. The connection between carcinoma and prostatic hypertrophy has long been disputed. Certain it is that the hypertrophied prostate very rarely takes on malignant change, and equally certain is it that carcinoma may occur in a gland to all appearances unaffected by hypertrophy. Yet many observers have attempted to prove the epithelial proliferation of hypertrophy a fertile soil for malignant changes. Thus Albarran and Hallé[1] examined 100 hypertrophied prostates, and among these found 14 that showed small areas of typical cancerous tissue.

Neoplasms of the prostate may run their whole course, extending to the neighbouring organs, causing metastases and death without involving the entire gland, though it is more common for the gland to be entirely involved early in the disease. The growth spreads rapidly by extension to the bladder wall and the prostatic urethra. Rectum, vesicles, ureter, and anterior urethra are sometimes invaded. The retroperitoneal and mesenteric glands are involved early, the inguinal glands later. Bone metastases are especially common. Von Frisch mentions von Recklinghausen's 5 cases of insignificant primary prostatic cancer with extensive secondary bone involvement.

Symptoms.—Unfortunately, cancer of the prostate is rarely recognised until the disease is well advanced. Indeed, von Recklinghausen's cases show that the primary prostatic disease may be overlooked even at a time when the secondary growths have assumed alarming proportions. Two other facts tend to confuse the diagnosis. In the first place, the prostate is commonly attacked by malignant disease late in life, and at first causes slight symptoms which the patient refers to advancing age or to hypertrophy of the prostate, if he possesses the dangerous "little knowledge," and which may deceive even the surgeon. In the second place, the progress of the disease is often nothing less than furious. Before the patient realizes he is sick the growth fairly fills the pelvis. It is this characteristic that has earned for the disease Guyon's title of *carcinose prostato-pelvienne.*

In children the initial symptom of the disease is most often an obstruction to urination; but adults commonly complain of severe *pain* long before there is any urinary difficulty. This pain has several striking characteristics. Though it may at first occur only during urination, it soon becomes continuous. The pain is quite severe. It is increased by urination and defecation, but never ceases entirely. It is concentrated in the perineum or the rectum, and thence radiates to the genitals, the hypogastrium, and the loins, in which last place it may be especially severe. It also causes reflex sciatica, and bilateral sciatica is especially suggestive of cancer of the prostate. These

[1] Guyon's Annales, 1900, xviii, 113, 225.

painful symptoms are characteristic of the early stages of the disease, and, apparently, are due to tension of the dense prostatic capsule. After this has been broken through the typical pain ceases, and there is left only dysuria from such retention or inflammation as may be present.

Slight *hematuria*, either at the beginning or at the end of urination, occurs in one quarter of the cases. In the later stages of the disease, when urethra and bladder are both the seat of malignant fungous ulcerations, copious hematuria is common. *Obstructive and inflammatory symptoms* are quite those of hypertrophy of the prostate; and towards the end constant straining urination, with foul bloody urine, is the most distressing symptom. Edema of the extremities and genitals, and cancerous cachexia are encountered in the terminal stages of the disease.

The growth commonly progresses with the greatest rapidity, and the patient usually dies within a year of the first appearance of symptoms. But, exceptionally, the new growth remains stationary or progresses but slowly for many months. Fenwick[1] makes a special class of these and compares them with mammary scirrhus. They may last for as long as three years.

Diagnosis.—The symptoms suggestive of cancer of the prostate are encountered only when the disease is sufficiently advanced to be distinguished by rectal examination, and upon this the diagnosis rests. In a pronounced case the cachectic condition, the dysuria, the foul, bloody urine, and the enlarged inguinal glands only require a cursory rectal examination to confirm the diagnosis. The finger, as soon as it passes the internal sphincter, abuts upon an enormous hard, nodular tumour on the anterior rectal wall. Perhaps the rectum itself is ulcerated.

But in the beginning cases the diagnosis may be no easy matter. The growth, as felt from the rectum, assumes one of two forms: it is either a circumscribed nodule in one of the lateral lobes, remarkably hard, though not necessarily prominent, or it is a less hard, irregular infiltration of the whole gland, which cannot be distinguished from simple hypertrophy, except, perhaps, by the characteristic pain, until it has attained an ominous size, given rise to secondary glandular enlargements in the groin and along the iliac vessels, and begun to invade the bladder and the periprostatic tissues.

The differential diagnosis between carcinoma and hypertrophy is often impossible in the earlier stages of the disease (see above). Cancer of the base of the bladder may be distinguished from cancer

---

[1] Edinb. Med. J., 1899, vi, 16.

of the prostate by delineating the normal prostate below the vesical growth, by observation of the urethral length, which is not increased unless the cancer is prostatic, and by cystoscopy, which shows an intravesical growth, but commonly fails to make out a prostatic one.

Treatment.—Extirpation of the prostate has been done 8 times (von Frisch). Five of the patients died within two months, 2 survived nine months (Czerny, Verhoogen), and 1 fourteen months (Billroth); but all these died of recurrence. Such a record discourages the hope of radical cure by the knife. Indeed, the well-known rapidity with which secondary glandular involvement takes place precludes expectation of any very brilliant results in this direction. Yet partial prostatectomy has given results which, if not brilliant, are at least slightly encouraging. Two of von Frisch's cases (middle lobe) remained well one year, and a case operated upon by Socin for sarcoma of the right lobe remained well two years.

Palliative treatment is almost equally futile. In the early stages, sedatives, tonics, and the catheter (if there is retention) may relieve the symptoms somewhat. Later, opium, suprapubic cystotomy, as for cancer of the bladder (p. 422), and colostomy, as soon as the rectum becomes ulcerated or obstructed, are the chief elements of palliative treatment.

CHAPTER XXI

THE BLADDER: ANATOMY, PHYSIOLOGY, EXAMINATION—EXSTROPHY OF THE BLADDER

ANATOMY

The bladder is a muscular sac lying, in the male, between the rectum and the pubes when empty, and distending, when full, into an oval bag occupying more or less of the hypogastrium (Fig. 86). Its position is fixed below by the urethra, by the pelvic fascia, which, after lining the cavity of the true pelvis, is reflected upward and lost on the bladder and rectum (as pubo-prostatic and inferior vesical ligaments), and by the recto-vesical fascia, which binds the prostate and the neck of the bladder to the rectum. The muscular tissue of the organ is covered on the outside by peritoneum, on the inside by mucous membrane. Above and on the sides the peritoneum covers the bladder, but is attached loosely, especially at the base, so as to offer no obstacle to any change in shape or position of the viscus.

A knowledge of the peritoneal reflections upon the bladder is essential to a correct understanding of the operations of epicystotomy and suprapubic aspiration. When the bladder is empty it lies contracted behind the pubes; the peritoneum leaves the abdominal walls at the symphysis, and passes at once to the bladder, over which it is spread, and thence reflected upon the rectum from the base of the bladder, so that, when the latter is absolutely or even partially empty no trocar or aspirating needle may reach it from the anterior abdominal wall without traversing the peritoneal cavity.

Very different, however, is the condition of the viscus when distended. Then, as its cavity fills up, the peritoneum is carried with it. In this way the distended bladder carries up the peritoneum in front, so that in extreme retention a distance of 2 to 5 cm., or even more, above the symphysis becomes bare of peritoneum. Hence the election of the region immediately above the pubes for aspiration and the necessity of filling the bladder before attempting suprapubic cystotomy. The relation of the peritoneum to the bladder also varies behind. When the viscus is distended the peritoneum barely reaches the blind ends of the seminal vesicles; when empty it descends between them almost to the prostate.

The *shape* of the bladder varies with age. The bladder of an infant is ovoidal in shape with its long axis running downward and

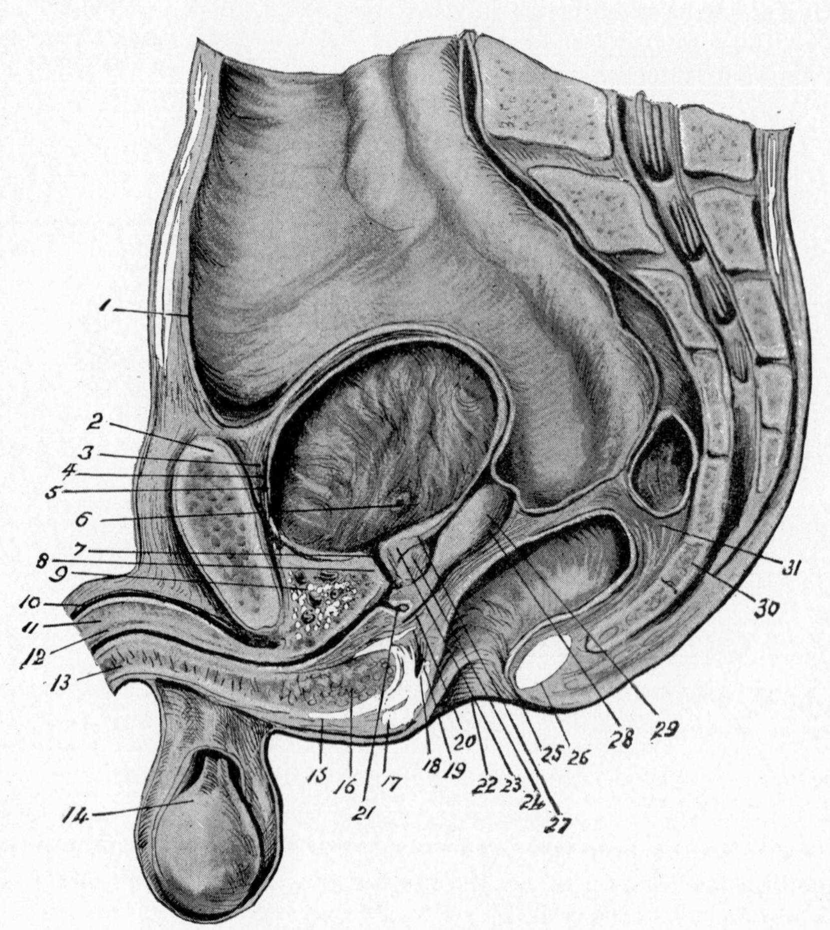

FIG. 86.—MEDIAN SECTION OF A FROZEN MALE SUBJECT.

The small intestine is removed. *1*, peritoneum; *6*, opening of the ureters; *8*, internal sphincter vesicæ; *9*, external sphincter, with the compressor urethræ muscle; *10*, dorsal vein of the penis; *15*, bulbo-cavernosus muscle; *16*, bulb of the urethra; *17*, sphincter ani; *21*, utricle; *24*, isthmus of prostate; *29*, seminal vesicles. (Henle.)

a little forward and its apex at the urethral orifice. It lies when full almost entirely out of the pelvis. As age advances the bladder sinks into the pelvis, assumes an almost spherical shape when filled, and possesses a flattened floor in the region of the trigone. Later still the *bas fond* appears with its attendant ills (p. 259).

The *muscle* of the bladder is composed of three coats—external, middle, and internal. The external or longitudinal coat consists of numerous fibres running from the prostate up over the fundus, where they are met by a similar set of fibres from the anterior surface. On the place of meeting there is often a swirl or "cowlick" of muscle fibres (Versari [1]). Over the sides of the organ the longitudinal layer is thin and unimportant. Its fibres are closely connected with the

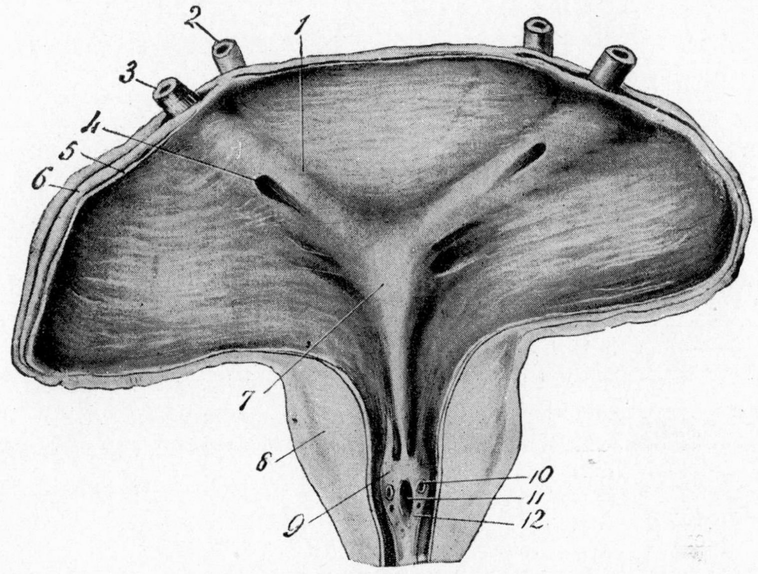

Fig. 87.—Lower Part of the Male Bladder, with the Beginning of the Urethra. Exposed by incising the anterior wall and laying it open. *3*, ureter; *4*, opening of the ureter; *2*, vas deferens; *9*, colliculus seminalis; *7*, centre of trigone; *8*, section of prostate; *10*, orifice of the common ejaculatory duct; *11*, opening of utricle; *12*, mouths of prostatic gland-ducts; *1*, interureteric fold. (Henle.)

prostate and the deep layer of the recto-vesical fascia, and intermingle with the deeper laye of the bladder muscle. The middle layer forms the bulk of the vesical muscle. Its fibres are densely interlaced and have a generally circular character. The internal layer of muscle consists of a few scattering bundles of longitudinal fibres, so irregular and inconspicuous that some anatomists deny their existence.

The *trigone* is a part of the bladder wall deserving special mention. It is a triangular region with sides some 2 cm. long lying between the orifices of the urethra and the two ureters (Fig. 87).

[1] Guyon's Annales, 1897, xv, 1089.

The muscle here is denser than elsewhere in the organ. A few fibres derived from the longitudinal coats of the ureters and urethra spread over its internal surface. A bundle of these fibres running along the base of the triangle is known as the muscle of Bell. The dense muscle tissue of the trigone has been declared by Kalischer to be part of the internal urethral sphincter (p. 240). This interpretation, though novel and startling, is very ably supported by its author.

The *mucous membrane* of the bladder is of a pale salmon colour, remarkably insensitive in health, covered by a stratified pavement epithelium, and lying in folds when the bladder is contracted, except over the trigone, where it is always smooth. The glands are not numerous, except on the trigone and near the neck. They are exceedingly small, and composed of clusters of simple follicles. The coats of the bladder are united by connective tissue, which is everywhere loose, except at the trigone.

The bladder is arbitrarily described as having four sides—anterior, posterior, and two lateral. These four sides meet above in the *fundus*, below and in front in the *neck*, which is the urethral orifice. The trigone and surrounding portions of the posterior wall are spoken of as the *floor*. The ureters pierce the floor of the bladder obliquely and open at the angles of the trigone (p. 469).

The *arteries* of the bladder are the superior, middle, and inferior vesical. They anastomose freely. The *veins* are numerous and lie in three planes—the subserous, the intermuscular, and the submucous. They anastomose freely with one another and with the prostatic plexus, and the plexus of Santorini above the neck of the bladder. They empty into the hypogastric veins. The *lymphatics* of the bladder wall were overlooked by the older anatomists, but their existence has been repeatedly verified of late years. They run chiefly beneath the mucous membrane and empty into several small groups of glands lying about the bladder itself and thence into the iliac glands along the internal and common iliac vessels. These iliac glands are commonly infected by vesical neoplasms. The lumbar glands are less frequently involved, the inguinal glands very rarely (Pasteau[1]).

The fetal bladder is connected with the allantois by the *urachus*, and this canal, closing at the time of birth, persists as a fibrous, subperitoneal cord connecting the fundus of the bladder with the umbilicus. This canal very exceptionally remains patent throughout the whole or a part of its length.

---

[1] État du système lymphatique dans les maladies de la vessie et de la prostate, Paris, 1898, p. 48.

PHYSIOLOGY

Capacity.—The capacity of the bladder is physiological, not anatomical (Guyon). Although in actual size the healthy bladders of different individuals do not differ materially, the actual capacity of the organ depends upon its sensitiveness, and this sensitiveness varies at different times and with different individuals. The physiological capacity of the bladder, the amount of urine an ordinary bladder holds when the desire to urinate is first felt, is about 250 c. c. (8 ounces).

Sensitiveness.—The healthy bladder is quite insensitive to touch, but very sensitive to tension. Thus a sound may be poked about in the bladder and cause no sensation whatever except in the prostatic urethra. On the other hand, the torture of "holding water" requires no comment. The sensitiveness of the bladder may be diminished by habit; beer-guzzlers and diabetics do not urinate more often than those who pass perhaps only half as much urine. The sensitiveness is, on the other hand, increased by nervousness and by inflammation.

Absorption.—Although the point is disputed, it is probable that the mucous membrane of the healthy bladder is practically as impervious as the skin. But fluids are rapidly absorbed through the mucous membrane of the posterior urethra, and also through the bladder epithelium when inflamed.

Contraction: Urination.—"Man urinates with his bladder, not with his urethra," says Guyon; but, though all are agreed thus far, there are diverse explanations of the mechanism of urination. (*Cf.* Rehfisch,[1] Ultzmann,[2] Guyon,[3] Versari.[4]) The known facts upon which we may depend are: 1. The vesical sensitiveness to tension. 2. The more marked sensitiveness of the posterior urethra, and the desire to urinate and the sensation of urination provoked by passing an instrument into it. 3. The presence of only one voluntary muscle to guard the outlet—viz., the external sphincter or cut-off muscle. 4. The incontinence of urine that results from distortion of or injury to the internal sphincter. Upon these may be built up the following plausible theory: The internal sphincter is the true guardian of the bladder. It remains closed, or at least sufficiently contracted to keep the urine out of the prostatic urethra while the bladder slowly fills. When the bladder has become distended to its physio-

---

[1] Virchow's Archiv, 1897, cl, 111.

[2] Deutsche Chir., v. Billroth. u. Lücke, 1890, lii, 8.

[3] Leçons cliniques, 1ière édition, 1896, ii, 379.

[4] *Op. cit.*

logical capacity the desire to urinate is felt, the bladder begins to contract, and, by means of a reflex carried out in the lumbar portion of the cord and comparable to similar reflexes in the other hollow viscera, as it contracts its sphincter opens and the urine penetrates the posterior urethra. A sharper desire to urinate is felt, and if this is acceded to by voluntary relaxation of the external sphincter, the bladder slowly contracts and empties its contents through the open channel, the last drops being ejaculated by the piston-stroke spasm of the deep urethra, or the stream cut off by a sharp contraction of the voluntary muscle. But if the desire to urinate is not acceded to, the outflow of urine is prevented by a conscious, voluntary contraction of the external sphincter and the desire for a time passes over, perhaps because the internal sphincter closes again, drives the few drops back into the bladder, and holds out a while longer. Then the desire returns, each time more imperiously, until it is satisfied.

EXAMINATION OF THE BLADDER

In most cases examination of the bladder is confined to examination of its contents. The patient is made to urinate in two glasses (p. 83), and from the contents of the second glass the nature of the contents of the bladder is inferred and some estimate of its condition obtained. To ascertain the *capacity* of the bladder a warm solution of boric acid is slowly introduced through a catheter until the bladder can hold no more. The amount of *residual urine* is learned by making the patient urinate, and then measuring the amount of urine obtained by catheter. The strength of the bladder muscle, the presence or absence of *atony*, is learned by watching the force of the stream thrown from the penis or the catheter. Special manipulations are employed to determine the presence of stone, tumour, rupture, distention, etc. The only instrument besides the catheter that is applicable to diagnosis of most bladder diseases is the cystoscope.

Cystoscopy

Cystoscopy is inspection of the interior of the bladder. Without entering into the historical aspect of the subject we may say that cystoscopy is performed to-day by two varieties of instruments. The one, a German product, perfected by Nitze, Leiter, and Casper, consists of an instrument shaped more or less like a metal elbowed catheter. In its beak is a small electric lamp connected through the shaft with a battery, and in its shaft an optical apparatus by means of which the operator, looking into the butt of the instrument, sees through a window near the beak the surrounding objects illumined by the light of the incandescent lamp. The other form of instrument we owe to Dr. Howard Kelly. It consists of a straight metallic tube into which the operator looks by means of reflected light (Chetwood has adapted his urethroscopic lamp to Kelly's instrument in a very satisfactory manner). This instrument, which is employed with the patient in the knee-chest position and the bladder filled with air, is admirably adapted to the female, but not generally applicable to the male bladder, and therefore requires no description here. We may confine our attention to the first class of instruments.

Choice of Instrument.—For a simple cystoscope I know none better than the old Leiter. Its beak is too long and angular, its shaft too short—defects which are overcome in Fenwick's modified instrument (Fig. 88)—but the inside of a bladder can be seen better

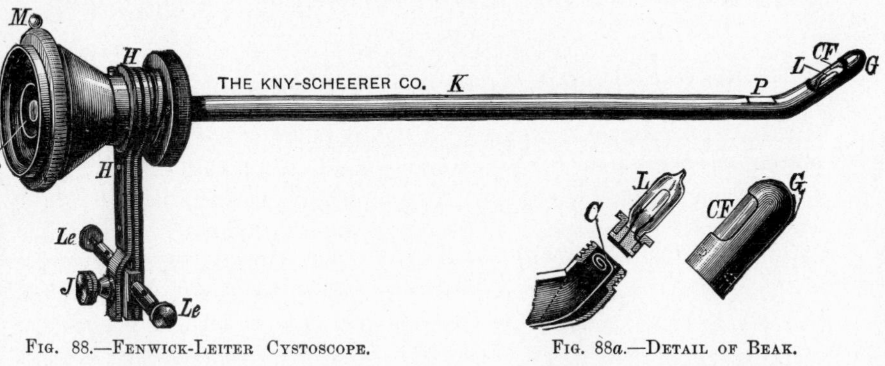

FIG. 88.—FENWICK-LEITER CYSTOSCOPE. *Le*, electrical connections; *Tf*, telescope; *P*, prism; *L*, lamp.

FIG. 88*a*.—DETAIL OF BEAK. *L*, lamp; *C*, connecting wire; *G*, metal hood; *CF*, window.

through it than through any of the newer instruments that have come into my hands (Nitze's, Albarran's, Casper's), with the exception of Nitze's photographic cystoscope, which is too large for general use. For an irrigating cystoscope the choice lies between Nitze's and Albarran's, and perhaps Boisseau de Rocher's new megaloscope, which I have not employed. For ureteral catheterization I prefer Nitze's instrument to Casper's or Albarran's. I have found no advantage in the various aërocystoscopes.

When the cystoscope was first introduced great pains were taken to show how two instruments were necessary for the inspection of the whole bladder, one with the window on the concave, and one with it on the convex side. Experience has shown that a satisfactory inspection may be made with the former kind alone, and the latter instrument (the original Nitze No. 2) is but little employed. The operating cystoscope of Nitze I have never employed, nor has it gained any wide popularity.

Cystoscopic batteries are obtainable of every important electrical company. To use the street current a rheostat must be interposed.

Preparation for Cystoscopy.—The instrument is prepared by soaking several hours in a 5% carbolic-acid solution, after which it is carefully washed with sterilized water before using. The newer instruments may be boiled.

The patient requires no great preparation unless his prostate is sensitive or his bladder inflamed. In the former case the gentle passage of sounds at intervals of three or four days for several weeks before the operation may materially blunt the prostatic sensibility. In the latter case it is proper to attack the inflammation in the hope of clarifying the contents of the bladder before employing the cystoscope. It is also prudent to administer urotropin for three or four days before operating to diminish the danger of infection and of urethral chill (p. 373).

Cystoscopy may almost always be performed under local anesthesia, and accordingly some local anesthetic is injected into the posterior urethra and bladder a few minutes before operating. The bladder is first washed out until the fluid returns clear of pus or blood, then 150 c. c. of 1% cocain solution is injected into the bladder and a few minutes later 10 drops of a 5% solution are instilled into the posterior urethra.[1] The patient is then made to remove his trousers and drawers and placed upon an ordinary gynecological office table with his buttocks on a low cushion and his feet spread apart and in the foot-rests. All is then ready for the operation. (The remote possibility of cocain-poisoning must be borne in mind. It happened once in my experience.)

The Operation.—The cystoscope is attached to the battery and the electricity slowly turned on until the lamp is at a white heat. Noting the amount of current necessary, the electricity is turned off, and the cystoscope, greased with a soluble lubricant, such as glycerin or lubrichondrin, is slowly introduced into the bladder. The instrument enters like a steel sound, but as it has a short beak it is often

---

[1] Eucain B. has not proved as satisfactory in my hands for bladder use as cocain. Nirvanin has a disagreeable property of irritating for a few moments before it anesthetizes. Guyon employs as an anesthetic injection into the rectum, forty-five minutes before operating—

℞	Antipyrin	gm. 150
	Laudanum	gtt. x
	Water	gm. 100

PLATE IV

Fig. 1, tubercular cystitis; primary stage. (Cystoscope I.) Numerous minute ecchymoses, surrounded by a hyperemic spot; many ramified vessels.

Fig. 2, partial hypertrophy of the prostate. (Cystoscope II.) Enlarged median lobe, projecting into the bladder.

Fig. 3, marked bilateral hypertrophy of the prostate; trabecular bladder. (Cystoscope II.)

Fig. 4, trabecular bladder; diverticulum of the lateral wall. (Cystoscope I.)

Fig. 5, encysted multiple stones—four only are shown. (Cystoscope I.)

Fig. 6, pin fixed in the anterior wall of the bladder, near its vertex; shadow on opposite wall. (Cystoscope I.)

Fig. 7, silk ligature adherent to the wall of the bladder; it projects from a red papilla (granulation tissue). (Cystoscope I.)

Fig. 8, two fragments of stone which remained in the bladder after lithotrity; in the larger one the nucleus of uric acid is seen. (Cystoscope I.)

PLATE IV

Fig. 1, tubercular cystitis; primary stage. (Cystoscope I.) Numerous minute ecchymoses, surrounded by a hyperemic spot; many ramified vessels.

Fig. 2, partial hypertrophy of the prostate. (Cystoscope II.) Enlarged median lobe, projecting into the bladder.

Fig. 3, marked bilateral hypertrophy of the prostate; trabecular bladder. (Cystoscope II.)

Fig. 4, trabecular bladder; diverticulum of the lateral wall. (Cystoscope I.)

Fig. 5, encysted multiple stones—four only are shown. (Cystoscope I.)

Fig. 6, pin fixed in the anterior wall of the bladder, near its vertex; shadow on opposite wall. (Cystoscope I.)

Fig. 7, silk ligature adherent to the wall of the bladder; it projects from a red papilla (granulation tissue). (Cystoscope I.)

Fig. 8, two fragments of stone which remained in the bladder after lithotrity; in the larger one the nucleus of uric acid is seen. (Cystoscope I.)

PLATE IV.

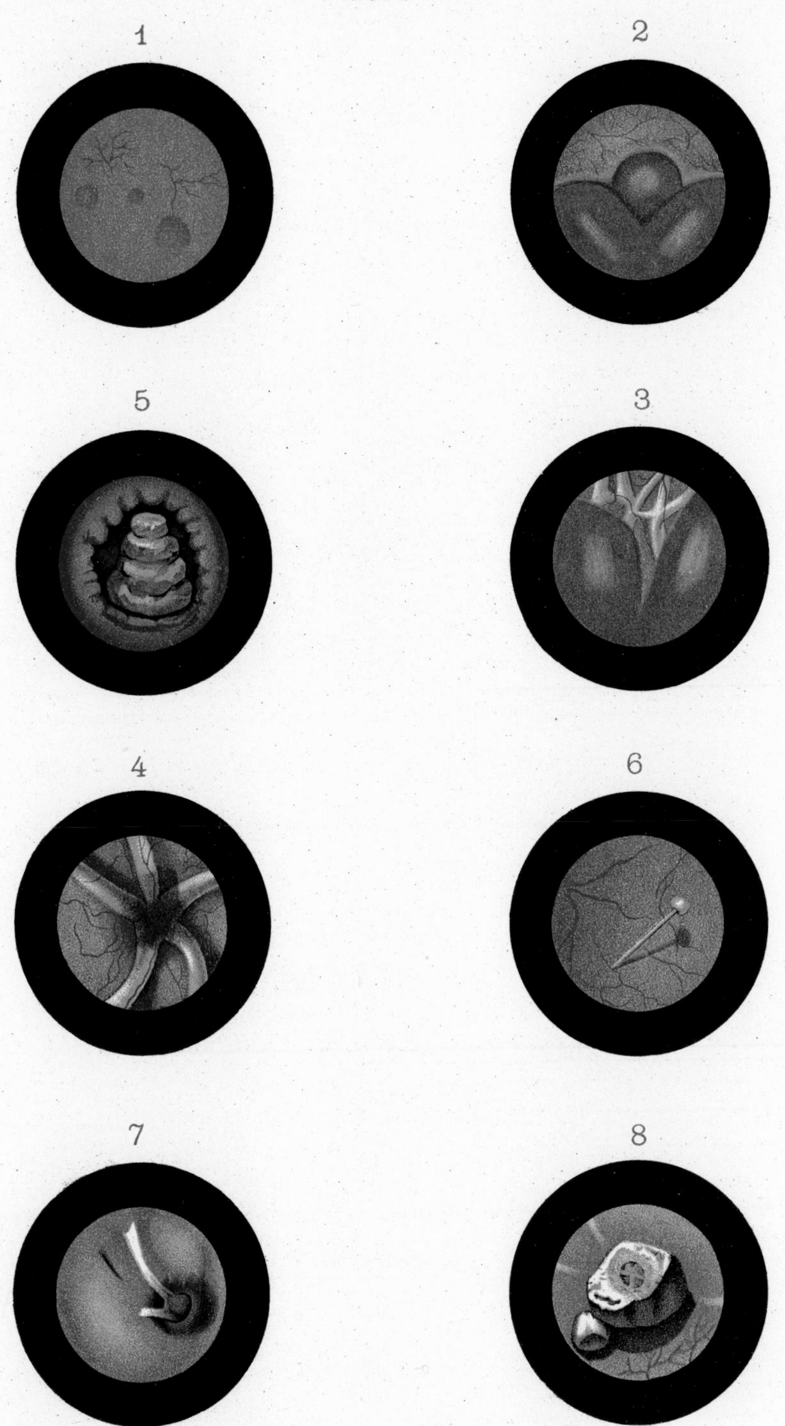

CYSTOSCOPIC PICTURES.

necessary to lift it into the membranous urethra by pressure on the perineum. Once in the bladder it may be freely moved forward and backward and rotated on its long axis, but this long axis should always be kept in the sagittal plane of the patient, except for the slight inclination allowable and necessary to catheterize the ureters. With the instrument well in the bladder the electric current is again turned on to the necessary strength and the beak of the instrument rotated so as to face the floor of the bladder. The surgeon then looks into the instrument and deliberately withdraws it until a dark-red crescent appears upon the scene. This is the neck of the bladder. Withdraw the instrument a trifle further and everything disappears from view; further withdrawal is impeded, and the patient complains of pain. If the neck of the bladder is normal it appears as a clear-cut crescent. If inflamed it appears nodular and velvety. If there is contraction or hypertrophy of the prostate, the neck of the bladder is deformed (Plate IV, Figs. 2, 3). Having carefully observed the lower part of the neck of the bladder, the cystoscope is pushed slowly backward in the median line. The salmon tint of the bladder wall passes through the field, here and there crossed by a vessel or interrupted by a fold of mucous membrane.

When the fundus is reached the instrument is turned 45 degrees to one side and the return trip is made. On this trip the ureteral opening should be seen. It may be recognised as an oblique slit or a slight prominence of the bladder wall, and if watched for a moment it will be seen to gather itself up and emit a spurt of urine. This may be visibly purulent or bloody. Thus the examination is continued all the way around until the beak of the instrument is turned downward again. It is best to begin and end the examination upon the floor of the bladder, since it is there that the diseases for which the surgeon seeks—tubercle, neoplasm, and stone—are almost always found. I shall not delay to describe the appearance of the normal and the abnormal bladder. The figures in Plate IV show the common abnormal pictures, but a few minutes of practical cystoscopy will teach more about these things than can be learned from hours of study. I need only remark that in order to see an object to the best advantage it must be brought as near as possible to the window of the cystoscope.

At the end of the examination the light is turned out and the instrument extracted. The patient is then instructed to empty his bladder. The organ is once again washed with boric-acid solution in order to empty it of all the cocain, and an instillation of 1:1,500 nitrate-of-silver solution given to forestall infection and to minimize congestion.

The three essentials commonly insisted upon for the proper performance of a cystoscopy are:

1. A urethra large enough to admit the cystoscope.

2. A bladder not too contracted to contain the necessary 150 c. c. of fluid.

3. A clear medium. This is the condition most difficult to fulfil. Unless there is profuse intravesical bleeding the contents of the organ can readily enough be made clear, but they will not remain so. Whether the case is one of tubercle, tumour, or stone, bleeding is a prominent feature, and the cystoscopic manipulations promptly evoke the bleeding. There are two ways of avoiding this difficulty. The first is to know in a general way what you expect to see, and to go straight for it and get a good view of it before it is obscured by the hemorrhage. The other way is to use an irrigating cystoscope, to wash the prism clean, and dilute the muddied contents of the bladder. This latter expedient is deemed the more scientific. I must confess to having found the former more practical.[1]

Indications.—Many surgeons constantly employ the cystoscope for the diagnosis of hypertrophy of the prostate, stone in the bladder, and cystitis. I do not consider it a proper routine method of diagnosis for any of these conditions. They may be better determined by other means. In tuberculosis the cystoscope should never be introduced except to decide a question of operation. The only indications for cystoscopy that I recognise beyond this are ureteral catheterization (p. 472), tumour (p. 419), and, in obscure cases, for a diagnosis.

Contra-indications.—In the presence of any acute inflammation cystoscopy is certainly contra-indicated. Chronic cystitis and inflammation, hypertrophy and tumour of the prostate, while they do not absolutely contra-indicate cystoscopy, make it a difficult and rather harmful operation. Cystoscopy irritates tubercular cases even more than do other local measures.

CONGENITAL ANOMALIES OF THE BLADDER

Double bladder, a condition in which the bladder is either divided into lateral halves by a central partition, or gives off one or two large lateral cavities, or is divided by a transverse partition, is very rare. The anomaly is a curious one and has a certain clinical significance in that it may give rise to troubles similar to those

---

[1] The injection of a solution of adrenalin (1: 2,000) serves to prevent hemorrhage in urine segregation (p. 476), and the same solution may be employed in simple cystoscopy.

caused by acquired diverticula (p. 342), with which, indeed, it is often confused. *Absence of the bladder* is also very rare.

Exstrophy of the Bladder

Exstrophy or extroversion of the bladder (ectopia vesicæ) is far more common in the male than in the female. Thus of the 49 cases collected by Pousson,[1] 37 were men and 12 women. In the female it is of less importance, as it may be more easily concealed, and does not prevent performance of the sexual act. Cases of pregnancy and successful delivery at term are recorded. The subject will be considered here, however, only in relation to the male.

The deformity is an arrest of development in the median line analogous to hare-lip, and is found in different degrees. In a type case the lower part of the front wall of the abdomen and the front wall of the bladder are absent. The pubic bones are more or less widely separated from one another, their ends being united by a strong band of fibrous tissue. The posterior wall of the bladder, pressed out by the intestines, forms a mottled, red, tomato-like tumour, occupying the position of the symphysis pubis. Inguinal hernia of one or both sides is not uncommonly present, either partial or extending down into the scrotum, which is usually normal, containing the testicles. The penis is rudimentary, and affected by complete epispadias. The ureters are sometimes greatly dilated, forming, as it were, rudimentary bladders. The pathology and etiology are given in detail by Connell.[2]

The above description applies to a type case. There may be variations in the absence of herniæ, in a normal union of the pubic bones, in the amount of the protrusion, etc. Ordinarily in the adult the mass reaches the size of the palm of the hand. With complete exstrophy there is also always complete epispadias. A condition analogous to exstrophy may exist where the bony union of the pelvis is lacking, but the anterior walls of the abdomen and bladder are perfect. Here there is a sort of hernia of the bladder forward. In such cases there is always some analogous condition of the external organs of generation.

In exstrophy of the bladder the patient's condition is miserable indeed. The mucous membrane covering the protruded posterior wall of the everted bladder is inflamed, thickened, ulcerated, and covered by decomposing stringy mucus of alkaline reaction, similar to that found in vesical catarrh. From the orifices of the ureters,

---

[1] Guyon's Annales, 1888, vi. 94, 155, 244, 337, 409, 471, 536, 615.

[2] J. Am. Med. Ass'n, 1901, xxxvi, 637.

which can be readily seen by pressing back the protruded mass, there constantly distils a limpid, acid urine. This at once becomes alkalinized by contact with the inflamed mucous membrane of the bladder, and goes into rapid decomposition, wetting the patient's linen and keeping him constantly surrounded by an atmosphere of ammoniacal, fetid gases, making him disgusting to himself and intolerable to his friends. The integument of the abdomen and thighs becomes excoriated and inflamed. The friction of garments in walking only serves to aggravate the existing difficulties, and the sufferer is in a truly pitiable condition.

By pressing back the inflamed bladder a small prostate is exposed, lying at the angle of the penis and the vesical tumour, and upon it the verumontanum and the ejaculatory ducts may be plainly seen. These patients have erotic fancies and seminal emissions, but they are incapable of full erection or of perfect sexual intercourse.

Patients with exstrophy of the bladder have been useful to science in facilitating experiments upon the rapidity of the appearance in the urine of substances taken into the stomach. Thus it has been found that asparagus affects the urine in eight and a half, turpentine in four and a half minutes, etc. (salts much more quickly). Furthermore, we have here positive evidence of the fact that the secretions forming on the surface of an inflamed bladder are alkaline, and that the urine coming down healthily acid from the kidneys, on reaching the bladder is at once alkalinized and promptly decomposed. Hence the rule to give alkalies to correct alkaline urine where such alkalinity is due to bladder inflammation, since by this means the urine is rendered less acid and irritating as it comes from the kidney. Moreover, the possibility of years of severe vesical catarrh without any ascending infection of the kidney enforces the lesson that the ureteral sphincters are the true guardians of the kidneys, and that ascending infection does not occur unless these portals are forced by the back pressure of urinary retention. Yet in the long run the inflammation of the exstrophied bladder does extend up the ureters to the kidneys and the patient thus usually meets his death.

Treatment.—*Palliative* treatment consists in wearing an appropriate urinal. No urinal can be well arranged for an infant or a young child, and at this time vaselin, hot water, and dusting powder are our only arms against the disease. In later life Earle's urinal may be worn. It consists of a metallic shield, preferably of silver, sufficiently bulged to contain the protruding vesical wall without coming into contact with it. The edge is rounded off so as to make for itself, by pressure, a deep groove around the vesical tumour. From its lower part, which is slightly bellied downward, extends a tube upon which is fitted a long, flat rubber bag, to be worn strapped to the thigh, and to serve as a reservoir for the urine.

The bottom of the bag terminates in a metallic screw, which can be removed to allow the urine to drain off. The metallic shield above is held in place by a truss, which serves at the same time (Fig. 89) to retain any hernial projections in the groin. The instrument may be kept clean by a weak solution of permanganate of potash. While wearing it the patient is preserved from any friction. All the urine is collected as it flows, and a considerable degree of comfort is thus obtained.

Radical treatment is obtained by operation. Unfortunately the most radical operations never result in a perfect *restitutio ad integrum.* Yet they are all, in a sense, radical. Three varieties of operation may be recognised—

1. Obliteration of the bladder.
2. The formation of a new bladder.
3. Diversion of the stream of urine.

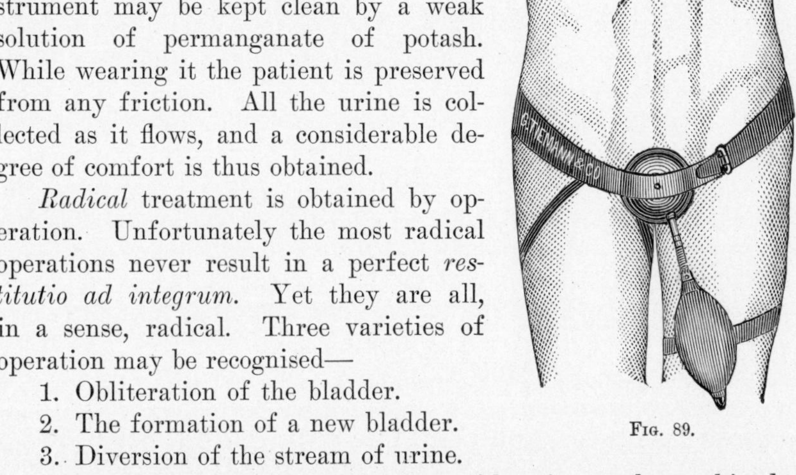

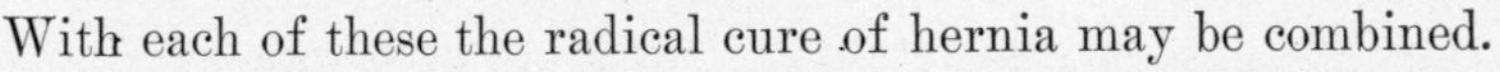

Fig. 89.

With each of these the radical cure of hernia may be combined.

1. *Obliteration of the Bladder* (Sonnenberg [1]).—This operation attempts but little. The mucous membrane of the bladder, or the whole bladder wall, is removed, and some attempt is made by skin-grafting or flap-raising to bring the abdominal wall together and so to remove the large raw surface of the bladder and to substitute scar or skin in its place. The ureters, with the mucous membrane around their orifices, are displaced downward and sutured to the end of the penile groove, which may be closed previously or simultaneously by one of the operations for epispadias (p. 22). Thus the object of the operation is to improve the patient's condition to the extent of leaving him with a manageable incontinence by removing the sore and stinking bladder. The operation, though by no means simple or always successful, has no immediate mortality.

2. *The Formation of a New Bladder* (Autoplastic Method).—Operations of this class should not be performed on children younger than five. This operation is the ideal one, but it is an ideal that has not been realized in practice; for the few patients who can be classed as satisfactory retain their urine only for some twenty minutes to an

[1] Berlin. klin. Wochenschr., 1882, xix, 471.

hour, and even these are but a small proportion of the unfortunates who, after their three, four, five, or more operations, have proved total failures. Several improvements in the technic have been recently suggested, but until some one shall produce a sphincter for the bladder the patient's capacity to hold his urine after operation will be entirely a matter of chance.

The operations may be described as—

a. Suture of the bladder itself.

b. The flap operation.

c. Closing the symphysis.

As a preliminary to operation urotropin should be administered to keep the urine sweet, and ureteral catheters should be introduced to keep the wound dry.

The ideal method theoretically is to dissect up the bladder wall, to turn it over, and to suture it so as practically to form a new bladder. There are two causes of failure. In the first place the bladder is so contracted that there is scarcely any tissue to work on. Pousson [1] has in some measure overcome this by boldly entering the peritoneal cavity, inverting the bladder, peritoneal coat and all, and then closing off the general peritoneal cavity (but he reports only one case, and that a failure). In the second place, in spite of ureteral catheters and constant changes of dressings, urine gets into the wound, which granulates instead of healing, with the result that the sutures tear out in the great majority of cases.

The flap operation has been developed by the ingenuity of Roux, Thiersch, Pancoast, Ayres, Holmes, and many others. (*Cf.* Pousson.) One or two flaps taken from the surrounding skin are turned in to form the anterior wall of the bladder, and the raw surface thus left is covered in as far as possible by other flaps. This operation often succeeds after many partial failures, but the hairs that ultimately grow from the inverted skin become encrusted with phosphates, and the patient finds his partial relief not worth the having. Recent experimenters have suggested filling in the gap with a segment of the gut (Tizzoni and Poggi, Enderlen [2]), and this operation has been performed once successfully on a man by Rutkowski,[3] whose patient eight weeks after operation could retain 25 c. c. of urine. The defect in the bladder wall in this case was not a large one. The gut used was the ileum, which was left attached to its mesentery. Manifestly such an operation is not without its dangers both immediate and remote. A simpler procedure, suggested by Mundel,[4] con-

[1] Guyon's Annales, 1898, xvi, 1223.
[2] Deutsche Zeitschr. f. Chir., 1900, lv, 50.
[3] Centralbl. f. Chir., 1899, xxvi, 473.
[4] Annals of Surgery, 1899, xxx, 715.

sists of elevating a flap from the abdominal wall and grafting to its raw surface the bladder wall of a sheep. After this graft has adhered it is swung over the bladder. This operation commends itself by its simplicity.

Attempts at closing the symphysis in order to diminish the gap to be covered over, and at the same time to attempt the formation of a sphincter, have not been very successful. Trendelenburg applies a belt, hoping by its pressure to approximate the bones, and if this fails he opens the sacro-iliac synchondrosis on each side. This operation is not applicable to children over eight years of age, and its results have been quite universally unsatisfactory, though Delagénière [1] reports a case in which after seven supplementary operations he obtained a radical cure and a satisfactory sphincter. Berg [2] has employed osteotomy of both iliac bones with rather better success. Not enough work has been done along any of these osteoplastic lines for broad conclusions to be laid down as to their results.

3. *Diversion of the stream of urine*, by means of ureteral implantation into the loin or the bowel, has long been a favourite but dangerous operation. Implantation into the loin may be condemned unreservedly (p. 496).

Numerous successful implantations of the ureters into the bowel have shown that the lower intestinal tract is in no way irritated by the urine and that the bowel readily retains the fluid from four to six hours. Yet the danger of ascending infection is here greatest of all. Much has been done to diminish this danger by transplanting the two ureters with the surrounding structures of the trigone in one piece (Maydl). But all of these operations are difficult and dangerous (the description of them belongs to the surgery of the ureter, p. 498). Frank's suggestion of a vesico-rectal anastomosis has given happy results when tried upon dogs.

Choice of Treatment.—Palliative treatment is always unsatisfactory, yet it may be employed by those who object to operation, for operative treatment is almost equally unsatisfactory. We still await the genius who shall give us a reasonably safe and certain cure for this condition. Most of the autoplastic methods are safe, but their results are scarcely worth the having. Maydl's operation does not give much better results. If the patient is cured by this operation he holds his urine from four to six hours, a result boasted by no other procedure. Yet the operation is a serious one. Its 13% reported mortality is probably an underestimate. It is impossible yet to judge how long the kidneys will withstand infection. But, such as it is, Maydl's operation is the best we have.

[1] Revue de Chir., 1900, xxii, 413. [2] Brit. Med. J., 1900, ii, 1168.

CHAPTER XXII

DISEASES OF THE BLADDER: HERNIA; HYPERTROPHY AND ATROPHY; ATONY AND PARALYSIS; RETENTION AND INCONTINENCE OF URINE; INJURIES

HERNIA OF THE BLADDER (CYSTOCELE)

CYSTOCELE is a disease that confronts the abdominal surgeon rather than the genito-urinary practitioner. It is scarcely recognisable except during herniotomy, and its whole clinical interest centres on the diagnosis of the condition before the bladder is injured by the knife, and on its remedies in case it is so injured.

Abdominal, inguinal (scrotal, sometimes on both sides), crural, perineal, and ischiatic cystocele, and cystocele through the foramen ovale (Lentin), have been noted. In women vaginal cystocele and femoral cystocele are most common; in men, inguinal. Thus among 22 femoral cystoceles collected by Gibson[1] 16 occurred in women, while 70 among his 77 cases of inguinal cystocele occurred in men. Lotheissen[2] collected 113 cases of inguinal cystocele in men and only 11 in women. He believes that cystocele occurs in 3% of all inguinal herniæ, although the usual estimate is from 1% to 2%. Inguinal cystocele is extraperitoneal in 69.2% of cases, paraperitoneal ("mixed") in 24.2%, and intraperitoneal in only 6.6%. As extraperitoneal cystocele is met with only in direct inguinal herniæ, it is in this class of cases that cystocele is to be especially looked for.

Cystocele is especially common between the ages of 30 and 60. Its pathogenesis, depending partly upon the hernial traction, partly upon dilatation of the bladder, has been studied by Lotheissen, Lambret,[3] Cheesman,[4] and Alessandri.[5]

Diagnosis.—The diagnosis is rarely made before operation. The suspected presence of cystocele is verified by the introduction of a sound into the bladder.

---

[1] Med. Record, 1897, li, 401.
[2] Brüns Beiträge, 1898, xx, 727.
[3] Bull. méd., 1899, xiii, i, 397.
[4] Med. Record, 1901, lix, 985.
[5] Guyon's Annales, 1901, xix, 25, 153, and 325.

Treatment.—The proper treatment of cystocele is herniotomy. If the cystocele is extraperitoneal, it may not be easy to close the abdominal wall firmly over it. Unintentional incision of the bladder during herniotomy is rather a grave complication. Lotheissen collected 65 such cases with 18 deaths. If the condition of the patient permits, the bladder should be closed by one or two layers of Lembert sutures, the efficacy of the line of suture tested by intra-vesical injection, and the radical cure completed. At the end of the operation a catheter should be tied into the urethra. If the patient's condition does not warrant the delay necessary to accomplish a satisfactory suture of the bladder, the organ may be fixed in the external wound after the manner of treatment of a strangulated hernia, and its closure deferred.

HYPERTROPHY OF THE BLADDER

Hypertrophy of the bladder has already been mentioned as a result of stricture of the urethra and hypertrophy of the prostate. Although many authors recognise a spontaneous hypertrophy of old age, clinically, at least, hypertrophy of the bladder is never spontaneous. It is the result of an obstacle to the free outflow of urine through the urethra, or, much less frequently, of severe prolonged inflammation with little obstruction (i. e., stone or tubercle). It is the physiological massing of forces to overwhelm the obstruction or to drive out the irritation. Hypertrophy is contrary to atrophy inasmuch as the former indicates that the bladder is keeping up its fight, the latter that it has been conquered.

Varieties.—Hypertrophy of the bladder may be concentric or excentric. In the former case the bladder is said to be contracted, in the latter dilated. A *contracted bladder* results rather from irritation than from obstruction. It is the reaction of a vigorous organ to constant calls to urinate when the obstruction to the outflow of urine is slight in proportion to the strength of the bladder (e. g., many strictures in relatively young subjects), or absent (e. g., stone, tubercle), or quite overshadowed by the intensity of the inflammation (e. g., some prostatics). The intensely inflamed mucous membrane will not permit more than a very few ounces of urine to accumulate in the bladder, and the muscle, incessantly summoned to expel these few ounces, finally hypertrophies so that the anatomical as well as the physiological capacity of the bladder is reduced to 100 or 200 c. c., and after the irritant (e. g., stone) has been removed, the concentric hypertrophy persists for many months and is never entirely overcome.

Excentric hypertrophy of the bladder results from obstruction rather than from irritation. The muscle is not called upon to expel small accumulations of urine frequently, but to expel large quantities completely. The effort of contraction leaves its sensibility dulled rather than aroused, and it submits to constantly increasing dilatation before rousing itself to the supreme effort. Meanwhile that effort begins to fail, the urine is not all expelled, and the accumulated residual urine adds its constant weight to dilate the organ more and more. The outcome is *atony*. However hypertrophied the muscle, it fights a losing battle, it gradually weakens, becomes more and more atonied, and finally, if the obstruction continues long enough, becomes almost completely atrophied.

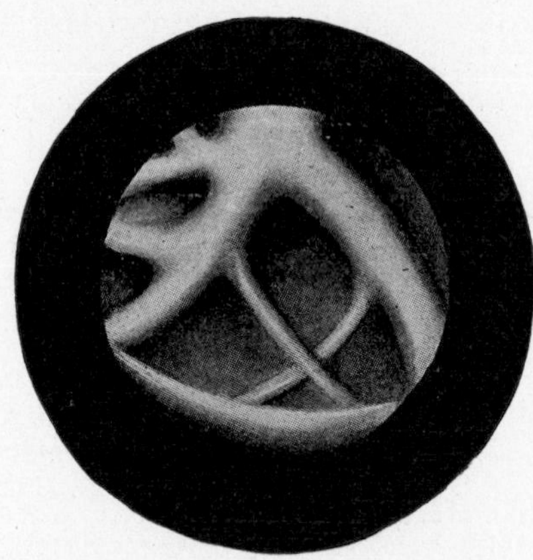

Fig. 90.—Cystoscopic View of Trabeculæ (Nitze).

Morbid Anatomy.—Although hypertrophy of the bladder occurs in two forms clinically distinct, and showing the one a contracted bladder, the other a dilated one, yet the essential lesions are quite the same in either case. The wall of the bladder is much thickened; its inner surface is thrown into deep folds by distinct bands of hypertrophied muscular fibres (Fig. 90). Between these raised bands the mucous membrane sinks in little pocket-like depressions. If the process is an old one these pockets may be found quite deep among the muscular fibres (*vessie à cellules, sacculated bladder*) (Fig. 91). These pockets may

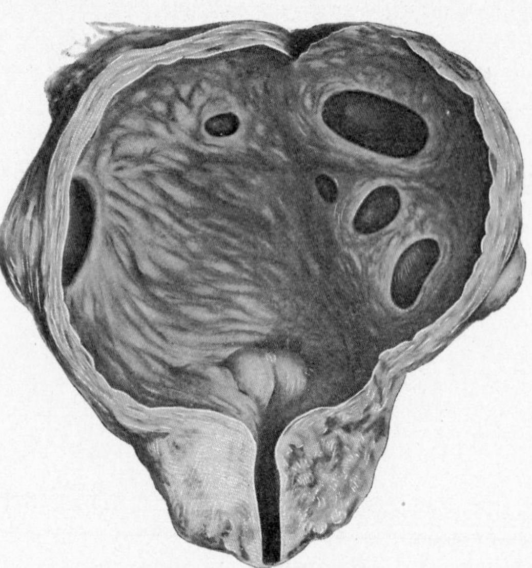

Fig. 91.—Sacculated Bladder.
Due to prostatic retention.

be so deep as to contain their own special residual urine, in which case their walls may be ulcerated and they often contain phosphatic stones (*encysted stone*) (Plate IV, Fig. 5). Indeed, the walls of such a sac may finally push themselves quite through the muscular coat of the bladder. The sac then enlarges indefinitely. Its walls are composed merely of the mucous membrane, a thin connective-tissue layer, and the peritoneum. Such a sac, divested of the muscular coat of the bladder, is known as a *diverticulum.* Diverticula have been known to exceed the bladder itself in size.

Microscopically the mucous membrane is seen to be inflamed, thickened, and infiltrated. The muscle of the bladder is greatly hypertrophied, but it is everywhere infiltrated with fibrous tissue, and the actual increase in thickness of the bladder wall is seen to be a fibrous degenerative change rather than a muscular compensation. The older the patient the greater the proportion of fibrous tissue present. These changes have been explained by the French school as a senile sclerosis of the bladder, a part of the general *sclérose urinaire* to which they attribute so many ills. Doubtless there is some measure of truth in this theory; but doubtless, too, the presence of the fibrous tissue is rather an expression of deep-seated inflammation, and an evidence that the bladder is losing ground in its fight; that the worn-out muscle is becoming more and more fibrous with the advance of age—in short, that it is wearing out. The various inflammatory changes associated with hypertrophy of the bladder need not arrest our attention here.

Symptoms.—There are no special symptoms of vesical hypertrophy. It is only a phase of some urinary disease. The contracted, irritable, concentrically hypertrophied organ declares itself by its constant irritability and inability to retain any great quantity of fluid. The patient, dilated, perhaps atonied organ, affected with excentric hypertrophy, shows quite opposite characteristics.

Treatment.—The treatment of hypertrophy of the bladder is the removal of its obstructive and inflammatory causes.

ATROPHY OF THE BLADDER

In rare cases in reduced, soft-fibred, debilitated individuals the bladder may be found weak and thin, apparently atrophied in all its coats, and liable to rupture. Atrophy of the bladder is the terminal phase of excentric hypertrophy (see above), when the fibrous elements have entirely replaced the muscle and have been stretched until the bladder is a mere bag. Such a complete atrophy is extremely rare.

ATONY OF THE BLADDER

Atony of the bladder is, as the name implies, simply a lack of tone in the organ. It is muscular paresis, and is to be clearly distinguished from paralysis, an affection of central and not of local origin. Truly, a stretched muscle which will not contract is paralyzed; but, to avoid confusion, the term atony must be retained, paralysis being only spoken of where there is nerve lesion. In old age every bladder suffers in a mild degree from what may be called physiological atony. A healthy boy can throw a stream from his bladder to a much greater distance than he can when he becomes an adult, even taking into consideration the increased size of the prostate and the enlarged calibre of the urethra, and the same remark holds true of adult life when compared with healthy old age. The bladder, being accustomed to a constant, slight distention, measurably loses its expulsive power with advancing age. Besides this physiological atony, however, there is a pathological form due to overstretching of the muscular coats, either gradual and continued (see above) or sudden and extreme (retention).

Any one may observe the phenomenon of atony in his own person. If the urine be voluntarily retained for some hours after the bladder is full and the natural desire felt, it is necessary, when an attempt is made at passing water, to wait some time, perhaps several minutes, before the stream begins to flow. When it comes, it commences very gradually, and without force, getting stronger as the flow continues; finally, the last drops dribble slowly away. This is the mildest pathological degree of atony, and is caused by temporary paresis of the overstretched bladder. In men of sedentary habits, or in those engrossed with absorbing occupations (students, actors), where the calls of nature are habitually disregarded, this slight degree of atony, often reproduced, may finally lead to permanent lack of the expulsive power. Rarely actual retention may come on, starting in voluntary retention, the bladder having lost its tone so far as to refuse to contract when the opportunity offers. This atony resulting from voluntary retention is, however, rare, and comparatively unimportant. The atony met with clinically occurs with excentric hypertrophy of the bladder (see above) secondary to urethral obstruction, usually by hypertrophy of the prostate.

Symptoms and Treatment.—The symptoms of atony are those already described under the head of chronic complete retention (p. 265). An acute atony may follow a severe acute retention. The *treatment* is that of the exciting cause. The atony itself will disappear partly or entirely, even though it has existed several years, if the obstruction to urination is completely removed.

PARALYSIS OF THE BLADDER

As atony is common, so is true paralysis of the bladder rare. It occurs only in connection with nerve-lesion, or rarely as a functional nervous affection (reflex urinary paralysis, Brown-Séquard). The causes of paralysis of the bladder are brain disease attended by hemiplegia (rare), partial paralysis from reflected peripheral nervous irritation acting through the spine (exceedingly infrequent), any disease or affection of the spinal cord or nerves (inflammatory, apoplectic, syphilitic, diphtheritic, cancerous, from pressure, Pott's disease, fracture of spine, tumour), especially if such spinal disease be attended by paraplegia, partial or complete. This latter set of causes, which may be summed up in the one word, paraplegia, is by far the most active and efficient. Vesical paralysis may come on gradually, as sometimes in Pott's disease and in certain syphilitic paraplegiæ, or (most commonly) suddenly. In the former case the bladder discharges its contents more feebly from day to day, the change perhaps taking place so gradually that the patient does not notice it. Soon some of the urine is retained, only an excess over a certain fixed quantity being voided.

The paralysis may remain partial or (together with the retention) it may become complete. Very rarely there is paralysis of all the muscles, and true incontinence results; but this is so exceptional that it may be said not to occur. Most commonly, as the paraplegia comes on suddenly, so also does the vesical paralysis, and a bladder, at a given moment perfectly healthy, immediately becomes incapable of contraction. Retention ensues, the urine overdistends the bladder and then overflows, dribbling away. The bladder then becomes inflamed, ulcerated, calculous. It is in some such deplorable condition as this that it usually first receives surgical notice and attention, whereas the whole list of symptoms might have been avoided (except the loss of contractile power) by the application of the proper preventives of cystitis at the proper time.

Treatment.—When a patient, from any cause, becomes wholly or partly paraplegic, his bladder should not be allowed to become distended. The catheter should be passed as soon as the retention is recognised, and reintroduced 3 or 4 times a day, each catheterization being conducted with the most minute antiseptic precautions. Precise, even exaggerated precautions must be taken. The catheter should be boiled, the surgeon's hands scrubbed, the patient's penis washed, and his fossa navicularis irrigated before the operation, and afterward a few drops of 1:2,000 nitrate-of-silver solution should be left in the posterior urethra and bladder. Urotropin should also be administered. Yet in spite of the most detailed precautions the prognosis is bad; the bladder ultimately becomes infected, as a rule, the kidneys are soon involved, and death is hastened by these complications.

If the patient is not seen until stagnation and overflow have occurred, it is more difficult to keep down the inflammatory outbreak, but the sooner this is attempted the more chance is there of success. After catarrh of the bladder is once established, the treatment becomes mainly palliative; but even here much can be done by the systematic, regular use of the catheter, with thorough washing of the bladder, as in chronic cystitis (p. 395).

RETENTION OF URINE

When, after an attempt at urination, a certain amount of urine remains in the bladder there is said to be partial retention of urine. If no urine at all can be passed, the bladder being full, there is complete retention. This may be caused by any urethral obstruction—inflammatory, spasmodic, or organic—or by paralysis of the bladder. The chief causes of retention of urine are hypertrophy of the prostate, contracture of the neck of the bladder, stricture and spasm of the urethra. The retention caused by hypertrophy of the prostate is the most important of all, and covers, in its various forms, every variety of retention. Guyon [1] recognises an acute complete retention, and three forms of incomplete retention—viz., acute incomplete retention (with distention—amounting clinically to an acute complete retention—and without distention), chronic incomplete retention without distention, and chronic incomplete retention with distention. This last condition is commonly spoken of as chronic complete retention. The retention is not actually complete, for there is overflow; yet the bladder is always absolutely full and distended. These varieties of retention, their causes, symptoms, and consequences, are described with the disease to which they usually owe their origin—i. e., hypertrophy of the prostate.

Diagnosis.—Acute complete retention of urine is often confounded with suppression of urine. In the former case the urine comes down to the bladder but cannot escape from it; in the latter no urine is manufactured by the kidneys. In either case no urine

---

[1] Leçons cliniques, 3ième édition, 1894, i, 162 *et seq.*

is passed; but with retention the bladder is full, with suppression it is empty.

In suppression there is always resonance over the pubes; in retention, always flatness. The bladder may often be seen and felt, filling up the hypogastrium, perhaps reaching to the navel. Pressure upon it usually causes a desire to urinate. Fluctuation may be made out between the finger in the rectum and the hand upon the hypogastric tumour. The bladder will not burst from retention of urine, unless it be previously ulcerated or subjected to mechanical violence when full (a fall or a blow); after it has been distended for a time, a certain amount of dribbling will take place through almost any obstruction. From the effect of violence, or if the urethra be ulcerated or sensibly weakened behind a stricture, extravasation of urine may occur through the urethral walls.

Treatment.—The treatment has been already considered in relation to stricture and prostatic disease.

INCONTINENCE OF URINE

Incontinence of urine, or enuresis, is that condition in which the urine flows involuntarily out of the bladder as soon as it flows in. Incontinence must be distinguished from overflow. In each instance there is a continual involuntary dribbling; but in the one case the bladder is always empty, in the other it is always full. Enuresis shows that the vessel leaks; overflow shows that the outflow pipe is obstructed. In the adult male dribbling of urine signifies overflow in 9 cases out of 10. With true incontinence the urine flows away without any pain or desire to urinate. Imperative urination, when the inflamed bladder contracts every few minutes with a force that the cut-off muscle cannot oppose, is often spoken of as false incontinence.

Incontinence in Adults.—Stagnation with overflow and false incontinence have been already considered. True incontinence depends upon—

1. Asymmetrical hypertrophy of the prostate, where, after the collection of a little urine, the rest trickles away, there being no distention of the bladder (p. 263).

2. Post-operative enuresis, resulting from overcutting the internal vesical sphincter (p. 308).

3. Paralysis of the sphincter muscle of the bladder (p. 345).

4. Tuberculosis of the neck of the bladder (p. 402).

The treatment of these conditions is detailed elsewhere. It is advisable that the patient should wear a urinal.

Incontinence in Children.—Infants have little or no control over their urination, especially at night, but after they leave off diapers they are expected to stop wetting the bed. There are doubtless few children who fulfil this expectation entirely. Up to the age of five or six an occasional accident may occur to the most normal child. But this is not enuresis. The true nocturnal enuresis of children—for it is only exceptionally diurnal—is not noticed, as a rule, until the child is five or six years old. Then he begins to wet his bed quite regularly, perhaps two or three times every night. He may also lose his urine involuntarily by day, and very rarely the incontinence occurs only by day and not by night.

Etiology.—While the enuresis of childhood may be symptomatic, it is usually idiopathic. Symptomatic incontinence may be due to tuberculosis or stone at the neck of the bladder, or to spinal disease, or it may be a reflex disturbance aroused by congenital stricture, by tight or adherent prepuce, etc. But the majority of cases are idiopathic, and due to a neurotic taint. Such children are, as a rule, shy, overgrown, pale creatures. They are often intelligent and given to quiet reading rather than to boisterous play. The tendency to enuresis often runs through the whole family, and the elders may show other neuroses. Even symptomatic cases often show a neurotic element.

Prognosis.—The prognosis is good. Even the most persistent cases recover spontaneously at the advent of puberty, so that while nothing is more common than enuresis in a child, nothing is more unusual than enuresis in an adult.

Treatment.—Symptomatic incontinence may be eliminated by a thorough examination of the urine, the prepuce, and the meatus, and an exploration of the urethra. The child's habits should be inquired into with an eye to indolence, masturbation, and mental overexertion. Such faults must be corrected, and a life in the open air, with plenty of exercise and not overmuch study, must be insisted upon. Good habits should be encouraged by awakening the child to pass water late at night and early in the morning, using moral suasion, and avoiding the use of fluids towards evening. Besides these means, absolute benefit may be expected from belladonna, commencing at a small dose, perhaps $\frac{1}{10}$ of a grain of the extract, if the child is very young, and increasing gradually until some of the poisonous effects of the drug are noticed. A tonic of strychnin and iron may be useful. Guyon considers faradization quite specific when the urethral muscles are relaxed. He places one electrode in the membranous urethra, the other over the pubes. If the deep urethra is hyperesthetic (which is unusual) instillations of nitrate of silver will do good.

Stumpf has obtained good results by making the child sleep with its head low and its pelvis elevated. Phillips gives antipyrin and arsenic. Perlis reports 156 cases treated with rhus aromatica. He employs the fluid extract and in some cases increases the daily dose to gtt. lxxx. Recovery occurred in 102 cases. Thirteen were unimproved.

Another means which has been employed is sealing the prepuce at night with a drop of collodion. Mechanical appliances, encircling the penis or pressing upon the perineum, have the disadvantage of tending to beget a habit of handling the parts. Hypnotics should never be employed. The results of treatment cannot be predicted with any confidence; but, when all other means fail, tonics and hygiene succeed.

WOUNDS OF THE BLADDER

Wounds of the bladder are not common, since the position of the organ protects it from ordinary accidents, inclosed as it is, when in a state of relaxation, by the bony pelvis. Excepting the violence done by instruments in lithotomy, possibly in lithotrity, or during other operations, the bladder is but little liable to injury except when overdistended. It may be perforated by a fragment of bone in fracture of the pelvis. Rising above the symphysis pubis it becomes exposed to incised, punctured, and gunshot wounds. Wounds of the bladder are exceedingly dangerous to life without being necessarily fatal. Bullets and fragments of shell have entered the bladder without producing fatal consequences,[1] and there formed nuclei for calculus, as have also portions of bone.[2] Surgical wounds aside, Bartels [3] was unable to find among 405 reported wounds of the bladder any incised wound. Lacerations of the bladder not communicating with the external wound are, clinically, ruptures.

Symptoms and Prognosis.—The symptoms of wounds of the bladder are comparable to those of rupture (plus an external wound). The *prognosis* depends upon the presence and severity of the complications, the availability of surgical assistance, and the position of the rupture, whether it is intraperitoneal or extraperitoneal. Bartels collected 131 cases of intraperitoneal wounds, of which only 1 survived, while of 373 extraperitoneal wounds only 85 died.

[1] I have recorded in the New York Journal of Medicine, May, 1865, the case of an adult whose bladder was perforated by a bullet during the New York riots in July, 1863, terminating in complete recovery.—Van Buren.

[2] Consult P. Maltrait, Traumatismes de la vessie, Paris, 1881.

[3] Arch. f. klin. Chir., 1877, xxii, 519, 715.

Modern surgery would give a far better prognosis for intraperitoneal wounds.

Treatment.—The ideal treatment is immediate incision, suture of the bladder, and packing of the external wound to prevent infection and secondary infiltration. Nothing less than this could be expected to save a patient with an intraperitoneal wound of his bladder, and extraperitoneal injuries are certainly best treated in this way. But if the case is not seen until infiltration has set in, wide incisions, irrigation, and drainage are necessary.

RUPTURE OF THE BLADDER

A bladder, when overdistended by urine, may be ruptured by external violence, and this especially if it be atrophied or thinned by disease, ulceration, or otherwise; or the accident may occasionally happen by the accumulation of urine alone without any recognisable external violence, as in case of stricture. (The empty bladder is never ruptured.) Such a spontaneous rupture is undoubtedly attributable to muscular contraction.

Clinically speaking, the most frequent cause of rupture of the bladder is a fall, the bladder being overdistended. Imperforate urethra is an efficient cause in the fetus. Ulceration and atony are predisposing factors. Among the exciting traumatic causes, falls, blows, and crushing injuries, with or without fracture of the pelvis, or even appreciable injury to the soft parts, may be mentioned. The patient is usually intoxicated at the time of injury, the alcohol predisposing him to rupture of the bladder in a threefold way—viz., by causing the bladder to fill rapidly, by obtunding its sensibility, and by making the injury possible. The rupture may be intraperitoneal or extraperitoneal. Subperitoneal rupture, in which the fundus of the bladder is torn without lacerating the peritoneum, need not be distinguished, for it either remains extraperitoneal or becomes intraperitoneal. *Intraperitoneal* rupture is the more frequent variety. It is caused by a blow upon the hypogastrium bursting the distended organ as a blow bursts a paper bag. There are often no associated lesions. It has been surmised that the fundus yields to the distending force not through any weakness of the bladder wall at that point, but because the intestines give way before it, while below the bladder is supported by the bony pelvis. *Extraperitoneal rupture* is almost always associated with fracture of the pelvis. Mitchell[1] has collected 90 cases, of which 36% occurred on the anterior surface, and

[1] Annals of Surgery, 1898, xxvii, 151.

most of the others about the neck. Rupture of the sides or base is commonly intraperitoneal.

Symptoms.—The symptoms are sudden occurrence of intense pain in the abdomen (perhaps masked by alcoholism) with urgent desire to pass water, while attempts to urinate are usually, but not always, ineffective. Ordinarily the patient from the first is unable to walk. There are local pain, tenderness, and usually tenesmus, with the passage of no urine or of only a few drops of bloody fluid. Collapse soon follows. Death may occur in this stage, or the patient reacts and passes into a state of acute peritonitis or infiltration. If he survives the acute attack, the symptoms merge into those of local peritonitis, constant and often ineffectual desire to urinate being still a prominent symptom. The infiltration may extend up into the loin and down the thigh even to the knee.

Diagnosis.—If rupture of the bladder is suspected, the catheter is introduced. If the rupture is large no fluid at all, or only a little bloody urine may be obtained. Rarely the urine is quite clear. To confirm the diagnosis a known quantity (200 c. c.) of salt solution is introduced into the bladder and withdrawn. If only a portion of the fluid returns, there is rupture. If all returns, there may still be rupture, but cystoscopy should eliminate the doubt. Air may be employed for this test if salt solution is unavailable, for chemicals should not be injected. Moreover, the surgeon should be prepared tô follow up the examination by immediate operation if rupture is discovered, since this instrumentation is calculated to spread urine and infection broadcast throughout the peritoneum or the cellular tissues. A speedy diagnosis, whether from the symptoms, by injection, or by cystoscopy, is imperative. For this reason Alexander[1] disapproves of the injection test, considering it a waste of time.

If the pelvis is fractured, the rupture is probably extraperitoneal. Otherwise it is probably intraperitoneal. Evidence of infiltration along the anterior wall of the rectum or above the pubes points to an extraperitoneal focus, while grave systemic disturbance and general abdominal distention and tenderness point to invasion of the peritoneum.

Prognosis.—Among Mitchell's 90 cases of extraperitoneal rupture of the bladder 37 were operated upon and 24 of these died (64.9%); while of the 53 treated expectantly 51 died (96.2%). Sieur[2] collected 34 cases of intraperitoneal rupture, all operated upon, with the following results:

---

[1] Annals of Surgery, 1901, xxxiv, 209.

[2] Archiv. gen. de méd., 1894, i, 129.

Operation.	Cases.	Cured.	Died.	Mortality.
Within 12 hours	13	8	5	38.4 per cent.
12 to 24 hours	10	3	7	70 "
24 to 62 hours	11	3	8	72.7 "
Total	34	14	20	58.8 "

Without operation practically all would have died.

These statistics encourage early operation so markedly as to call for no comment. Doubtless the relatively low post-operative mortality of intraperitoneal (58.8%)[1] as compared to extraperitoneal rupture (64.9%) may be due to the fact that the immediate gravity of the peritoneal cases enforces early operation, while the slower progress of extraperitoneal ruptures encourage ill-advised delay.

Treatment.—When the diagnosis is established there is no treatment other than immediate operation; when it is in doubt an exploratory operation affords the quickest and surest means of reaching a conclusion that must be reached quickly if at all. The only contra-indications to operation are shock and grave visceral injuries, and if an infusion of salt solution improves the general condition the operation should be performed even in shock.

The first incision should open the peritoneal cavity through the median line. If an intraperitoneal tear is encountered, it is closed over with a layer of Lembert sutures in the bladder wall, and another in the peritoneum. All accumulations of fluid are then gently mopped up, and if the urine is infected the whole lower part of the peritoneal cavity is copiously irrigated with salt solution. If the urine is known to be clean this lavage may be omitted. Meanwhile the strength of the suture line is tested by filling the bladder with salt solution. If any escapes, the leaky portion of the wound is protected by additional sutures. This test is most essential. In 4 cases mentioned by Walsham[2] the cause of death was leakage through the sutured bladder wound. The abdominal wound is then closed with a single wick of gauze running to the point of rupture. A catheter is tied into the bladder until the seventh day.

If the peritoneum proves to be untorn, the abdominal wound is closed and the bladder opened through a small suprapubic incision (p. 460). If the hole in the bladder is found presenting, it is sutured, tested, and the external wound drained. But if the rupture is situated at the bladder neck or at some other inaccessible point, it may be treated by suture or left untouched, and drainage may be established through the abdominal wall and the urethra or the perineum.

[1] Or 51%, according to Alexander's figures.

[2] Univ. Med. J., 1895, iii, 200.

CHAPTER XXIII

ETIOLOGY OF INFLAMMATIONS OF THE UPPER URINARY TRACT—BACTERIURIA: ITS NATURE, SYMPTOMS, DIAGNOSIS, AND TREATMENT

THE upper urinary tract consists of the kidneys and their ureters, the bladder, and the posterior urethra. The cut-off muscle separates the upper from the lower tract. The former is inside the body, as it were, and is in its normal state entirely aseptic. The lower urinary tract—i. e., the anterior urethra—is in no way separated from the integument, and is always filled with the germs that flourish upon the surrounding parts.

Bacteria of the Healthy Anterior Urethra.[1]—The flora of the anterior urethra is subject to the widest variations. Among many non-pathogenic bacteria, such as are often found upon the skin, the urethra may also contain the bacillus coli, pyogenic staphylococci and streptococci, and the proteus vulgaris. The presence of these microbes is by no means constant. Indeed, in view of the fact that they cause no inflammation, and therefore get no hold upon the mucous membrane, and are being continually swept away by the stream of urine, it is small wonder that the urethral flora is subject to constant changes both in number and variety. Indeed, so great is the cleansing influence of the urinary stream that the urethral microbes are almost entirely confined to the balanitic portion of the canal. The microbes found in the normal bulbous urethra are few, and rarely pathogenic.

The anterior urethra becomes inflamed in one of three ways:

1. By the introduction into it of the gonococcus.

2. By injury to its wall (trauma, stricture, the congestion of sexual excess, retained catheter, stone, etc.).

3. By diversion of the stream of urine. Thus it may be noted that while a patient is urinating entirely through a hypogastric

[1] Lustgarten and Mannaberg, Vierteljahresschrift f. Derm. u. Syph., 1887. Rovsing, Die Blasenentzundungen, 1890. Melchior, Cystite et infection urinaire, Paris, 1895. Wassermann and Petit, Guyon's Annales, 1891, ix, 371.

wound he often complains of a mild urethral discharge which disappears as soon as urethral urination is resumed.

But the inflammations of the anterior urethra are taken up more fully in another section. Enough has been said of them here.

BACTERIURIA, CYSTITIS, AND PYELO-NEPHRITIS

Leaving aside prostatitis, the special characteristics of which have already been considered, the infections of the upper urinary tract are:

1. Infection of the urine with no appreciable lesion of the bladder or the kidneys—Bacteriuria.
2. Inflammation of the bladder—Cystitis.
3. Inflammation of the kidney, its pelvis, and the ureter—Pyelo-nephritis.

Inasmuch as the upper urinary tract is aseptic when in its normal condition, the three prime questions to be answered in regard to inflammations are:

1. What are the bacteria of urinary inflammations?
2. How do they obtain access to the urinary tract?
3. What are the accessory causes of inflammation?

Bacteria of Urinary Disease

Although the bacteriology of pyelo-nephritis has not been so thoroughly studied as that of cystitis and bacteriuria, the statistics of these latter two, collected by Albarran, Hallé, and Legrain,[1] probably express with fair accuracy the importance of the various microbes in all three varieties of urinary infection. These authors have collected 304 cases from the reports of Rovsing, Morelle, Denys, Reblaub, Krogius, Barlow, Melchior, and Bastianelli, and have classified the bacteria as *frequent* and *rare*. Their results may be tabulated as follows:

Frequent Bacteria

Bacillus coli—131 times (43%)—89 times in pure culture.

Staphylococcus pyogenes—70 times (23%).

Proteus of Hauser—26 times (8.5%).

Streptococcus pyogenes—15 times (5%).

Gonococcus—10 times (the authors think this figure unduly small).

Bacillus typhosus.

---

[1] Guyon's Annales, 1898, xvi, 1159.

Rare Bacteria

Pneumococcus, diplo-bacillus of Friedländer, bacillus longus ureæ (Rovsing), diplococcus ureæ liquefaciens (Melchior), and many others found in isolated cases by individual authorities. These rare bacteria possess no clinical interest, and require no description here.

The bacillus tuberculosis, it will be observed, has been omitted from the above classification, and its consideration is reserved for a subsequent chapter.

Bacillus coli (*Urobacillus non-liquefaciens, Coccobacillus ureæ pyogenes*).—This germ, the most common of all, has been investigated by every writer upon this subject, but with widely differing conclusions. While most authors have placed it among the most active causes of cystitis, Rovsing[1] finds that it never causes cystitis, though sometimes a slight pyelitis.[2] These opposing views can only be reconciled by admitting the personal equation, and by frankly recognising the fact that the virulence of this bacterium varies between wide limits. Numerous attested cases of cystitis prove it not always so innocent as Rovsing believes, while the ever-increasing number of reported cases of bacteriuria containing the bacillus coli in pure culture show that its venom has been overestimated in the opposite camp. On only one point are all agreed—viz., that the bacillus coli is not ammoniogenic; it causes *acid* cystitis, pyelitis, or bacteriuria.

Clinically the bacillus coli may be put down as almost the sole cause (the gonococcus and the tubercle bacillus excepted) of all urinary infections in which the urine remains acid. It is, as a rule, but slightly virulent. Without a predisposing factor—a fertile soil upon which to grow—it causes no infection whatever. When it takes root upon a slight lesion of the prostate or of the kidney (or its pelvis) it causes a bacteriuria or perhaps a very mild pyelitis. When assisted by retention (prostate, stricture, stone, or tumour) it causes a more severe inflammation which may do permanent damage to the kidney, but is not likely to arouse any very acute symptoms or to produce any deep-seated lesions in the bladder. The bacillus coli may be associated with other bacteria in inflammations of the most intense severity.

Pyogenic Staphylococci and Streptococci.—These bacteria effect the decomposition of urea with the formation of ammonia. They are the common causes of *alkaline* cystitis and pyelo-nephritis.

[1] Guyon's Annales, 1897, xv, 817, 1009, 1121, 1251, and 1898, xvi, 179, 278.

[2] Rovsing's position has been assailed by Melchior and by Albarran and Hallé (Guyon's Annales, 1898, xvi, 363, 388).

Their virulence is greater than that of the bacillus coli. Like it they do not set up or maintain any urinary affection unless aided by an accessory lesion, but they very rarely cause bacteriuria, and the alkaline cystitis or pyelitis caused by them is severe in its symptoms and grave in its consequences.

Proteus of Hauser (*Proteus vulgaris, Urobacillus liquefaciens septicus*).—Experiments on animals at the hands of Krogius, Schnitzler, Bastianelli, and Melchior have shown that an intense and even a fatal cystitis may be produced, without the assistance of any predisposing cause, by injecting into the bladder a pure culture of the proteus vulgaris.

Like the pyogenic cocci this bacterium decomposes urea and causes *alkaline* cystitis. Probably it cannot take root and flourish in man without the aid of a predisposing agent, but it is nevertheless the most virulent of the common bacteria of urinary infection. Yet it has been found once in a simple bacteriuria.

Gonococcus.—It has long been known clinically that a gonorrheal inflammation may extend from the anterior to the posterior urethra and thence to the bladder, and that the gonorrheal prostate may form a base whence repeated incursions into the bladder are quite possible. Yet the proof of the existence of gonococcal cystitis has been singularly slow in appearing, and the cases reported are remarkably few. Thus far we only know that the gonococcus alone, unaided by any predetermining cause, may cause an acute cystitis; that in such cystitis the urine is acid; and that this purely gonorrheal cystitis recovers or is replaced by a secondary mixed infection so that the gonococci, if still present, can no longer be found. Hence that striking clinical condition, acute gonorrheal cystitis, may be accepted as purely gonococcal in origin; while nearly all the subsequent chronic manifestations in the bladder are due to secondary infection by those bacilli coli and pyogenic cocci that everywhere follow in the wake of the gonococcus to perpetuate the inflammations inaugurated by it.

Bacillus Typhosus.—It is only within a few years that the importance of the bacillus typhosus in urinary infection has been appreciated. According to the recent studies of Richardson [1] and Gwyn,[2] typhoid bacilli appear in the urine during the second and third weeks of the fever. Typhoid bacteriuria occurs in from 15% to 30% of all cases of typhoid. Grave pyelo-nephritis is rare, and while the bacilli usually spontaneously disappear from the urine they may remain for

---

[1] J. of Exper. Med., 1898, iii, 349, and 1899, iv. J. of Mass. Ass'n of Boards of Health, 1899.

[2] Johns Hopkins Hosp. Bull., 1899, x, 109.

years. Typhoid bacilluria is peculiarly amenable to treatment. The urine is acid and closely resembles that of bacillus coli bacteriuria.

Routes of Invasion

Bacteria may reach the interior of the urinary tract by one of four routes (Rovsing):

1. From the urethra—ascending invasion.
2. From the kidney—descending invasion.
3. By irruption of a neighbouring focus.
4. By the circulation—indirect invasion.

Scientists are still at odds as to the predominating importance of any one route over any other. For the first observers, Pasteur, Bouchard, and others, the urethra was all important. Then Rovsing, Melchior, and Bastianelli, while still attributing the majority of cases to the urethra, recognised a renal origin for some cases. Albarran, Hallé, and Legrain hint that descending infection is more common than is generally believed. Infection through the blood or the lymphatic current has been made by most authors the special attribute of the tubercle bacillus, but Reymond [1] and Van Calcar [2] believe that the bacillus coli passes directly out of the rectum and in through the bladder when there is constipation or other intestinal obstruction. In the present state of our knowledge it is not possible to reconcile these opposing views, and in our consideration of the various routes of invasion it will be more practical to confine ourselves as strictly as possible to the clinical aspect of affairs.

Urethral or Ascending Invasion.—The three methods by which microbes may ascend from the urethra are:

1. Through instrumentation.
2. By extension upward of a urethral inflammation.
3. By spontaneous ascension of the urethral bacteria.

1. The passage of an instrument into a clean bladder is a frequent cause of cystitis. The gentle passage of a smooth, soft, clean instrument through a normal canal into a healthy bladder never causes cystitis. Perhaps bacteria are carried into the bladder by every instrument. Perhaps numerous pathogenic germs are often introduced in this manner. But experiment and experience unite to proclaim that the healthy bladder is thoroughly able to sweep itself clean of these enemies. Whether the germs come from a dirty catheter, or from an inflamed or a normal urethra, the bladder may be absolutely protected from them by the prophylactic injection of nitrate of silver (p. 218). But this is not enough. The bladder may

---

[1] Guyon's Annales, 1893, xi, 253 and 343.

[2] *Ibid.*, 1899, xvii, 1253.

be thus protected, but not so the posterior urethra. Not to mention the gonococcus, any of the specific bacteria enumerated above can take root in the prostatic portion of the canal if only the soil is sufficiently harrowed to receive the seed. Contusion or abrasion by the rough passage of an instrument often suffices, and if the bacteria are at hand, if a posterior urethritis is lighted up, if this posterior urethritis extends to the bladder and even to the kidneys, the heavy, rough, unskilled hand of the surgeon is to blame. No man with a general experience can fail to see that an infinite gentleness with a modicum of cleanliness spares the posterior urethra many woes into which it is plunged by the proud possessor of an infinite cleanliness with only a modicum of gentleness. It is not for me to depreciate cleanliness—the cleaner you are the better; but, if I may be allowed the phrase, the gentler you are the best. A gentle catheterization followed by an antiseptic irrigation does not cause any inflammation, unless the prostate is already inflamed or considerably congested, unless the vesical powers of resistance are greatly lowered, or unless there are gonococci about.

2. Infection of the urine by direct extension of an anterior urethritis backward is met with clinically only in gonorrhea and stricture.

3. Whether the bacteria of the uninflamed anterior urethra can ascend to the bladder in face of the urinary stream is a question not yet definitely decided. Certainly they may ascend a short distance along the anterior urethra, for they have been found, in a certain proportion of cases, at varying depths in the canal. Paladino-Blandini[1] found that if pure cultures of the staphylococcus aureus, the bacillus typhosus, and the "bacillus of green pus" were placed within the meatus urinarius of the guinea-pig, these bacteria could usually be found in the kidney at the end of twenty-four hours in the male, and at the end of forty-eight hours in the female. These experiments suggest that perhaps even immobile bacteria may travel against the urinary stream in small numbers, at least, and that the bladder and even the kidney may thus be invaded at any time. But before accepting such a theory, with all its startling possibilities, we must await confirmation of Paladino-Blandini's experiments by other observers.

With stricture of the urethra the combination of obstruction and infection is particularly favourable to the ascent of bacteria and the production of inflammation.

Renal or Descending Invasion.—Without stopping to debate the question whether or not the healthy kidney can transmit liv-

[1] Guyon's Annales, 1900, xviii, 1009.

ing bacteria in any numbers without injury to its secreting structure, we may accept as proved clinically, notably in the case of the typhoid bacillus, the fact that bacteria may enter the urine in great numbers from a kidney clinically sound. There is strong evidence for the belief that in the course of the various infectious diseases, even in tuberculosis, bacteria are commonly transmitted by the kidneys without leaving any appreciable trace of their passage through those organs. When the kidneys are inflamed their bacterial output is still less doubtful.

It has been shown, moreover, by Carle, Posner and Lewin, Lesage and Macaigne (*cf.* Melchior, Rovsing, Van Calcar, Albarran, Hallé, and Legrain), that any coprostasis or constipation enhances the virulence of the bacillus coli in the intestine and causes these germs to leave the intestine in great numbers. A certain number of these bacteria reach the urine, presumably by excretion from the kidney. It is the prevailing tendency nowadays to attribute the spontaneous infection of prostatics to this cause, and hence great stress is laid upon keeping their bowels clear to avoid this possible source of danger. Direct extension of a parietal inflammation from kidney to ureter and from ureter to bladder occurs only in tuberculosis.

Irruption of a Neighbouring Focus.—Apart from those self-explanatory cases in which a fistulous or an exstrophied bladder becomes infected, the opening of an extraneous abscess into the urinary channels is rare. Perinephritic, perityphlitic, and, in the female, pelvic abscesses, may so rupture.

Invasion from the Circulation.—In spite of the contentions of Van Calcar and a few others, the great body of authors is united in denying that bacteria reach the urinary channels by emigrating from the general blood stream through the wall of ureter or bladder. It is generally admitted that only the tubercle bacillus may gain access from the lymphatics.

Accessory Causes of Inflammation

From a consideration of the facts briefly noted in the preceding paragraphs one is tempted to wonder not that the urinary organs become infected, but that they escape the infection that forever threatens them both from above and from below. If every infectious disease, every inflammation, every constipation sends its myriad of bacteria through the kidneys; if every colony of germs deposited within the meatus sends its scouts upward as far as the kidney, it requires some stretch of the imagination to call the upper urinary tract aseptic, and it encourages a belief in the bountiful dispensations of Providence to find that the bladder and kidneys are not perpetually inflamed. Yet there is another equally important side to the picture. We have seen the perpetual incursions of the enemy: let us look at the measures Nature has taken to repel them—or, to use a more striking metaphor—we have seen the perpetual sowing of the seed: let us now consider the soil, its natural fertility, and the means by which it is rendered more or less fertile, remembering that however rich the seed it cannot grow upon a barren spot.

In its normal condition the urinary tract is an unfavourable soil. The walls of the channels are smooth, protected by a thick layer of epithelium, and constantly irrigated by the urinary stream. It is probable that the renal epithelium possesses a bactericidal power, and it is quite possible that the vesical epithelium possesses the same power to a less extent (Van Calcar). Certainly the bladder shows a marvellous resistance to infection so long as its mechanical functions are not interfered with. Many and many a man lives for years with a kidney pouring down a continual stream of foul pus and bacteria into his bladder, and yet, so long as that organ can perform its functions properly, so long as there is no obstruction to urination, the bladder suffers even less from the putrid stream flowing through it than would the integument under similar circumstances. But let an obstruction to urination arise, let the bladder become overstrained and congested in its fight against a stricture, let a pool of residual urine collect behind a hypertrophied prostate or a contracted neck, and inflammation at once results.

We have seen that most bacteria are not of themselves able to cause a urinary inflammation. Indeed, the gonococcus and the tubercle bacillus are quite unique in their capacity for causing an inflammation without any accessory lesions, and yet even they are not above availing themselves of accessory lesions when these exist. *No other bacterium can take root and multiply in the urinary tract unless the soil upon which it flourishes is congested.* Congestion is the plough that prepares the soil to receive the seed. This congestion may be acute or chronic. If acute it may be perpetuated by the bacteria once they have lodged. It appears under several clinical forms, of which the chief ones may be enumerated.

Bacteriuria is commonly perpetuated by a renal or a prostatic congestion (p. 364).

Cystitis is usually kept up by the congestion of retention (prostatic hypertrophy, stricture) or of stone or tumour. It may be set up by trauma.

Pyelo-nephritis is usually kept up by the congestion of retention, stone, or tumour. It may be set up by trauma.

The predisposing causes of bacteriuria are so special that they are best considered in the section devoted to that disease. The predisposing causes of cystitis and pyelo-nephritis are retention, stone, and tumour. That stone and tumour should cause congestion, ulceration, and in various ways undermine the resistance of the epithelium is no strange matter. But these conditions are special and none too common, while retention of urine is such an all-pervading cause of inflammation that it must be broadly though briefly considered here.

Retention.—The cause of retention of urine is commonly a urethral obstruction, and the urethral obstruction is commonly due to organic stricture, to contracture of the neck of the bladder, or to hypertrophy of the prostate. It is true that "stricture and prostate" does not cover all the ground. Thus retention may be due to vesical paralysis without any obstruction whatever, or the obstruction may be ureteral and not urethral (but such an obstruction gives special symptoms), or even if the obstruction be urethral, it may be due to a thousand things—to congenital tightness of prepuce or meatus, to stone, to spasm, to tumour; but, allowing all these exceptions, it is my belief that 95% of all cases of retention are due to urethral stricture, to contracture of the neck of the bladder, or to prostatic hypertrophy. These are the cases that we meet in practice, with a well-defined set of congestive and inflammatory symptoms affecting the upper urinary organs throughout.

Effect upon the Bladder.—The first effect of any urethral obstruction is that the bladder has to strain in order to empty itself. This strain implies congestion, and as the obstruction in the cases with which we are dealing is always chronic and usually progressive, so is the strain and with it the congestion, chronic and progressive. The bladder is pushed to the last extremity. In struggling to overcome the obstruction it undergoes compensatory hypertrophy (p. 341); it gives all its reserve force to this end, and if other enemies appear in the shape of an invading horde of bacteria it is no longer in so fit a condition to expel them as it should be. Yet it usually escapes infection until its muscle has been sufficiently overcome to permit the accumulation of a pool of residual urine. This is the burden that cannot be borne. The bacteria now arriving find a safe harbour in the residual pool. Here they settle and multiply. They have leisure to work at the congested bladder wall, and if they are ammoniogenic the irritating changes they produce in the urine aggravate the state of affairs to a marked degree. Clinically a chronic alkaline cystitis is infinitely more severe than a chronic acid cystitis, unless that cystitis be tubercular.

From this brief review it will be observed that the *bacteria are not the most essential agents of infection.* They can do no harm in the urinary tract until some adventitious cause comes to prepare the soil for their growth. Unless the predisposing cause is there no inflammation can occur. While the predisposing cause persists an inflammation may indeed be cured, but there is no assurance that it will not relapse. So long as the predisposing cause exists there is danger. To cure the patient absolutely and permanently of his inflammation the predisposing cause must be removed. This done, the bladder will quickly dispose of the bacteria. This is the quintessence of urinary therapeutics: *to prevent inflammation avoid trauma; to cure inflammation relieve retention.*

Effect upon the Kidneys.—The effects of retention upon the kidneys may be summed up briefly. These organs become congested with the bladder, partly by a reflex nervous mechanism, but chiefly by the heightened urinary pressure transmitted from the bladder to the ureter, the pelvis and the kidney itself. In these cases of "stricture and prostate" that we are studying the pressure increases slowly through a space of weeks or months. Hence there is commonly little or no distention of ureters or kidneys until absolute retention is reached. But all the while there is a chronic congestion, causing in the ureters an inflammatory sclerosis comparable on a small scale to that met with in the bladder, while in the kidney the sclerosis resulting from long-continued congestion takes the form of a chronic nephritis (p. 555). The kidneys are thus permanently damaged. A certain proportion of the excreting epithelium is destroyed, and the remainder is forced to excessive work by this very loss. Thus congestion is piled on congestion and the kidneys are as ready as the bladder to become bacterially inflamed. If now an inflammation flares up in the residuum of the *bas fond*, the kidney falls an easy prey to it. Yet even here evidence of a conservative effort on the part of the kidneys is not wanting. The kidney does not—it has been already noted—become dilated until the state of chronic complete retention has been reached, and it is a noteworthy, clinical fact that until the kidney becomes so dilated and pouched that it has its own *bas fond* it does not usually become infected by ammoniogenic bacteria. It may fall a prey to bacillus coli infection of a light catarrhal sort in its early days of congestion, but it is not attacked by the bacteria of ammoniacal cystitis until it provides a special nook for their multiplication. Thus we frequently encounter cases of the most violent ammoniacal cystitis complicated by pyelonephritis, it is true, but acid pyelo-nephritis of a comparatively benign character. Occasionally the reverse of the picture is seen: a pouched, suppurating, disintegrated kidney pouring its multitude of bacteria through the bladder, which latter is affected little or not at all, because it is fully able to empty itself.

Instrumentation.—Rough instrumentation may, by bruising the neck of the bladder, light up a prostatitis and perhaps some cystitis; but the cystitis is only caused indirectly and will be of short duration unless some other cause of inflammation steps in to perpetuate it. The cystitis caused by instrumentation in cases of stricture or of hypertrophied prostate is started by the instrument and perpetuated by the retention. Other forms of trauma rarely figure in the etiology of urinary inflammation.

BACTERIURIA

The one form of urinary infection that does not lend itself readily to classification is bacteriuria—the presence of great numbers of bacteria in the urine without obvious parietal lesion. It can scarcely be termed an infection of the urine without any lesion of kidney, bladder, or prostate. Such a theory, though it has been generally accepted, is opposed to all that we know of urinary bacteriology. We know that the simple injection of bacillus coli into the bladder does not cause bacteriuria. We know that the simple passage of bacillus coli, even in great numbers, from the kidney does not cause bacteriuria. We know that bacteriuria is often only an initial or a terminal phase of cystitis or pyelo-nephritis. We know, finally, that in many cases the bacteriuria may be temporarily conquered by vigorous treatment only to reappear again as soon as the treatment is remitted. In view of these facts it is not possible to accept the old theory that bacteriuria is due to the presence in the urine of a microbe which multiplies so fast that it is not swept away by the urinary stream. On the contrary, we can only conclude that bacteriuria is a collective term covering several different conditions whose salient characteristic is the rapid multiplication of bacteria, so that they swarm in the urine and are associated with little or no pus to indicate the existence of the local inflammation from which they take their origin. It is not just to restrict the term bacteriuria to those cases in which the urine contains no demonstrable pus whatever, for a little pus may appear in one specimen of urine and be absent from the next.

Bacteriuria has been studied at length by Roberts,[1] Krogius,[2] Rovsing,[3] Jeanbrau,[4] Gassman,[5] and others.

---

[1] Brit. Med. J., 1881, ii, 623.
[2] Guyon's Annales, 1894, xii, 196.
[3] *Ibid.*, 1897, xv, 910.
[4] Gaz. des hôp., 1899, lxxii, 653.
[5] Guyon's Annales, 1900, xviii, 148.

Etiology.—*Bacteria.*—The bacterial agent in this condition is usually the bacillus coli, less frequently the staphylococcus or the bacillus typhosus. Jeanbrau has collected 67 cases with bacterial reports. In 56 (83.5%) cases the bacillus coli was found, in 7 cases the staphylococcus, and in the remaining cases the proteus, the streptococcus, the bacillus subtilis, and a large coccus. The bacillus typhosus does not appear in this list, but from what we are learning of the frequency of bacteriuria during typhoid fever and the possibility of its continuance, one may foresee that the typhoid bacillus will figure prominently in the statistics of the future.

Route of Invasion.—Jeanbrau has collected 29 cases of ascending invasion, chiefly attributed to urethritis, prostatitis, and catheterism. Renal invasion has not been clearly established in any great number of cases. Yet all typhoid bacteriuria must be of renal origin, as are also many of the bacillus coli cases. Invasion through a fistula or from a neighbouring pelvic abscess is too rare to be clinically notable.

Predisposing Causes.—In the pathogenesis of bacteriuria three salient facts may be observed:

1. The absence of cystitis (proved every time the cystoscope was employed).

2. The presence in many cases of the symptoms or signs of nephritis or pyelitis (22 cases in Jeanbrau's tables), of prostatitis, or of prostatic hypertrophy (19 cases), of urethritis or stricture (5 cases), of incontinence of urine (2 cases), of vesiculitis, etc.

The predisposing causes of cystitis and pyelitis are notable for their relative unimportance here. Retention was observed only 8 times, stone and tumour but 5 times. But bacteriuria is oftenest associated with an inflammation of the kidney or the prostate. In other words, *bacteriuria is usually the expression of a catarrhal prostatitis or pyelo-nephritis*, though it may be the expression of a catarrh of any part of the urinary tract, provided only that the parietal lesion is sufficiently slight and the bacterium sufficiently prolific.

When bacteriuria originates in the prostate or bladder it is said to be partial or vesical. The urine in the ureters and kidney pelves is perfectly clear. But when bacteriuria originates in the kidney the whole of the urine is bacterial; there is total bacteriuria.

The association of bacteriuria with incontinence of urine has been noticed by several authors. It is an open question whether the bacteriuria causes the incontinence or the incontinence the bacteriuria. When the incontinence is due to a spinal lesion the bacteriuria may very fairly be attributed to the weakened resistance of the urinary organs to infection.

Symptoms.—*The Urine.*—The urine of bacteriuria is hazy. It contains no gross particles or cloud of pus, but seems to be filled with the finest sort of a white powder. In a strong light the urine has a peculiar opalescence. Its reaction is acid in the great majority of cases. Its peculiar sickening odour has been compared to that of a mouse or a dead fish. No deposit occurs on standing, nor is the haze affected by heat or chemicals unless albumin is present. The centrifuge affects the cloudiness but little, and throws down only the merest trace of a deposit. A microbic sediment may be obtained by adding equal parts of absolute alcohol to the urine and then centrifuging (Hallé).

Examination under the microscope of a drop of urine obtained from the bottom of a centrifuge tube reveals innumerable bacteria, usually the squirming bacillus coli, intermingled with a few epithelia and leukocytes, with perhaps casts and blood-cells and crystals.

The urine may be albuminous. It is rarely phosphatic.

Course of the Disease.—The urinary signs just described are the only essential characteristics of bacteriuria. In many cases there are no subjective symptoms whatever. The symptoms, when there are any, are those of the underlying prostatitis, pyelo-nephritis, etc. Thus bacteriuria may appear under many different forms. It may be the initial or the terminal stage of pyelitis, cystitis, or urethritis. It may be the most striking symptom of prostatitis or vesiculitis. It may result from typhoidal or other infection. Yet amid these and other clinical types there are two forms of bacteriuria so prominent clinically as to overshadow all other types of the disease. These are the pyelo-nephritic type and the prostatic type.

Pyelo-nephritic Type.—The course of the disease is that of a pyelo-nephritis. It may occur during a typhoid fever, during pregnancy, as a result of a general infection, of a diarrhea, or of a chronic constipation. The urine is acid, albuminous, bacterial. The disease is, in fact, a catarrhal pyelo-nephritis (p. 567).

Prostatic Type.—There may or may not be prostatic hypertrophy. The disease is often the terminal stage of an acute gonorrhea. There may be fistula or stricture. The urine is not albuminous unless it contains blood. It may be acid, containing bacillus coli, or alkaline, containing staphylococci or streptococci.[1] The symptoms are those of prostatitis or vesiculitis, and the bacterium is found in the expressed secretions of the prostate and vesicles. In fact, the course of the disease is that of a prostatitis or a vesiculitis, modified only by

---

[1] In only one case (Pedenko) were staphylococci found to be the cause of pyelo-nephritic bacteriuria.

the fact that the bacteriuria is for a longer or shorter time the prominent symptom.

Diagnosis.—If the urine is uniformly hazy, and that haze is cleared neither by chemicals, nor by the centrifuge, nor by standing, and there is no purulent deposit, bacteriuria is present. Bacteriuria may be suspected by the urinary appearance and odour. It can be diagnosed only by the centrifuge (which fails to clear the urine) and the microscope (which shows what little deposit there is to be almost entirely bacterial).

The distinction between pyelo-nephritic and prostatic bacteriuria may not be easy in a given case. Indeed, the two doubtless often coexist. Yet an alkaline bacteriuria is almost invariably prostatic, a bacteriuria following gonorrhea or due to instrumentation or to stricture is probably prostatic. A bacteriuria occurring during the course of a prostatitis or of a prostatic hypertrophy is doubtless prostatic. Finally, the expressed prostatic secretion (after urethral and vesical irrigation) will be found to contain the incriminated bacteria in great numbers if the bacteriuria is prostatic.

On the other hand, if the bacteriuria is pyelo-nephritic, the urine is acid and contains casts and albumin, and the clinical picture of pyelo-nephritis may be discerned.

Treatment.—Bacteriuria may continue indefinitely if left untreated, but unless of long standing it is usually very amenable to treatment. The treatment is that of pyelo-nephritis or of prostatitis, or, if no underlying lesion can be determined, the treatment is by urotropin and diluents (p. 373). Typhoid bacteriuria, for example, almost always yields readily to this treatment.

CHAPTER XXIV

THE TREATMENT OF URINARY INFECTIONS AND INFLAMMATIONS

So closely connected and so often confused are bacteriuria, cystitis, and pyelo-nephritis, and so many points of treatment do they possess in common, that it is convenient to group here their general therapeutic features, and to refer back to them in the succeeding chapters in such a way as to impress upon the surgeon the necessity of taking a broad view of the whole field. Thus, without losing sight of the particular details proper to each case and to each disease, he may appreciate what might be termed the Principles of Urinary Therapeusis applicable alike to the prevention and the cure of inflammation of the upper urinary tract. The subject may be subdivided into Prophylaxis, Palliative Treatment, and Radical Treatment.

Prophylaxis

Clinically speaking, the prevention of urinary infection presents itself under three aspects:

1. The prevention of spontaneous infection when some disease of the urinary organs (notably prostatic retention) renders them especially liable to become inflamed.

2. The prevention of infection from urethral instruments.

3. The prevention of infection during or after operations upon the urinary organs.

1. The Prevention of Spontaneous Infection.—Since spontaneous infection of the urinary organs does not occur unless these organs are made vulnerable by the action of some predisposing cause (p. 359), the ideal preventive is the removal of such a cause. Thus the removal of stone, stricture, or tumour safeguards the bladder and kidneys absolutely. But in many cases, notably in prostatic hypertrophy, such radical treatment may well seem more formidable than the disease itself. Then the patient must be forewarned of the constant danger of infection, and forearmed against it by instructing him in the rules of what we have elsewhere termed Prostatic Hygiene. He must model his every movement on the avoidance of congestion and excess by moderation in diet, exercise, and exposure, by regulation of the bowels, by regular catheterization, if necessary, and with it urinary antisepsis. The details of this manner of life have already been considered (p. 275).

2. **The Prevention of Catheteral Infection.**—If there is one disease to which the term surgical is attached with opprobrium—viz., the surgical kidney—it is because of the gross carelessness shown by many surgeons in urethral instrumentation. Catheterism is such a vulgar operation and the bladder and kidneys resist infection so sturdily, that many a surgeon never learns to be gentle and soon forgets to be clean—for in the urethra cleanliness is next to gentleness—so that when he encounters a bladder or a kidney whose resistance is weakened, he omits the necessary precautions, and if a surgical kidney results from his catheterism it results indeed from his own act. The precautions with which urethral instrumentation should be surrounded—cleanliness before operation, gentleness during it, and antisepsis after it—have been detailed (p. 218). As we have suggested, these precautions may often be disregarded with impunity. If the urinary channels are entirely healthy, the *gentle* introduction of a catheter will do no harm in 99 cases out of 100 even though scant attention be paid to cleanliness. If the anterior urethra is inflamed an indiscreet catheterism will result in prostatitis and epididymitis far oftener than in cystitis. A clumsy or rough maneuvre will have the same result. But if there is predisposing disease, retention, paralysis, stone, or tumour, the minutest precautions often fail to prevent infection of the bladder and kidneys. In these cases every detail of gentleness, cleanliness, and antisepsis must be observed, not forgetting the so-called urinary antiseptics (p. 372).

3. **The Prevention of Operative Infection.**—The antiseptic principles governing the surgery of the urinary organs are not quite those of general surgery. The urologist bases his hopes of a clean wound chiefly upon efficient drainage. The general surgeon depends upon absolute cleanliness. Both drainage and cleanliness are essential. Yet of the two *drainage* is the more important. The majority of urinary operations, notably the operations for stricture, prostate, and surgical kidney, are performed almost solely for the purpose of re-establishing or maintaining the urinary right of way, and the constant practice of dealing with organs bathed in a flow of purulent urine tends to beget a certain scorn for a minute asepsis. So many cases do well under the coarsest asepsis that one is tempted to forget that they may do better under an aseptic *régime*. The detail of drainage belongs to each special operation.

Asepsis and antisepsis are of secondary importance to drainage, inasmuch as drainage is the essence of the operation and cannot be dispensed with, whereas in many cases it is possible to neglect a strict asepsis. Yet asepsis and antisepsis are of the first importance in that they are essential to some operations, beneficial in all, and absolutely necessary to the surgeon's instinct. Unless the surgeon is accustomed to keeping his fingers clean in all operations he cannot be depended upon to keep them clean in any. Therefore the usual rules for clean hands, clean instruments, and a clean patient must be observed in urinary operations as much as in any others. But besides the surgical asepsis a urinary antisepsis must be observed. If the urine is befouled, as it so often is, every effort must be made to clear it before operation as far as the nature of the case admits, and even if the urine is not infected it is advantageous to render it antiseptic in order that it may exert a bactericidal effect upon the wound after operation. The urinary antiseptics that may be depended upon to accomplish this are enumerated below. Urotropin is the best of them, since it produces the strongest antiseptic effect upon the urine, and since it seems clinically to prevent post-operative suppression and urinary fever better than any other drug.

Besides this urinary antisepsis by the administration of drugs much good may be done by local antisepsis in the bladder (p. 371).

Palliative Treatment

In the treatment of infection of the urinary tract some measures are employed purely for the purpose of alleviating symptoms. Many others, however, hold an intermediate position, as it were. They are sometimes palliative, sometimes curative. Thus the cure of a bacteriuria may often be accomplished by means that would only alleviate a chronic cystitis. Again, a cystitis behind a hypertrophied prostate may perhaps be effectually cured by urinary antiseptics, yet so long as the prostatic obstruction is not removed the imminent danger of relapse remains, and in course of time the inflammation will doubtless recur, so that the cure is often only a temporary one—a palliation, not an absolute cure.

Thus I prefer to class as palliative measures all forms of treatment that have for their object the reduction of inflammation, even though they may in certain cases effect complete and permanent abolition of the disease. These palliative measures may be classed as—

1. Anodynes, Balsamics, Alkalies.
2. Local Urinary Antiseptics.
3. General Urinary Antiseptics.
4. Diluents.

1. **Anodynes, Balsamics, Alkalies.**—**Anodynes.**—Whatever pain is associated with renal inflammations is not caused by any concentration or acidity of the urine. But the pain of cystitis is often considerably increased by a concentrated irritating urine, and the pains of urethritis even more so. The anodynes employed, whether by rectum, by mouth, or locally, are discussed elsewhere (p. 114). But of all the drugs employed to relieve these pains anodynes are the least desirable. They exercise no beneficial influence except by giving rest and allaying spasm. In acute conditions it may be necessary to use them, but in chronic conditions they should be studiously avoided, and used if at all only with the constant purpose of dropping them at the earliest possible moment.

Balsamics.—Balsamics are far more useful. They exhibit marked antiseptic and anodyne qualities in inflammations of the urethra and prostate, but they are of little use in inflammations of the urinary organs. Renal inflammations are not modified by them, and vesical inflammations are only influenced inasmuch as the prostate shares in the disease. Hence the cystitis of gonorrhea or of hypertrophy of the prostate is more influenced by balsamics, as a rule, than any other form of the disease. Their virtues have been discussed (p. 115).

Alkalies.—Alkalies have a more direct bearing upon the urinary organs proper. They render service in the treatment of all forms of cystitis, (1) by overcoming hyperacidity of the urine; (2) by diluting the urine by virtue of their diuretic properties; (3) by a slight antiseptic influence. The advantage of reducing the urinary acidity is notable even in alkaline cystitis, for, unless there is ammoniacal pyelitis as well (which is unusual), the urine when it reaches the bladder is always sufficiently acid to irritate the inflamed mucous membrane with which it comes in contact. Neutralization of this acidity eliminates the irritation without increasing any tendency to ammoniacal inflammation which may exist. Indeed, the feeble antiseptic property of the alkalies helps to diminish the inflammation of any mucous membrane with which they come in contact. The diuretic property of the alkalies is further useful in preventing undue concentration of the urine and in assuring a free urinary outflow. The special properties of the alkalies most frequently used have been considered elsewhere (p. 113).

To sum up: Anodynes, balsamics, and alkalies are useful in the treatment of urethritis, prostatitis, and cystitis. Their purpose is to lessen the disagreeable symptoms of these diseases and to render the urine innocuous. The more chronic the inflammation the less serviceable are these remedies. They may sometimes effect a cure, but are usually relied upon merely as adjuvants to local treatment.

2. **Local Urinary Antiseptics.**—Topical applications to the urethra and bladder have long been employed in the treatment of inflammations of these organs. Recently lavage of the inflamed kidney pelvis has been advocated. Although enthusiastically supported by certain surgeons it has not yet passed the experimental stage (p. 479). We shall therefore confine our remarks to those antiseptics that have been found useful in the bladder.

Nitrate of Silver.—Of the older applications nitrate of silver is the best, and among the newer ones it stands in the first rank. It is employed by instillation (p. 133) or by irrigation (p. 122). Whatever the method employed, the strength of the solution should be carefully graduated according to the sensitiveness of the patient. Some patients cannot endure nitrate of silver except after a prolonged course of preparatory treatment. The prevailing practice of disregarding the patient's sensitiveness and burning him cruelly with each injection cannot be too strongly condemned. Tubercular cystitis is made worse by nitrate of silver.

Irrigations are chiefly employed for the general cystitis of prostate, stone, or tumour. Instillations are generally more serviceable in posterior urethritis and in acute cystitis. When irrigations are employed the first strength should be between 1: 24,000 and 1: 16,000. If the patient bears this well, the treatment is repeated daily, or on alternate days, increasing the strength of the solution by about one third each time. This course is followed as long as the urine is rendered clearer and while the symptoms are diminishing. But any evidence of irritation, whether by an increase in the intensity of the symptoms or in the quantity of pus, is a signal that the dose is too strong or too frequently repeated. The next irrigation should be postponed a day and administered in less strength than the last; or it may seem wise to change to another remedy, or to administer an anodyne, and temporarily to desist from all local treatment. Although the tissues grow quite rapidly tolerant of stronger solutions, the action of these solutions cannot but be intense and the tissues require a longer time to react. Thus, solutions of 1: 6,000 should not be employed oftener than every other day, nor solutions of 1: 3,000 oftener than twice a week. Many patients cannot go higher than 1: 4,000, while others take 1: 1,000 without serious protest.

Instillations may begin between 1: 2,000 and 1: 1,200. They are employed every other day or twice a week. Two or three visits are usually required to accustom the urethra to the drug, which may then be run up rapidly to 1% or even 5%, when a maximum effect may be expected.

In acute gonorrheal cystitis no local application compares with an instillation of nitrate of silver (p. 139). In other forms of acute cystitis I have not found it remarkably efficient. In chronic cystitis of any kind it is one of the best of local applications (p. 393).

Protargol.—Of the newer synthetic silver salts protargol seems the most useful. I have employed citrate of silver, argonin, and argentamin, but with unsatisfactory results. Protargol is most useful in the urethra (p. 135); but it may be used in the bladder when nitrate of silver is too irritating. The dose by instillation is from 1% up to 20%, beginning at the low figure; by irrigation from 0.5% to 10%.

Potassium Permanganate.—This drug is to the urethra what the silver salts are to the bladder. In the latter organ potassium permanganate may be employed when nitrate of silver irritates. It is especially useful in acute cystitis when the silver instillation fails. It is employed only by irrigation. I have used it in strengths varying from 1: 8,000 to 1: 4,000.

Boric Acid.—Boric acid is very mildly aseptic; it has no very specific action upon the bladder, and yet it holds a place in bladder lavage from which it will not be easily dislodged. This is on account of its entire innocuousness. It may be placed in the hands of the patient with the assurance that it will do him a definite good and can do him no harm. As far as I know, it is the only wash that can be intrusted to the stupidest patient with entire safety. The reason of this is that even in saturated solution it is entirely unirritating. The saturated (4%) solution is always employed. About 10 grammes of the crystalline boric acid (pulverized boric acid dissolves less rapidly) is mixed with 200 c. c. of hot water. After stirring for a minute or so the residue is allowed to sink to the bottom and the solution is ready in sufficiently accurate strength for all practical purposes.

The ease with which the boric-acid solution is prepared makes it superior to salicylic-acid solution, Thiersch's solution, or physiological salt solution. I use it for all mechanical irrigating, for the purpose of cleansing the bladder and filling it for cystoscopy, stone-searching, etc. It is also most useful for the daily prophylactic irrigation of prostatics. It will not cure cystitis, but it helps to prevent it.

The numerous local remedies not mentioned above, of which thallin sulphate and mercurol are the most important, are useful chiefly in inflammations of the urethra and of the prostate (p. 134). Corrosive sublimate is useful only in tubercular cystitis (p. 406). Carbolic acid is not suited to vesical irrigations.

3. **General Urinary Antiseptics.**—Thus far we have been concerned with remedies whose sphere of influence does not extend

above the bladder. The last two classes with which we shall deal relate chiefly to renal inflammations, though their influence may be marked in inflammation of the bladder as well.

Under the term general urinary antiseptics I mean to include those remedies which when administered by the mouth produce such change in the urine as to render it a germicidal fluid. The number of drugs that exercise this influence in some slight degree is doubtless very great. Several of the alkalies and most of the balsamics already enumerated give the urine some antiseptic properties; but the urinary antisepsis of these drugs is overshadowed by the stronger influence of certain remedies about to be described. The four chief ones are urotropin, salol, benzoic acid, and boric acid.

Urotropin.—Hexamethylenetetramin, the ammonium salt of formaldehyd, is the most valuable drug we possess for combating pyelo-nephritis and many other urinary diseases. Unfortunately it is sold only under such trade names as urotropin, cystogen, and aminoform. The drug was introduced to the profession by Nicolaier,[1] and it is to him that we owe most of our knowledge of its chemical, physical, and physiological properties. The most notable characteristics of urotropin are:

1. Its action is entirely confined to the urinary organs. (In a few cases I have known it to interfere somewhat with digestion.)

2. Its action upon the urinary organs is due in large part to its splitting up under the influence of the urinary acids, with the result that formaldehyd is liberated in the urine.

3. Its alleged effects are five: antiseptic, irritant, antiphosphatic, antiuric, and diuretic.

Antiseptic Effects.—Urotropin is the best urinary bactericide we possess. Yet it is not infallible. Sometimes it will even fail when other urinary antiseptics will succeed, and it will often fail unless used undestandingly, its merits appreciated, its deficiencies recognised, and its limitations defined.

Urotropin is employed in bacteriuria, in pyelo-nephritis, in cystitis, and in posterior urethritis. In the treatment of total *bacteriuria* urotropin is invaluable. It prevents and controls almost all cases of typhoid bacilluria (p. 366) and pyelitic coli bacilluria. It may be necessary to employ it to the limit of toleration, even in doses of 3 to 6 grammes a day, in order to control an existing catarrhal pyelo-nephritis; but once the bacilli have been driven from the urine they may be kept away by smaller doses, which, however, may

---

[1] Centralbl. f. d. med. Wiss., 1894, xxxii, 897. Zeitschr. f. klin. Med., 1899, xxxviii, 350.

have to be continued for many weeks in order to prevent recurrence. In vesical bacteriuria urotropin is a useful adjuvant to local treatment, but in such cases local remedies must be depended upon to effect the cure. In suppurative *pyelo-nephritis* the germicidal virtues of urotropin are again of the utmost value. Suppurative pyelo-nephritis is commonly encountered only after it has reached a chronic state, and hence little good may be expected to accrue from the high initial doses that prove so useful in overcoming catarrhal pyelo-nephritis. On the other hand, I recall at least 4 or 5 cases in which renal suppuration of long standing and some severity has been controlled by small doses of urotropin, 0.5 to 2 grammes a day, administered for several months.

The treatment of *cystitis* and *posterior urethritis* by urotropin does not at first sight seem entirely rational. The drug, though antiseptic, is distinctly irritating, and is therefore less likely to be beneficial than balsamics and anodynes. In straightforward cases of chronic posterior urethritis, and in cases of acute cystitis it has been my experience that urotropin does more harm than good. My happiest experiences with the drug in this connection have been (*a*) in preventing the occurrence of cystitis in old men reduced to catheter life and in the prevention of catheteral and operative infection in general, (*b*) in preventing the occurrence of urethral chill or suppression of urine after the passage of sounds as well as after urethrotomies, cystotomies, and other operations on the urinary organs, and (*c*) in conquering that irritable form of posterior urethritis that flies to chills and swelled testicles every time any attempt is made at local treatment. The singular freedom from post-operative chill and suppression enjoyed by my patients since I began employing urotropin as a prophylactic has led me to use it as a matter of routine. I administer two or three 0.5-gramme tablets the day before the passage of a sound in stricture cases (p. 218) and the same dose for two days before every operation upon the urinary organs. As urotropin is found in the urine for two or three days after its administration I do not feel called upon to resume its use until the second day after operation. I have related elsewhere [1] several striking examples of the action of urotropin in the conditions enumerated above.

Irritant Effects.—The dosage of urotropin is determined chiefly by its irritating properties, which vary with each individual, and with the same individual at different times. The irritation manifests itself under two forms: (1) Irritation of the neck of the bladder and (2) cauterization of wound surfaces. The *irritation of the neck of*

[1] Phila. Med. J., 1900, vi, 606.

the bladder is much the more important. This it is that marks the limits of tolerance to the drug. All observers are agreed that the more water drunk with urotropin—i. e., the greater the urinary dilution—the less likely it is to irritate. I have known 1.5 grammes a day to cause an intense strangury within twenty-four hours. Yet I have had a patient take 4 and 5 grammes of urotropin a day for weeks together without any ill effects, and Nicolaier states that certain individuals can take 6 to 10 grammes a day. The underlying cause of these peculiarities is not known, but they are a warning always to begin administering the drug in small quantities, not to increase the dose without at the same time increasing the amount of water imbibed, and to recognise that in some cases the limit of tolerance may be reached before the limit of efficiency is attained, in which case the drug must be given up. Yet such cases are quite exceptional.

Happily there is another not less interesting side of the question. A certain mild irritant effect produced by the drug upon the kidneys [1] and the neck of the bladder is probably the cause of its efficiency in certain cases. Thus a light renal stimulation may well be one element in the prevention of chill and acute suppression by this drug, and I have attributed the few cures of posterior urethritis that I have obtained by the use of urotropin to a similar stimulating effect upon the neck of the bladder.

An evidence of urotropin irritation that may not be overlooked is its effect upon the urine. If the urine is hazy with bacteria (e. g., in a case of light pyelo-nephritis or bacteriuria) and urotropin is employed in sufficient quantity to clear the urine of them, the irritation may be, and often is, sufficient to provoke an epithelial desquamation and flow of pus that clouds the fluid quite as much as before. To the casual eye there is no notable change in the urine. Yet the desired effect has been attained: the urine has been cleared of its bacteria, and is now clouded with the epithelial and purulent exudate due to mechanical irritation. If this fact is overlooked and the drug pushed vigorously, the irritation will increase and the bacteriuria apparently grow worse instead of better. The distinction, therefore, between pyuria and bacteriuria is a cardinal one, the neglect of which may lead the surgeon sadly astray. Of the several more or less accurate tests for establishing this distinction the test by centrifuge and microscope is easily the best. The supposedly bacterial urine is centrifuged for three minutes at about 250 revolu-

[1] Nicolaier has produced albuminuria and hematuria in rabbits and dogs by the administration of large doses of urotropin.

tions a minute. If the haze is bacterial the fluid remains hazy, while whatever pus is present will be found collected at the bottom of the tube. But if the urine has been cleared of bacteria the centrifuge renders the urine completely clean and sparkling, while what was before a haze is now a sediment. This sediment, if examined under the microscope, is found largely epithelial if due to the irritation of urotropin, largely purulent if due to inflammation. In the treatment of bacteriuria, therefore, it must be remembered that the effect of treatment often cannot be discerned without the aid of the centrifuge and microscope, and it is a safe rule in practice to gauge the progress of the case chiefly on this showing.

A very rare mishap, which has occurred once in my practice, is the *cauterization of a wound* in the bladder by the urine containing urotropin.[1] I have seen no similar case reported, and should hesitate to lay stress on this isolated fact were it not for the importance of the inference if correct (and its plausibility is manifest). This I need scarcely insist upon. If the surgeon at any time encounter a case whose operative wound instead of healing becomes covered with a leathery slough and seems daily less likely to heal, and if this result is due to urotropin, he must recognise the fact and eliminate the cause immediately. The theory that urotropin may be the cause of this sloughing seems plausible to me from my experience with similar sloughing that I have seen occur in wounds treated with formaldehyd.

Antiphosphatic and Antiuric Effects.—Although not germane to the subject of urinary antisepsis, the antiphosphatic and antiuric effects of urotropin merit a word here. Curiously enough urotropin was at first praised as a uric-acid solvent rather than as a disinfectant. German authorities have insisted that urotropinized urine is an excellent uric-acid solvent at the body temperature. It will even dissolve uric-acid calculi *in vitro*. Casper also insists upon its value in phosphaturia. According to this author, not only do the phosphates disappear from the urine while the urotropin is being administered, but the phosphaturic tendency is also permanently overcome if the administration of the drug is continued for a sufficient length of time. I have not been able to verify this claim.

Diuretic Effects.—Authorities do not agree on the subject of diuresis by urotropin. In most cases it is certainly not markedly diuretic, yet severe post-operative suppression is sometimes immediately relieved by it. In this connection a case in Dr. Chetwood's practice merits quotation.

---

[1] *Cf.* Phila. Med. J., *loc. cit.*

"Mr. A. B., about forty, submitted to an external urethrotomy for stricture. During the twenty-four hours following operation he passed but 2 or 3 ounces of urine. His temperature rose to 105° F., his pulse was tumultuous and irregular, and he was apparently about to die of acute suppression of urine. Urotropin was then administered (0.5 gramme *q. i. d*) and within twenty-four hours the floodgates were opened, the temperature and pulse came down, and for two or three days all went well. Then, to test its efficacy, the urotropin was withdrawn. Within a day the urinary excretion became much less and temperature and pulse ran high again. Again the urotropin was administered, kidneys, temperature, and pulse promptly reacted, and the convalescence thereafter was uneventful."

No more striking example of diuresis could be desired. I have seen similar effects in other cases, but only when the kidneys were acutely congested. This diuresis is due, I believe, to the mildly stimulating effect of the urotropin upon the kidneys. When these organs are normal or chronically congested (e. g., in chronic uremia) the diuresis produced by urotropin is insignificant. In acute congestion I have found it most notable.

Résumé.—I recognise that the above description of the qualities of urotropin is not in accord with the teachings of many of the best authorities. It is founded, however, on a large clinical experience extending over several years, and if I do not accept urotropin as an appropriate drug for the routine treatment of gonorrhea, chronic urethritis, and cystitis, it is because I have been unable to convince myself of its constant efficiency in these maladies. The following facts I can vouch for from my own experience:

1. In total bacteriuria and in light pyelo-nephritis urotropin seems almost a specific.
2. To prove effective in these diseases it may have to be administered in high doses until the urine is practically clear of bacteria, after which smaller doses may suffice.
3. The progress of the cure can be judged only by constant recourse to the centrifuge and microscope.
4. The dose must not be sufficient to cause irritation of the neck of the bladder.
5. The possibility of such an irritation cannot be overlooked, even when very small doses are employed.
6. In diseases of the bladder and the prostate urotropin may often be depended upon to prevent inflammation, but is only of secondary importance in controlling it, and may even be positively harmful.

7. In the treatment and prophylaxis of the various forms of urinary septicemia and urethral chill urotropin is often most useful.

8. Its routine employment both before and after operations on the urinary passages is indicated.

9. The urine containing urotropin occasionally has an escharotic effect upon wounds, which may constitute a contra-indication to its employment.

10. Urotropin is an admirable diuretic in post-operative suppression.

Salol.—Salol is commonly placed second in the list of urinary antiseptics. This drug is disintegrated in the upper intestine into its component salicylic and carbolic acids. These antiseptics are absorbed into the system and excreted in the urine, where they exert their antiseptic action. But in order to obtain any very definite antiseptic effect on the urine as much as 3 or 4 grammes a day must usually be administered. This is a large dose for any stomach to bear, and as the patients for whom the drug is likely to be most serviceable are often urinary dyspeptics (p. 565), the stomach rebels before the drug does any good. When well borne, however, the effects of salol are excellent. It has not the immediate bactericidal effect of urotropin, but may be employed as a prophylactic against cystitis or in the treatment of any inflammation of the urinary organs when urotropin fails. It does not irritate the neck of the bladder, but when given in overdose produces the smoky urine of carbolic-acid poisoning.

Benzoic Acid.—Benzoic acid and the benzoates of sodium and ammonium are employed, as a rule, under the vague impression that they acidify the urine, and thereby antagonize ammoniacal cystitis. Happily the practice is sounder than the theory. As Dr. William Ashhurst [1] has shown in experiments with the sodium salt, its effects are:

"I. An inconstant diuretic action, accompanied by a slight diminution of the acidity of the urine.

"II. A retardation or absolute prevention of alkaline fermentation.

"III. An action in nature germicidal or inhibitory to the growth of certain micro-organisms either within the bladder or when introduced into the urine after voiding, these susceptible organisms including especially those which tend to produce the alkaline fermentation, but which develop in the urine while it is still acid."

Thus the administration of sodium benzoate diminishes instead

[1] Phila. Med. J., 1900, v, 457.

of increasing the acidity of normal urine, and maintains the urinary acidity only by opposing ammoniacal fermentation. Hence it is solely a urinary antiseptic. In strength it ranks a little below salol, but is rather more digestible than that salt. Dose: 3 to 6 grammes a day.

Boric Acid.—Boric acid and borax (sodium biborate) are both employed as urinary antiseptics, but their strength is less than that of the above-mentioned drugs. Two or 3 grammes a day may be administered.

4. **Diluents.**—Diluents are all-important in the treatment of every inflammation of the urinary tract. They diminish the density of the urine not by lessening the output of solids but by increasing the watery excretion of the kidneys. Thus their primary action is upon the kidneys. These organs are stimulated to a free physiological action, and any tendency to congestion or inflammation in them is minimized or entirely overcome. The urine itself is rendered more bland, its crystalline contents more fully dissolved, its acidity or alkalinity lessened. The flow of urine is increased, less time is given for bacterial proliferation in the pelvis of the kidney, and the bladder is scoured by more frequent acts of micturition. Thus the sum of the action of diluents is: (1) Diminution of any kidney congestion that may exist, (2) diminution of the irritating properties of the urine, and (3) increased irrigation of the inflamed cavities.

Dilution of the urine—diuresis—may be obtained either by administering drugs that increase the excretion of water through the kidneys or by increasing the amount of water drunk by the patient. It is convenient for our present purpose to divide diuretics into three classes:

1. Medical diuretics: drugs that are admirably diuretic in various diseases of the kidneys, but for one reason or another are not useful in inflammations of the urinary tract, except for their effect upon the kidneys. Such are digitalis, calomel, sodio-salicylate of theobromin (diuretin), broom, squill, pilocarpin, gin, etc.

2. Diuretic drugs that are useful in certain urinary inflammations—viz., the alkalies, especially potassium acetate, urotropin and the balsamics.

3. Water, the great diuretic.

Diluent Drugs.—All of the medical diuretics referred to above are of value for their effect upon the kidneys. They may be absolutely essential to the treatment of certain cases complicated by grave organic changes in the renal parenchyma; but for their simple diluent effect they are not employed, since the alkalies, the balsamics, urotropin, etc., have an equal diuretic effect combined with some medicinal effect upon the inflamed surfaces of the urinary tract. But, after all, water is the diluent upon which we depend most.

Diluent Waters.—There are waters and waters. Some are diluent and some not, entirely apart from their chemical ingredients. The general test which may be applied to any given water consists in drinking it freely and noting whether it lies heavy on the stomach. The water that can be drunk in greatest quantity without overloading the stomach is in practice the best diluent. Thus rain water is more diluent than well water, as a rule; still water more than charged water; alkaline more than acid water. Yet, quite apart from these broad properties, some waters are more diluent than others, quite as gin is more diluent than brandy, and beer more diuretic to some persons than to others, and for reasons equally obscure. For ordinary dilution of the urine, such as is a part of the treatment of every one of the inflammations in question, rain water or reaerated (not charged) distilled water suffices, if drunk freely up to 3 or 4 pints a day. For more marked dilution, such as is useful in the treatment of bacteriuria and pyelo-nephritis, Poland water, or any of the alkaline or lithia waters may be employed. In some cases, notably in acute or severe pyelo-nephritis, in obstinate bacteriuria, and in partial or total suppression of urine, post-operative or other, the greatest possible diuresis is required. Apart from drugs, such as potassium acetate, urotropin, etc., the best means I have found of overcoming these conditions is the use of Suwannee water. This water is more diluent than any other with which I am familiar. Like all mineral waters it is most efficient at its own spring, where as much as 5 gallons have been drunk in a day by one man. Stafford water is said to be equally good.

Radical Treatment

The radical treatment of any inflammation of the urinary organs is the removal of that predisposing retention, irritation, or congestion, which gives the bacteria their opportunity to attack the tissues. This implies special treatment for each special disorder. At the same time the palliative measures must be applied in order to help allay the inflammation. The cure of an inflammation by palliative measures alone, without recourse to radical treatment, is too often only temporizing with the main issue.

CHAPTER XXV

CYSTITIS

Classifications.—The inflammations of the bladder are reducible to a very small number of clinical types, though each of these types has many variations. Authorities differ so widely in their classifications of cystites that an accepted classification can hardly be said to exist. The following simple scheme will suffice for our purposes:

Non-bacterial Cystitis....	Traumatic.	
	Chemical.	
Bacterial Cystitis: Simple	Acute.	
	Chronic	Acid.
		Alkaline.
	Interstitial.	
Tubercular Cystitis.......	Pericystitis.	

The non-bacterial cases will be dismissed briefly. Tubercular cystitis is considered in a subsequent chapter.

NON-BACTERIAL CYSTITIS

Non-bacterial cystitis is the natural reaction of the vesical mucous membrane to a mechanical or a chemical irritant.

Traumatic Cystitis.—A mild cystitis or irritability of the bladder, as it is often called, may be caused by the passage of concentrated urine containing phosphates, urates, or oxalates. There is more or less urinary frequency and distress, and besides the crystals the urine contains a certain amount of pus. The so-called gouty or rheumatic cystitis is of this nature.

A more severe inflammation without infection is commonly caused by stone in the bladder (p. 435) and by rough instrumentation. In such cases there may be much tenesmus and distress together with an abundance of blood and pus in the urine.

Treatment.—The irritation due to concentrated urine may be dispelled by diluting the urine and correcting the cause of the urinary concentration. Urinary dilution may be obtained by cutting down the patient's nitrogenous foods and instituting a course of diuretic waters. To prevent a recurrence of the trouble, the patient's gouty, rheumatic, neurotic, or dyspeptic tendency must be appropriately treated. The use of the hot rectal douche (p. 131), or of deep urethral instillations (p. 218), or the administration of a urinary sedative or alkalinizer (p. 370) may be useful.

For phosphaturia dilute hydrochloric acid, gtt. v to xv *t. i. d.* in water, is often serviceable. Urotropin has also been found useful (p. 373).

For the irritation of stone, its removal is the logical treatment.

The cystitis caused by instrumentation is not a cystitis at all, but a traumatic prostatitis, which may or may not become bacterial and extend to the bladder (p. 357).

Chemical Cystitis.—Any strong irritant entering the healthy bladder, whether from above or below, causes cystitis. The intense strangury caused by the administration of cantharides has acquired an undeserved notoriety on account of the alleged sexual excitement accompanying it. As a matter of fact, the acute prostatic congestion induced by this drug is said to cause priapism, but the sensations of the patient in this condition are anything but pleasant. Rehn, and later Lichtenstein,[1] have called attention to a similar strangury occurring in coal-tar workers, apparently due to inhalation of irritating vapours. Rehn believes that sarcoma of the bladder occurs in some of these cases. The irritation due to urotropin is more important, since that drug is so freely used nowadays (p. 374).

While hyperacid urine is somewhat irritating to the bladder, ammoniacal urine is far more so, and the reason why an ammoniacal cystitis is likely to be so much more intense than an acid cystitis is doubtless for this very reason—that the ammonia adds fuel to the fire of bacterial attack.

Cystitis may equally be caused by irritants introduced through the urethra. Nitrate of silver is so often used in concentrated solution that it bears an unenviable notoriety in this regard.

Treatment.—Removal of the cause constitutes the essence of treatment. To allay the irritation the sedative remedies employed in bacterial cystitis may be used.

SIMPLE BACTERIAL CYSTITIS

This is the disease that is generally spoken of as cystitis. It may be acute or chronic, superficial or interstitial.

---

[1] Deutsche med. Wochenschr., 1898, xxiv, 709.

Etiology

The etiology of cystitis has been considered in the preceding chapter. The conclusions therein reached may be summed up as follows:

I. Bacteria may reach the bladder (1) from the urethra, (2) from the kidney, and less often (3) by irruption of a neighbouring focus of inflammation, and (4) from the blood or the lymph vessels.

II. Bacteria reaching the bladder will not cause any inflammation of that organ unless there is congestion due to (1) retention, (2) trauma by instruments, stone, or foreign body, (3) disease of the bladder wall, such as neoplasm, tubercle, or simple ulcer, or (4) unless the disease extends directly to the bladder from the neighbouring tissues, the ureter or the urethra (gonorrheal cystitis), or (5) unless the bladder is paralyzed.

III. A cystitis thus begun will disappear spontaneously unless it is perpetuated by some of the accessory causes enumerated. Of these causes the most common, clinically, is retention, which retention is almost always caused by stricture of the urethra, hypertrophy of the prostate, or contracture of the neck of the bladder.

IV. Acid cystitis is caused by the bacillus coli, the tubercular bacillus, the typhoid bacillus, or the gonococcus. Alkaline cystitis is due to staphylococcus, streptococcus, or proteus infection.

Guyon, recognising the importance of the accessory cause, has described—

1. Gonorrheal cystitis.
2. Tubercular cystitis.
3. Calculous cystitis.
4. Cystitis of stricture.
5. Cystitis of prostatics.
6. Cystitis of neoplasm.
7. Cystitis in women.
8. Painful cystitis.
9. Membranous cystitis.

This division, which does not pretend to be scientific, has no practical indication. On the contrary, so long a series based on etiological (1, 2, 3, 4, 5, 6, 7), symptomatic (8), and pathological (9) factors is anything but lucid. For our present purposes we may at once eliminate gonorrheal cystitis (p. 74), tubercular cystitis (p. 402), and the cystitis of women. The striking features of the cystitis of stone (p. 435), of stricture (p. 184), of prostatics (p. 266), and of neoplasm (p. 417) are due in each case to the etiological factor. The resultant inflammation of the bladder is much the same. In any case it may be acute or chronic, acid or ammoniacal, superficial or interstitial. Painful cystitis and membranous cystitis may be dismissed with reference to their special features.

Thus it seems advantageous, while recognising the influence of predisposing causes and special characteristics in modifying the course of the disease, to describe cystitis, not as a variable condition, but as an entirely typical inflammation with certain characteristics to distinguish it, however much it may be modified by accessory circumstances.

Morbid Anatomy

The lesions of cystitis are usually unevenly distributed over the bladder. Indeed, in many acute or mild chronic cases the lesions are entirely confined to the neck of the bladder and the trigone. This so-called inflammation of the neck of the bladder is commonly due to some prostatic inflammation, which latter must be attacked in order to cure the "inflammation of the neck." It may be noted here that in every acute cystitis and in every chronic cystitis of long standing the prostatic urethra as well as the bladder is inflamed, and the vesical inflammation is most intense about the neck and the trigone, unless some special feature of the disease (tumour, stone, pouch) produces a distinct focus of more intense inflammation elsewhere in the organ.

Acute Cystitis.—At first there is a sharp congestion most marked about the trigone and the neck, or entirely confined to that region. The mucous membrane is swollen and bright red in colour. The capillaries are dilated, the epithelial cells swollen. Then the epithelial cells begin to desquamate. The angry crimson of the mucous membrane is blotched by petechiæ, its gloss is lost, and here and there minute vesicles or abscesses appear. After these break small ulcers remain. If the acute condition persists the muscular and peritoneal coats may become inflamed.

The urine is filled with epithelium, pus, and red blood-cells.

Chronic Cystitis.—The *mucous membrane* is irregularly thickened and dense. Its surface is rough, red or gray in colour, perhaps mottled by purple or brownish blotches left by submucous hemorrhages. Here and there may be seen areas of ulceration and granulation. Sometimes the granulations grow to be distinct little villosities several millimetres long. The ulcerations may extend deep into the substance of the organ and communicate (rarely) with abscesses in the muscular tissue. In long-standing cases the epithelium may become cornified in spots, the superficial epithelia being replaced by dense shiny scales resembling the horny layers of the skin (*leukoplasia vesicæ*).

The microscope shows multiplication of the epithelial layers and desquamation of the superficial cells. All the tissues are infiltrated with new connective tissue. The vessels are congested and hypertrophied.

The general irregularities of the mucous membrane depend upon the changes in the muscular tissue.

The *muscle* of the bladder is usually hypertrophied. The whole bladder wall is thickened, and individual bundles of muscle stand out in bold relief under the mucous membrane, throwing it into numerous folds. In long-standing cases the mucous membrane forms cellules and pouches between these folds. The varieties of hypertrophy and atrophy have been described (p. 341).

The microscope shows an *interstitial cystitis,* more or less marked according to the age and intensity of the superficial lesions. The muscular bundles are separated and infiltrated by new connective tissue. The hypertrophy of the muscle is evidently more apparent than real (p. 343). In extreme cases almost all the muscle is replaced by fibrous tissues. Abscesses are rare.

Pericystitis.—The changes that occur in the connective tissue surrounding the bladder are usually of a protective character. An intense chronic cystitis often provokes a thickening of the perivesical tissue and of the peritoneum. Less frequently a diffuse fibrolipoma occurs, comparable to the perirenal fibro-lipoma (p. 540), and like it protective in character. In such cases the fibrous masses may often be felt through the rectum, and I have known them to be mistaken for cancer of the prostate until cystotomy showed the prostate to be normal and the whole bladder to be thickened. When there is much pericystitis the bladder is usually found in a state of concentric hypertrophy with fibrous, undistensible walls.

Suppurative pericystitis is usually due to rupture of the bladder.

Abscess.—Abscess of the bladder is rare. Small abscesses of the mucous membrane may run their course unnoticed. Abscesses within the wall of the bladder may begin in some infected interstitial focus or in a pocket of the mucous membrane. They burst into the bladder, leaving deep necrotic pockets, which may continue to suppurate indefinitely, or lead to perforation of the wall of the bladder. Purulent venous thrombosis has been seen.

Membranous Cystitis.[1]—*Exfoliation of the mucous membrane,* partial or complete, may occur as the result of an intense cystitis or of trauma. It is rarely seen except as a complication of prolonged and difficult parturition.

---

[1] *Cf.* Harrison, Twentieth Century Practice, i, 264. Fenwick, Lancet, 1894, i, 209.

True *diphtheritic cystitis* is so rare that its etiology is not well understood. It is encountered in connection with intense ammoniacal cystitis; but whether the intensity of the inflammation is the cause or the effect of the false membrane is not entirely clear. There may be small shreds or a cast of the greater part or the whole of the bladder. The membrane may even extend up the ureters to the kidney. The only clinical features of the disease are: (1) Intense ammoniacal cystitis; (2) fetid urine; (3) the expulsion of the false membranes, and (4) the necessity of cystotomy to relieve the tormented bladder and to extract the membranes.

Symptoms

The three characteristic symptoms of cystitis are:

1. Pus in the urine—Pyuria.
2. Frequency of urination—Pollakiuria.
3. Pain, notably pain with urination—Dysuria.

While pain, frequency, and pus are certainly characteristic of cystitis, they may also be caused by pyelitis. Moreover, in mild chronic cases the frequency and pain are not at all notable; the pyuria is the only definite symptom. There are other symptoms of cystitis, notably certain urinary changes, but these are special to certain forms of the disease and will be discussed with them.

Pyuria.—Whenever there is cystitis pus may be found in greater or less quantity in the urine. To distinguish that the pus comes from the bladder the two-glass test must be employed. An ounce or two of urine (the first flow) is passed into a glass beaker, the remainder (the second flow) into a similar vessel. The first flow shows the contents of the bladder combined with the washings from the urethra. The second flow shows the contents of the bladder to all intents undiluted. Pus in the urine causes a general cloudiness, which after standing settles to the bottom, leaving the supernatant fluid relatively or absolutely clear. The cloudiness cannot be dispelled by heat or chemicals. The addition of liquor potassæ to the urine causes the pus to agglomerate into flocculent gelatinous particles that are quite characteristic. The pus cells may also be recognised under the microscope. Unless there is some pus in the second flow of urine there can be no cystitis. Yet the presence of pus does not prove that there is cystitis (p. 391).

Frequency of Urination.—Except in very mild cases, or in case of retention or suppression of urine, frequency of urination is a constant symptom of cystitis. It is a fair index of the severity of the inflammation. In mild cases the patient urinates every three hours or so by day and empties his bladder only once or twice during the night. On the other hand, a patient suffering from acute cystitis spends day and night in urinating. The calls to urinate occur every ten or fifteen minutes, and, if not obeyed, result in the expulsion of the contents of the bladder, no matter how much the patient strains to retain his water. This is the so-called false incontinence, quite different from true incontinence (p. 347). Frequency of urination is by no means pathognomonic of cystitis. It may be purely neurotic, or due to stone, to prostatitis, to hypertrophy of the prostate, etc. The frequency due to prostatic hypertrophy is chiefly nocturnal; that due to cystitis or to stone is usually diurnal.

Pain.—The pain of cystitis (unless there is abscess) is due to the presence of urine in the bladder. If there is no retention the pain is intermittent. If there is retention the pain is constant or remittent. It is most severe at the time of urination, and in the milder cases it is felt only at that time (dysuria). It is felt chiefly in the glans penis and the perineum. It may radiate along the under surface of the penis, up the rectum, to hypogastrium, groin, hip, testicle, thigh, or loin. When the inflammation runs high there is often a continuous ache in the perineum, the hypogastrium, or the hip. With the dysuria there is an irritative cramp or spasm of the bladder and its sphincter as the last drops of urine are passed and for a few moments thereafter (tenesmus). The patient strains away after the bladder is empty, thus markedly adding to the irritation already present. There may be a sympathetic tenesmus of the rectum excited by the urinary straining, sometimes with most unpleasant results.

Systemic Disturbance.—Though patients suffering from cystitis often exhibit such symptoms as chills, fever, sleeplessness, anorexia, and loss of flesh and strength, these symptoms are not directly referable to the inflammation of the bladder. All the febrile symptoms are due either to inflammation of the prostate or to implication of the kidneys, and the loss of appetite, sleep, and strength is due to the distressing symptoms of pain, dysuria, and tenesmus.

Having thus briefly summed up the chief symptoms common to all forms of cystitis we pass to a consideration of the types of the disease—viz., acute cystitis, chronic acid cystitis, chronic ammoniacal cystitis, interstitial cystitis, and pericystitis.

Course of the Disease

Acute Cystitis.—Excepting the acute cystitis of mechanical or chemical origin (p. 381) and the acute exacerbations that occur during the course of a chronic inflammation of the bladder, acute cystitis is always of gonorrheal origin. This *acute gonorrheal cystitis* may be accepted as a type of all acute cystitis, since it is the most acute as well as the most common of all. It may or may not be due to the gonococcus. It occurs during a gonorrhea, during severe simple urethritis, or even during gleet—if the gleet depend upon stricture—by direct continuation of the inflammation backward upon the mucous membrane. The inflammation is confined to the region of the neck, and does not attack the body of the bladder.

It rarely appears until after the first week of a gonorrhea, and is commonest during the third week, when the inflammation has reached the posterior urethra. It is frequently seen in practice as a result of simple extension of inflammation later in the course of the disease. Often, however, a second or provoking cause has been in action, and without its assistance the complication of gonorrheal cystitis might have been escaped. These provoking causes are anything which will irritate the urethra: alcoholic beverages, sexual intercourse, abortive treatment of gonorrhea, catheterism, jolting, violent or sometimes even moderate exercise. Any of these causes may light up a cystitis of the vesical neck in any patient with urethritis.

The symptoms of gonorrheal cystitis vary from a hardly appreciable irritability—with congestion—up to the very highest grade these symptoms (of irritability) can assume, with a tenesmus so constant as to amount to actual incontinence, the patient voiding a few drops of blood or milky fluid every few minutes. The tenesmus is particularly painful, although the mere passage of urine is often attended by great pain. A noteworthy feature of gonorrheal cystitis is the absence of general phenomena. Fever is sometimes inappreciable, and rarely runs high. Anxiety, *malaise*, and nervous distress are, however, disproportionately prominent. Constipation is habitual. The urethral discharge becomes greatly lessened, or even disappears on the advent of the bladder symptoms; as the latter disappear, however, the former returns. Gonorrheal cystitis varies in duration from a few days, in abortive cases, up to many weeks, and sometimes leaves permanent trouble behind in the pelvis of the kidney, in the prostate, or in the seminal vesicle. It is not followed by chronic cystitis unless retention, stone, or tumour perpetuates the inflammation.

The Urine.—The urine of acute cystitis is usually acid, thickly purulent throughout and often bloody. If an attack of acute cystitis occurs during the course of a chronic ammoniacal inflammation the urine remains ammoniacal, but the other symptoms are the same as described above. Chemical examination reveals the presence of albumin derived from the blood in the urine. The microscope shows great quantities of pus cells and bacteria with a variable number of red blood cells and desquamated epithelia.

Chronic Cystitis.—Chronic cystitis is very common, so much so that there are few diseases of the lower urinary passages of which it does not form a part. Chronic cystitis, moreover (unlike many other chronic inflammations), rarely commences as an acute disease, but is chronic from the first. It never occurs as an idiopathic affection, but is invariably a secondary result arising from other morbid conditions of the urinary passages (p. 359). Once started, it does not tend to get well spontaneously, but to become slowly and steadily worse. Fortunately, its causes are well known, and most of them easy of demonstration. Many of these can be removed, and with them the chronic inflammation which they keep up. Some cases are incurable on account of permanent structural alterations in the bladder walls, or because the cause cannot be reached. All, however, may be benefited by careful and judicious management, and there are few abnormal conditions of the body whose amelioration is more satisfactory to the surgeon, or more grateful to the sufferer.

The symptoms of chronic cystitis resemble those of the acute form, in a degree proportionate to the grade of the inflammatory process. They are often complicated by retention (p. 346), by atony (p. 344) or hypertrophy of the bladder (p. 341), by stone, by tubercle, by tumour (pp. 402, 417), etc. There may only be slightly increased frequency of urination, with slight cloudiness of the fluid, in very chronic cases; or the calls may be very frequent, and the pains excessive, varied, and constant, as in the acute disease. In fact, chronic cystitis is liable at any time to be lighted up into an acute state by the continued action of its own cause, or by the supervention of other causes (cold, violent exercise, abuse of alcohol, acid urine, instrumentation, etc.). Between these acute attacks the symptoms of the disease are so slight that the patient may fancy himself well, and rejoice over the fancied cure while the spark of future and worse inflammation is yet smouldering within him. Even the surgeon might be deceived by such a case were it not for the persistent urinary evidence of disease.

The Urine.—The urine in chronic cystitis is clouded by pus and bacteria. It is rarely bloody unless there is tubercle, stone, or cancer. It may be acid or alkaline.

Chronic Acid Cystitis.—When the urine is acid and the cystitis chronic the vesical inflammation is usually mild (unless it be tubercular). The amount of pus in the urine is not great, and the subjective symptoms are slight or entirely absent. This form of cystitis is often encountered with hypertrophy of the prostate, associated with slight pyelo-nephritis. The inflammation, though mild, is usually quite unconquerable, except by removal of the prostatic obstruction. The dangers connected with it are: (1) The pyelo-nephritis, and (2) the development of ammoniacal cystitis, and it is against these that the treatment is chiefly directed. The acid cystitis may be controlled by intelligent treatment, and, if the kidneys are protected and alkaline fermentation prevented, the patient gets along very well at the expense of systematic local treatment, which he is, as a rule, quite ready to accept in lieu of an operation calculated to relieve all his sufferings. (See Treatment.)

Chronic Alkaline Cystitis.—This form of chronic cystitis is of serious import. Its severity is usually in marked contrast with the mildness of a chronic acid cystitis. Urination is frequent and painful, the urine foul and ammoniacal (it may be only slightly alkaline) and filled with clots of ropy muco-pus mingled with crystals of triple phosphates and often tinged with blood. A complicating pyelonephritis is as common as with acid cystitis; but the symptoms of the bladder inflammation are far less tolerable and often no less difficult to control. Unless checked by appropriate treatment the disease tends to grow more severe by successive attacks of acute inflammation, until, finally, the patient succumbs, worn out by his ceaseless agony. The kidneys give out after a time, and it is through them that the patient usually meets his end (p. 553).

Interstitial Cystitis.—During interstitial cystitis the bladder gradually contracts down, undergoing concentric hypertrophy, its walls thicken enormously, possibly reaching the thickness of an inch. Abscess may form in them; the cavity becomes nearly obliterated, perhaps down to 25 c. c.; incontinence ensues; the mass, like a hard, smooth, wooden ball, may be felt in the hypogastrium, or from the rectum. It is not necessarily very sensitive to pressure, and is smooth and of even hardness on its surface. This condition of bladder disease is not curable. The bladder walls cannot be redilated. But removal of its cause will make life bearable for the patient by relieving the pain, even though he still has to urinate frequently.

Diagnosis

Acute Cystitis.—This can be confounded only with acute prostatitis, from which it may be differentiated by rectal touch, which detects a hot, throbbing, swollen prostate in the one case, nothing of the sort in the other.

Chronic Cystitis.—It is a common error to label every case of pyuria "cystitis." This is most fallacious. There may be pus in the urine for years and yet no cystitis. Indeed, the three characteristic symptoms—pain, pus, and frequency—are again and again due to

PLATE V

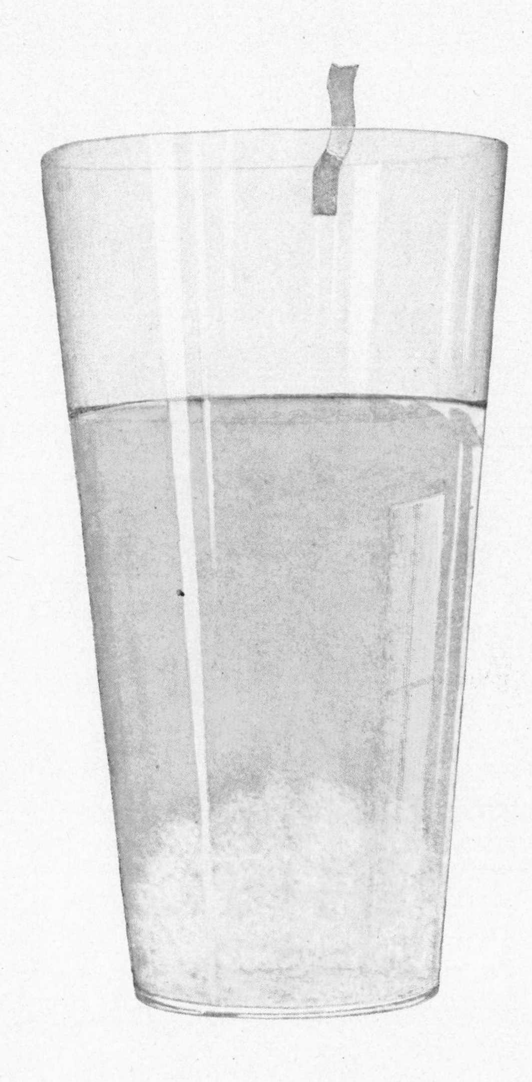

such widely divergent causes as pyelo-nephritis, prostatitis, and vesiculitis without the presence of any cystitis whatever. Another source of misapprehension is the fact that the inflammation of the bladder is often only an element of the inflammation of the whole urinary tract, in which case its treatment, whether successful or not, has little bearing on the far more important inflammation of the renal pelvis. The surgeon must therefore face two difficult problems of diagnosis:

1. The existence or the absence of cystitis, and
2. The presence or the absence of pyelo-nephritis, prostatitis, and vesiculitis.

The existence of cystitis may oftentimes be affirmed with certainty without any very searching examination. Thus the clinical features of the cystitis of stone or tumour, or of severe chronic ammoniacal cystitis, are usually quite unmistakable. But, on the other hand, there are a great number of cases showing acid or alkaline urine and more or less characteristic symptoms of cystitis that are not inflammations of the bladder at all. So deceptive are these cases that they may mislead the most expert. Thus Rovsing refuses to accept the diagnosis of cystitis unless it is confirmed by a cystoscopic examination. This is all very well from the bacteriologist's point of view, but for the clinician the cystoscope can have no charms; for if a cystitis does exist no manipulation is better calculated than cystoscopy to aggravate the symptoms of the disease. Yet, like many other diseases of the urinary organs, cystitis can only be diagnosed by its physical signs; its symptoms are often most misleading. The physical signs of cystitis are found chiefly in the urine. *When there is cystitis the urine is always purulent throughout* in both the first and the second flow (p. 83). Again, *when the urine is ammoniacal there is always cystitis.* But pyuria does not always indicate cystitis, and ammoniacal cystitis may often be accompanied by pyelitis and other lesions, the diagnosis of which is most important. Indeed, *when the urine is purulent and acid, pyelitis must always be suspected.* Finally, *a chronic pyuria, in the absence of retention, stone, tubercle, or tumour, is always due to prostatitis or to pyelitis, never to cystitis.*

Differential Diagnosis

Although the differential diagnosis between pyelo-nephritis and cystitis rests largely on an understanding of the signs of the former disease, there are certain striking points of differentiation that may be brought out by a careful urinary examination and merit discussion here, inasmuch as pyelo-nephritis is mistaken for cystitis far more often than cystitis is mistaken for pyelo-nephritis. This confusion arises chiefly from the fact that the two inflammations often exist together, in which case the more acute symptoms of the less important cystitis blind the surgeon to the existence of a pyelonephritis which, in the long run, will do the patient far more harm than will his bladder lesion. A less frequent cause of confusion is the fact that a diseased kidney sometimes produces symptoms of cystitis when the bladder is entirely sound (p. 571). The surgeon, confronted with a case whose symptoms are pyuria and dysuria, may struggle for months to heal an uninflamed bladder, overlooking, all the while, a pus kidney that stares him in the face. Every surgeon who has had any experience with renal diseases has met such cases, and probably has sometimes been deceived himself. The distinguishing feature of *renal pus* is that it *sinks to the bottom of the glass and there forms a compact level base like sand* (Plate IX). *Bladder pus,* on the contrary, *forms a billowy, fluffy deposit, and often* does not sink fully to the bottom of the glass, but *remains more or less suspended in the fluid* (Plate V).

When cystitis and pyelitis exist together (Plate VI) a very simple test suffices to distinguish them. After the patient has urinated in two glasses his bladder is gently irrigated with a hot boric-acid solution until the fluid returns clear. On withdrawing the catheter the anterior urethra is also flushed with the solution. An hour later the urine is withdrawn with a catheter (in order to avoid possible prostatic contamination), and if it is then as purulent as before, the pus comes from the kidney. This test fails if catheterization causes bleeding or if a clean return flow cannot be obtained from the wash. The remittent character of renal pyuria, as well as the chemical and microscopical characteristics of kidney urine will be commented upon elsewhere (p. 558). Suffice it to say that an expert physiological chemist can always distinguish pyelo-nephritis from cystitis by the presence or the absence of bladder epithelia on the one hand, and albumin, casts, deficient excretion of solids, and renal and pelvis epithelia on the other.

Prostatitis and vesiculitis are distinguished by an examination of their secretions expressed by rectal touch as well as by the sensation imparted to the finger in the rectum (p. 89). Tubercular cystitis is distinguished by its marked peculiarities (p. 404).

Prognosis

Acute cystitis recovers spontaneously or under treatment, or becomes chronic. *Chronic cystitis* is curable with its predisposing cause (retention, stone, tumour) or even without it. Thus many cases of cystitis due to prostatic obstruction are cured though the

PLATE VI

THE URINE OF SEVERE ALKALINE CYSTITIS COMPLICATED BY SUPPURATIVE PYELO-NEPHRITIS

The urine is alkaline and muddy when passed. On standing it becomes somewhat clearer; but always remains hazy with bacteria; while at the bottom there settles a rolling mucous cloud, underneath which is the flat sandy bottom of renal pus.

PLATE VI

THE URINE OF SEVERE ALKALINE CYSTITIS COMPLICATED BY SUPPURATIVE PYELO-NEPHRITIS

The urine is alkaline and muddy when passed. On standing it becomes somewhat clearer, but always remains hazy with bacteria; while at the bottom there settles a rolling mucous cloud, underneath which is the flat sandy bottom of renal pus.

PLATE VI

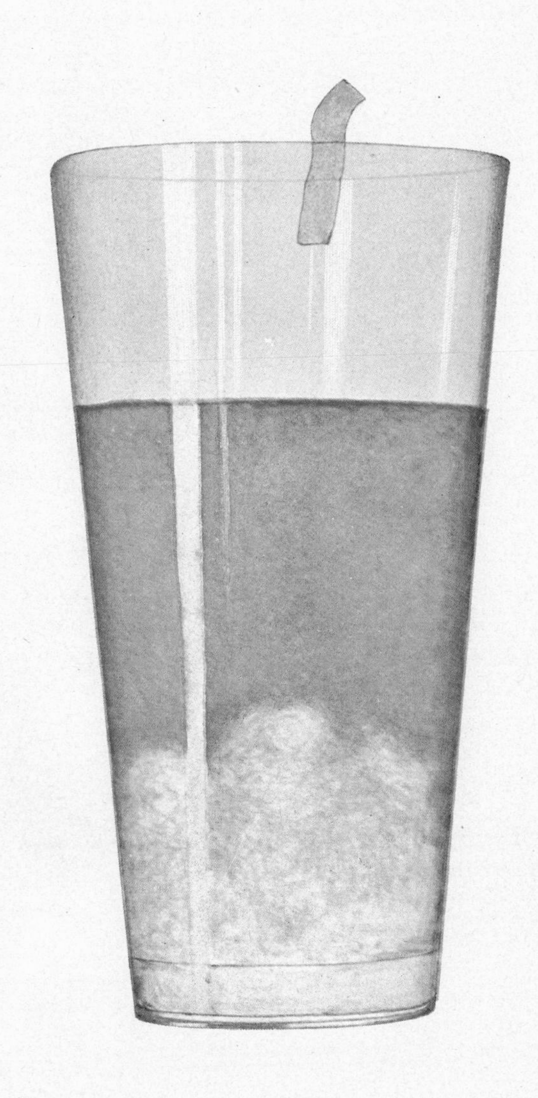

obstruction remains. But they are always in danger of relapse until the predisposing cause is removed.

The danger to life from cystitis itself is not great. Rupture of the bladder, interstitial and perivesical suppuration and peritonitis are remote possibilities. As long as the kidneys remain sound the patient's life is safe. But when the infection once reaches them the prognosis darkens (p. 362).

Treatment

Prophylaxis.—Prevention of cystitis is an important element in the treatment of gonorrhea, prostatitis, stricture, hypertrophy of the prostate, bladder, stone, and tumour, as well as in every passage of an instrument into the bladder. It requires no special notice here.

Treatment of Acute Cystitis.—Acute gonorrheal cystitis is the type of all acute inflammations of the bladder, and the treatment of the gonorrheal inflammation (p. 139) is that of all the others. Nitrate-of-silver instillations are not so efficacious in the non-specific inflammations. If there be any removable cause (catheter tied into the bladder) it should be taken away. If the cause be stone or a foreign body, no attempt should be made to remove it until the intensity of the inflammation has been quieted. If cantharides, turpentine, or cubeb is being taken by the patient, it should be discontinued during the acute stage of the affection, to be resumed in the subacute stage. Copaiba sometimes works wonderfully well in quieting acute symptoms, but it cannot be relied upon. Asparagus should not be eaten by a patient with acute cystitis; common salt, strong coffee, and lemon-juice should also be avoided. There is no occasion for any local or general abstraction of blood, but the measures detailed at pp. 110–112 should be studiously enforced. If the cystitis be a strangury from cantharides, plenty of opium—or camphor in emulsion—and a very free use of diluents, must be relied upon. In all cases repeated use of a full hot bath or a hot hip bath has a soothing effect. The rectum should be kept free by copious warm enemata, and opiates should be given by the rectum, not by the mouth. Absolute rest, with the hips raised, and alkaline diluents, suffice in mild cases. If abscess form in or around the walls of the bladder, an opening should be made externally through the hypogastrium, the rectum, or the perineum at the earliest possible moment, to prevent perforation and infiltration.

Treatment of Chronic Cystitis.—The peculiarity of chronic cystitis, depending, as it always does, upon some other morbid condition, renders its special description unsatisfactory, and begets a necessity for constant reference to the other affections which underlie it.

A reference to the pages devoted to the treatment of the inflammation of the urinary tract in general (pp. 367 to 380), and to the sections on those diseases with which cystitis is especially associated, notably prostatic hypertrophy, stricture, and stone, will give a better foundation for the treatment of the disease than anything that can be said here. In general, the radical treatment of chronic cystitis consists in removal of its cause. If the cause is not removable, or if it has been removed, the treatment is palliative. Attention to the general health, the urinary hygiene, the condition of the bowels, and the quality of the urine constitutes the essential background, the passive part of the cure, as it were, while the active work is performed locally.

The Urine must be Modified.—Its specific gravity should be kept below 1.020—below 1.015, if possible. This object is attained by making the patient drink plenty of water. Some balsamic, such as oil of wintergreen, eucalyptus, sandal-wood, or turpentine, is administered, together with an alkali. The addition of a urinary antiseptic is especially valuable in prostatic cases, and may be useful in any event. These internal remedies are conveniently put up in soft capsules, each capsule containing a dose. Favourite combinations are:

℞ Ol. santal. flav. .... 10 grammes
Potass. citrat. .... 5 "
M. Fiant caps. moll. No. XV.
Sig.—One capsule after each meal.

℞ Salol
Oleoresin. cubeb.
Copaiba, Para } .... āā 5 grammes
Pepsin .... q. s.
M. Fiant caps. moll. No. XV.
Sig.—One capsule after each meal.

℞ Ol. santal. flav.
Oleoresin. saw palmetto } .... āā 5 grammes
M. Fiant caps. moll. No. XX.
Sig.—One capsule after each meal.

℞ Urotropin .... 5 grammes
Ol. santal. flav. .... 10 "
M. Fiant caps. moll. No. XX.
Sig.—One capsule after each meal.

Any number of similar prescriptions may be devised. None of them is specific, and I hesitate to lay down any rules for their administration. I am inclined to use urotropin if there is any fever and whenever the kidneys are threatened, and I am never satisfied with any preparation that disagrees with the patient's stomach. It often seems beneficial to change the prescription once or twice a month unless the patient is doing peculiarly well.

Hygiene must not be Forgotten.—The patient must be made to understand the various dangers to be avoided—alcohol, sexual excess, exposure to cold, overexercise, overeating, etc. (p. 275). Some patients are far more sensitive to those influences than others; and older men, especially prostatics, are the most sensitive. But each patient is a law unto himself, and must find out by his own experience those liberties in which he may indulge and those he must avoid. The surgeon can only help him by general suggestions and careful watching.

The Local Treatment is the most Important.—This is the active, efficient part of the treatment from which a cure is expected; it must be systematic and intelligent. The more acute or recent the inflammation the more advantage there is in using instillations and in pushing the strength of the solution to the limit of toleration. These cases must be managed by the surgeon himself. I have had most success with nitrate of silver, protargol, and permanganate of potash. Chronic, long-standing cases often cannot be cured unless the cause of inflammation is removed. Ammoniacal inflammation may sometimes be overcome by vigorous local treatment, and the attempt should always be made, as the patient is far safer with chronic acid cystitis than with chronic alkaline inflammation. In most of these chronic cases, however—they are practically all due to prostatic hypertrophy, to stone, or to contracture of the neck of the bladder—the surgeon must be satisfied to hold the disease in check as best he may. The patient is taught to use his own catheter systematically, and instructed in the use of a boric-acid solution for irrigation (p. 281). Any acute phenomena may usually be allayed by a few irrigations with stronger solutions at the hands of the surgeon.

To estimate the results of treatment we have a reliable index in the urine. Months of practice are required before the surgeon is able to estimate the import of urinary showing; but once he has become expert, a glance suffices to tell him whether the patient is better or worse for his last treatment. The two-glass test is always to be used (p. 83) and the contents of the second glass especially noted. If the patient's symptoms are acute or his general condition low, these, too, should react to the treatment; but in the majority of chronic cases the symptoms are so mild that the results of treatment show chiefly, if not entirely, in the urine.

Cystostomy.—Drainage of the bladder by means of a suprapubic or a perineal incision is employed for the relief of inveterate cystitis when other palliative measures fail and the symptoms are too intense to be borne. When the cause of the cystitis is an inoperable tumour, permanent drainage by a suprapubic opening is the only available relief (p. 422). Also, in certain cases of sacculated bladder, interstitial cystitis, and pericystitis, prolonged suprapubic drainage gives the organ the physiological rest it requires in order to rally the forces left to it. If these conditions are not known to exist cystostomy may still be performed, but it must be recognised to be an exploratory, not a palliative operation, undertaken for the discovery and removal of the cause of cystitis, not merely for the relief of symptoms. Even if there is interstitial cystitis or pericystitis, an essential part of their operative relief is usually the removal of the urethral obstruction to which the inflammation is primarily due.

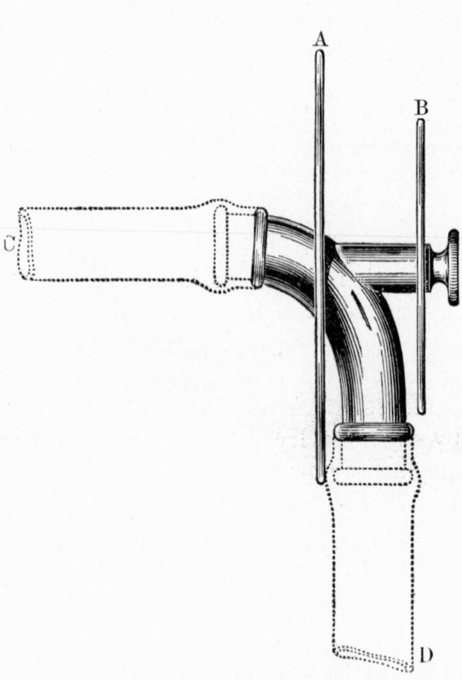

Fig. 92.—Permanent Suprapubic Drainage-tube. *A*, plate fitting against abdomen; *B*, plate to go inside of belt; *C*, rubber tube into bladder; *D*, rubber tube to urinal.

The choice between the suprapubic (p. 459) and the perineal (p. 457) route cannot be decided categorically. The safety with which suprapubic cystostomy may be performed in these surgical days, and the excellent opportunity for inspection and palpation of the bladder which this route affords, make the operation above the bone the surgeon's choice in most cases. But urethral obstruction of one sort or another is such a constant cause of chronic cystitis that I have a strong leaning towards the perineal operation, which gives, if anything, better drainage than does the suprapubic route, and through which any form of urethral obstruction, stricture, hypertrophied prostate, or contracture of the neck of the bladder may be removed. A thorough digital exploration may also be made from the perineum, but inspection of the interior of the bladder is not possible. In any case, if the perineal or the suprapubic opening proves unsatisfactory, a counter opening may be made with little added risk. The suprapubic route is better suited for permanent drainage. Of the many forms of tube employed to keep the fistula open I have derived the most satisfaction from the one figured herewith (Figs. 92, 93). It may be made of silver or hard rubber. The tube must be of a sufficient calibre to carry off thick mucus and clots. A short rubber drainage-tube is slipped over the extremity *A*, and this is introduced through the fistula into the bladder. The tube is held in place by a home-made washable belt passing outside the smaller disk (not between the two), and tight enough to press the inner disk firmly against the skin, so that no urine can escape outside of the tube. Continuous drainage may be maintained by attaching the outer end of the tube to a leg urinal. If the bladder will contain a little fluid, it is more convenient to cork the tube and allow "hypogastric urination" only at stated intervals. All attempts at obtaining a muscular hypogastric orifice are foredoomed to failure. The corked tube is the best we have. If no tube is employed the fistula narrows down to a dribbling hole which is entirely unmanageable.

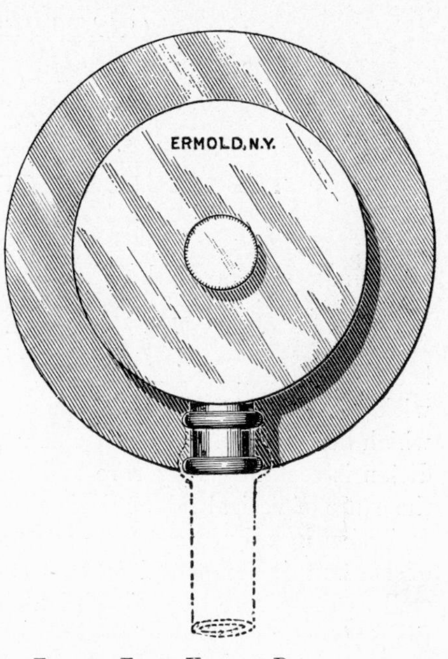

Fig. 93.—Front View of Drainage-tube.

Treatment of Interstitial Cystitis and Pericystitis.—Interstitial cystitis and pericystitis are usually evidence of a neglected chronic cystitis. The adequate treatment of the inflamed mucous membrane will prevent inflammation of the underlying tissues. Even after interstitial cystitis and pericystitis have appeared much may be accomplished by palliative measures; but oftener operation will be necessary. Cystostomy releases the bladder from the slavery of incessant straining and gives it a needed rest. Perivesical abscesses are to be opened wherever they point. After a suprapubic tube has been worn for some weeks or months the bladder may be ready to resume its functions, and the suprapubic fistula may be allowed to close.

CHAPTER XXVI

SIMPLE AND TUBERCULOUS ULCERATION OF THE BLADDER

TUBERCULOSIS OF THE BLADDER

Etiology

Tuberculosis of the bladder is almost always secondary to a tubercular lesion elsewhere in the genital or the urinary organs. Like these lesions it is commonest in the young adult, though it has been observed in the infant and the aged. It may be primary. Fenwick [1] recognises a distinct type of multiple tubercles in the bladder which he thinks characteristic of a primary invasion. But this condition is certainly very rare and the clinician is justified in seeking the cause of vesical tuberculosis elsewhere in the genito-urinary tract. Infection usually comes from the prostate or the kidney—I leave out of account instrumental infection, in which I put small faith, as well as those rare cases in which the bladder may be infected from the peritoneum (Bryson [2]) or from some other neighbouring organ—and is probably usually carried by the lymphatics. Some writers believe that when there is a tubercular focus in the kidney and the urine is laden with tubercle bacilli, an infection of the bladder often occurs from these bacilli in the urine. Allowing a stone in the bladder or some inflammation or injury of that organ as a predisposing cause, the assumption may be granted; but in those cases which this theory is called upon to explain—viz., the common descending ulceration about the mouth of one ureter—it does not seem entirely adequate. Moullin [3] has elaborated a theory fully in accord with our knowledge of the general tendencies of tubercular disease and more in accord with the clinical facts. According to this author, the trigone and base of the bladder contain a submucous network of lymphatics which are intimately related to other lymphatics similarly

[1] Ulceration of the Bladder, London, 1900.

[2] Morrow's System of Genito-urinary Diseases, etc., 1893, i, 846.

[3] Inflammation of the Bladder and Urinary Fever, 1898.

situated in the ureter, kidney, and prostate. Thus a tubercular inflammation of the kidney may extend along the ureter until it reaches the bladder, or it may leap from the kidney to the bladder, breaking out in few intervening spots or in none. Similarly it may extend from the prostate or from one part of the bladder to another; but whether these extensions of the disease leave large intervening areas of healthy mucous membrane or not, the bacteria travel from the old focus to the new one chiefly, if not wholly, through the lymphatics. The influence of an antecedent inflammation in preparing the soil for the tubercular bacillus is very striking in those cases which begin as acute gonorrhea, drag on as chronic gleet, and terminate in frank tuberculosis of the prostate or the trigone.

Most recent writers upon this subject incline to the belief that the bladder is more frequently involved by a descending process from the kidney than by an ascending one from the prostate; but, however this may be, there are two forms of vesical tuberculosis, each one showing distinct evidence of the origin of the disease. The one, ulceration at or about the neck of the bladder, points to a primary focus in the prostate; the other, an ulcer surrounding one ureteral orifice, points to a tuberculosis of the corresponding kidney. Mixed and irregular forms, of which there are not many, may arise from either source.

Morbid Anatomy

The bladder, like every other organ, may be involved in a general miliary tuberculosis. Apart from this phenomenon of purely pathological interest, the bladder infected by tuberculosis may present two clinical aspects. There may be simply a number of discrete tubercles developed immediately beneath the epithelium, or, as the result of the breaking down of one or more of these tubercles, tuberculous ulcers may appear. The tubercles evince an acute condition, the ulcers, a long-standing malady. The two often coexist.

The tubercles appear as minute whitish areas, the size of a pinhead, surrounded by an area of congestion (Plate IV, Fig. 1). They are usually grouped together over irregular areas of the bladder wall, while between them the mucous membrane is red, swollen, and velvety. Thus a diffuse vesical tuberculosis gives the whole mucous membrane this congested, velvety appearance. Although the tubercles may be seen, and sometimes even felt, through the unbroken epithelium, the initial deposit occurs, as Coplin[1] has justly remarked, not in the epithelium, but in the subepithelial connective tissue.

The tubercular ulcer "is singularly round and discoid. . . .

[1] J. of Cut. and Gen.-Urin. Dis., 1898, xvi, 557.

Even the confluent ulcers rapidly lose the isthmus which at one time partly separated them and quickly assume a roundish outline. The floor of the ulcer is shaggy, of a dirty yellowish colour. It is uneven in contour. . . . Commonly the ulcer does not become larger than 1 or 2 cm., or about the size of a 5-cent piece. The floor of the ulcer is the submucosa containing considerable embryonic tissue. In some instances and at a few points in any ulcer the muscular wall may be exposed. . . . I think extension into the muscular wall must be rather infrequent. . . . The edges are elevated and slightly undermined . . . hard to the touch . . . extremely muscular" (Coplin).

The above description, written from the point of view of the pathologist, is entirely in accord with the clinical findings. I have never known perforation of the bladder to occur, though I have followed many cases for years. Senn,[1] however, makes a point of the danger of perforation. Coplin suggests that perforation, which he believes very exceptional, may be due to a mixed infection. The great irritability of the bladder—its characteristic inability to retain more than a few ounces—is due at first to the great sensitiveness of the tubercular lesions, later to an actual infiltration and contracture of the muscular walls—a sort of concentric hypertrophy.

The distribution of the lesions may be irregular, but the centre of trouble is always in the trigone or about the mouths of the ureters. Thence the tubercles, ulcers, and congestion spread slowly to all parts of the organ by lymphatic extension, by direct growth and coalition of the ulcerated tubercles, and perhaps by contact, an ulcer of one surface giving rise to a secondary ulcer on the opposite surface by actual contact with the mucous membrane.

In the more acute forms of the disease the tubercles, the ulcers, and the lesions of simple cystitis are variously combined. But in the commoner chronic cases the disease assumes one of two forms. If the infection comes from one kidney the bladder lesions are entirely confined to the neighbourhood of the corresponding ureteral orifice. Ulcerations and tubercles are closely grouped around this point as a centre. If, on the other hand, the disease begins in the prostate, the neck of the bladder bears the brunt of the inflammation. The mucous membrane here becomes congested, thickened, and ulcerated until the condition is almost an exact counterpart of a simple contracture of the neck of the bladder. In perineal section, with cutting down of the contractured orifice, I have sometimes been unable to detect by eye or finger any difference between the simple and the tubercular inflammation (p. 317).

---

[1] Tuberculosis of the Genito-Urinary Organs, 1898, p. 188.

Direct extension of the inflammation from or to the lower part of the ureter and the posterior urethra is common. Extension to the anterior urethra is rare.

Symptoms

Vesical tuberculosis is simply a specialized inflammation of the bladder with characteristics so little distinct that many of the most pathognomonic among them have been determined only within the last twenty years. The course of the disease is varied and often obscure. Sometimes the symptoms are quite characteristic, but the final diagnostic test rests always with the discovery of the tubercle bacillus in the urine.

Onset.—The disease, beginning usually during the course of a renal or prostatic tuberculosis or of a chronic gleet, declares itself first by one of two symptoms, hematuria or irritability of the bladder. This onset may be spontaneous or provoked by the use of instruments in the urethra. Whether bleeding or irritability comes first the other soon follows.

Hematuria.—The hematuria of tuberculosis is usually quite characteristic. It is a prominent symptom of the disease first and last. It differs from the hematuria of stone in being influenced little, if at all, by jolting or exercise, and it is only in exceptional cases a free hemorrhage, such as is common with neoplasms. The first bleeding noticed by the patient is often the exudation of a few drops of pure blood at the end of the urinary act. The blood is squeezed, as it were, from the base and neck of the bladder by its own contraction. This *terminal hematuria* is usually accompanied by some terminal pain and spasm and is strongly suggestive of tuberculosis, though it may occur with any severe congestion about the neck of the bladder. The next urine passed is usually red with blood, and so the bleeding continues for a few hours or days, and then apparently stops, to recur after an interval of days or weeks. In the meanwhile, however, the urine is not entirely clear of blood. Though not a bright red, it may still be smoky, and even when clean and sparkling the microscope will almost invariably detect a few red blood-cells in a centrifuged specimen, and a trace of albumin will also be found. So these bleedings recur, never profuse enough to fill the bladder with clots, growing perhaps more, perhaps less frequent, but never stopping entirely. They occur by night as well as by day; they are uninfluenced by exercise or by rest. As the disease progresses and its lesions spread the hemorrhages become, if anything, less profuse and more continuous. The urine gets to be hazy all the time, and contains a few small bright-red clots. The last few drops passed may be pure blood, but beyond this there is not likely to be any severe bleeding unless it is stirred up by the introduction of instruments into the bladder.

Irritability of the Bladder.—The characteristic irritability of the bladder—the frequency of urination and the pain accompanying the act—is often the earliest and always the most distressing symptom of tuberculosis. At first, the frequency of urination is not great, although there may be undue discomfort as soon as a few ounces of urine have collected in the bladder, and the pain is chiefly confined to the end of urination. As the bladder contracts down on the last drops of urine, as the terminal hematuria appears (if there is terminal hematuria), a sharp pain is felt in the perineum and often on the under surface of the penis at the peno-scrotal angle. Pain may also be felt in the glans penis and may radiate in various directions. The effect of this pain is to excite a tighter spasm of the bladder, and the result of this spasm is an increase in the pain, so that a good deal of pain and spasm persists after the last drop of urine has been expelled, leaving a soreness which may not pass off before another urinary act renews the wretched cycle. At first this terminal pain is only fairly constant, but later it accompanies every act of urination and grows more severe as the disease progresses.

After a short time, when ulcers have formed, or a mixed infection has occurred, another pain is felt, a pain before urinating, often an imperious and irresistible spasm which, if not immediately acceded to, will squirt a few drops of urine down the sufferer's thigh in spite of all his efforts to prevent it. The increased sensibility to pressure brings on some such spasm, more or less severe, as soon as a few ounces have entered the bladder; and what with this spasm before urinating and the more intense spasm afterward, what with the constantly decreasing capacity of the bladder and the increasing frequency of urination, the patient knows no peace day or night. The irritability of the bladder is even more strongly marked when instrumentation is attempted. Such are the bleeding and spasm aroused by almost any instrument or wash that the patient soon learns to dread the catheter and the searcher with all his soul. A special antipathy of the tubercular bladder to nitrate of silver is often a means of distinguishing tuberculosis from simple cystitis.

The Urine.—The urine of tubercular cystitis is acid. At first it may be clear or bloody. Later it is bloody, and often foul with the products of a suppurative cystitis ingrafted on the tubercular process either spontaneously or as the result of catheterization. But, however foul and ammoniacal, however full of shreds of bloody mucus and stringy clots the urine may be, its one striking characteristic is its continued acidity. It is by no means impossible for the urine of a mixed infection to be alkaline when passed as a result of the predominance of pyogenic cocci; but, clinically, alkaline urine is most exceptional in tuberculosis, however violent the mixed infection. The urine may be only slightly acid, though it is usually strongly so, but acid it is; and this persistent acidity, in face of the ammoniacal odour and the foul muco-pus so characteristic of alkaline cystitis, is often one of the most suggestive features of the disease.

Chemical analysis of the urine usually reveals albumin in considerable quantity derived from the red blood-cells, or perhaps in part from the kidney.

The microscope shows red blood-cells and bladder epithelium. A diligent search for casts must be made, for, if found, they suggest the existence of a renal lesion, presumably tubercular.

The Tubercle Bacillus.—The most important part of the urinary examination is the search for the tubercle bacillus. The final diagnosis often depends upon the discovery of this bacterium, and the present knowledge of our more expert urinalists is, happily, such as to afford an almost perfect analysis of its presence or absence. Unfortunately, however, the practitioner who has not a skilled bacteriologist at his call, or whose patient cannot afford the expense entailed, must make his diagnosis either from the clinical aspects of the case alone (see below) or from such an examination as can be conducted without any great technical skill and without any laboratory. To such I can only urge the necessity of depending upon the clinical aspects of the case, the presence or absence of a tubercular tendency, of other tubercular lesions, or of a characteristic symptom-complex, rather than upon the unfamiliar use of delicate scientific manipulations. Every man to his own calling. The trained clinician is quite as likely to diagnose a vesical tuberculosis correctly by clinical methods as the scientist is by scientific methods. As Thomas A. Edison, the greatest living clinician in another science, has said, "I could guess closer than those men could calculate."

But for those who have laboratory facilities and a sufficient scientific training there are adequate methods. The special difficulties to be overcome in searching for tubercle bacilli in the urine are: (*a*) The small number of bacilli present in the urine, (*b*) the danger of mistaking the smegma bacillus for the tubercular bacillus.

In order to make a thorough examination of the urine for tubercular bacilli the specimens employed should be passed into a sterilized vessel and submitted to the centrifuge. Thus external contagion is prevented and the bacteria are concentrated. When the urine is quite clear sedimentation of the bacilli is favoured by the addition of a small quantity of clear egg albumin which entraps them and carries them to the bottom of the centrifuge tube. The sediment is then examined by means of fixing and staining and cultivation, or by injection into guinea-pigs. Of the three methods the first two—viz., staining and cultivation—are rapid and accurate if properly performed by an expert. But they present many difficulties and liabilities to error, and cannot be carried through satisfactorily, except by a bacteriologist especially trained in the methods of distinguishing between the tubercle and the smegma bacillus. Koenig, Bunge, and many others have been led astray by the alleged discovery of the tubercle bacillus in urine. Hence, the guinea-pig test, though slow, is the appropriate one for all but the most skilled. The injection of sedimented urine and the post-mortem examination of the animal several weeks later require no special description here.

The ordinary staining methods by which the tubercle bacillus is readily distinguished in sputum do not avail to distinguish it from the smegma bacillus in the urine. A full exposition of the difficulties surrounding this work with an explanation of the means devised to overcome these difficulties is detailed by Sondern.[1] I have not attempted to employ these special methods myself, but I can vouch for the accurate results obtained by Dr. Sondern.

Other Symptoms.—Among the other symptoms due to tubercular cystitis a partial incontinence of urine from spasm or from ulceration of the neck of the bladder is notable. Mixed infection adds pyuria to the hematuria, and phosphatic stone may be formed and multiply the patient's agonies. The symptoms of involvement of the other genito-urinary organs are, sooner or later, important, and the rapid pulse, hectic fever, and general deterioration characteristic of this disease may be distinguished in advanced cases.

Diagnosis

Familiarity with the symptom-complex just laid down, together with the discovery of tubercular lesions elsewhere in the body, may be depended upon to establish the diagnosis in many cases. A family history of tuberculosis may also be elicited.

Differential Diagnosis.—The evident features about the disease, early or late, are bleeding and irritability. It may be confused with simple cystitis, stone, tumour, contracture of the neck of the bladder, and renal tuberculosis. From *simple cystitis* it is distinguished by the preponderance of hemorrhage and irritability, by the special antipathy of the tubercular bladder to nitrate of silver, by

---

[1] Jacobi Festschrift, 1900, p. 484.

the evidence of tuberculosis elsewhere in the body, and by the discovery of the tubercle bacillus in the urine. *Stone in the bladder* often gives rise to symptoms closely resembling tuberculosis; the searcher establishes the diagnosis. *Tumour* is not often confused with tuberculosis, but excessive irritability from the former, or excessive hemorrhage from the latter may make them seem very much akin. *Contracture of the neck of the bladder* may (pp. 317, 400), as we have seen, be either simple or tubercular. The symptoms of the two resemble each other so closely that one of our best-known genito-urinary surgeons habitually confounds them. Evidence of tuberculosis elsewhere in the body, or the discovery of the tubercle bacillus in the urine is absolutely essential to convict any one with a contracted vesical neck of being tubercular. *Renal tuberculosis* often gives symptoms purely referable to the bladder (p. 602). The cystoscope may be required for a diagnosis.

Method of Examination.—In the examination of a patient with tubercular cystitis the nature of the disease may be first suspected from the symptoms, the history, or the evidence of tuberculosis in the testicles, prostate, or lungs, or from the general tubercular aspect of the patient. If this is the case every effort should be made to establish the diagnosis without introducing any instrument into the bladder. This can often be done, and the patient's gratitude well earned. But if the surgeon inclines to operative treatment (which I do not), if there is question of stone or of renal lesion, or if the idea of tuberculosis does not cross the surgeon's mind, instruments may be employed. The use of any instrument in the tubercular bladder is likely to be followed by considerable prolonged spasm, which can be minimized only by gentleness. The searcher must be used (p. 436) if stone is suspected. The cystoscope I have employed but rarely. General anesthesia is usually required to overcome the vesical spasm and bleeding, and the diagnosis of renal tuberculosis can usually be made without cystoscopy. In only one condition is the cystoscope absolutely essential—viz., when removal of a tubercular kidney is contemplated. Cystoscopy is then essential to determine the condition of the bladder and permit catheterization of the opposite ureter (p. 472). It is notable that if the bladder lesion is confined to the neighbourhood of the ureteral mouth it will usually heal after nephrectomy, and is no contra-indication to the operation.

Urinary examination and detection of the tubercle bacillus are always part of the routine examination. I have employed the tuberculin test, but I consider the febrile reaction which it causes an unwarranted strain upon the system.

Prognosis

The course of the disease is irregular and slow. The symptoms grow worse year by year; but the disease may last a long time—I know of one man who is no worse now than he was twenty years ago, though he has had a violent tuberculosis of the bladder all that time—since it is not in itself fatal, though it may well render life unendurable. When death occurs this is due to renal or pulmonary involvement, and upon the implication of these vital organs depends the prognosis. Recovery is possible, though rare.

Treatment

Conservative treatment of tuberculosis of the bladder has given far better results than any of the radical procedures that have been employed. It must be the surgeon's aim to let the bladder entirely alone, if possible, and to confine his treatment to the climatic, hygienic, dietetic, and tonic treatment appropriate to tuberculosis of any organ. Whatever local or operative treatment has to be undertaken, hygiene is always the backbone of a cure. Among tonics, cod-liver oil, creosote, and guaiacol hold their accustomed places. Guyon favours an iodoform pill. Vaughan[1] and Chetwood have achieved cures by the use of nuclein in 5% solution hypodermically (3 grammes daily), by the stomach (4 grammes daily), and in the advanced stages as an intravesical injection (50% solution). I have had good results from ichthyol and ichthalbin administered internally. Balsamics and alkalies may be employed to modify the urine and to soothe the bladder. Urinary antiseptics are useless and likely to prove irritating.

Local Treatment.—In the early stages of the disease local treatment is absolutely contra-indicated. It only irritates the bladder and provokes ulceration of the tubercles.

When the disease is well advanced some treatment is usually necessary to control the vesical spasm. Local treatment is employed for this purpose, often with great success, but only according to certain well-defined rules. In the first place, gentleness is more essential here than in any other form of urinary disease. In the second place, irrigations must not be used. They are very badly borne by the sensitive bladder and do no more good than instillations. In the third place, nitrate of silver, boric acid, and permanganate of potash, so soothing to simple cystitis, cannot be employed in tubercular cystitis on account of the violent reaction they provoke even in

[1] Med. News, 1894, lxv, 657, 675.

very weak solution—this is especially true of the silver salts. Finally, the best rule for local treatment is to use the drug that gives the most comfort, regardless of any curative powers it may possess.

The favourite topical applications of various authors may be briefly enumerated. Guyon employs corrosive sublimate, beginning at a strength of 1:20,000 and running up very slowly to 1:10,000 or 1:5,000, or to whatever strength is well borne. Collin employs the following:

℞ Pulv. iodoform........................	1 gramme
Guaiacol...............................	5 grammes
Ol. oliv. steril.........................	100 "

Chetwood has used 25% to 100% solutions of guaiacol valerianate in olive oil, and 3% to 12% watery solutions of thallin sulphate. Both Senn and Horwitz suggest trichlorid of iodin in 0.2% to 0.5% solution, and the former also employs the familiar 10% iodoform-glycerin emulsion. Cumston has employed lactic acid (5%).

Of all these remedies, the ones I have found most soothing are sublimate, guaiacol valerianate, and thallin. Of these, the former two are the more healing, but one is forced to use thallin when nothing else gives relief. The instillations should be repeated 2 or 3 times a week. Improvement is always slow, but when a local application is benefiting the patient he is quick to recognise the relief and hails it with delight.

Operative Treatment.—Hygiene and local treatment may fail—they often do. The indications for operation are: 1. To relieve symptoms by establishing continuous drainage and so allowing the bladder to rest. 2. To cure the disease by topical applications. 3. To remove the diseased tissue by cautery, curette, or knife. The last indication can seldom be acted upon. It is very rarely possible to remove all the diseased tissue, since the primary focus is usually in some adjacent organ and the oldest bladder lesions are about the trigone, where they can least well be excised. Moreover, an operative failure entails dire results. The patient may be relieved of his dysuria, but he is condemned to a permanent tubercular fistula. If the operation has been performed as a last resort, with this permanent fistulization in view, the patient may well be content to put up with it; but if he finds himself, without any warning, condemned for life to a foul fistula, a leg urinal, and a filthy bed, his gratitude to the surgeon will be slight indeed. Hence early operation is not indicated; there is too much to lose and too little chance of gain. It is generally conceded that operation is required only when local treatment has failed completely and the patient is unable to endure his agony. Then the prospects may be clearly set before him: the slight chance of permanent cure, the possibility, the advantages and the disadvantages of permanent fistula. If the patient is willing to risk everything on the chance of improving his condition, the surgeon may then proceed with a clear conscience to do what he can.

The selection of operation must be left to the surgeon's judgment. If the patient is far gone with renal or pulmonary disease a simple suprapubic cystotomy (p. 459), with permanent drainage, will give the best results. It will suppress his pains at the cost of a continuous drainage—an exchange he is glad to make.

Apart from those ulcerations about the ureter that may be expected to disappear after nephrectomy (p. 608), there are two forms of tuberculosis that may demand operation while the patient is still in excellent health and before any signs of tuberculosis have been detected elsewhere in the body. The localized vesical tuberculosis may be disseminated more or less generally over the mucous membrane, or it may consist of an isolated process, commonly at or near the neck of the bladder. Under these circumstances, if the dysuria is quite uncontrollable, suprapubic or perineal cystotomy may be performed. Most surgeons prefer the suprapubic route, some the perineal. Once in the bladder the surgeon may be sorely tempted to excise or to scrape away the focus of disease. Extirpation of the whole mucous membrane has even been resorted to (Delagénière [1]), while such lesser operations as excision of an ulcer or cutting down the neck of the bladder are frequently performed. The results have been unalluring. In a few cases the excision of tubercular ulcerations has effected a cure, but in many the vesical tuberculosis has relapsed and the spread of the disease in other organs has been unchecked. Any interference with a tubercular vesical neck is likely to result most disastrously in permanent incontinence, and perhaps in permanent tubercular perineal fistula. Dr. Chetwood has obtained rather more encouraging results with his perineal galvano-cauterization, but the method is as yet experimental in this respect. On the whole, an attempt to extirpate an isolated tubercular focus in the mucous membrane of the bladder may be successful, but the chances are strongly against it.

On the other hand, excellent results have been obtained by medication of the bladder through the suprapubic wound. The bladder may be irrigated daily with the iodoform, guaiacol, or sublimate solutions described above. The result may be disappointing, yet such treatment often alleviates the symptoms and may effect a cure.

---

[1] Guyon's Annales, 1896, xiv, 59.

SIMPLE ULCER OF THE BLADDER

There are five kinds of vesical ulcers:

1. **Tubercular Ulcers.**

2. **Malignant Ulcers.**

3. **Inflammatory Ulcerations.**—These have no clinical significance. They consist of exfoliations and superficial exulcerations of the mucous membrane occurring in the course of an acute or a chronic cystitis.

4. **Traumatic Ulcers.**—These result from stone or are post-partum complications. The bladder wall having been crushed during parturition by forceps or by the child's head, a part of it may slough away.

5. **Simple Ulcers.**—These ulcers, known also as idiopathic, embolic, and perforating ulcers, are met with from time to time. Bartleet,[1] Wyeth,[2] and Johnston [3] have reported cases, and Güterbock [4] mentions the subject; but Hurry Fenwick [5] has considered the subject most intimately. While confessing the extreme infrequency of the condition, and admitting that it can only be distinguished from tubercular ulceration by the absence of tubercle bacilli from the urine (a perilous criterion), the absence of any other evidence of tubercular disease, and the ultimate recovery of the patient (though a tubercular ulcer may heal spontaneously), he maintains, nevertheless, that the simple ulcer of the bladder is a distinct clinical entity. "There is usually only one ulcer. . . . Its size rarely exceeds that of a shilling, and its situation is nearly always to the inner side of the ureteric orifice. . . . It usually affects the tissues of the posterior wall and does not actually encroach upon the trigone." Fenwick compares this ulcer to the simple ulcer of the stomach, and mentions one case of perforation.

The *symptoms* are comparable to those of tuberculosis; but the pains are alleviated by all forms of irrigation, instead of being made worse. The *prognosis* is good. A *cure* may be effected by curetting.

---

[1] Lancet, 1876, i, 210.

[2] N. Y. Med. J., 1892, lv, 582.

[3] Brit. Med. J., 1893, i, 1003.

[4] Die Krankheiten der Harnblase, 1890, p. 375.

[5] Brit. Med. J., 1896, i, 1133; also Ulceration of the Bladder, London, 1900.

CHAPTER XXVII

TUMOURS OF THE BLADDER—VARICOSE VEINS—URACHUS CYST AND FISTULA—VESICO-INTESTINAL FISTULA

TUMOURS

Varieties

The great majority of tumours of the bladder are of epithelial origin. These tumours begin habitually as benign papillomatous growths, but soon undergo malignant (carcinomatous) degeneration. Next in frequency come the connective-tissue growths, fibroma, myxoma, and sarcoma, and the mixed tumours, fibromyxoma and myxosarcoma. Isolated examples of other neoplasms have been recorded, such as leiomyoma,[1] rhabdomyoma,[2] angioma,[3] nævus,[4] chondroma,[3] epithelioma, and adenoma. Epithelial, dermoid, and hydatid cysts have also been observed.

Etiology

No more is known about the pathogenesis of tumours of the bladder than about that of any other tumours. It has been surmised that a papillary tumour might originate from the hypertrophied formations met with in chronic cystitis, and the rare epithelioma is said to arise from the cornified epithelium (leukoplasia) produced by the same disease. In confirmation of this theory are the reports of Lichtenstein [5] and Wendel [6] concerning epithelial tumours resulting from cystitis due to anilin dyes. On the other hand, tumours of the bladder are clinically the cause, not the result, of inflammation.

---

[1] Terrier and Hartmann, Revue de chir., 1895, xv, 181. Ramsay, Phila. Med. J., 1900, vi, 43, 86.

[2] Livio, Rivista clinica, 1887, xxvi, 42. Pavone, Guyon's Annales, 1899, xvii, 68.

[3] Albarran, Tumeurs de la vessie, Paris, 1891. Langhans, Virchow's Archiv, 1879, lxxv, 291.

[4] Arbuthnot Lane, Brit. Med. J., 1895, i, 1093.

[5] Deutsche med. Wochenschr., 1898, xxiv, 709.

[6] J. Amer. Med. Ass'n, 1900, xxxiv, 1256.

PLATE VII

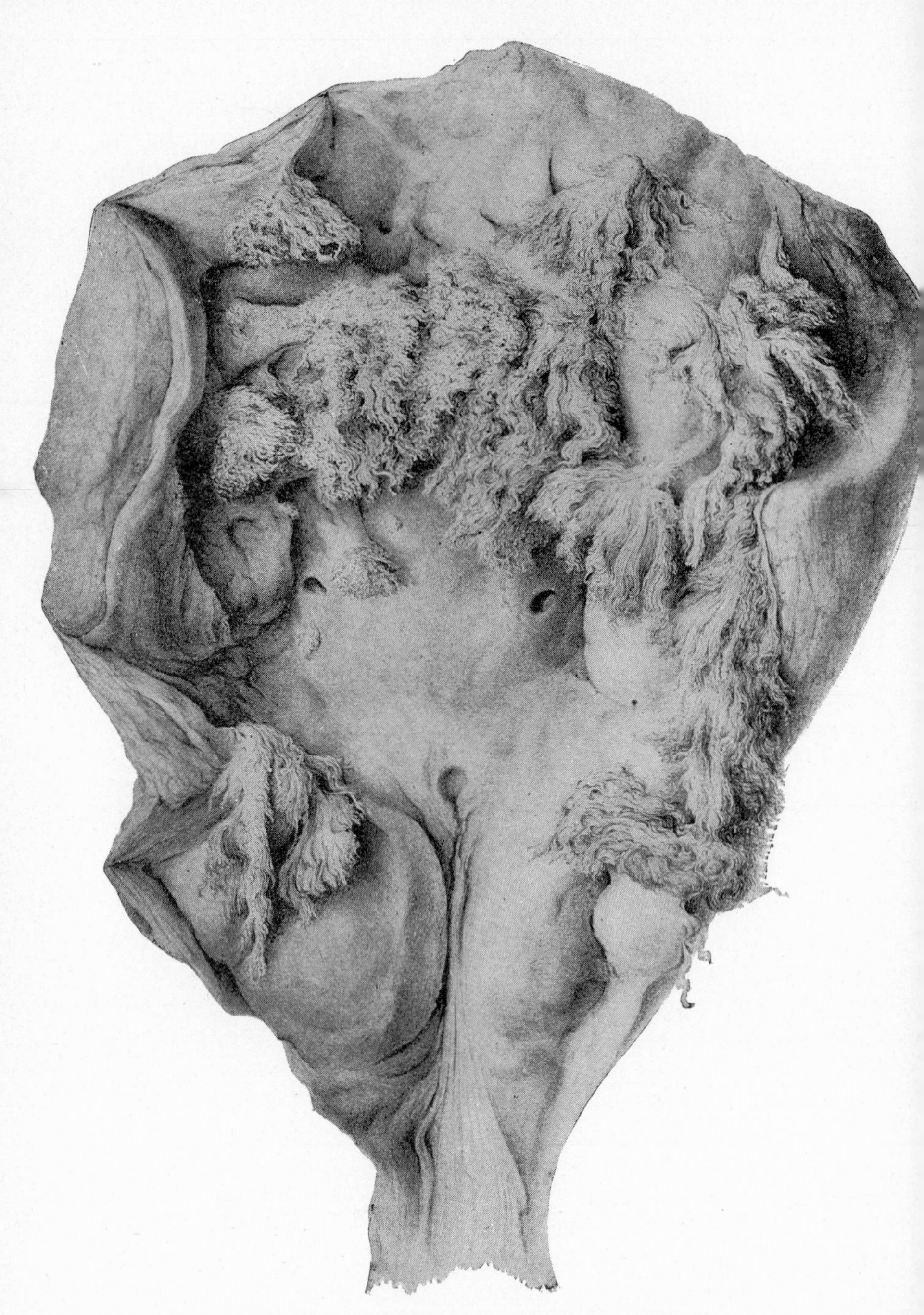

MULTIPLE VILLOUS PAPILLOMA OF THE BLADDER.
HISTOLOGICALLY: TRUE BENIGN PAPILLOMA (Albarran).

Age and Sex.—Men suffer from tumours of the bladder at least twice, perhaps thrice, as often as women. Of 99 cases of bladder cancer collected by Nason,[1] 78 occurred in men. Tumours have been met with at all ages, but the great preponderance of carcinoma makes the decades between thirty and sixty the most prolific of neoplasms.

Multiplicity.—From 25% (Albarran) to 40% (Fenwick[2]) of tumours of the bladder are multiple. This multiplicity is due chiefly to the contact inoculation of the epithelial tumours. The growth seems to give rise to secondary deposits in that part of the vesical mucous membrane that comes in contact with it when the bladder is empty.

Situation.—The commonest point of origin for tumours of the bladder is the immediate neighbourhood of the ureteral orifices. They are fairly frequent about the neck of the bladder, but show no special affinity for the remainder of the trigone. A point of great importance in the cystoscopic diagnosis of neoplasms is the fact that the primary tumour is almost always found in the lower half of the bladder. The upper half is involved frequently enough, but only by extension or contact inoculation from the original growth. So rare are primary tumours confined to the upper half that the possibility of their occurrence in that region is commonly overlooked.

Morbid Anatomy

Epithelial Tumours.—We may overlook the rare epithelioma and adenoma—the latter usually a prostatic growth—to concentrate our attention upon the commonest of all bladder tumours, the papilloma and the carcinoma.

Papilloma (*Villous Tumour, Papillary Fibroma, Fimbriated Papilloma*).—This neoplasm has been gracefully described by Thompson[3] as follows:

" The most obvious characteristic of the growth is a structure in which the vesical mucous membrane is developed into fine papillæ, which consist of long fimbriated processes of extreme tenuity, and usually form a group arising from a small circumscribed base (Plate VII). This last-named part contains other and more solid structure than that which enters into the papillæ themselves. Sometimes the processes are almost single, thread-like forms arranged side by side, and undivided for a considerable distance; others are bifid, generally more compound still; some may be described as digitate, and occasionally the processes radiate and suggest forms resembling those of leaves. Immersed in fluid, the long fimbriated growths float out

---

[1] Brit. Med. J., 1901, i, 1199. [2] Lancet, 1888, i, 473.
[3] Tumours of the Bladder, London, 1884, p. 57.

like slender-leaved aquatic plants in deep water, and when removed to air collapse and form a soft mass resembling a small strawberry." The villi are composed of capillary loops covered by several layers

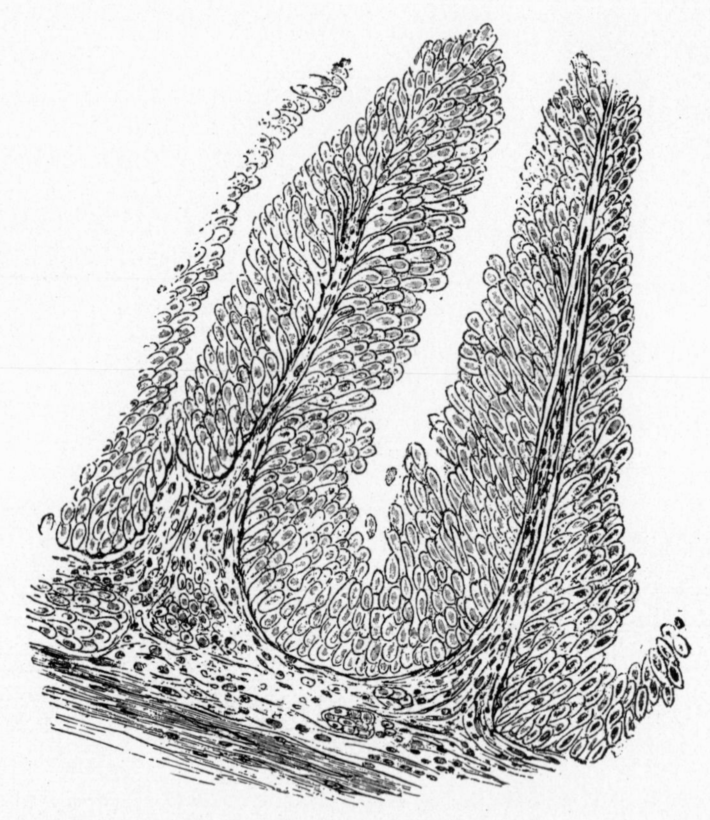

Fig. 94.—Fimbriated Papilloma, showing Two of the Slender Papillomatous Processes or so-called "Villi" (from Thompson).

of columnar epithelium (Fig. 94). The "more solid structure" of the pedicle contains the muscular, fibrous, and vascular elements of the bladder wall. Exceptionally, independent villi spring from the wall of the bladder itself, or the pedicle is short and broad, giving the growth a sessile appearance.

Carcinoma.—Lobular, alveolar, reticular carcinoma, myo-carcinoma, adeno-carcinoma, and cylindroma have been described (*cf.* Albarran). Without entering into the minute pathology of these varieties we may be satisfied to divide carcinomata into 3 clinical types: 1. Primary carcinoma. 2. Degenerated papilloma. 3. Secondary carcinoma. Of the last variety nothing need be said. Of the other two the former occurs as an infiltration of the vesical wall. It is a sessile

PLATE VIII

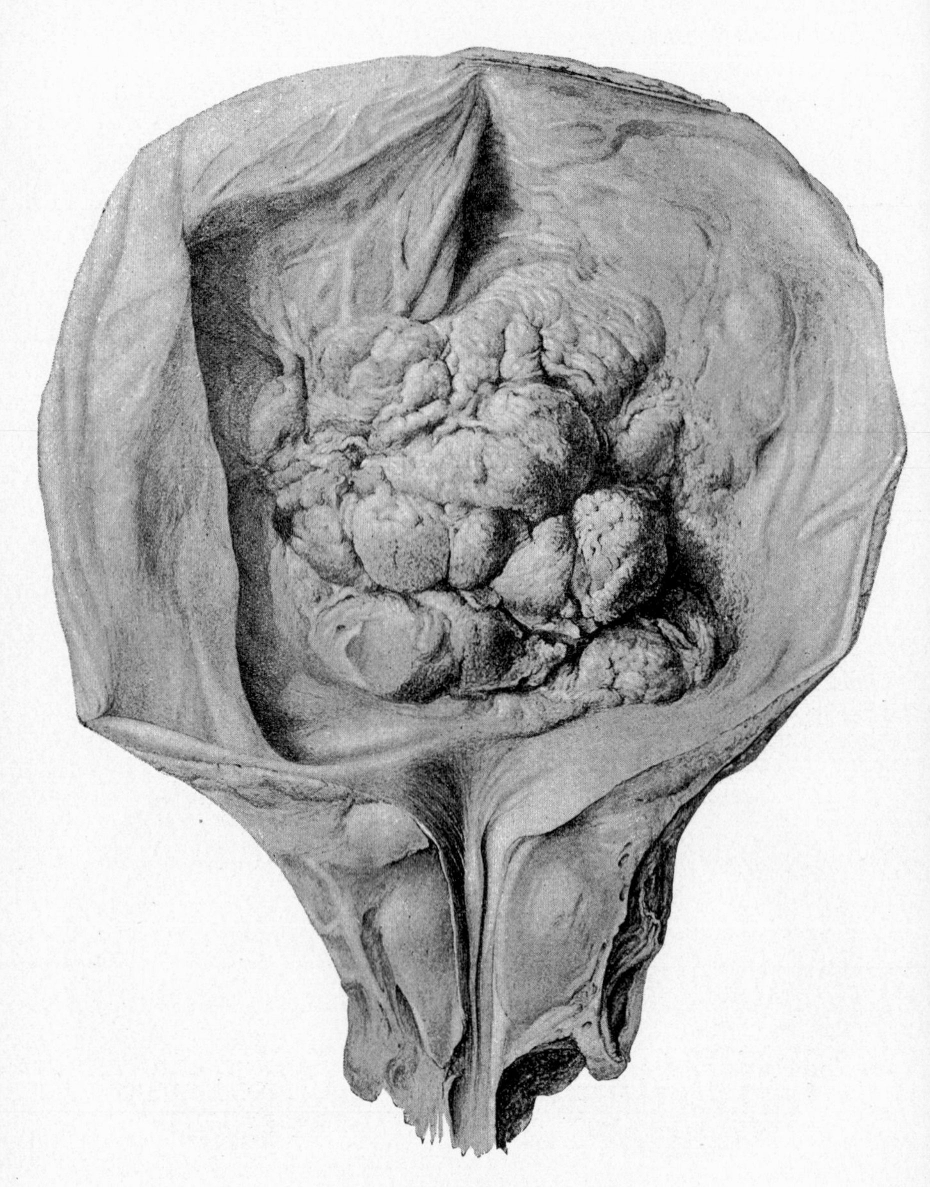

CARCINOMA OF THE BLADDER.

HISTOLOGICALLY: EPITHELIAL CANCER (Albarran).

tumour projecting more or less into the bladder (Plate VIII). Its surface is fungating (Fig. 95), often necrotic, ulcerated, and covered with adherent lime salts. Its base extends deep into the muscle of the organ. On the other hand, the degenerated papilloma (papillary carcinoma) has no very fixed character. It may appear to be a pure papilloma until the microscope reveals areas of carcinomatous degeneration in the pedicle (Figs. 96, 97). In a more advanced stage the tumour retains the superficial aspects of a papilloma, but the base, broad, hard, and infiltrating, is clearly cancerous.

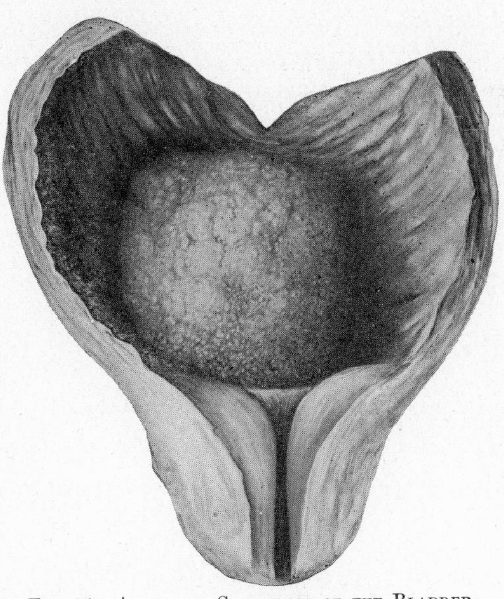

Fig. 95.—Alveolar Carcinoma of the Bladder.

The older authors, and some recent ones too, recognise a class of *relapsing papilloma*, with no special limitations, but possessing the common characteristic of recurring soon after an apparently complete removal.

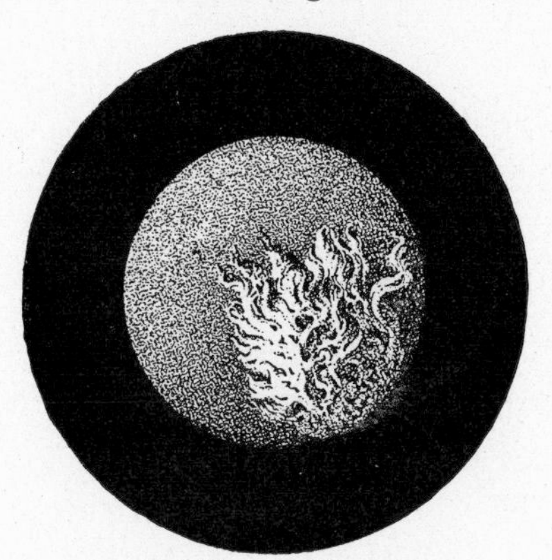

Fig. 96.—Villous Epithelioma (from Albarran).

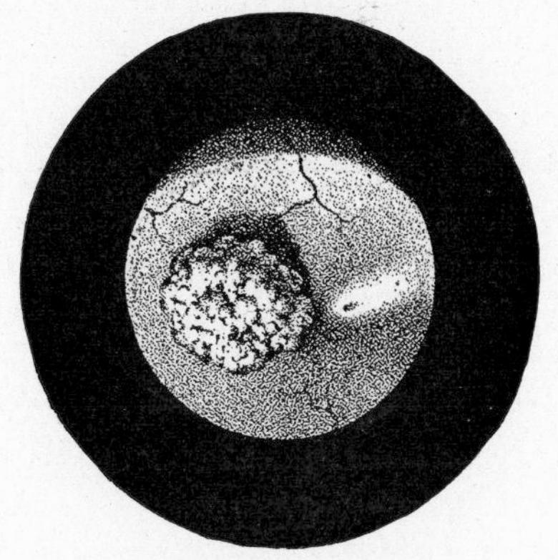

Fig. 97.—Lobulated Epithelioma (from Albarran).

Such a fact admits of only one explanation: the tumour was not completely removed in the first place. This failure may be due (*a*) to overlooking some papillomatous filament distinct from the main tumour or (*b*) to mistaking a carcinoma for a papilloma. The latter is the graver, and, unfortunately, the commoner error. Two conditions favour it. The carcinomatous degeneration may have only just begun, the tumour being still a pure papilloma to all appearances, and this malignant change, commencing in the pedicle, spreads as rapidly towards the base of the tumour as towards its periphery. In frank carcinomata the malignant epithelial infiltration is commonly found to extend 1 to 2 cm. into the muscular wall of the bladder beyond the area of manifest induration; and so in these cases the malignant change has often reached the muscle wall by the time the tumour is removed, and therefore this most dangerous portion of the neoplasm is overlooked and left behind unless a wide section of apparently normal muscle is excised. The prevention of this oversight—the elimination of that form of relapsing papilloma which ultimately declares its malignant character—is one of the ideals of genito-urinary surgery.

Albarran deserves the credit of explaining these transition tumours and relapsing papilloma. He showed that practically all these tumours of doubtful nature are carcinomatous, wholly or in part. Thus, among 132 vesical tumours examined, he found 100 carcinomata against 24 papillomata, a conclusion quite the reverse of what had previously been held. Guyon's aphorism expresses the same idea: "We still await in our practice the papillomata encountered in statistics."

Propagation.—Papilloma is apparently propagated only by the contact inoculation alluded to above. Carcinoma is propagated in 3 ways: (*a*) By contact inoculation, (*b*) by infiltration of the surrounding tissues, and (*c*) by lymphatic invasion.

A broad distinction may be laid down between the rapidity of dissemination in vesical and in prostatic growths. The former, whether carcinoma or sarcoma, progress slowly, remain for years confined to the bladder, and but rarely give rise to metastatic growths of any clinical importance. Pasteau[1] has shown that the glands along the iliac vessels are enlarged in 43% of all sessile tumours of the bladder and in 85% of infiltrated tumours; but the infection gets little further than this: the patient dies of secondary functional and inflammatory disturbances of the urinary organs. Prostatic growths, on the contrary, are disseminated throughout the pelvis with frightful rapidity, giving rise to the *carcinose prostato-pelvienne* of Guyon (p. 321). The reason for this relatively slow dissemination of vesi-

---

[1] État du système lymphatique dans les maladies de la vessie et de la prostate, Paris, 1898, pp. 46, 52.

cal tumours is not clear. It was originally attributed to the absence of lymphatics from the bladder, later to their fewness, and recently to the presence of the perivesical fibro-lipomatous inflammation which commonly occurs as a barrier to the extension of a neoplasm, as is the case in interstitial cystitis (p. 385). Though these theories are not by any means fully explanatory, the fact that bladder neoplasms grow slowly remains true.

Secondary Lesions.—Any tumour of the bladder may undergo fatty, granular, colloidal (malignant), or calcareous degeneration. It may also become inflamed, ulcerated, or encrusted with salts of lime. Perforation of the bowel and of the peritoneum are exceptional.

The secondary changes in the urinary organs are of greater importance. The tumour acts in very much the same way as a hypertrophied prostate. It offers a point of least resistance for the origin of cystitis, and, sooner or later, it obstructs the orifice of the urethra and interferes with the contractions of the bladder, thus setting up the long train of secondary phenomena of retention with infection—cystitis, atony, pyelo-nephritis (p. 265)—terminating only with the patient's death.

Other Tumours.—The other tumours of the bladder are not sufficiently frequent to require more than a summary consideration.

Sarcoma.—Round-celled, spindle-celled, mixed-celled, lympho-sarcoma, fibro-sarcoma, myosarcoma, myxosarcoma, alveolar, giant-celled, telangiectasic, and chondrosarcoma are described. The tumour usually encroaches but little on the cavity of the bladder. It appears either as a hard sessile growth or an intramural infiltration. Its surface may be smooth, papillary, or ulcerated.

Myxoma (*Polyp*).—Pure myxoma is exceedingly rare. The growth is usually a fibromyxoma or a myxosarcoma. The surface of the tumour is lobular and smooth, resembling polypus of other regions.

Fibroma.—Pure fibroma is very rare. The tumour being benign, usually small, and of firm texture, passes unnoticed during life, unless, as in Qahoubian's [1] case, it grows large enough to interfere with micturition.

Myoma.[2]—This tumour is benign, may be intravesical, interstitial, or subserous, and, like the fibroma, passes unnoticed unless it interferes with the mechanism of urination.

Cysts.—Several varieties of cysts occur in cystitis. They have no clinical significance. Urachus cysts receive special consideration at the end of this chapter. Albarran describes a cystadenoma.

---

[1] Guyon's Annales, 1897, xv, 839. [2] *Cf.* Ramsay, Phila. Med. J., 1900, vi, 43, 86.

Dermoid cysts occasionally occur in the wall of the bladder. They are diagnosed only when, after rupture, hair from them is passed in the urine. This symptom, pilimiction, is pathognomonic.

Echinococcus cysts [1] grow in the pelvis and burst into the bladder. They very rarely develop primarily in the bladder wall.

Symptoms

Hemorrhage.—The first, the last, and often the only symptom of a tumour of the bladder is hemorrhage. In general, the more villous the tumour the more profuse the bleeding. Hence with such tumours as myoma and fibroma, the surface of which is often covered with a normal mucous membrane, there may be no hemorrhage whatever.

The characteristic hemorrhage of a neoplasm, whether renal or vesical, begins without cause or warning, continues copious and painless, unaffected by rest, diet, or medication, and ceases, as it begins, without apparent rhyme or reason. Its cessation may leave the urine entirely normal and the patient lulled into a false sense of security by what he considers his happy escape from a perilous condition. A profuse hemorrhage of this character is almost pathognomonic of neoplasm. Yet bleeding from a tumour may not be characteristic. It may be mild and continuous, associated with cystitis evoked by instrumentation, or amenable to treatment. It may not be the initial symptom. In short, it may assume any form. But to be characteristic it must be spontaneous, profuse, unalterable, and unaccompanied by any other symptom.

Usually the hemorrhage grows more severe and recurs more frequently as the disease progresses. But this is by no means always the case. There may be intervals of years between the hemorrhages; indeed Albarran cites a few cases in which the hemorrhage stopped entirely after spontaneous detachment of the growth.

Hemorrhage from neoplasm of the bladder may be excited by the introduction of any instrument (especially a metal one) into that organ, and when thus produced it assumes its characteristics of profusion, painlessness (except for the passage of clots), resistance to treatment, and spontaneous cessation.

Pain and Dysuria.—These symptoms usually appear some days, weeks, or months after the first hemorrhage. Exceptionally, pain and dysuria precede the bleeding. This is alleged to occur most frequently in sarcoma. Pain may be evoked by the passage of clots; it may be due to cystitis, to obstruction of the urethra, or to the interfer-

[1] Deutsche Chir. v. Billroth u. Lücke, 1890, lii, 305.

ence of the bladder muscle by the tumour itself. Sharp, lancinating pains also arise spontaneously from malignant growths.

Retention.—The passage of urine may be suddenly arrested by a large clot or by the tumour. In the former case, a few moments of spasm and straining will usually expel the clot; but if the tumour itself obstructs the internal orifice of the urethra, the condition resembles prostatic hypertrophy. All the familiar forms of acute and chronic retention, with or without infection, are encountered. The sudden shutting off of the stream, which is a characteristic symptom of stone, may be due to tumour. Thus Nitze had a patient whose stream would be suddenly obstructed unless he urinated while lying on his back. Tumours in the region of the ureteral orifice sometimes obstruct that duct partially or completely. On the whole, however, retention is an unimportant feature of the disease.

Cystitis.—The course of the disease is commonly divided into two stages (1) before infection, (2) after infection. Yet there may be cystitis before the first symptom of tumour appears. At one time or another inflammation of the bladder is sure to occur. The tumour itself is a point of least resistance. The blood from it is an excellent culture medium. Instruments introduced into the bladder often bring germs with them, and thus in one way or another, at one time or another, cystitis occurs. When once the tumour has become inflamed there is little hope of overcoming the inflammation except by removing the tumour; and if this is not done early in the disease the inflammation persists, spreads to the kidney, and is largely instrumental in the patient's final taking off.

The symptoms of cystitis due to tumour of the bladder are often most distressing. The dysuria is usually severe, and small quantities of foul urine full of pus and blood are passed with infinite pain and straining.

Course of the Disease.—Among 140 cases collected by Albarran the *first symptom* was hematuria in 109 (78%), dysuria in 10 (7%), cystitis in 5, pollakiuria in 5, and in the remainder, various combinations of hemorrhage (in 10), dysuria (in 7), cystitis (in 2), retention (in 2), the passage of shreds and once the extrusion of the tumour from the urethra (in the female).

During the first period of the disease, before infection occurs, the symptoms are extremely mild. The dysuria is rarely severe, and, were it not for the hemorrhages that occur from time to time, the patient would give little thought to his urinary organs. These hemorrhages are rarely so profuse as to cause any grave anemia. This condition continues for months or years. The patient's general health is excellent, and if he is shy he may bear his bleeding in silence and come to the surgeon only after cystitis has set in.

When cystitis occurs the symptoms promptly become more aggravated, and the patient, exhausted by the loss of blood and distressed by the constant spasm of his bladder, grows rapidly weaker. Albarran alleges that a sudden turn from the simple bleeding of papilloma to the lancinating pains and rapid cachexia of carcinoma can sometimes be made out. I confess that the progress of carcinoma has seemed to me almost as slow and mild as that of papilloma. I have several times watched patients pass years of comfort with a typical carcinoma of the base of the bladder. I should put the average duration of life with any malignant tumour of the bladder at from three to five years. A papilloma may last many years before it degenerates—as nearly all of them do in the long run—into carcinoma.

The Urine.—The appearance of the urine depends upon whether cystitis or hemorrhage is present at the time of examination. Between whiles it may be entirely normal, or there may be microscopical and chemical evidence of hemorrhage—viz., the presence of red blood cells and albumin. When cystitis exists there is commonly some hemorrhage as well, so that the urine contains both pus and blood.

The urine may also be searched for shreds of tumour tissue. These are especially common with papillomatous growths. They sometimes are as large as a pea, resemble blood clots in appearance, and are easily overlooked. If found, they confirm the diagnosis of tumour, but do not denote the character of the growth, since simple papillæ may sprout from almost any tumour of the bladder. Watson [1] lays much stress on the discovery of "a more or less abundant sediment, in which are found large numbers of epithelial cells of great variety of shapes with large nuclei."

Casts and albumin from the kidney may appear in the urine, whether the tumour is in the bladder or the kidney.

Diagnosis

The suggestion of tumour of the bladder usually comes from a typical hemorrhage (see above). Such a hemorrhage may, however, be caused by a neoplasm of the kidney, or it may be a spontaneous renal hemorrhage of obscure origin. There are several fine points of distinction between a renal and a vesical hemorrhage, as given in the table on the opposite page, but the best criterion is the cystoscope.

---

[1] Morrow's System of Gen.-Urin. Dis., 1893, i, 577.

Differential Table of Hematuria

Tubercle.	Stone.	Bladder tumour.	Kidney.
1. Slight and remittent at first.	Same.	Profuse and intermittent.	....
2.	....	Clots large.	Clots small, if any.
3. Blood bright or maroon.	Same.	Same.	Blood usually dark.
4. Little affected by exercise.	Brought on by exercise.	Little affected.	....
5. May be produced by instrumentation.	Same.	Same.	Unaffected.
6. Associated with characteristic pain.	Same.	No pain at first.	....

Cystoscopy.—Of all the instrumental manipulations employed in the diagnosis of tumours of the bladder, cystoscopy stands first, for it alone indicates the presence, the nature—as far as that can be determined—the location, and the number of tumours. The last point is especially important. Many small villous tumours, which may be distinctly seen floating in the urine (Fig. 96), are almost undiscoverable when the bladder is opened and a digital or a visual examination made of its empty cavity. Unless, therefore, the exact location of every villous papilla is definitely determined by cystoscopy previous to operation, some one of them may be overlooked. The relapse which inevitably results from such an oversight exposes the patient to renewed danger of carcinomatous change as well as to the inconvenience of a second operation.

There are only two contra-indications to cystoscopy. Hemorrhage may be so free as to make it impossible to gain any accurate data, even with the irrigating cystoscope, or the bladder may be so irritable as to frustrate the operation. In the former case a few days' delay, in the latter a general anesthetic, make the cystoscopy practicable.

The technic of cystoscopy has already been described (p. 330). Some authors insist on the advantages of the irrigating cystoscope for this work; they hold, with reason, that the hemorrhage often quickly obscures the field of vision. Yet I have not found that the irrigating device is of any great assistance in clearing the contents of the bladder.

In examining the bladder for tumour two things must be borne in mind: First, the tumour (if there is one) will be found, in almost every case, near the orifice of one or the other ureter or of the urethra; second, the tumours are multiple in a fair proportion of cases, and a complete cystoscopy should include a minute inspection of every portion of the bladder. Such an inspection is often impossible on account of the hemorrhage.

The characteristics of the different tumours, as seen by cystoscope or during operation, have already been described (Figs. 96 and 97).

Recto-abdominal Palpation.—Bimanual examination, with the patient in the dorsal or the knee-chest position, often affords valuable information about the nature of the growth. A papilloma or a small hard tumour cannot be felt, but any considerable infiltration of the base of the bladder is readily distinguished. Such an infiltration is definite evidence of the malignant character of the growth, and makes its successful extirpation impossible with the surgical means at our command. In making this examination the prostate gland should be delineated by the finger in order that a growth in the bladder wall may be clearly distinguished from one in the prostate.

The Stone-searcher.—When cystoscopy is impossible Thompson's searcher may be depended upon to give some evidence of the presence and nature of the growth. A large, hard tumour may be distinctly felt by this instrument, a villous growth will be made to bleed freely by its contact, and any considerable area of infiltration is distinguished by its rough, unyielding character.

Cystotomy.—Exploratory cystotomy should be performed above the pubes, not in the perineum (as suggested by Sir Henry Thompson twenty years ago), and the operation, like an exploratory abdominal section, should be performed for the purpose of removing the growth, if any is formed, rather than for a mere diagnosis.

Differential Diagnosis.—It is often impossible to distinguish between a benign and a malignant papilloma of the bladder. In general, infiltration of the bladder wall, solidity of structure, and a duration of more than two or three years may be looked upon as suggestive of malignancy. On the other hand, villosity, pedunculation, and a short history favour benignity.

The distinction between neoplasm, on the one hand, and stone, pericystitis, and hypertrophy of the prostate, simple or malignant, on the other, is made by the cystoscope and recto-abdominal touch, as described above.

Treatment

Palliative Treatment.—If there is any possibility that the tumour is benign, palliative treatment is entirely inappropriate. The tumour should be dealt with surgically and at once. The patient must be encouraged to submit to immediate operation on the ground that delay may prove fatal. Yet before undertaking operation it may be necessary, even in these cases, to check hemorrhage or to alleviate cystitis.

The Treatment of Hemorrhage.—It is customary when the patient is bleeding freely from a tumour of the bladder to put him to bed and to restrict his diet. I am not sure that either measure is particularly efficacious; but I am sure that beyond this we tread on uncertain ground. The internal administration of the fluid extract of *senecio-aureus*, in 2 c. c. doses 3 times a day, has given Dr. Chetwood very fortunate results. *Oil of turpentine*, so efficacious in kidney hemorrhage, has no certain value here, nor do I put any faith in other astringents administered by the mouth. In one case I have employed saturated solutions of *gelatin* with the idea of increasing the coagulability of the blood with no great success. Local measures are equally unreliable. *Silver nitrate* is praised by Thompson, and it certainly has a temporary hemostatic effect. *Alum* (2%) is equally good. Solutions of the *suprarenal extract* are somewhat irritating and produce only the most ephemeral results. A hot solution of gelatin seemed to do good at my hands in one case. *Antipyrin* has been praised. But, as a matter of fact, one of the features of the bleeding is its defiance of all medication. A desperate hemorrhage requires *cystotomy*.

The evacuation of clots may cause trouble. They are best evacuated by a large woven or metal catheter; a Bigelow evacuator is even better if the growth is not at the neck of the bladder. Through this instrument very hot (115°) salt solution or alum (0.25%) is injected repeatedly. If a clot obstructs the eye of the instrument it is drawn out by aspiration with a piston syringe. The bladder is thus emptied by repeated irrigations and aspirations. I do not care to use hydrogen peroxid in the bladder. It is irritating, the passage of the bubbles causes considerable spasm, and it is but little more efficient in disintegrating clots than is the hot salt solution.

The Treatment of Cystitis.—As in hypertrophy of the prostate, so in neoplasm of the bladder, the best way to treat cystitis is to prevent it. The *prophylactic measures* are the same in either case—viz., urinary antisepsis, and, if necessary, systematic catheterization (p. 278). There is this difference, however, that if the neoplasm is at the neck of the bladder, the passage of the instrument may do more harm than the evacuation does good. In this event the bladder is best let alone. *The cure* of an existing cystitis is quite as arduous a task as the checking of a hemorrhage. Any local medication excites the bleeding, while general treatment is of as little use here as in any other form of cystitis. The only course to follow is to administer whatever general treatment seems to suit the patient best and to use as much local treatment as circumstances permit. As a matter of fact, the unendurable dysuria of cystitis forms one of the chief indications for *palliative cystostomy* (p. 395). I have been forced to this expedient a number of times, and have always found it most serviceable. Simultaneous scraping or cauterization of the growth may be of material aid in ameliorating the symptoms and checking the cause of the disease for a time.

Operative Treatment.—Palliative suprapubic cystostomy is the operation suited to all desperate and incurable cases. Even though no pretence is made of eradicating the disease the patient's life is prolonged by the very fact that he is relieved of his worst symptoms. I have at present under my care a striking example of the value of this operation. Before operation the patient weighed 120 pounds, and was tortured day and night by incessant straining. Within six months after operation he gained 25 pounds, although the tumour, which was only curetted, was a typical villous carcinoma.

The radical operations employed for tumour of the bladder may be reduced to 4 types:

1. Intravesical excision.
2. Excision after cystotomy.
3. Resection of the bladder.
4. Extirpation of the bladder.

1. **Intravesical Excision.**—This may be performed upon the female bladder through the dilated urethra. But upon the male it must be performed by means of an operating cystoscope, such as Nitze[1] employs. The operation is performed as follows: A cystoscope is introduced into the bladder and the location and other characteristics of the tumour are observed. Then a specially devised electro-cautery snare is thrown about the base of the tumour. The current is turned on, the peduncle burned through, and the stump recauterized. The hemorrhage is slight. In the course of time the tumour is voided through the urethra.

According to Nitze, the instruments required for this operation number 15 at the very least; snares, cauteries, cystoscopes, etc., and no little skill is required as well. Moreover, the operation is manifestly suited only to small tumours, and, while it is true that the tumours most likely to elude the surgeon's eye when the suprapubic operation is undertaken are the very ones that are most conveniently dealt with by this process, it is small wonder that even the 31 operations without a death reported by Nitze have brought him few imitators.

2. **Excision after Cystotomy.**—This and the other operations about to be described are all performed through an epicystotomy

---

[1] Centralbl. f. d. Krankh. d. Harn. u. Sex. Org., 1896, vii, 377, 469, 601.

wound (p. 459). The bladder is opened in the usual manner by a vertical incision, and the wound in the abdominal wall enlarged, if necessary, by a transverse cut at its lower extremity. A previous cystoscopy has shown the surgeon the exact position of the tumour, which he now searches for with his finger, and draws into the wound by a volsella forceps or a Guyon clamp. A clearer field of operation may be obtained by putting the patient into the Trendelenburg position before proceeding to excise the tumour. This may be done in one of several ways. If the tumour is distinctly pedunculated, it is convenient to burn it away close to the bladder wall with the Paquelin or the galvano-cautery, or Watson's cautery clamp may be employed. For that form of papilloma which grows as a bunch of tufts from a circumscribed area of the mucous membrane, the best operation is a thorough curetting, with subsequent cauterization of the bleeding points. The advantage of using the cautery to check bleeding is obvious. But this treatment is not entirely appropriate to the excision of sessile or frankly malignant infiltrating tumours. These require resection of the bladder wall.

After the tumours have been burned away, a final minute search is made over the bladder wall with the aid of a headlight or mirror (Fenwick employs a tubular speculum to keep the field dry, both in the search and in operating), and any other growths that are thus found are treated similarly. The suprapubic wound is then closed by Gibson's suture (p. 463) about a drainage-tube. There are no special features in the after-treatment.

3. **Resection of the Bladder.**—Resection of that part of the bladder wall surrounding a tumour is essential in the removal of every sessile or infiltrating growth of the bladder (except the myomata), whether it is frankly malignant or not. Papillomata that are apparently benign in character and have stout peduncles require excision or thorough cauterization of the surrounding mucous membrane. But if the tumour is truly sessile, or if there is any evidence whatever of infiltration of the bladder wall, a section of the whole thickness of this muscle must be excised, including an area of apparently normal tissue 1 cm. beyond the limit of induration.

If the tumour lies on the upper or the lateral wall of the bladder the operation is comparatively simple. Peritoneum is stripped away if possible, the requisite section removed, and the gap sutured with two layers of catgut, the one buried for the muscle, the other for the mucous membrane. If the tumour is conveniently situated, the suture may be re-enforced by a layer of subperitoneal Lembert stitches. A wick of gauze may be inserted between the peritoneum and the incision in the bladder wall to avert infiltration. Free drainage of the suprapubic wound is essential.

If the peritoneum is adherent to the bladder it may be more convenient, after irrigating the viscus thoroughly and packing it with iodoform gauze, to open the peritoneum boldly and excise the section of the bladder from without.

Unfortunately, the great majority of vesical tumours spring from the base of the bladder, from that portion of the organ, namely, which is least accessible, and where free removal of the growth is impeded by the presence of the ureters, the prostate, and the urethra. The rectal colpeurynter is useful in these cases both to force the field of operation up into the wound, and, by pressing upon the pelvic plexus of veins, to control the hemorrhage, which is always considerable. If the growth encroaches upon the mouth of a ureter that duct may be transplanted to the fundus of the bladder (p. 493), although this protracts the operation and increases its peril.

If it is expected that the edges of the wound can be approximated, the incision is best performed with the knife. The burst of bleeding from the cut bladder may be disregarded for the moment, since it is best controlled by the sutures themselves. But if it is foreseen that the section removed from the walls of the bladder will leave too wide a gap to be closed by suture, the incision is more conveniently made with a thermo-cautery heated only to a cherry red. The incision then bleeds relatively little, and such bleeding as does occur may be controlled by forceps, suture, or further cauterizations. The wound is then approximated as far as possible and the raw surfaces left to granulate.

At the close of the operation the bladder may be left empty or it may be packed with iodoform gauze. With our present knowledge of the innocuousness of the ureteral catheter it would seem proper to catheterize both ureters, and thus to divert the stream of urine from the bladder for the first forty-eight hours after operation. Unless this is done the bladder must be gently washed twice a day after operation with hot salt or boric-acid solution. The only special features of the after-treatment are the prevention of hemorrhage and rupture of the bladder. Both of these dangers must be foreseen at the time of operation and prevented by adequate suturing. A general oozing, which often occurs and may assume alarming proportions, is best prevented or controlled by irrigation with a hot 25% alum solution.

4. **Extirpation of the Bladder.**—Total extirpation of the bladder is a most formidable operation, the results of which have been ex-

tremely unsatisfactory. Tuffier and Dujardin [1] review the first 9 operations, including 1 of their own. Of these, only 4 survived. The operation was performed 3 times on the male with only 1 recovery, which case died seven months later. Of the 6 females operated upon, 3 survived, and 1 was known to have been alive three years later. The authors conclude: "We believe that total cystectomy is rarely indicated. It should never be attempted except on a patient strong enough to undergo a shock which is always considerable. Moreover, the tumour must have invaded the vesical tissues so extensively as to make partial extirpation impracticable. Finally, there must be no malignant secondary deposits, as they would render the eradication of the disease incomplete, and therefore illusory." Unfortunately such a combination of widespread local lesion and absence of secondary deposits is not met with clinically. The operation itself is one before which any surgeon may quail. The uretero-rectal implantation which it involves is almost certain to bring about the patient's death within a few months or years. It is quite incredible that there should be no secondary glandular involvements, and quite impossible that these deposits should all be removed. The severity of the operation is attested by its recorded mortality, while its futility is manifest. On the other hand, palliative cystostomy does not subject the patient to any inordinate risk, leaves him fully as comfortable, and assures him quite as long a life as does the more radical procedure. Mann [2] and Bovée [3] take a less pessimistic view of the results of extirpation.

Results of Operation.—Motz [4] has collected the records of 55 cases operated upon at Necker. Of these, 35 had been operated upon three years or more before. Ten only survived; and of the 18 cases of epithelioma only 1 was alive at the end of three years. Nine papillomata gave 4 relapses and 2 operative deaths. Albarran counted 36 cures in 48 operations for benign tumour and 23 cures in 97 operations for malignant growth. Clado collected 49 cures in 62 operations for benign tumours and only 28 cures in 111 operations for malignant disease. Even these statistics are optimistic. Papilloma, myoma, and pure fibroma are undoubtedly curable, but malignant disease is almost sure to prove fatal, however small the growth, however radical the operation. I believe that in these cases cystostomy gives more satisfaction to the patient than any resection of the bladder, unless the tumour is entirely circumscribed and its indurated base no more than 2 cm. across.

---

[1] Revue de chir., 1898, xviii, 277.
[2] American Medicine, 1901, ii, 55.
[3] *Ibid.*, 1901, ii, 59.
[4] Guyon's Annales, 1899, xvii, 1212.

CONDITIONS RESEMBLING TUMOURS OF THE BLADDER

Under this title it is convenient to classify three dissimilar conditions which have nothing in common except their extreme rarity and no connection with tumours of the bladder except a clinical resemblance.

Varicose Veins of the Bladder

A few cases have been reported which showed only one symptom—i. e., a spontaneous, profuse, uncontrollable hemorrhage of the bladder, which hemorrhage was found to arise from a ruptured varicose vein lying immediately under the mucous membrane. The diagnosis was made either by cystoscopy as the hemorrhage was ceasing, or by suprapubic cystotomy undertaken for the relief of the hemorrhage, as in Dr. Ellsworth Elliot's case. If the hemorrhage does not stop spontaneously the only treatment is cystotomy with ligature or cauterization of the bleeding point.

Urachus Cyst, or Fistula

Towards the middle months of intra-uterine life the urachus (the canal connecting the bladder with the umbilicus) becomes obliterated. Exceptionally, it remains patent throughout or at one extremity. This patency gives rise to a urachus cyst,[1] or fistula,[2] as the case may be. Urachus cyst is exceedingly rare. I have seen one in an adult which formed a large, irregular, fluctuating, hypogastric tumour. Occasionally a sacculated bladder simulates urachus cyst.

Urachus fistula is commonly a congenital condition and is usually caused by urethral obstruction. Certain cases of persistent permeability of the urachus without any obstruction of the natural urinary passages are quite inexplicable. The urachus may open in adult life as a result of urethral obstruction, but doubtless this does not occur unless there has been some congenital defect in the closure of the canal. Urachus fistula may be distinguished from fistulæ resulting from the bursting of an abscess or from malignant infiltration.

The treatment of urachus cyst, or fistula, consists in the excision of the canal or cyst after the urethral obstruction has been removed. Indeed, some fistulæ have been closed by merely removing the obstruction and cauterizing the canal by injections of alcohol or other irritants.

---

[1] Phila. Med. J., 1899, iii, 830.

[2] Delore, Guyon's Annales, 1899, xvii, 962. Jahn, Beitrag z. klin. Chir., 1900, xxvi, 323.

Intestinal Fistula

Vesico-intestinal fistula may be traumatic, ulcerative, cancerous, tubercular, or congenital. Congenital fistula is very rare. Ninety-five reported cases of acquired vesico-intestinal fistula in man have been collected by Chavannaz.[1] Of these, 13 were traumatic, 29 ulcerative (from stone, abscess, etc.), 19 cancerous, 7 tubercular, and 27 unclassified. The fistula usually opens into the rectum (43 cases) or into the sigmoid flexure (14 cases), but it may open into almost any part of the intestine, even the appendix vermiformis. The fistula may be short and direct, but in fully 25% of the cases there is an intermediate suppurating cavity between the vesical and the intestinal orifice.

Symptoms.—The most notable symptom of vesico-intestinal fistula is the passage of gas from the urethra (*pneumaturia*). This symptom is always present and is always noted by the patient. The urine may also be passed partly or wholly by the bowel, and when the opening is large feces may enter the bladder and issue with the urine. Cystitis is inevitable.

Diagnosis.—As a rule the diagnosis may be made from the presence of pneumaturia, although gas may be evolved by fermentation within the bladder itself. Thus the intravesical action of the yeast fungus upon saccharine urine has been known to cause pneumaturia, and I have seen two obscure cases in which the presence of gas could not be accounted for. If the evidences of bladder disease do not sufficiently confirm the diagnosis of fistula, an injection of methylene-blue solution into the bladder will decide the question by transuding through the fistula and appearing in the dejecta. The position of the fistula may be estimated by cystoscopy, by rectal touch, and, if necessary, by the rectal speculum.

Prognosis.—The prognosis depends on the nature of the fistula. Traumatic fistulæ often heal spontaneously if the bladder is kept clean and the urethra clear. Tubercular and malignant fistulæ will not heal.

Treatment.—Palliative treatment consists of daily irrigation of the bladder and bowel. Traumatic and ulcerative strictures that do not heal kindly may be stimulated by rectal injections of alcohol or of the ethereal solution of hydrogen peroxid (p. 129). Palliative operation consists in colostomy. This is the only appropriate treatment for incurable fistula. Temporary colostomy is also employed as a preliminary to the attempt at radical cure. Palliative colostomy

---

[1] Guyon's Annales, 1897, xv, 1176, 1287, and 1898, xvi, 85, 203.

has been performed 11 times. Seven patients survived the operation one month; but of these, only 4 lived out the year and only 2 survived three years.

A radical cure may be attempted in several ways. Chavannaz reports 3 cures by dilating the fistula and scraping its rectal extremity. Suprapubic section and suture of the vesical end of the fistula improved 1 case. Inasmuch as fistulæ between the bladder and intestine above the rectum are almost all either tubercular or malignant, they are only susceptible of palliation by colostomy. Vesico-rectal fistulæ may be operated upon by the methods employed in the treatment of urethro-rectal fistulæ (p. 247).

CHAPTER XXVIII

URINARY CALCULUS—VARIETIES—ETIOLOGY—VESICAL CALCULUS—MORBID ANATOMY—SYMPTOMS—DIAGNOSIS—TREATMENT OTHER THAN RADICAL

URINARY CALCULUS

A URINARY stone, or calculus, is a body resembling a stone in its general characteristics, and formed of crystalline urinary salts (exceptionally of other substances) held together by viscid organic matter, and showing, microscopically or to the naked eye, a laminated structure.

All true calculi are composed of a nucleus, single or multiple, and layers more or less concentric of the same or of another material arranged around it (Figs. 98, 99, 100). This is the case for large as well as for microscopic calculi, even for those requiring a magnifying power of 250 diameters (Beale) to make out their lamination. This fact of lamination alone differentiates calculus from gravel, the latter being crystalline dust or concretions of crystals more or less large, but not possessed of definite structural arrangement.

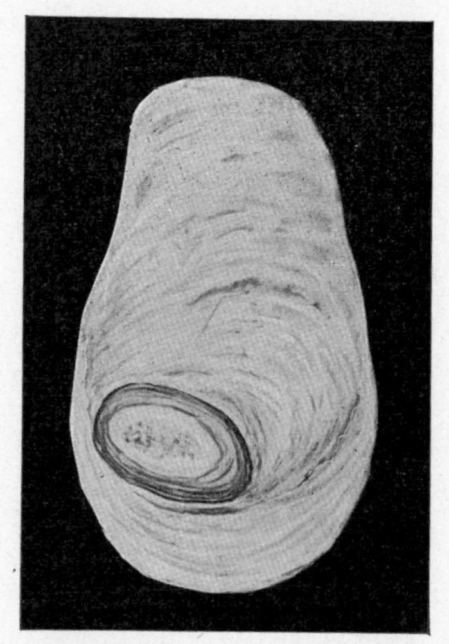

FIG. 98.—SECTION OF A PHOSPHATIC STONE, SHOWING EXCENTRIC DEVELOPMENT.

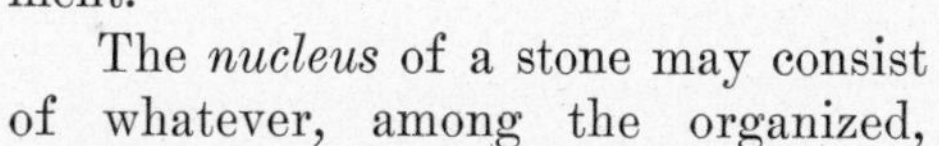

The *nucleus* of a stone may consist of whatever, among the organized, crystalline, or earthy constituents of normal or pathological urine, is capable of concreting into a more or less solid mass; or it may be a foreign substance either coming from within the body or introduced from without. The nucleus is usually in the centre of the stone (Figs. 99, 101). An unusual excentric development is shown in Fig. 98.

The calculus takes its distinguishing title from the salt or salts which enter chiefly into its composition. Thus a phosphatic stone is usually accepted as a stone composed apparently of phosphates, though it may have a nucleus of some other salt (Fig. 101). The classification of stones according to the nature of their nuclei would have its advantages, but it is clinically impracticable.

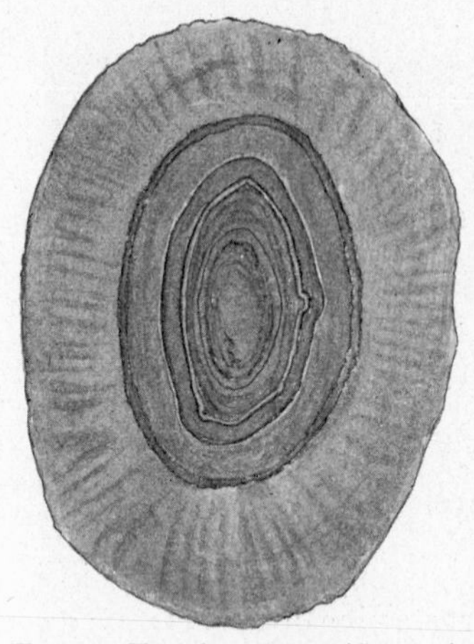

FIG. 99.—URIC-ACID STONE (SECTION). The marked central lamination suggests a preponderance of uric acid, while the more amorphous periphery shows an intermixture here of urates.

VARIETIES

The more refined and obscure points relative to the varieties of stone and their pathogenesis cannot be dwelt upon here. I have considered the subject at length in another place.[1] All stones come under one of the following groups:

Primary stone, which develops in an acid urine without any antecedent inflammation, may consist of uric acid, urate of soda, lime, or potash, oxalate of lime, cystin, xanthin, carbonate of lime, crystalline phosphate of lime, or indigo.

Secondary stone, which develops in an alkaline urine as the result of inflammation, may consist of ammonio-magnesium phosphate (triple phosphate), amorphous phosphate of lime, tricalcic phosphate, urate of ammonia, or urostealith.

Among the primary stones only those composed of uric acid, oxalate of lime, and urates are common; the other varieties are extremely rare. Secondary stones are commonly formed of mixed phosphates, very rarely of urate of ammonia or urostealith. Primary calculi are usually formed of the same substance throughout, while secondary phosphatic calculi are often found about a primary stone as a nucleus. While the proportions vary in different countries, uric acid forms the nucleus of from 50% to 80% of all stones.

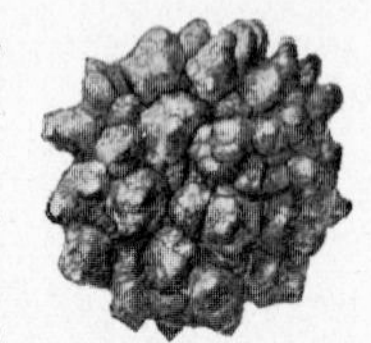

FIG. 100.—OXALATE OF LIME (MULBERRY) STONE.

Uric Acid.—Uric-acid stone is the most common in the human subject. It may be mixed intimately or in layers with urates, oxalate of lime, or phosphates. It does not attain a very great size, and may be single or multiple. In structure it is either laminated or amorphous.

---

[1] Internat. Encycl. of Surgery (Ashhurst), vol. vi, p. 145.

The laminated uric-acid stone is of a dark reddish-brown colour, very hard and heavy. When cut and polished it resembles an agate,

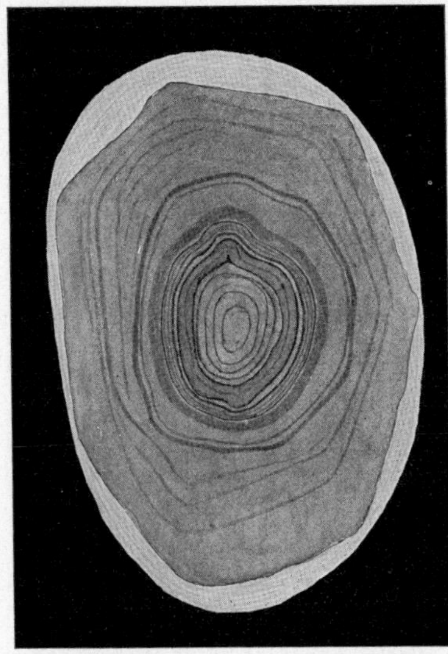

Fig. 101.—Section of Stone of Mixed Uric Acid and Oxalate of Lime, coated with Phosphates.

Such a stone would pass for phosphatic on inspection.

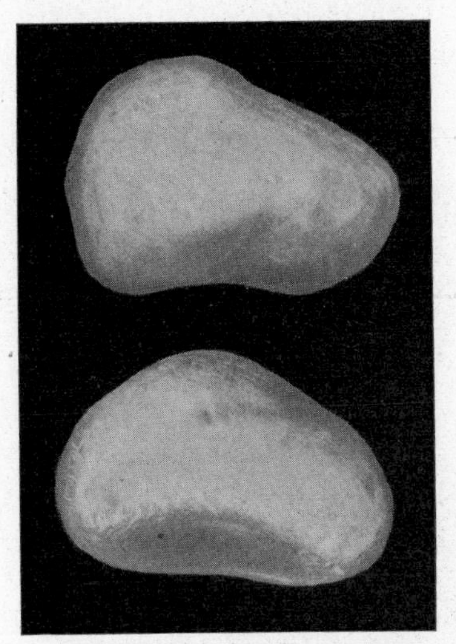

Fig. 102.—Multiple Phosphatic Stones (Natural Size).

The irregular shape is due to friction. (There were 6 similar stones in this case.)

displaying a concentric arrangement of irregularly curved lines of slightly varying colour and thickness (Fig. 99). The amorphous variety is much less common. It is rather soft, gritty looking, and comparatively structureless on section. It is of a reddish-yellow colour and composed chiefly of urates, and hence is commonly known as urate stone.

Oxalate.—Oxalate of limestone is commonly single, blackish-brown in colour, and very hard. It is usually covered with blunted asperities, whence it has acquired the name of mulberry calculus (Fig. 100). Upon section it shows undulating laminæ, which may vary widely in colour, as there is often an admixture of uric acid or phosphates in the composition of this stone (Fig. 101).

Phosphate.—Mixed phosphatic or fusible calculus is the common secondary calculus. It may grow to an enormous size, and may be single or multiple (Figs. 101, 102, 103). It forms around a primary calculus, a blood clot, or a foreign body. It is granular, soft, light in weight, and of a dirty white colour. It may be amorphous or laminated.

The other forms of calculi are so rare as to require no special mention. Cystinuria has a medical rather than a surgical interest. (*Cf.* Cohn [1] and Moréigne.[2])

Etiology

The causes of stone formation are extremely obscure. Secondary (phosphatic) stones are known to result from the changes in the urine commonly known as alkaline fermentation. Such calculi are frequent in old men suffering from the cystitis of prostatic hypertrophy, and are less frequently met with as the result of other forms of inflammation. But the etiology of primary calculus is most obscure. Primary stones are very uncommon in women. The negro is said to be singularly exempt, and there are two periods of life during which they are most frequently found—viz., in the first two and in the fifth decades of life. But the most notable feature of the occurrence of primary stone is its great frequency in certain localities and its comparative rarity in others. Thus India leads the list with hundreds of operations a year. Egypt, perhaps, comes second, and North America is, as a whole, comparatively exempt. Yet in certain parts of India primary calculus is quite as rare as it is with us, and it has also been observed that the tendency to stone among the inhabitants of a certain district seems to increase or decrease regularly over a long period of years. To explain these vagaries various theories have been adduced. The influence of climate, the soil, the water, the civilization of the inhabitants, as affecting their occupations, the diet, especially the amount of salt habitually taken—all of these and various other factors have been implicated.

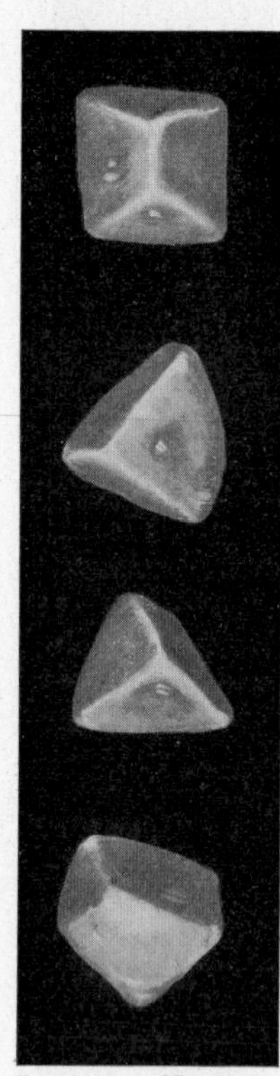

Fig. 103. — Multiple Small Phosphatic Stones (Natural Size). These stones are selected from a group of 33 similar ones. These small stones show sharp faceting from friction.

There is some evidence of a hereditary tendency to stone formation closely allied to the uric-acid diathesis. Indeed, the predisposing cause of primary stone is undoubtedly the presence of crystals in the urine. Without crystals there can be no calculus, yet the urine may contain crystals for years and no stone form.

[1] Berl. klin. Woch., 1899, xxxvi, 503.

[2] Guyon's Annales, 1899, xvii, 803, 910.

A notable example is the phosphaturia so common in the young. It may continue for years, and the urine may be so thick with phosphates that the terminal drops, if they fall upon the patient's shoe, give the effect of a splash of mortar. Yet phosphatic stone is never due to this phosphaturia. In point of fact, the microscope reveals that a urinary calculus is made up, not of the sharp-pointed crystals so commonly seen in the urine, but of rounded masses, showing neither angles nor polarity, and consisting of an amorphous collection of granules of a urinary salt embedded in a structureless, albuminous substance. If true crystals appear, they occur simply as foreign bodies entrapped in the stone. Rainey and Ord have conclusively shown that the determining cause of calculus is the increased density of the urine and the presence of colloid substances in solution, in conjunction with an excess of urinary salts; for "a crystalloid is deposited from solution in the presence of a colloid," and crystals introduced into a colloidal solution are disintegrated and re-formed by simple, molecular coalescence. Thus the nucleus of a stone is always laid down in an albuminous substance. A blood clot, a foreign body surrounded by the muco-pus which it stirs up by its presence, are common examples—and once the nucleus has formed, it is always in such a foreign body surrounded by albuminous matter that new layers of stone are constantly being formed.

The rate of growth of a stone must vary greatly, and although it would be most interesting to be able to estimate by the size of a calculus how long it had existed, such an estimate cannot be made with any accuracy. Thus it is known that phosphatic stones grow, as a rule, much faster than primary ones, and yet I have removed a uric-acid calculus weighing 2 ounces from a boy nine years old, and a hair-pin from a girl's bladder (in which it had remained for more than a year), which was encrusted with less than a dram of phosphates.

VESICAL CALCULUS

Number and Shape.—Single calculi are generally rounded or ovoidal in shape (Figs. 98, 99, 100, 101). When a calculus is unusually elongated it is suggestive of the presence of several nuclei or of a foreign body. Calculi formed about foreign bodies are always phosphatic (Fig. 122).

Multiple calculi are usually phosphatic, less frequently urates. In general, their number bears an inverse relation to their size. When few in number they influence one another's shape and grow to be many-sided rather than rounded (Figs. 102, 103). Hence when a stone passed spontaneously presents one or more flat sides or facets, the presence of other stones in the bladder (or kidney) may be inferred.

Fantastic dumb-bell and other shapes are assumed by encysted calculi (Fig. 104), part of the stone taking the shape of the pocket which contains it, while the remainder protrudes irregularly into the vesical cavity.

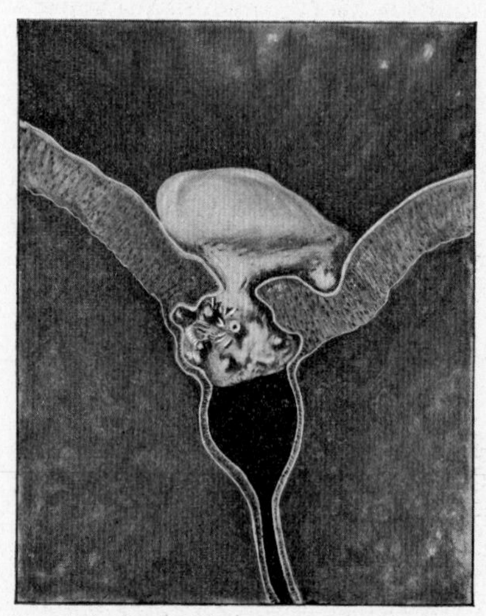

Fig. 104.—Stone Encysted in the Orifice of the Ureter.

Size.—Partly on account of the infrequency of stone, partly on account of the surgeon's omnipresence, large stones are rarely seen in this day and in this country. The largest stone in my collection weighs 5 ounces. Dr. Thomas Smith[1] removed a stone weighing 24½ ounces, and Lieutenant-Colonel Bamker[2] one weighing 25 ounces. Both were phosphatic.

Morbid Anatomy

The changes which the calculus itself undergoes have been noted above, except the rare phenomenon of spontaneous fracture. Spontaneous fracture is apparently due to long-continued dilution of the urine, which weakens the colloidal framework of the stone sufficiently to permit it to break into pieces. This rare phenomenon has been taken advantage of by the purveyors of various lithia waters. The claim that any water or drug will infallibly, or even probably, cause spontaneous fracture of stone is not based on any very good theory, and is not supported by experience. Moreover, when the calculus does break it is not to be expected that all the fragments will be expelled. One or more will remain in the bladder, and around these as nuclei new stones will form.

The changes in the bladder caused by the presence of stone are primarily congestion, secondarily inflammation. The little hard calculus rolling about over the mucous membrane of the bladder keeps that tissue in a constant state of irritation and congestion, which manifests itself in hemorrhage and pain—the early symptoms of stone. Sooner or later infection occurs upon the *locus minoris resistentiæ* and the cystitis of stone adds its pyuria and dysuria to the signs of irritation.

---

[1] Lancet, 1886, ii, 244.

[2] Med. Record, 1900, lviii, 637.

As the stone grows larger it tends more and more to settle in one particular spot, which it ulcerates and gradually distends as a niche or pocket into which the stone fits quite accurately. Hence it is very useful in the operation of litholapaxy to determine the exact spot in which the stone is first found, for the broken fragments usually show a decided tendency to gravitate to that spot in preference to any other. The favourite position for a stone in the bladder is in the *bas fond* immediately behind the neck of the bladder. Exceptionally, the stone rests in a diverticulum of the bladder or sends out prolongations into the ureter or the urethra.

Rupture of the bladder or the urethra containing a stone is exceptional, and is usually due to the abscess formation which itself is rare.

Symptoms

There is no symptom, no set of symptoms, absolutely and invariably pathognomonic of stone in the bladder, except the physical signs elicited by the surgeon's examination. Yet there is a certain group of symptoms which is very suggestive of stone. Chief among these are frequency of urination, pain, and hematuria, occurring by day and increased by exercise.

Frequency of Urination and Pain.—The pollakiuria and dysuria of stone are usually intense. They appear early in the disease and are the patient's chief complaint from beginning to end. The characteristic distress is absent during the night while the patient lies quietly on his back, and during the day so long as he is still. But every jolt induces spasm. When walking the patient moves slowly and gingerly, almost on tip-toes. Riding over a rough road or in a railroad train, or even walking downstairs, is misery. The pains are situated chiefly in the glans penis, along the pendulous urethra, and in the perineum. The desire to urinate is quite irresistible. Such is the distress, sometimes mild, sometimes severe, caused by the mere presence of the stone. As a result of some extra exertion or an acute infection, the patient, from time to time, has what is known as a *fit of the stone*. During this time his pains are greatly intensified. He may have to urinate as often as every ten or fifteen minutes day and night, so that he spends his time in one long spasm.

As the stone grows larger and the cystitis more intense these paroxysms become more and more frequent. They exhaust the patient's strength, and during them he resembles a woman in the second stage of labour. In children, prolapse of the rectum and involuntary defecation are common results of this straining; while adults complain of hemorrhoids, pass blood by the rectum, and during the paroxysms suffer from unavoidable escape of intestinal flatus and often of feces. When there is considerable prostatic hypertrophy or the stone is encysted, there is less tendency to dysuria, so that even with intense cystitis the paroxysms may be neither frequent nor severe.

Hematuria.—Hematuria, like the characteristic dysuria, is traumatic in origin, and is, during the first stages of the disease, only aroused by some jolt. It is usually associated with dysuria, and the hemorrhage, though profuse, is usually short-lived. Later in the disease the perpetual straining due to cystitis may make the hematuria quite continuous.

Stoppage.—Sudden stoppage of the urinary stream is a symptom of stone which is peculiarly characteristic though not very common. It is caused by the stone rolling into the vesical orifice and plugging it like a ball-valve. Striking cases, like that of Sir Henry Thompson, whose patient could urinate only while lying on his back, are most uncommon. Prostatics with stone do not show this symptom, and it may be caused by prostatic or vesical tumour.

In children certain special symptoms are associated with stone, notably priapism and a tendency to pull at the prepuce, with a resultant lengthening of that tissue.

Certain reflex pains in the back, testicle, eye, and sole of the foot (pododynia) are among the infrequent symptoms of stone in the bladder.

Course of the Disease.—Although a stone may lie quiescent in the bladder for many months, it usually begins to set up irritation before long. There may be a history of renal colic or of the introduction of some foreign substance into the bladder; there may be a long history of chronic cystitis, or there may be no suggestion of how the stone began. Then, after a longer or shorter time, appear the characteristic dysuria and hematuria, more or less clearly marked. Later, if there is no cystitis already, infection occurs, and leads gradually, by repeated attacks of greater frequency and intensity, to the perpetual spasm described above.

Diagnosis

Every case of painful or hemorrhagic cystitis should be searched for stone. Although the subjective symptoms just described may be absolutely characteristic, in most cases they are confused and ill-described by the patient, so that the only means of making the diagnosis clear is to search.

Sounding or Searching for Stone.—Many different ways have been suggested to prove the existence of stone in the bladder. Among these the cystoscope and the X-ray have grown in favour of late. The cystoscope is fallacious even in the hands of the most expert.

Stones, as seen through it, have been mistaken for tumours and prostatic outgrowths, and its use is often difficult as well as painful, on account of the bleeding and the excessive sensitiveness of the neck of the bladder. The X-rays are even less accurate. In contrast with these methods by which the surgeon endeavours to see the stone, are the old proved methods of touch. Nothing is so characteristic, so entirely unmistakable as the click of a stone against a searcher. It is alleged that the stone may be so covered with mucus as not to click, and that a stone in a saccule of the bladder or behind a hypertrophied prostate cannot be touched by the searcher. I can only say that, in a lifelong experience, I know of several cases whose stones I have overlooked; but in every one of these I either did not make the attempt or was unable to introduce a searcher. Once only have I found a small, untouched stone behind a large prostate a few weeks after a supposedly successful litholapaxy. Yet I have often touched stone after others had failed to do so, and must believe that the searcher is a no more accurate means of diagnosis than any other instrument, unless guided by a practised hand. I have been able to identify a stone by its impact against a soft-rubber catheter, and I have often employed in the final search, after litholapaxy, a Bigelow aspirator

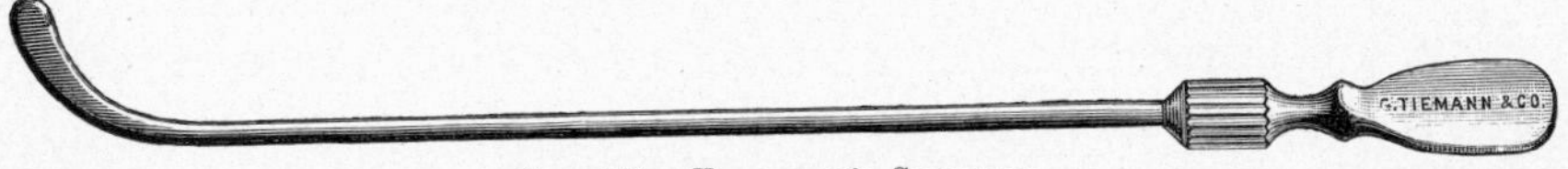

FIG. 105.—THOMPSON'S SEARCHER.

(p. 449) in the hope of obtaining a click from a very small fragment. But for routine use there is no instrument so well borne by the patient, so easily and quickly manipulated by the surgeon, and so accurate in its results as the Thompson searcher (Fig. 105). The addition of a sounding-board, a stethoscope, a microphone, or a wax covering only detracts from the simplicity of the operation.

To *sound for stone*, the patient is placed upon a table or a firm couch, lying upon his back, with the shoulders low and the pelvis raised upon a hair cushion or some other solid support, so that it may be several inches higher than the shoulders.[1] The thighs and legs are extended and lie flat. The bladder should, when possible, contain about 100 c. c. of fluid, either the patient's urine or a warm boric-acid solution. The difficulty is not to recognise the stone when it is touched, but to touch it at all if the bladder is capacious; for it

[1] If the stone is movable and the bladder contains fluid, when the pelvis is raised higher than the shoulders the stone will roll away from the tender neck of the bladder and rest at the fundus behind the trigone, where it is most easily found.

may elude all search when the bladder is full, and may be covered by the loose folds of the viscus and out of reach when the bladder is empty. Hence not less than 100 nor more than 175 c. c. of fluid should be injected. It is best not to make the examination during a fit of the stone; but if the bladder is excessively irritable or the patient is nervous—and particularly for a second search after one negative exploration—it is wiser to use general anesthesia than to risk failure without it.

The surgeon, standing at the patient's right side, introduces the searcher gently, making its heel slide along the membranous urethra and the floor of the prostatic sinus, and aiding its passage through these segments of the urethra by depressing with his left hand the skin over the pubes, so as to relax the suspensory ligament of the penis. In some cases the whole search is made less painful by keeping the ligament thus relaxed throughout the entire proceeding. When the heel of the searcher enters the bladder it should be carried gently down the inclined plane formed by the base of the bladder until arrested. Most often the stone will be struck at this point. If not, then the toe of the searcher should be gently rotated as far as it will go, first towards one and then towards the other side of the bladder. Next, the searcher is drawn forward, well inclined to one side, and by rotating the cylindrical handle gentle taps are given to the wall of the bladder along the entire side as far forward as the instrument can be drawn. It is then slid back to the fundus along the course it has just traversed. This double passage is repeated on the other side of the bladder. Next, the beak of the sound is reversed, and the whole floor of the bladder is swept by to-and-fro lateral motions of the tip, as it is brought forward to the vesical neck and carried back again to the fundus. If encysted or adherent stone is suspected, the fundus may be more fully examined by flexing the thighs to relax the abdominal muscles, and sweeping the bladder with the sound while counterpressure is made above the pubes.

Should a stone be touched, the bulbous tip of the searcher passed over its surface will indicate whether it is rough or smooth. The character of the click produced by tapping the stone gives a clew to its composition, a dull, low-pitched sound indicating a soft stone, probably phosphatic, while a clear, high-pitched click indicates an acid stone.

To ascertain the size of the stone, the tip of the searcher is tapped along its surface from one end to the other, and the distance traversed is estimated roughly by the length of shaft introduced or withdrawn. During operation the size of the stone may be estimated more accurately by grasping it in the lithotrite and carrying it up to the abdominal wall, where it may sometimes be outlined by the fingers.

The number of stones present cannot be very accurately made out. If the searcher clicks to one side and then to the other, two stones may be assumed to be present; and if at the beginning of litholapaxy a stone grasped by the lithotrite can be made to click on one or both sides, there are two or three stones present. No accurate calculation can be made beyond this except by lithotomy.

The operation of sounding should always be terminated by an instillation or irrigation of nitrate of silver, and if the patient is much irritated he should be kept in bed for a day or two thereafter. The surgeon should not hesitate to desist without having reached an absolutely satisfactory conclusion, for the most skilful surgeons have failed to find stone. If the searcher alone fails the examination may be completed under general anesthesia with searcher and aspirator or cystoscope, in which case the patient should be prepared to undergo immediate operation if the stone is found. If he will not accept this alternative, he may be given palliative treatment, the possible presence of stone being always kept in mind, until either his improvement shows that stone is not present, or the persistence of his symptoms forces him to accept operation.

Prognosis

Unless the stone is small enough to be viable through the urethra, there is only one prognosis—it will certainly remain, and the symptoms will inevitably grow more severe until it is removed by operation. I have never known any of the so-called solvent treatments of stone to be of the slightest use. They do not check the growth of the stone, they do not ameliorate the cystitis, they do not cause spontaneous fracture.

The prognosis as to recurrence is referred to in connection with the preventive treatment.

Treatment of Stone other than Radical

Preventive Treatment.—Efforts may be made looking towards the prevention of stone formation in two directions: (*a*) In correcting an inherited or a diathetic tendency to acid primary stone formation, when this is known to exist; (*b*) in overcoming local physical conditions whose continuance threatens stone as a secondary symptom—alkaline, secondary stone.

(*a*) *When lithiasis exists, when a patient constantly passes acid concentrated urine more or less charged with crystals, when he has already passed one kidney stone and fears the formation of another, what may be done to aid him?*

I need not here discuss the colloidal theory, because that theory has not yet reached the practical stage. The scientific writings of Ord and Carter are full of suggestion, but another master must teach us how to apply them.

Practically the best that can be done at present may be accomplished by—

1. Dietetics.
2. Exercise.
3. Encouraging elimination by other avenues.
4. Diluting the urine constantly.
5. Use of solvents, and attempts to dilute the colloids.

But over and above all this the diagnosis of stone in the kidney must be made, for if a stone remains there it is quite fatuous to attempt to prevent the formation of others in the bladder.

1. **Diet.**—Thompson, who has given this matter much attention, believes that uric-acid formation lies essentially in the liver, and that it is by correcting disease of that organ that we may hope to overcome the diathesis. He adopts, in the main, the Carlsbad notions, and cuts off sugar, fat, and alcohol, rather than the meats. In truth, such a dietary usually proves more effective than the old-fashioned one, which interdicted nitrogenized food because uric acid is a nitrogenized product, overlooking the fact that there is necessarily enough nitrogen eliminated every day in the urine to supply unlimited uric acid, given the colloidal and other conditions upon which the formation of calculus depends.

Practically, then, it is found that a proper diet consists of meat, poultry, fish, eggs, bread, and all the cereals, all the fruits and roots, green vegetables and salads, with butter and milk in moderation—though the last sometimes keeps up uric-acid tendencies. If any of the above-mentioned articles prove hard to digest, that fact alone is sufficient to condemn it in the individual case.

Sugar is harmful; most wines and liquors are pernicious; sometimes a little light wine is allowable, or gin or old whisky in selected cases. Heller showed that an exclusive diet of rye bread caused all uric acid to disappear from the urine, this substance being replaced by hippuric acid, a solution of which is a natural solvent of uric acid.

2. **Exercise.**—Exercise, probably by improving digestion and giving plenty of oxygen to the blood and tissues, is a factor of such generally recognised value in preventing uric-acid formation that its mention alone is required: discussion is unnecessary.

3. **Encouraging Elimination.**—The liver has a large share in uric-acid formation, and, by preventing its becoming what is called torpid, a long stride is made in the preventive treatment of stone. The action of the bowels should therefore be closely attended to. Added to this, a course of Glauber's salts may be given occasionally, or small, graded, prolonged courses of the sulphate-of-soda bitter waters (Hunyadi, Friederichshall). Garrod[1] speaks strongly in favour of long courses of the benzoates of sodium and potassium for the purpose of acting as uric-acid solvents.

4. **Dilution.**—Many persons prone to discharge uric acid and urates in excess and to have concentrated urine, are not free drinkers of water, and for such persons some good may be done by encouraging them to take a glass of water between meals and another on retiring. This renders the urine by so much the more dilute, and thus militates against precipitation of the urinary salts. Filtered rain-water is better than ordinary water for this purpose. Distilled water is excellent, and some of the unaërated mineral-spring waters, such as Wildungen, Poland, Bethesda, better still; after being charged with carbonic-acid gas, their diuretic property is much lessened.

5. **Solvents.**—A quick way to dissolve acids in the urine is to administer alkaline medicines, particularly those that also have a diuretic effect, such as the acetate or the citrate of potash. Here belong also all the alkaline salts and the alkaline mineral waters. As a preventive of stone formation, the alkaline method is defective in that it is by no means essential, and in many instances, if long continued, it finally ceases to act, or may have the further harmful effect of disturbing digestion, and sometimes directly causing anemia. When alkaline medicines are given, it must be remembered that they produce their maximum effect if administered about two hours after the end of a meal. The borocitrate of magnesia in about 1-gramme doses, 3 times a day, is well borne if a long course of alkaline medicine is desired.

The so-called uric-acid solvents are more satisfactory. They have the advantage of being better borne by the stomach and of acting best when given in interrupted courses—a month of medication followed by a month of rest. Urotropin, piperazin, and uricedin are useful. They need not be taken for a lifetime, but only during those periods when the urinary specific gravity and acidity run high.

Crystals of oxalate of lime do not cease to appear under an alkaline course. They constantly occur in connection with phosphaturia. Dilute mineral acids, nerve tonics, bitters, exercise, and air are the

---

[1] Lancet, 1883, i, 670.

best means with which to fight this tendency. Beale believes that the free use of carbonate of ammonium will prevent cystin formations.

To dilute the colloids, which seem to preside over crystallization, all that at present can be done is to keep the urine dilute and bland, and the digestion perfect, to prevent catarrhal conditions of the stomach and intestine, and to avert feverishness from whatever cause. Whether hydrangea is valuable or not I have not yet decided. Cider habitually used seems to help.

To sum up, my directions to patients are habitually as follows: 1. Eat lightly. Take meat but once a day. Eschew sweet foods, fried foods, and, above all, such foods as interfere with digestion. 2. Drink no wines but white wines; no liquors but gin and whisky—these in moderation. Drink plenty of water (any flat mineral water will do, and the patient will drink it more faithfully because it comes in bottles). 3. Exercise freely at all times, and in the open air. 4. Keep the bowels regular. 5. Alkalies or solvents I prescribe with little hope that the patient will continue to use them.

(*b*) *The preventive measures useful against secondary phosphatic stone formation* are better known and more certain of success. No amount of phosphates in the urine can cause secondary alkaline phosphatic stone. This is due always to inflammation somewhere along the urinary tract. Therefore, the means of prevention of secondary stone include the surgical treatment of all obstructive urethral disease (stricture, enlarged prostate), the removal of tumours and foreign bodies, the relief of residual urine by the timely employment of the catheter, and the treatment of vesical catarrh by irrigation, medicated injections, etc. In short, if stagnation can be prevented stone can be prevented. Old prostatics, who will not submit to radical operation, but are satisfied to carry about a pool of residual urine in a trabeculated, sacculated bladder—these are the men who return year after year for the aspiration of phosphatic stones.

The Electrolytic Treatment of Stone.—Although the electric current influences crystallization, and although Bouvier-Demortiers, Dumas, Prévost, and Erckmann have shown that stone may be pierced and disintegrated by the galvanic current, yet the method is a failure for all practical purposes, and not worthy of adoption under any known circumstances.

The Solvent Treatment of Stone.—Since Pliny's ashes of snail-shells even to the present day, the wise and the foolish alike have searched unceasingly for something which, taken by the mouth, might be capable of dissolving a stone in the kidney or the bladder, and the substance has not been found. The Joanna Stephens remedies worked wonders in the last century, until Parliament bought the secret for £5,000, after which they quickly fell into disuse and are now forgotten. Each of the four patients, whose cures were attested by the trustees appointed by Government to investigate the matter, died with stone in the bladder, as proved by autopsy.

The most serious efforts of modern times to dissolve small acid stone (in the kidney) by medicine taken into the stomach are those of Roberts [1] and Garrod,[2] of England, and they are most praiseworthy. The former uses long courses of the citrate of potash (3 grammes every three to four hours), substituting bicarbonate if the citrate proves too diuretic; the latter uses the same salts of lithium in a smaller dose.

Beale [3] uses carbonate of ammonium to prevent cystin precipitation (3 grammes 3 times a day in 1 case) for three years.

All these efforts are in the right direction, but there is little hope of effecting any serious good with them if the stone is large enough to be worthy of the name.

The Palliative Treatment of Stone.—In cases unfit for operation a judicious combination of alkalies, rest, milk diet, anodynes, and tonics, addressed to the individual needs of the case, aided by catheterization, vesical irrigation, and medicated injections, may be appropriate.

---

[1] Urinary and Renal Diseases, 2d American edition, 1872, pp. 298–321.

[2] Lancet, 1883, i, 669.

[3] *Ibid.*, 1884, ii, 363.

CHAPTER XXIX

VESICAL CALCULUS—RADICAL TREATMENT—FOREIGN BODIES IN THE BLADDER

It has always been customary among writers upon the subject of the treatment of stone to weigh minutely the advantages and disadvantages of the various operations, as well as the propriety of subjecting certain cases to any operation. The lapse of time has brought theory and experience no nearer together. Each operation still has its supporters, and doubtless always will have. But, thanks to Bigelow and Lister, thanks to the modern perfection of operative technic, the difference of opinion, which seems bound to persist, almost narrows itself down to a matter of taste. The general surgeon who interferes but rarely with the bladder cannot fail to prefer the generous drainage and clear field afforded by the suprapubic operation. On the other hand, the surgeon who has been educated in the deft maneuvres of litholapaxy will subject almost every case to that operation. If the statistics of the two operations are not identical, they are equally good in this respect at least: the surgeon who is unskilled in litholapaxy will have a higher mortality and more complications from that operation than from simple suprapubic cystotomy, while the skilled lithotritist will be able to assure his patients more rapid and comfortable cure than they could expect from lithotomy, with absolutely no danger of death in properly selected cases. In short, the situation may be summed up as follows: *Suprapubic lithotomy exposes the patient to more dangers and inconveniences than does litholapaxy. Yet lithotomy is appropriate to all cases, which litholapaxy is not; while litholapaxy requires a special training, which lithotomy does not.*

The facts upon which these views are founded will be developed in the following sections. We need dwell upon only three operations —viz., litholapaxy, perineal lithotomy (or litholapaxy), and suprapubic lithotomy. Lithotrity is dead, having disappeared from surgery as its brilliant child and successor, litholapaxy, established its claims. Similarly, perineal litholapaxy has replaced the lateral operation and all other devices for extracting large stones through the perineum.

LITHOLAPAXY

Of all the operations that are or have been employed in the treatment of stone in the bladder, litholapaxy when properly performed is generally conceded to be the safest and most brilliant. In support of this proposition it is only necessary to adduce the authority of Cabot and Chismore in this country, of Thompson and Harrison in England, of Guyon in France, and of the entire school of Indian surgeons who alone see more cases of stone than all the rest of the world put together. No age is a bar to litholapaxy. Any stone may be crushed if it can be caught in the jaws of the lithotrite. It is alleged that the stone may be too hard for the lithotrite to break, but I have not met such a case. The size of the stone may constitute a contra-indication to litholapaxy. The crushing of a large stone is always a tedious and protracted operation, and I am not prepared to agree entirely with Freyer,[1] who once continued the operation for two hours in order to remove a large stone. Such a stone would, I believe, be more safely relieved by the knife. These and the other contra-indications to litholapaxy may be summed up briefly:

1. Cases complicated by prostatic hypertrophy, in which—
   a. Instruments cannot be introduced,
   b. The stone cannot be grasped, or
   c. The condition of the bladder and prostate is such as to indicate cystotomy or prostatectomy, the stone aside.
2. Cases complicated by cystitis so severe as to resist all attempts to ameliorate it. Such cases will usually show some obstruction at the neck of the bladder, which is best dealt with by perineal section.
3. Cases complicated by stricture, impassable or resilient, or with such urgent symptoms that there is no time for dilatation.
4. Cases complicated by tumour of the bladder.
5. Cases of encysted or adherent stone.
6. Cases of stone formation around a foreign body, the extraction of which through the urethra would be difficult or impossible.
7. Large or hard stones, as remarked above.
8. Cases of general sepsis or uremia, in which rapidity of operation and thorough drainage are the only important points.

This formidable list covers practically but a small percentage of

---

[1] Litholapaxy, 1896, p. 62.

cases. Cabot[1] adds such contra-indications as certain cases of false passage, ankylosed hip, and recurrent stone, yet argues strongly in favour of the crushing operation. Harrison, in his latest report of 110 stone operations, gives 101 litholapaxies, and I find in my own records 198 operations with 157 litholapaxies. Fully nine tenths of the cases not amenable to crushing are excepted on account of the necessity of drainage or the condition of the prostate. I venture to reproduce a recent summing up of my views[2] on the subject of the treatment of stone complicating enlargement of the prostate.

1. When stone complicates enlarged prostate, if the condition of the latter be such that were the stone absent no operation would be called for, then the whole question is to be solved by deciding whether the obstructive quality of the prostatic enlargement, the size of the bar, the depth of the *bas fond*, the irritability of the prostatic urethra, and its resentment of instrumental interference—whether any of these factors be sufficiently accentuated to make litholapaxy impossible, or to make it possible only at the expense of leaving the patient (as to his subjective symptoms) worse than before. If such conditions do obtain, then the stone should be removed by the knife.

2. In short, the main matter is one of diagnosis by the searcher, the cystoscope, rectal touch, and the tentative testing of the prostatic urethra with instruments.

3. The mere size of the prostate is not a factor in the problem.

4. The size or position of the stone is not a factor, unless the stone is encysted, or too large for the lithotrite to grasp, or formed about a foreign body. The smallness alone of the stone is relatively an argument against litholapaxy, since the symptoms in such a condition must be ascribed to the prostate rather than to the foreign body.

5. If lithotomy be performed the suprapubic route should be elected, since this opens the door for more perfect work and permits the surgeon to remove obstructions, such as third lobe, interstitial growths, outstanding horse-collar enlargement, bar, and to lower the vesical end of the urethral floor, thus accomplishing all that could be done by a more extensive prostatectomy, without very seriously increasing the operative risk.

6. Finally, here as elsewhere in surgery, the only safe practical guide is surgical judgment based upon diagnosis, and guided by experience.

Preparation of Patient.—If when first seen the patient is suffering from an acute cystitis, he should be put to bed and kept there until the attack subsides under treatment. If unaffected by

---

[1] Bull. Johns Hopkins Univ., 1900. [2] Trans. Med. Soc., State of New York, 1898.

treatment, litholapaxy may still be performed, though I confess a preference for the perineal cutting operation.

If the cystitis is not extremely acute, preparation for litholapaxy need occupy but forty-eight hours, while the patient is freely flushed with some bland diuretic water and, if possible, accustomed to a milk diet. During this time I administer 0.5 gramme of urotropin thrice a day, and prefer to have the patient in bed. The night before operation the intestinal tract should be cleared, and it is well to irrigate the bladder twice a day with boric-acid solution in order to reduce infection as far as possible. It is well to estimate the calibre of the urethra by the introduction of a blunt sound or a bulbous bougie. The usual catharsis and bath should precede operation. I have entirely abandoned the use of quinin and other antipyretics. Shaving the pubes and perineum is unnecessary, and antiseptics applied to the skin over an infected bladder only make of it a whited sepulchre. *Antisepsis must terminate the operation, not precede it.*

Instruments Required.—Besides the usual tables, rubber cloths, basins, towels, etc., I carry the following outfit to all litholapaxies:

One searcher.
Three lithotrites, at least.
Two aspirators, and at least 2 tubes.
One sound—full size for the individual.
One rubber catheter.
One large piston syringe (150 grammes).
The apparatus for making the two solutions I employ—viz., 2% boric acid and 1:4,000 nitrate of silver.[1]

Nearly every operator of prominence has his own lithotrite, and many have devised washing-bottles and special tubes. With any form of apparatus the operation may be done, and with more or less rapidity and success, according to the deftness of the surgeon. On these different questions it is impossible to enter freely here, as it is impracticable to describe all the instruments employed at various hands. I shall only describe the instruments which I employ, and touch briefly upon the more notable points of those commonly used by other operators.

Lithotrites.—The lithotrite (Fig. 106) may be called upon in any operation to perform two very different functions—viz., to crush a stone of some size and perhaps of great hardness, and to catch and

[1] For this purpose a small bottle of 10% nitrate-of-silver solution, a dropper, small and large graduates, and a box of boric-acid crystals form an adequate outfit. One gramme of the silver solution to 400 (approximately 10 minims to 8 ounces) of water make a 1:4,000 nitrate-of-silver solution.

crush small crumbling fragments that are only just too large for aspiration. For the former purpose a heavy, powerful lithotrite with a fenestrated female blade (Fig. 107) is required, while for the latter I prefer a lighter instrument with a solid female blade of a broad duck-bill shape. A complete outfit should include these and several intermediate varieties of lithotrites, as the surgeon's judgment dictates. Small lithotrites are made for children.

The powerful lithotrite should possess several characteristics: (1) The male blade must fit entirely within the fenestrated female blade: this minimizes the danger of catching the bladder wall; (2) the male blade when screwed home should pass quite through the female blade: an instrument thus constructed cannot become clogged; (3) the wheel (Fig. 108) or globe (Fig.

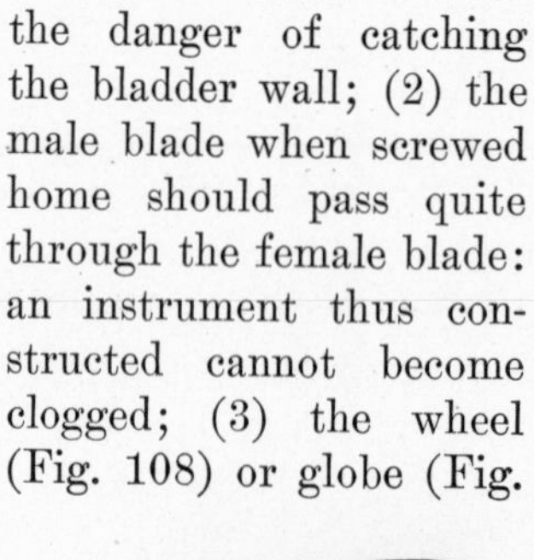

Fig. 106.

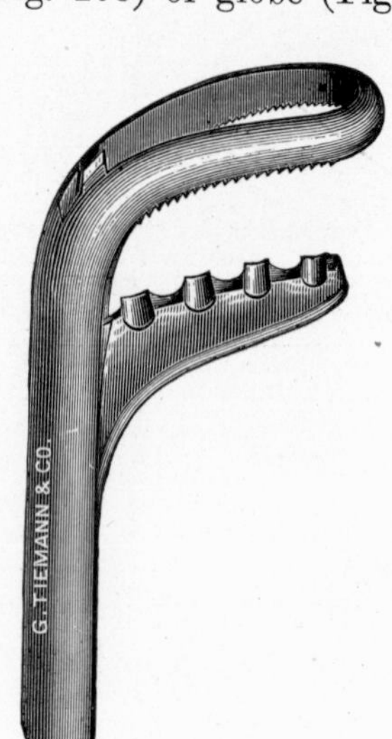

Fig. 107.

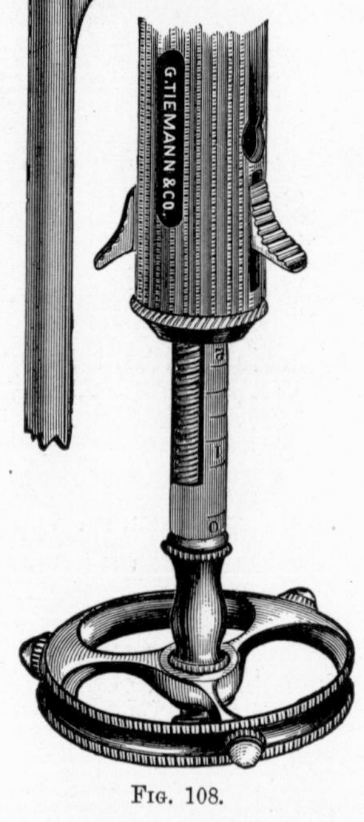

Fig. 108.

106) handle of the instrument must be large enough to afford firm purchase for the surgeon's hand (instrument makers have a tendency to neglect this point upon which the utility of the instrument largely depends); (4) the catch for adjusting the screw action should be sufficiently prominent to be worked without the least difficulty. In my

instrument (a modification of Réliquet's) the catch is saddle-shaped (Fig. 108). Bigelow's lithotrite (Figs. 106, 109) has a forward curve at the toe of the female blade which assists its passage over an enlarged prostate, but carries the bite of the instrument away from the wall of the bladder so that it cannot crush small fragments. Chismore had added to his lithotrite an automatic hammer such as dentists use, and with it claims to crush the hardest and largest stones with scarcely any effort.

For small, soft fragments a flat-bladed, duck-bill instrument is useful. This instrument should only be employed towards the end of the operation. The non-fenestrated blade has a tendency to clog, but this instrument will, in my hand, pick up fragments that no other lithotrite will catch. For small, hard fragments I employ a light, small-bladed fenestrated instrument.

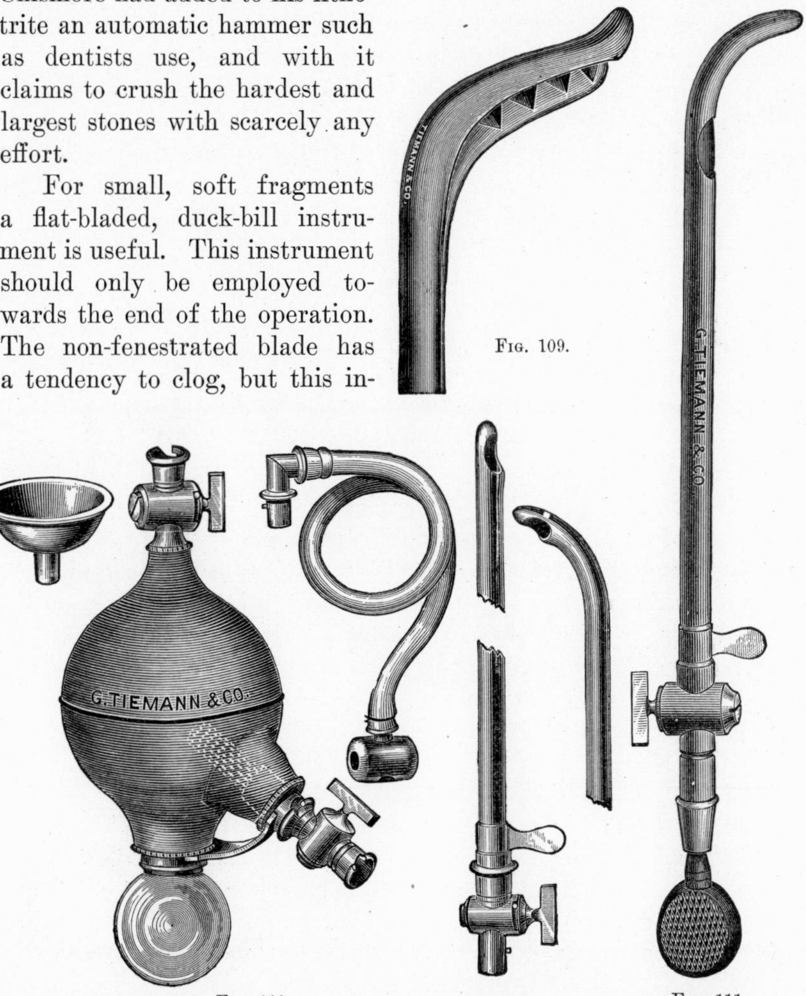

Fig. 109.

Fig. 110.

Fig. 111.

The Aspirator.—The aspirator or washing-bottle of Bigelow (Fig. 110), as now perfected, I prefer to any other. The aspirating lithotrite of Chismore I have employed but once, and cannot say that I found it advantageous.

Washing-tubes.—Bigelow's tubes (Fig. 110) are equal to any others. The large terminal eye, when placed just within the vesical orifice, acts quite as thoroughly as can any straight tube. Although I formerly used a straight tube I have abandoned it. Its introduction causes a great deal of bruising and it has no special advantages. Guyon's tube, which has two eyes, is excellent to search for the last fragment, for the water rushing through its two eyes causes more commotion of the contents of the bladder than occurs with any single-eyed instrument. But in my hands it seems more liable to catch the bladder wall, and therefore I rarely use it. To catch the last fragment I prefer a tube of my own (Fig. 111), which is, for all purposes of introduction, a short curved sound. Its eye is on the concave side of the junction, between shaft and beak, and is protected by an obturator. It has also a stop-cock in its shaft to prevent the escape of fluid from the bladder when the obturator is withdrawn. I find it most useful when introduced and turned beak downward. Its tip then depresses the floor of the bladder into a dependent pouch whose contents are readily aspirated into the eye which overhangs it.

Anesthesia.—Small stones may be aspirated whole or crushed and aspirated from a tolerant bladder without anesthesia. For the majority of cases I have found local anesthesia unsatisfactory. The patient usually suffers a good deal, and his straining may interfere very seriously with the manipulations. When local anesthesia is employed $\frac{1}{4}$ grain of morphin should be administered hypodermically and 2 ounces of whisky by mouth a quarter of an hour before operation. Five minutes later a few drops of a 10% solution of cocain or eucain-B are instilled into the posterior urethra. Five minutes after that 100 grammes of a 2% solution are injected into the bladder. Five minutes later the operation may commence.

This method has not given me any satisfaction, and the use of cocain is not without its dangers. I prefer general anesthesia. For short operations nitrous oxid suffices; longer ones require ether or chloroform.

The Operation.—This is litholapaxy—to catch the stone with an instrument passed through the urethra, to fragment it sufficiently for the detritus to pass out through a tube, and to suck out the *débris* by some suitable apparatus.

The patient is placed upon the operating table on his back with his feet widely separated and a sand-bag beneath his hips. He is then catheterized and 100 to 175 c. c. of warm boric-acid solution injected into the bladder. A lithotrite, selected in accordance with the size of the stone, is then introduced (Fig. 112). It may have to be assisted over the prostate by pressure on the perineum. Once in the bladder, the instrument is passed gently onward until its jaws touch the back wall. Then, gentle tappings along the side wall quickly indicate the position of the stone. When this is found, the jaws of the lithotrite are turned away from it, opened, returned while open over the spot where the stone was found, and, being gently closed, the stone will be grasped. The screw power is now thrown on by the aid of the button in the handle, and a half turn given

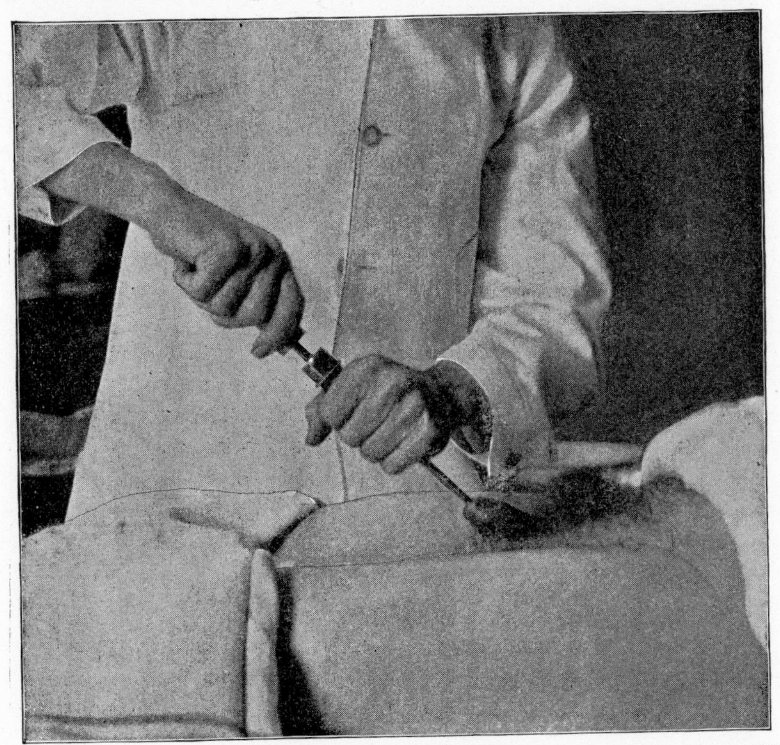

Fig. 112.—Showing the Manner of holding the Lithotrite when opening and shutting in the Search for Fragments.

to the screw. This fixes the stone. As the half turn is being given, the jaws of the lithotrite are to be gently moved away from the bladder-wall towards the centre of the bladder. If a portion of mucous membrane has been entrapped with the stone, the operator instantly appreciates it as an obstacle to the easy rotation of the shaft of the instrument. In such case the jaws are unlocked, the stone allowed to drop out, and another effort made to catch it more cleanly. If the instrument rotates freely to the centre of the bladder, the screw power is firmly applied and the stone fragmented. The large fragments fall on either side, and are easily picked up and again and again fragmented.

With a fenestrated instrument there is no occasion to stop to clear the jaws or to test them for clogging. The work goes evenly on until the operator infers that he has manufactured enough *débris* to make a creditable wash, and then a tube, as large as the urethra will admit, is introduced, the washing-bottle coupled, the stop-cock

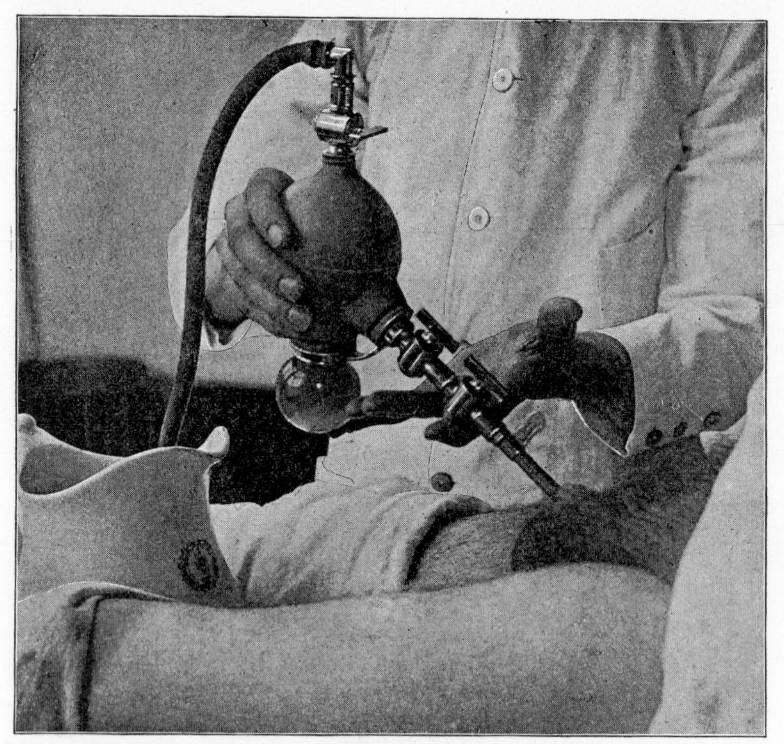

Fig. 113.—Showing the Manner of holding the Bulb. The Left Hand holds the Weight while the Right manipulates it.

turned, and by alternate compressions and relaxations of the bulb the fragments are sucked up into the bottle and fall into the receiver beneath (Fig. 113). Care must be taken to allow no air to enter the bladder. In the case of small tubes this is best averted by pausing in the introduction, when the eye is yet within the prostatic sinus, and filling the tube from a piston syringe. If the tube is large the bottle is simply coupled before the eye reaches the bladder; then, having turned on the stop-cock, the operator waits a moment until he hears the air which was contained in the tube bubble up within the bottle, there to remain out of harm's way in the air-space at the top. Now the bulb is compressed, the prostatic sinus is flooded, and the end of the tube, as it were, floated in through the open gate at the bladder's mouth.

If the tube becomes clogged by a fragment (which the competent operator at once recognises by the increased resistance to his pressure upon the bulb), a forcible compression of the latter will often dislodge the impacted body. Should this maneuvre fail, the bottle must be uncoupled and a catheter or other instrument run down the tube to drive out the impacted piece. Under no circumstances should a tube be withdrawn with a sharp fragment impacted in its eye, for the fragment will scratch if it does not tear the deep urethra and the result will be urethral fever if not abscess or infiltration.

The lithotrite is again introduced, some more *débris* made and removed, and so on until no further click of fragments can be heard as the water swashes in and out of the bladder either by the operator or by an assistant's ear placed against the hypogastrium. For this final search I use my tube (Fig. 111), sometimes supplementing it with Guyon's tube. The latter is especially liable to catch the wall of the bladder, and the unaccustomed ear may be deceived by the muffled, fluttering click thus produced. No description is adequate to distinguish the bladder click from the stone click, but a single experience should fix the distinction clearly in the surgeon's mind.

After the surgeon has thus satisfied himself that no fragment remains in the bladder, a catheter is again introduced and the boric-acid solution drained away. (There is no better criterion of the surgeon's skill than the colour of this solution. The more bloody it is the rougher has been the operation.) A few rapid washes suffice to clear the bladder of clots. The nitrate-of-silver solution (1: 4,000) is injected. As the last grammes are entering the catheter, the instrument is slowly withdrawn, so that the solution bathes the posterior and the anterior urethra. As soon as a few drops trickle from the meatus the catheter is reintroduced and the bladder emptied. The patient is then returned to his bed.

I know no operation of which the success depends so entirely upon the surgeon's skill and technic. What is most difficult to the novice is to crush the stone methodically and deliberately. The first catch and crush is usually easy, and perhaps in a given case it would be possible for an unskilled operator to make quick work of the larger fragments without any particular method; but long before the last fragment has been crushed such an operator will find himself pottering about in the bladder, never finding any considerable fragment, although the clicks upon the aspirators assure him that there is plenty of work left to do. This deadlock may continue quite indefinitely, and the only way to avoid it is to know in exactly what part of the bladder the stone tends to lie and in exactly what part of the bladder the beak of the lithotrite is. The practised surgeon learns these things from the very first touch, and appreciates also the general contour of the bladder, its trabeculæ, saccules, etc. But the neophyte's only hope is to go slowly. He learns by the first grasp whether the stone lies to the right or to the left, whether near the neck of the bladder or far from it, and, accordingly, he can check his tendency to wander fruitlessly about by directing the blades of his instrument to this spot where the larger fragments are almost sure to be found, or by closing the lithotrite and using it as a searcher. It is scarcely necessary to say that the lithotrite has no wider range of motion than any other urethral instrument. It may be pushed forward and backward; it may be rotated; the shaft may be elevated or depressed a few degrees, but any turn of the shaft towards the right or the left is quite unnecessary, and likely to be dangerous. It is also to be noted that when the lithotrite is touching the base of the bladder it is opened by pulling the male blade forward, while to open it near the neck of the bladder the female blade is pushed backward. It is in general easier and safer to crush the stone near the neck of the bladder, and the instinctive tendency of the beginner to let his instrument gravitate towards the fundus must be overcome.

When a fragment is peculiarly elusive it usually lies in some kind of a pocket, from which it may be extracted by rolling the patient to one side or the other, putting him in the Trendelenburg position, or simply by depressing the floor of the bladder with the open lithotrite and imparting a succession of short, sharp jars to the patient's pelvis until the stone rolls into the grasp of the instrument.

After-treatment.—The course of diuretic water and urotropin is resumed as soon as possible after operation. If the bladder is very irritable a catheter may be tied in (p. 210), but as a rule I prefer to let the patient urinate spontaneously, and only use a catheter in case of retention, and for a routine boric-acid wash twice a day. The irritability of the bladder the first few days may be controlled by morphin or by opium suppositories. Nitrate-of-silver injections or instillations afford great relief towards the end of the first week, but they are irritating during the first days.

I consider it unwise to let a patient—especially an old man—get up before a week has passed. He may seem well before that time, but his soreness may return and mild cystitis occur if he gets up too soon. I have in many exceptional instances turned my patient out on the second day, but I do not think well of this. I have indeed operated in my office several times under cocain—and with no anesthetic in the case of small stone—but this again only in exceptional cases.

The after-treatment cannot be considered complete until the patient has been searched for stone one month after the operation, nor can any assurance be given that no fragment has been left behind until this search has been performed. On this occasion the aspirator with a small tube is the best instrument to use. It is, however, more irritating than the searcher.

Complications.—Complications during Operation.—The difficulties most commonly encountered in finding and crushing the stone have already been noticed. It may happen that the stone cannot be crushed, either on account of its great size or hardness, or on account of its position in a small-mouthed pocket. In any such case litholapaxy must be given up and suprapubic lithotomy performed immediately if possible. Clogging is quite impossible with a fenestrated lithotrite.

The complication most to be feared is inability to crush and remove the last fragment. If there is much sacculation or trabeculation of the bladder the last fragment is most elusive, and, rather than protract the operation unduly, it may be preferable to postpone its completion to another time. This concession can only be made with reluctance, since it forfeits the most brilliant advantage of litholapaxy—viz., the entire removal of the stone. Spasm of the bladder is a most annoying feature of operations under local anesthesia, but is rarely troublesome when a general anesthetic is employed.

Post-operative Complications.—After litholapaxy all the complications may occur that are met with after the various operations upon the urinary tract, from catheterism upward: retention, hemorrhage, mild or pernicious urethral fever, cystitis, peri-urethral abscess, epididymitis, or even the graver complications, suppression, surgical kidney (pyelo-nephritis), possibly even pyemia and septicemia; but, as a rule, a careful operation has no sequence but a little temporary discomfort for a week or less, followed by cure.

Impacted fragments in the urethra, one of the horrors of old-fashioned lithotrity, should never occur with this operation. If the bladder is left empty of fragments such a complication is obviously impossible. Should it ever occur, the foreign body may be pushed back into the bladder or removed from the urethra with a Thompson's dilator, or by one of the methods already alluded to (p. 40). Hemorrhage is usually checked by the nitrate-of-silver wash. Should it be profuse and the bladder fill with clots, the easiest way to remove these is by the aspirator, using a small tube. Cystotomy is the last resort.

The commonest post-operative complications are those relating to the prostate and to the kidneys. If the prostate is enlarged and succulent it resents the rough handling to which it is unavoidably subjected and causes the patient much distress for the first few days. Epididymitis and abscess of the prostate are common complications of a litholapaxy roughly performed. But the most skilled hand cannot always prevent a prolonged post-operative prostatic inflammation which may make both patient and surgeon wish that perineal section had been performed. Less frequent, but far more dangerous, are the kidney complications. It is the old man with long-standing cystitis—perhaps one who has been often operated upon for stone—whose kidneys, worn out by retention and infection, are most likely to succumb. Lithotomy is much better suited to such cases, since the atonied, pouched bladder makes litholapaxy a very trying operation, while perineal section is quicker, provides better drainage, and permits removal of the prostatic obstruction causing the recurring stone. But it is vain to argue with these men; they are satisfied with the relief they are accustomed to obtain from litholapaxy and cannot be made to see its lurking dangers.

Relapse after litholapaxy may occur from one of three causes: (1) A fragment may be left by the operator; (2) a new stone may come down from the kidney; or (3) phosphatic reaccumulation may occur in an old catarrhal bladder. The first contingency is guarded against by the thorough search at the end of operation, and again a month later. The second is prevented by the hygienic rules already laid down, or is foreseen by establishing the presence of kidney stone. The third can be prevented only by lithotomy, and not always by that operation. Freyer states that he has had no relapses after litholapaxy, although he has performed it 610 times. I cannot pretend to have equalled this record, nor, I believe, can any other surgeon, but I am sure that litholapaxy, if properly performed, exposes the patient to no more danger of recurrence than does lithotomy, except inasmuch as lithotomy enables the surgeon to deal with obstructive conditions which cannot be reached by litholapaxy.

Statistics and Mortality.—Since no two surgeons recognise exactly the same indications for litholapaxy, no estimate of the mortality after this operation can be made without reference to the proportion of cases submitted to it. Thus I have had 18 deaths (9%) from 198 operations for stone in the bladder. Yet of my 157 litholapaxies I have only lost 7 (4%), and only 1 in my last 63 cases. That one was a prostatic who persuaded me against my judgment, after many days of argument, to crush his stone. He died uremic on the fourteenth day after operation. Had lithotomy been performed upon him I believe he would have lived. Indeed, every one of my deaths after litholapaxy has been caused either by suppression of urine or by chronic uremia. Every one of my patients who has died after being operated upon for stone was over sixty, except one who was fifty-eight years old. Hence I repeat that litholapaxy should have no mortality. The only cause of death after litholapaxy is the uremia to which old men with chronic retention are so liable; and these old men, in whom the danger of uremia may be foreseen, should be submitted, not to litholapaxy, but to lithotomy, in order to give them every chance that rapid operation and good drainage will afford.

PERINEAL LITHOTOMY AND LITHOLAPAXY

Although perineal lithotomy is of a most respectable antiquity, it has, in conjunction with the suprapubic operation, been cast into the shade by the remarkable results of litholapaxy. Indeed, it is doubtful whether the cutting operation can ever regain its prestige as regards the young. But recent perfections of the technic, notably our increasing knowledge of the advantage of galvano-cauterization of the prostate, our better appreciation of the danger of uremia and the means of avoiding it, and the various refinements of anesthesia and antisepsis, combine to make lithotomy preferable to litholapaxy in an ever-increasing proportion of cases. Lithotomy is to be employed, not only when it is impossible to crush a stone, but also when it is impracticable—i. e., when lithotomy would mean a quick, thorough operation as against a tedious incomplete litholapaxy.

The scope of perineal lithotomy has been greatly widened by the application of litholapaxy to it. By this means stones of any size may be removed through the perineum; but it is my personal preference to extract unduly large or hard stones, encysted and adherent stones, and stones complicated by tumour by the suprapubic route, reserving the perineal operation—lithotomy or litholapaxy, as the case may be—for those cases of prostatic hypertrophy complicated by stone in which the stone cannot be dealt with by the urethra, and the prostate can be dealt with through the perineum; especially if the condition of the kidneys is such as to make a speedy operation and good drainage of the utmost importance.

Lateral lithotomy I shall not describe; it has been replaced by perineal litholapaxy.

Preparation for Operation.—The patient is prepared as for any perineal section (p. 201), and the instruments are the same as those employed in external urethrotomy, with the addition of stone forceps (Fig. 114) and scoop (Fig. 115) and a set of litholapaxy instruments.

Fig. 114.
Lithotomy Forceps.

The Operation.—With the patient in the lithotomy position, a grooved staff is introduced into the urethra and pressed forward towards the perineum. The operator, seated on a low stool, punctures the perineum in the median line with a sharp scalpel, carrying it into the groove of the staff, making the external incision not more than an inch long. The surgeon's object is to open the membranous urethra, avoiding the bulb, for incision of the latter gives rise to annoying hemorrhage. It is therefore customary to guide the point of the scalpel by a finger (protected by a finger-cot) introduced into the rectum. With this finger the apex of the prostate is felt, and the scalpel is so introduced as to open the urethra just in front of this point, due care being taken not to open the rectum at the same time. Before removing the scalpel a blunt-pointed bistoury or Blizard knife is introduced alongside of it into the groove of the staff. The scalpel is withdrawn and staff and bistoury together pushed forward into the bladder. A female silver catheter is then introduced through the perineal wound and guided into the bladder along the staff. Immediately a spurt of urine assures the surgeon that he is not in a false passage. The catheter is then replaced by a grooved director and the staff removed. The surgeon then endeavours to introduce his finger, guided by the director, into the bladder. Any constricting bands are cut through. When a free passage has thus been made the director is removed. In the class of cases to which this operation is most appropriate the surgeon will now be confronted by a hypertrophied prostate or a contracted neck of the bladder. This must be dealt with according to his experience (p. 313).

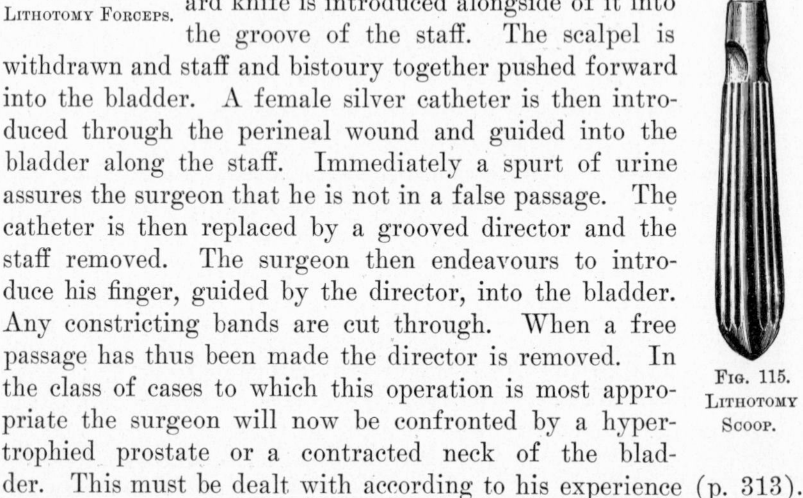

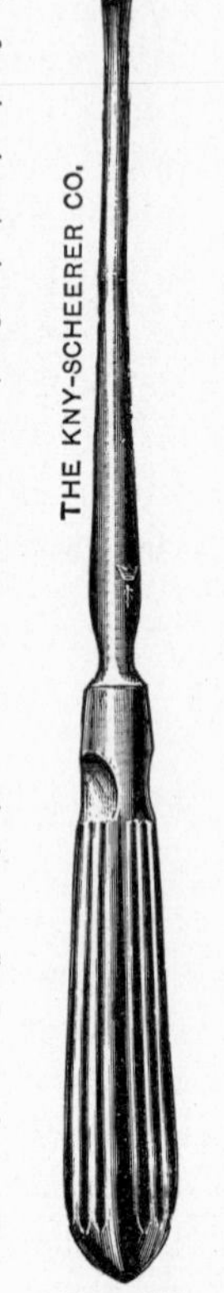

Fig. 115.
Lithotomy Scoop.

When the finger reaches the bladder it usually comes immediately upon the stone. This, if quite small, is extracted by the stone forceps; if large it is crushed and the fragments removed by forceps (Fig. 114) and scoop (Fig. 115), great care being exercised in the removal of angular pieces; or the entire stone may be reduced to fragments small enough to pass through the tube of the aspirator. A short, straight aspirating tube of large calibre (31 French) is useful for this purpose, and my tube for last fragments. Incision of the prostate, which forms part of the old operation for stone, is quite unnecessary, unless that organ is hypertrophied and requires incision for its own sake. Such incision allows much larger stones to be taken away whole; but it is preferable to crush large pieces and to remove them by the scoop or the aspirator. The crushing is effected by a strong lithotrite. Stones too large for such a lithotrite should be removed by suprapubic lithotomy. The operation is terminated by a nitrate-of-silver (1:4,000) wash, and a perineal tube is introduced (p. 204). The after-treatment is the same as for perineal prostatectomy (p. 306). There are no special dangers or complications connected with the removal of the stone. It is not always easy to crush or extract a stone lodged in some pocket tightly surrounded by a spasmodic bladder, and it is especially difficult to remove the last fragment behind a hypertrophied prostate. But if the prostate is dealt with at the same time, adequate drainage is assured, and any dust left behind may be expected to come away during the ensuing days with the irrigations.

SUPRAPUBIC LITHOTOMY

If in any case it is advantageous to see the whole bladder (cases of tumour, ulcer, or saccule), or if the stone is too hard to be crushed and too large to be handled by the perineal or the urethral route, the suprapubic operation should be performed.

The patient is prepared as usual by shaving, soap poultice, catharsis, and urotropin. The surgeon, his assistant, and the instruments are prepared as for any major operation.

Instruments.—The only special instrument employed in this operation is the colpeurynter (Fig. 116). This inflatable rubber bag is greased, introduced into the patient's rectum (after he is on the table), and inflated with some 300 c. c. of air or water. By this means the bladder is distinctly elevated out of the pelvis, and the space on its anterior wall uncovered by peritoneum is thus increased. But the assistance thus rendered is not often material. The practised surgeon can reach the bladder without the aid of the colpeurynter, and hence this ingenious device is little used. Several recorded cases of rupture of the bowel because of overinflation have not added to its popularity.

To the usual armamentarium of scalpels, forceps, scissors, retractors, sutures, etc., a catheter and a lithotomy forceps should be added. I employ a special retractor (Fig. 117) for the upper angle of the wound. Watson's lateral retractors I have never used.

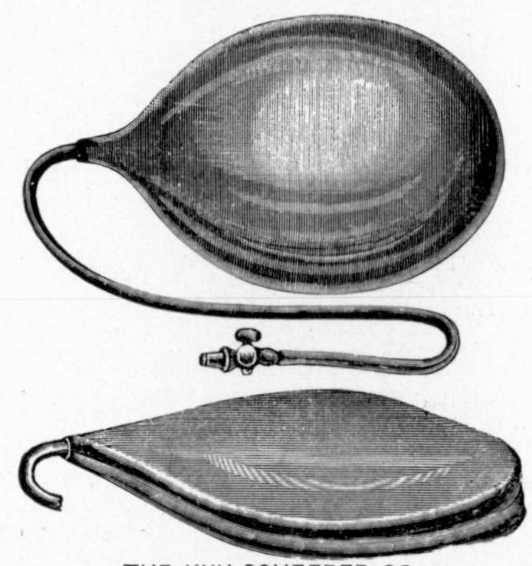

Fig. 116.—The Colpeurynter.

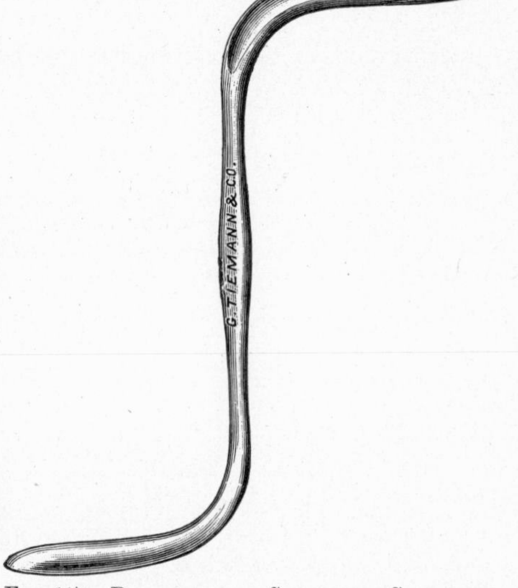

Fig. 117.—Retractor for Suprapubic Cystotomy.

The Operation.—The patient lies on his back. A slight elevation of the hips, or even a full Trendelenburg position, is sometimes useful for the purpose of bringing the contents of the pelvis up towards the abdominal wall.

The first step in the operation is the inflation of the bladder. Some 200–300 c. c. of boric-acid solution are injected through a catheter: more if the bladder is dilated, less if contracted. In order to retain this fluid a rubber catheter is tied around the penis. The removal of this should not be neglected lest it cause gangrene.

The Incision.—A transverse incision through the skin and the inner part of each rectus muscle, or even through the whole muscle, is sometimes employed and gives a larger field of operation than does any vertical incision. But it weakens the abdominal wall considerably and perhaps permanently if the wound is left open to suppurate, as it so often is. The vertical incision is, therefore, generally preferred, and if during the course of the operation more space is required, this incision may be made T-shaped by a transverse cut at its lower extremity. For ordinary purposes, then, a central incision about 3 inches long is made in the middle line, terminating at the pubic symphysis. The superficial fascia is cut through with the skin, the deep fascia more carefully. The sulcus between the recti muscles is sought, but, if not easily found, a central incision is made cleanly through the muscle parallel to its fibres. No separation of the muscles should be made except what is absolutely necessary, for such separation favours the extension of subsequent infiltration. Particularly is it desirable not to poke about with fingers or instruments in the prevesical space behind the symphysis. This is the most dangerous area after the operation, the one in which pus is most likely to form and be a source of complication.

After getting fairly through the muscles, a thin fascia is observed with yellow fat beneath it. This fascia is divided transversely, then the pulp of the finger is placed between the yellow layer of fat and the symphysis, and the fat is rolled upward towards the upper angle of the incision. This layer of yellow fat contains the peritoneum, which is not seen unless adherent, in which case it may be torn into.

Tearing the peritoneum is not an important accident. The wound is quickly sutured with fine catgut and kept out of the way in the upper angle of the incision during the remainder of the operation.

After the fat has been rolled up the bladder is exposed, covered with distended veins. With short-curved needles in a holder, a portion of the bladder is taken up in a broad loop on each side, the silk knotted in long loops, and these are used as retractors. Even though the veins be large they may be disregarded and the bladder boldly cut into between the ligature loops.

As soon as the bladder is opened the fluid gushes from it and it collapses. The penis ligature must now be removed (and the colpeurynter deflated and extracted). Now the bladder is freely opened, the finger enters, finds the stone, and rolls it into a suitable position. With a forceps it is easy to seize and extract any stone or foreign body and to inspect the inside of the organ by using a reflector or an electric light, or by adopting the Trendelenburg position.

The treatment of tumours and prostatic growths through a suprapubic incision has already been considered (pp. 303, 423). No treatment has yet been devised for saccules. Clarke,[1] who has had an unusually wide experience of these cases, states that after lithotomy the sac sometimes contracts down and gives no further trouble; but if its orifice is small and the sac itself large, independent drainage should be provided for it. He suggests the feasibility of perineal drainage, but admits that it has not been employed.

---

[1] Brit. Med. J., 1899, i, 1141.

Drainage.—After cystotomy some kind of drainage—be it suprapubic, perineal, or urethral—is essential. So long as continuous effectual drainage is established the route chosen makes little difference; but there is, as yet, no general agreement among surgeons as to what route possesses the most advantages. It is generally admitted that the suprapubic wound must not be closed unless the bladder is uninfected. In the majority of cases, therefore, suprapubic drainage must be employed. This usually suffices; but if the suprapubic wound is closed, or if any operation is performed upon the prostate, I habitually employ perineal drainage. Urethral drainage by the retained catheter I do not care for after operation, as such a catheter is too small to discharge clots freely. The perineal opening is no source of danger. I have devised a rapid and practically bloodless method of making it.

A large urethral staff is passed into the bladder. With a finger in the rectum as a guide (its tip placed upon the apex of the prostate), a straight bistoury is plunged into the perineum, passed in front of the anterior wall of the rectum and into the groove of the staff near the apex of the prostate. Now a long silver probe is prepared by having a stout silk thread tied through its eye, which thread is passed through the tip of a red rubber catheter, about size 35 French, and out through its lumen, and knotted inside the lumen so as not to pull through. This probe, a little curved at its tip, is passed along the blade of the knife as a guide into the urethra and bladder. The knife before withdrawal is made to enlarge the urethral wound sufficiently—about 1 cm.—and upon its withdrawal is made to cut and enlarge the perineal wound to about the same dimensions. A finger passed through the abdominal wound easily hooks up the probe, and by the aid of the string and the knot the catheter is drawn through the small punctured wound, which it accurately fits, arresting all hemorrhage by its own pressure.

Closure of the Wound.—When there is no cystitis the suprapubic wound may be closed entirely on condition that continuous drainage be provided through the perineum or the urethra. Many complicated methods of suturing the bladder have been devised, but as they assure no special security they may be dismissed. In suturing the suprapubic wound, or any other wound of the bladder, it is only necessary to avoid passing the sutures through the mucous membrane, to make them close enough and strong enough to close the wound completely, and to test the line of suture by inflating the bladder. The wound if once hermetically sealed to the passage of water or air may be depended upon to remain so. These rules are carried out in practice as follows:

1. Before suturing the bladder a perineal tube is inserted.

2. The bladder is then closed by a continuous suture of catgut or light chromicized gut passing only through the muscular coat.

3. This line of suture is tested by injecting fluid through the perineal tube.

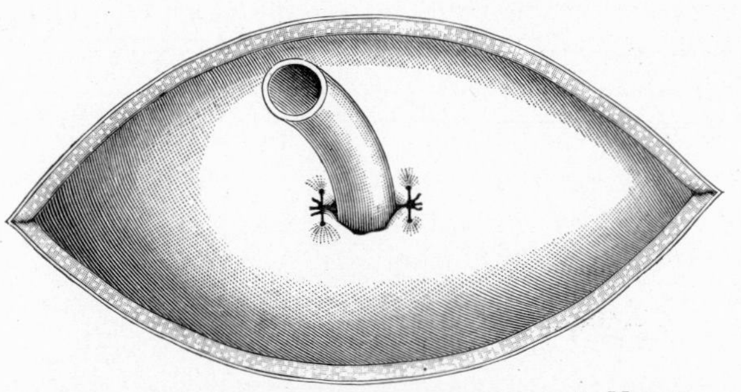

Fig. 118.—Drainage of the Bladder, Gibson's Method. Tube inserted and stitches employed to diminish size of opening.

4. Any weak spot is strengthened by an additional stitch and the whole may be further protected by Lembert sutures.

5. If there is any doubt in the surgeon's mind as to the possibility of infection or infiltration the abdominal wound is provided with a sufficient number of provisional sutures and packed. At the end of forty-eight hours the packing is removed and the sutures tied. Otherwise the abdominal wall is closed by a single set of transfixing sutures or in layers.

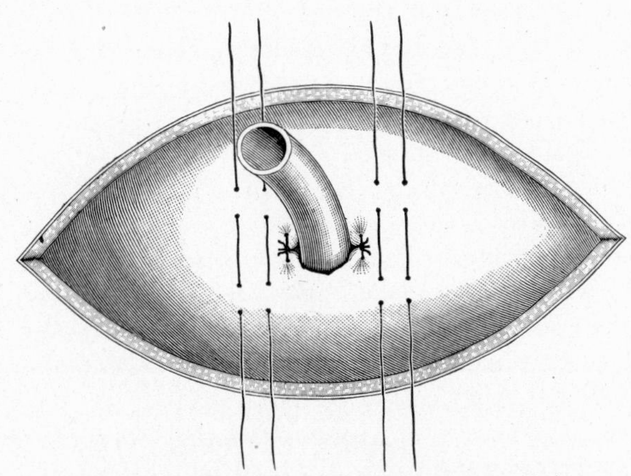

Fig. 119.—Drainage of the Bladder, Gibson's Method. First set of inversion sutures in place ready for tying.

But in the majority of cases, after all, the surgeon is unable or unwilling to dispense with suprapubic drainage. In infected cases he dares not close the suprapubic wound. In clean cases the advantage of closing the wound is the avoidance of a prolonged convalescence with an annoying, unmanageable suprapubic fistula. A recent suggestion by Gibson [1] will, if it fulfils its early promise, revolutionize our ideas upon this matter. The proposed operation is quite simple, being an adaptation of Kader's operation for gastrostomy. A drainage-tube is placed in the bladder wound, which is sutured close

[1] Med. Record, 1901, lix, 45.

about it (Fig. 118). Two inversion sutures are then introduced above and below the tube (Fig. 119); these are tied and a second row introduced (Fig. 120). The tying of these completes the closure of the bladder wall. As a result the tube is tightly hugged by the bladder so that no urine can escape around it, and the inversion is such (Fig. 121) that, when the tube is removed, the funnel-shaped opening is rapidly and permanently closed by the intravesical pressure.

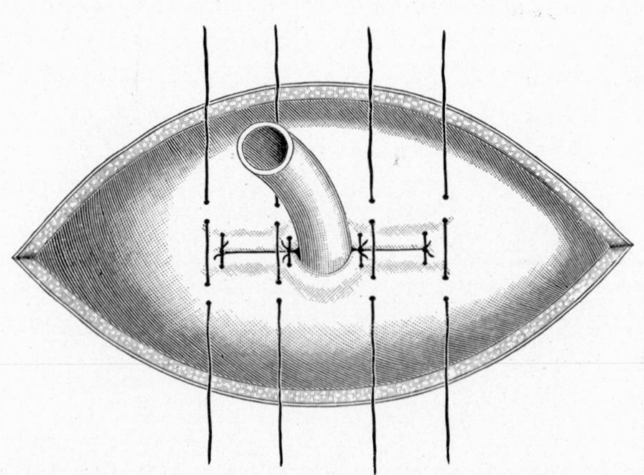

Fig. 120.—Drainage of the Bladder, Gibson's Method. First set of sutures tied, second set in place for tying.

I have not yet had the opportunity of testing this method thoroughly, but I have seen admirable results from it, not a drop of leakage occurring either while the tube was in place or after its removal. If such results can be depended upon from this method, the necessity of risking a complete closure of the bladder will be done away with; and in those cases where prolonged or permanent suprapubic drainage is necessary, the adoption of such a procedure will also do away with the leakage during the first weeks after operation while the wound is closing down about the drainage-tube. Indeed, the chief objection to suprapubic cystotomy is that, with the old methods it has been impossible in the majority of cases to obtain satisfactory drainage. With the double siphon of Guyon, as well as with the self-retaining catheter of Pezzer, it has been impossible to prevent a great deal of overflow alongside the tube. This overflow is often sufficient to soil the patient's dressings, linen, and bed-clothes many times a day and to keep him, at least for the first few days after

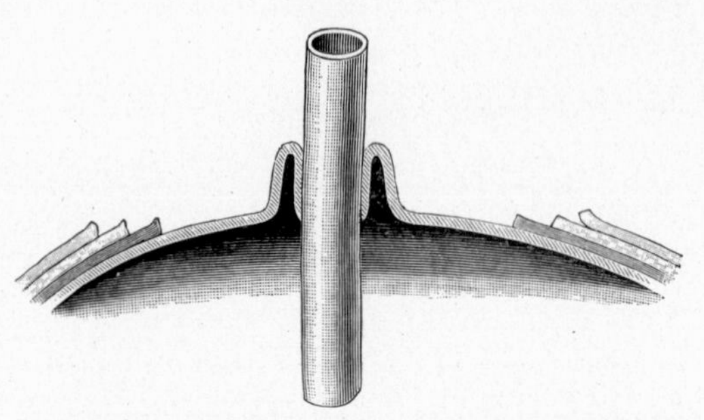

Fig. 121.—Drainage of the Bladder, Gibson's Method. Longitudinal section, showing bladder infolded by two sets of sutures.

operation, bathed in a pool of ammoniacal urine anything but aromatic. As suggested by Dr. Gibson, it would be well to use a double tube for drainage, one tube to be kept closed and used only for irrigation, in order that the other—the real drainage-tube—need not be disturbed.[1]

A metal tube for continuous drainage (Fig. 92) may be introduced at the time of operation or a few days thereafter.

After-treatment.—The dressings must be changed as often as they become soiled. The bladder should be irrigated at first twice a day, later once a day. If perineal drainage has been employed the tube is removed towards the end of the first week. The suprapubic wound need not be kept open longer than five days unless more prolonged drainage is demanded by the condition of the bladder.

Mortality and Statistics.—I have performed suprapubic lithotomy 19 times with 7 deaths (37%); and 20 perineal lithotomies with 5 deaths (25%). Of the 7 fatal suprapubic sections, 3 were prostatectomies and 3 were performed as a last resort after the failure of litholapaxy. Of the 5 fatal perineal cases, 2 were subsequent to futile litholapaxy. My preference for litholapaxy is almost entirely due to the fact that it is easier for the patient. It requires less preparation, less after-treatment, and insures the sufferer more comfort. But I see no reason why a lithotomy, whether suprapubic or perineal, performed on a comparatively healthy man should prove fatal. All of my patients that have died have been old men with foul bladders and *damaged kidneys*, and this was their weak spot, a weak spot even for litholapaxy. Four of my patients who died were distinctly uremic and 4 distinctly septic before operation. Of the remaining 4, 1 died of pyemia, the remaining 3 of uremia due to the operation; and all of them—not only those who died but a large proportion of those who did not die—were recognised to be in a condition where any surgical interference must be a matter of the gravest moment. But when a patient's symptoms are absolutely unbearable, when they are threatening to terminate his life, there is no choice. Something must be done to relieve him, and the bare chance that he may survive the operation must be taken; for even should it hasten his death, that is better than to leave him to continued misery leading certainly to a fatal termination.

---

[1] Intermittent siphonage has been found useful by Dawbarn (J. Am. Med. Ass'n, 1901, xxxvii, 1231) and others in order to encourage suprapubic drainage. Better results may be expected from the method, recently introduced in France, of continuous instillation of salt solution through a retained urethral catheter.

FOREIGN BODIES IN THE BLADDER

Besides the foreign bodies[1] which find their way into the bladder through wounds, or come down the ureters (renal calculi), a host of substances have been encountered in the bladder introduced through the urethra. All imaginable articles, such as pins, beads, stones, pieces of straw, heads of grain, glass tubing, pipe-stems, pencils, portions of chalk, wax, etc., have been found in the male bladder, introduced there through the urethra under the influence of morbid erotic fancies. In this way substances of every conceivable description which the orifice of the urethra will admit are introduced into the canal and again extracted, until, on some unlucky occasion, the object slips beyond the grasp and remains fixed in the deep urethra or the bladder. The patient's shame will often deter him from seeking relief; the foreign body may create no disturbance at first, and so he flatters himself that everything is all right, until, sooner or later, perhaps long after he has forgotten his boyish folly, symptoms of stone arise, and this when removed is found to have formed upon a nucleus introduced from without (Fig. 122).

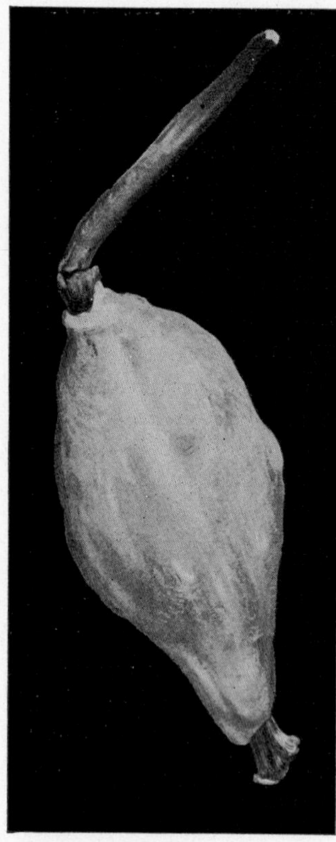

Fig. 122.—Phosphatic Calculus formed upon a Twig.

Not infrequently, however, a foreign body comes legitimately, as it were, into the bladder; dermoid cysts containing bones, teeth, and hair, may discharge into its cavity. The broken end of a catheter may constitute the foreign body, usually in cases where the individual is himself obliged to have frequent recourse to a catheter. The old-fashioned gutta-percha bougie has fallen into disfavour on account of its peculiar brittleness. Again, substances of all sorts—bone, seeds, etc.—may enter the bladder through fistulæ, while splinters, bullets, and bone may be lodged there traumatically.

The natural history of a foreign body in the bladder is that it

[1] *Cf.* Poulet, Foreign Bodies in Surgery, translation. N. Y., 1880, p. 145.

causes some irritation, becomes surrounded with mucus, and thus becomes a nucleus for stone. In this respect blood-clots, tumours, fragments of tumours, ulcers, and kidney stones act like foreign bodies, inasmuch as they may become centres of stone formation unless they are passed from the urethra.

Treatment.—If the foreign body be a portion of catheter or bougie, the patient will usually hasten to tell his troubles and demand relief. If, however, it be some other foreign body, he will probably demand relief from his cystitis, all the while denying any knowledge of its cause, even after the foreign body has been extracted. When the nature of the substance in the bladder has been learned, an attempt should be made at extraction, to prevent it from becoming a nucleus for stone. If there be much cystitis present, rest in bed, with demulcents and some anodyne, for several days before the operation, is advisable. Anything which will go into the urethra would come out again if it could be correctly seized and drawn upon in a correct line, with its point turned backward; consequently, an attempt should be made to reach all long bodies, such as pencils, and all small bodies by using a small lithotrite or other forceps designed for this special purpose, of which there are several varieties kept by instrument-makers. If the object be seized in a faulty diameter it may be released and caught again. This rule applies to portions of metallic catheters as well. It is exceedingly difficult to catch them correctly; soft catheters, however, are very easy to extract; they become doubled up, and may be withdrawn however caught. The difficulty in seizing a portion of soft catheter is that it cannot be felt on account of giving no click or grating against a metallic forceps; consequently, in the search for such a foreign body, the blades of the lithotrite have to be shut occasionally over different parts of the bladder surface, until the offending body is caught. Care must be exercised, of course, not to catch a fold of the bladder. The cystoscope is of assistance here.

Two substances, wax and glass, demand a special notice. The former becomes so soft at the temperature of the body that not only can it not be felt, but, if seized, can only be taken away piecemeal, and some portion is pretty sure to remain behind. As to glass and other brittle substances, the danger of injuring the bladder in attempts at extraction with forceps renders all such efforts, as a rule, unadvisable. Consequently, for all foreign bodies of wax or glass, and for all such as cannot be extracted after patient effort with the lithotrite, cystotomy should be performed, and this as early as possible, before the foreign body has had time to become encrusted with urinary salts. If for any reason the operation has to be postponed, the bladder should be washed daily in order to retard calculous deposit upon the nucleus. Dr. Douglas, of Rondout, N. Y., in cutting a patient to extract a piece of glass, fearing that pressure with his forceps might splinter it in the bladder during extraction, devised the ingenious expedient of covering the blades of his forceps with soft molasses candy, knowing that if any of this substance was left in the bladder it would melt and pass away. The device was fully successful.

CHAPTER XXX

ANATOMY, PHYSIOLOGY, AND EXAMINATION OF THE URETER

There are many diseases of the ureters, such as simple and tubercular ureteritis, renal colic, and stone in the ureter, that are too intimately bound up with the diseases of the kidney to be dealt with separately. They can only be touched upon in this section of the work, but will receive more generous mention with the kindred maladies of the kidney. As a matter of fact, the chief interest of ureteral surgery centres about the various operative procedures, exploratory and plastic, to which they are subjected, and to these the subsequent chapters will be chiefly devoted.

ANATOMY

The ureter is the excretory duct of the kidney. It is a fibro-muscular tube beginning as the funnel-shaped neck of the renal pelvis and terminating at the lateral angle of the trigone of the bladder. There is normally one ureter for each kidney. Each ureter is from 35 to 40 cm. (14 to 16 inches) long. The ureter is, when empty, a closed tube like the urethra. Its physiological calibre is that of a cylinder about 0.3 cm. ($\frac{1}{8}$ inch) in diameter. The lumen of the ureter is slightly constricted at three points: (1) A distinct narrowing at a point about 2 cm. from its upper extremity, (2) a slight narrowing where it crosses the brim of the pelvis, and (3) a muscular constriction at its entrance into the bladder.

Structure.—The ureter is composed of 3 coats: the fibrous, the muscular, and the mucous.

The *fibrous* external coat runs continuously from the fibrous envelope of the kidney and its pelvis to the bladder. It is a tough, glistening, elastic tissue.

The *muscular* coat consists of an external longitudinal and an internal circular layer of smooth muscle. It is well developed in both the ureter and the pelvis of the kidney. In the calices it thins out to a few stray fibres. At the vesical extremity of the ureter its muscle pierces that of the bladder and is continued as a band of fibres running along each edge of the trigone. Thus there is one band joining the two ureters (interureteric muscle) which sometimes raises a distinct transverse fold in the mucous membrane, while another thinner band of fibres runs from each ureter towards the neck of the bladder. The ureter possesses no proper sphincter. Its power of resisting regurgitation from the bladder is due to its oblique course through the muscular wall of the bladder, and to the constriction of the bladder muscle, which automatically closes the ureteral orifices as it contracts to force the urine into the urethra.

The *mucous membrane* of the ureter is smooth and thrown into longitudinal folds when the organ is collapsed. The epithelium consists of several superposed layers, the deeper ones conical or ovoidal, the superficial ones cuboidal or flattened. Though some expert microscopists claim to be able to distinguish the epithelium of the pelvis of the kidney from that of the ureter, most conservative observers confess their inability to make such a distinction, and do not even venture to assert that any given cells in the urine come from any part of the ureter or its pelvis unless the presumption is confirmed by other signs, notably the presence of renal casts and albumin.

Relations.—The ureter lies immediately behind the peritoneum throughout almost its whole length. It is firmly attached to this structure so that when the peritoneum is detached from the parietes it carries the ureter with it. When this dissection is performed by the finger the ureter may be identified as a cord interrupting the smooth yielding surface of the peritoneum within 3 cm. ($1\frac{1}{2}$ inches) of the spinal column. In the abdomen the ureter lies upon the psoas muscle and crosses the genito-crural nerve. It is in turn crossed by the spermatic (or ovarian) vessels. On the right side it lies close to the vena cava. At the brim of the pelvis it crosses the common iliac vessels at or near their termination. Thence it plunges down in a fold of peritoneum (posterior false ligament of the bladder), passes under the arch of the vas deferens, and lies external to it, entering the bladder wall close above the seminal vesicle and about 2 cm. from the median line. Thence it runs 2 cm. obliquely forward and inward through the bladder muscle and beneath the mucous membrane, and emerges at the angle of the trigone 3 cm. from its fellow and the same distance from the urethral orifice.

Topographical Anatomy.—The ureter, like the kidney, can very rarely be felt when in a normal state. When tender or enlarged, however, in a thin subject it may be traced almost from the kidney to the brim of the pelvis. In fleshy subjects it can only be felt at this latter point—viz., at the outer edge of the rectus muscle on a line joining the anterior spines of the ilia. Tenderness at this point can always be distinguished by palpation, and if the patient is not overfat an enlarged ureter can be rolled between the finger and the iliac artery. In the female pelvis the ureter is readily felt through the vaginal vault almost up to the pelvic brim. But in the male it is only in exceptional cases that tenderness or enlargement at the lower extremity of the ureter can be appreciated by rectal touch in the region just internal to the base of the seminal vesicle.

PHYSIOLOGY

The ureter transmits the urine from the kidney to the bladder partly through the force of gravity, but chiefly by its peristaltic action. Waves of contraction run along it quite as they do along the intestine, and as each wave reaches the bladder the ureteral orifice becomes slightly raised and tumefied, emits a little jet of urine, and then sinks back again. This is perhaps the most picturesque phenomenon observable through the cystoscope. The contractions of the two ureters are quite independent and not often synchronous. They recur irregularly every five, ten, or twenty seconds. Exceptionally the intervals are much longer.

Like the bladder, the ureter is insensitive to touch unless inflamed. But, like the bladder, it is extremely sensitive to distention—witness the agonizing pain of renal colic. Whether those obscure cases of renal colic attending the passage of concentrated crystalline urine (p. 631) are due to distention or to simple scratching of the ureteral walls it is impossible to say. Dr. Bryson has recently advanced the theory that pain of the upper third of the ureter is radiated to the kidney, pain of the middle third to the abdomen, and pain of the lower third to the bladder and urethra. While this may often be the case, I cannot accept the conclusion that the vesical pain of renal origin, which so often mystifies the most expert, is always due to an irritation at the lower end of the ureter. I believe that this pain is often due to a disturbance purely in the renal pelvis without any implication of the ureter.

EXAMINATION

The methods of examining the ureter are reducible to two: (1) Palpation; (2) urethral catheterization and its various modifications.

Palpation

The ureter may be palpated through the abdominal wall, through the rectum (the vagina in the female), or through an exploratory incision (p. 637).

Abdominal Palpation.—It is practically impossible to distinguish tenderness in the upper part of the ureter from tenderness in the kidney itself, and any ureteral swelling in the loin is overshadowed by the associated renal enlargement. In feeling for the ureter through the abdomen deep palpation is first employed at the point where the ureter crosses the pelvic brim. If the rounded tube can be made to slip under the finger here it may sometimes be followed, especially if tender, up the outer border of the rectus for a short distance; but unless greatly distended it becomes quite lost to abdominal palpation a few centimetres above the umbilicus.

Rectal Palpation.—When ureteral stone is suspected, rectal palpation should always be employed on the chance that a stone impacted in the lower end of the duct may thus be diagnosed. It is noteworthy that in one of Bishop's [1] cases a stone that could not be felt by vaginal touch was palpable through the rectum.

The ureter is felt for just above the seminal vesicle, about 1 cm. from the median line.

Vaginal Palpation.—As the ureters curve upward, outward, and backward around the cervix from the trigone of the bladder, they are readily palpable through the vaginal vault when diseased, and may also usually be felt when normal. The trigone of the bladder terminates at a point on the anterior vaginal wall about 2 cm. below the cervix. Each ureter may be traced outward and backward from this region as a firm cord. Recognition of the normal ureter by palpation requires considerable skill.

Ureteral Catheterization

It is interesting but quite unnecessary to dwell upon the various measures that have been suggested in former years for the purpose of collecting the urine of each kidney separately. Surgeons have long been awake to the utility of such a proceeding, and many very ingenious methods have been devised for obstructing one ureter while allowing the urine to flow freely from the other. The sum of them all was failure. The next step was to introduce a catheter directly into one or both ureters by means of some kind of a cystoscope (the attempt at catheterization without cystoscopy having

[1] Edinburgh Med. J., 1889, vi, 47.

proved futile). Latest has come Harris's ingenious device for dividing the bladder into two reservoirs from each of which the urine of one kidney may be drawn separately. We need only concern ourselves with these last two devices—catheterization and segregation.

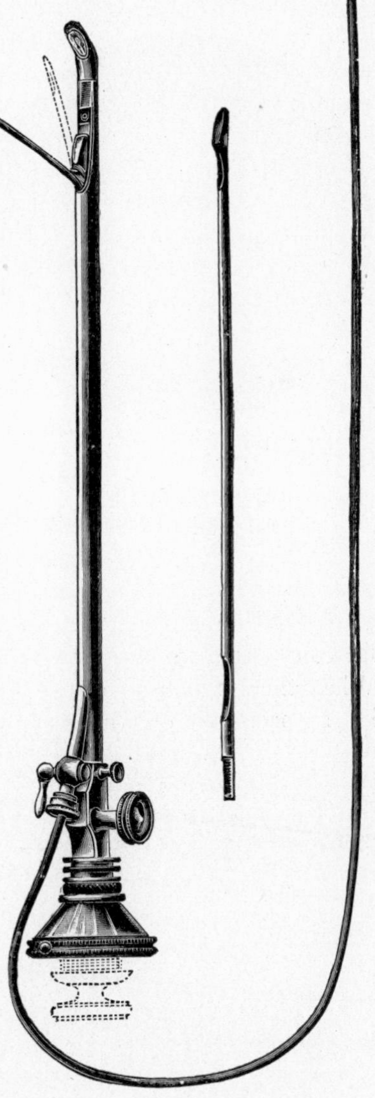

Fig. 123.

The ureteral catheter may be introduced by means of the so-called optical cystoscope (p. 330) or through the straight tube employed by Kelly. The latter apparatus is not generally applicable in the male and therefore merits no consideration here, although it may be said, by the way, that for simplicity and cleanliness it far surpasses the other method. In the female I always employ Kelly's tubes. Dr. Chetwood has fitted the lamp of his urethroscope to this instrument, and I have found the modification most useful.

For ureteral catheterization by the optical cystoscope patient and instrument are prepared as for cystoscopy, though general anesthesia is usually preferable here. The *choice of instruments* must lie with the surgeon. The three instruments most in favour at present are those of Casper, Albarran, and Nitze. I have employed Casper's instrument; but though it has several points of superiority, the optical apparatus is so poor that I prefer Nitze's new modification of Albarran's cystoscope (Fig. 123). Even this leaves much to be desired, and an improvement upon it will doubtless soon appear; but for the present it seems the best we have. A detailed description of the instrument is unnecessary. The manipulation of its simple mechanism can only be learned by practice.

Technic.—*To find the ureteral orifice* is the first point. As this is the most difficult part of the operation it should be undertaken with the utmost care and precision. The cystoscope is introduced (p. 332) and its beak turned directly downward. The light is then turned on and the instrument adjusted by pulling it out or pushing it in until the dark circle of the neck of the bladder intrudes upon the field of vision. It is then slowly rotated to an angle of 30° to 45° from the perpendicular. During this procedure the surgeon watches attentively every portion of the mucous membrane that comes into view. The mouth of the ureter may project prominently and unmistakably, or it may be quite invisible. Sometimes it appears as an oblique slit in the mucous membrane (Fig. 124), sometimes as a gaping crater. It may be flat upon the bladder wall or it may be distinctly elevated on a little mound. One of its most striking characteristics, one that often calls attention to it, is its intermittent muscular contraction which accompanies the ejection of a little jet of urine.

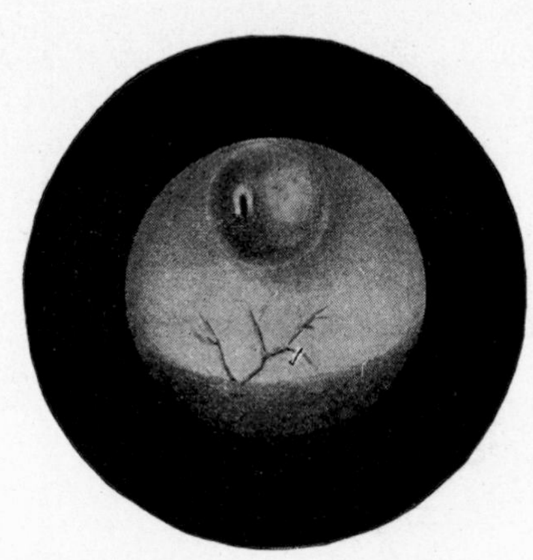

FIG. 124.—(NITZE.)

When the surgeon spies a point that he suspects is the mouth of the ureter, but of which he is not certain, he has only to wait until he sees the little slit gather itself together and eject the urine (Fig. 125), and by this he recognises it definitely. At the same time he will note whether the jet consists of limpid urine, of cloudy pus, or of dark blood.

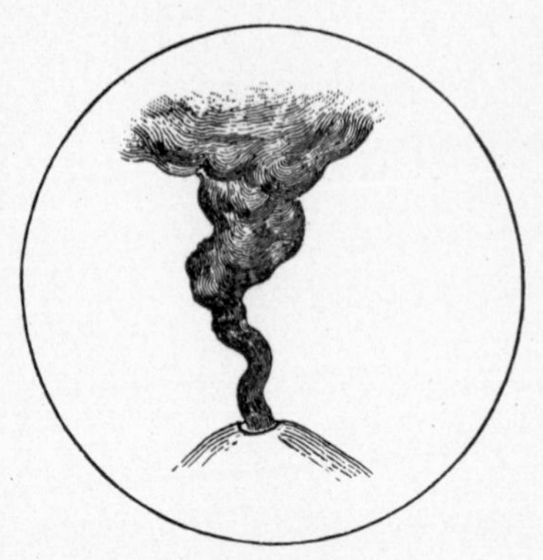

FIG. 125.

It may be no easy matter to find the ureteral orifice. If it is not found after a short search of ten minutes or so, the cystoscope may be extinguished and withdrawn and a greater quantity of fluid introduced on the chance that the orifice may have been hidden by a fold of mucous membrane. But, whatever difficulties may be encountered, they must be overcome by methodical gentleness. The operator who allows himself to become flurried is lost. There must be no haste, no aimless wandering about. If the ureter is to be found at all, it will be met with very near the neck of the bladder and not more than 2 cm. from the median line. It is useless to wander over a wider field.

To introduce the catheter may be impossible; but, as a rule, this depends solely upon finding the ureteral orifice. I have said that the finding of the ureter is the most difficult part of the operation, because when the ureter is once found and the cystoscope properly placed in relation to it, the catheter may then be introduced perfectly well unless there is some physical peculiarity of the case that makes the operation impossible. In other words, if the operation is possible at all its success depends more upon the discovery of the ureter and the proper position of the cystoscope than upon anything else. The position of the cystoscope should be such that the ureteral orifice is brought as near as possible to the lens. For this purpose the shaft of the instrument must be turned towards the ureter. Unless this is done the operation is incredibly difficult.

With the instrument thus closely approximated to the ureter, the catheter (which has been previously tested to prove that its lumen is clear) is pushed slowly into the cystoscope until it appears inside the bladder. The little director (if the Nitze instrument is used) is then elevated a trifle and the catheter again pushed forward. If it tends to pass beyond the ureteral orifice the director is turned up more sharply, or the instrument is withdrawn a trifle, and so by a series of trials, with the cystoscope always as near as possible to the ureteral orifice, the catheter is finally introduced. Success is not yet certain, but the difficult part of the task is now accomplished. The catheter is gently impelled onward until it has been introduced about 5 cm. into the ureter. This is far enough for a ureteral catheterization; for other purposes it may be necessary to introduce it further. The lamp of the cystoscope is extinguished and the instrument slowly extracted, great care being taken not to disturb the catheter. In order to avoid pushing the catheter too far into the bladder it is well to make a characteristic scratch upon it before beginning to extract the cystoscope, in order that there may be some means of knowing the exact point at which it should be fixed. The catheter is tied in like a filiform bougie and its end is carried into a small sterilized bottle which it is convenient to attach to the patient's thigh by means of adhesive plaster.

If the urine flows freely it should require not more than two hours to collect 25 c. c. of urine, which is all that is needed for the purposes of examination.

Urine Segregation.—I abstract a description of this instrument and its employment from the writings [1] of its inventor, Dr. M. L. Harris, of Chicago.

The chief part of the instrument (Fig. 126) might be described as a twin catheter, the shaft of which is inclosed in a metal sleeve. Each half of the double beak may be rotated outward independently. To the outer extremity of each half glass bottles may be attached to receive the urine, and a rectal lever is held to the shaft of the catheter by means of a fulcrum and spring. The whole instrument may be sterilized by boiling.

Anesthesia is obtained by injecting into the rectum—

℞		
℞	Antipyrin	1 gramme
	Tr. opii	1 c. c.
	Water	90 c. c.

This solution produces anesthesia of the floor of the bladder after thirty minutes, which time is employed in preparing for the operation.

The anterior and the posterior urethra are successively washed, and the bladder irrigated until the fluid returns clean. Then 60 c. c. of a 5% solution of suprarenal extract is injected into the bladder and allowed to remain there ten minutes. This is then drawn off, the bladder washed once more, and 15 to 20 c. c. of a 2% cocain solution is injected and allowed to remain in the bladder for six minutes.

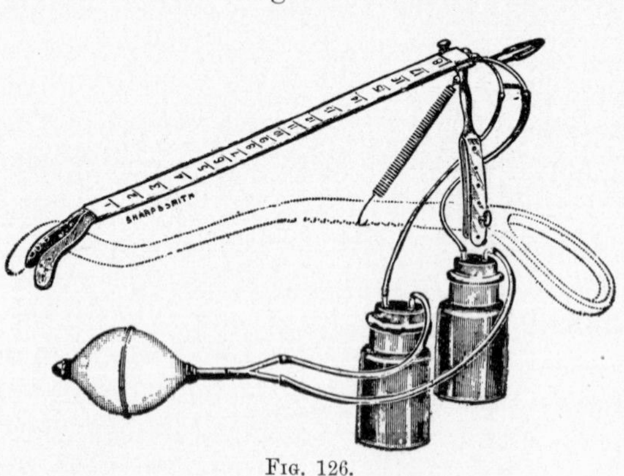

Fig. 126.

This is drained off, the bladder irrigated once again, and the patient is ready.

With the patient lying on his back, his knees drawn up, the lubricated catheter is introduced very gently until its beak is well within the bladder. During this time the outer ends of the catheter are attached to a short circuit of rubber tubing. The fulcrum crutch is attached to the shaft of the catheter some 2 or 3 cm. from its outer

[1] J. of the Am. Med. Ass'n, 1898, xxx, 236. Med. Record, 1899, lv, 457. Annals of Surgery, 1900, xxxii, 149.

extremity. Now the rectal lever is lubricated and introduced into the rectum. It is attached by the fulcrum and spring and carefully held in the median line (it has a tendency, before the catheter is turned down, to slip off sideways). Finally, each half of the catheter is rotated gently downward through an arc of 120°, or thereabouts, until it is felt to rest gently upon the floor of the bladder (too great a pressure might occlude the ureter). The whole instrument is then gently withdrawn until it rests against the neck of the bladder. The shaft of the rectal lever should now be in a line with the patient's body, the catheter inclined obliquely. With the instrument in this position, the end of the rectal lever projecting between the two catheters elevates the floor of the bladder into a ridge on each side of which is a pocket, each pocket drained by a separate catheter. The short-circuit tube is now removed and the fluid in the bladder allowed to drain off. It may be necessary to wait a few minutes until the instrument becomes filled with urine. Each curved tube is then attached to its own bottle; the straight tubes are connected again by the short-circuit tubing after the flow of urine has been started by a few gentle squeezes of the aspirating bulb. Vigorous aspiration is only harmful. It causes hemorrhage by sucking the mucous membrane into the instrument.

The instrument must usually be left in place for thirty minutes in order to obtain enough urine to examine. Harris estimates the normal functional capacity of the kidney at 0.16 c. c. of urine per minute per kilo of body weight. This is an average estimate as the urine descends intermittently. After the desired amount of urine has been obtained, the catheters are folded back, the rectal lever detached, the instrument extracted, and the operation closed by a final washing of the bladder.

Advantages and Disadvantages.—In attempting a comparison between the ureteral catheter and the urine segregator it must be remembered that the latter has a much more restricted range of usefulness than the former. The urine segregator has no therapeutic uses while the ureter catheter has many. The instruments can only be compared in the field of diagnosis. Even in this field comparison is not easy, for the surgeon who is accustomed to using the ureteral catheter will obtain better results from it, while he who is familiar with the segregator will find this the more useful. In general it may be said that the segregator is by far the easier instrument to use. Yet this is not said in order to encourage a careless handling of the instrument, for carelessness is more likely to cause the operator to fail than any other one thing. Two errors may be committed. The instrument may be so clumsily arranged that the watershed is not erected between the two catheters, and consequently the two kidney urines are not segregated: ordinary caution avoids this mistake. The second possible error is the rough introduction of the catheter, whereby the prostate or the bladder is made to bleed. This bleeding is the real bugbear of the operation. Repeated irrigation will cleanse the bladder of pus, but if once a hemorrhage is started irrigation only increases it. It is in order to prevent the small amount of hemorrhage which is almost inevitable that the suprarenal extract is employed in the bladder. There are certain conditions, such as intense cystitis, tumour, stone in the bladder, or prostatic hypertrophy of any size that make segregation impossible, either on account of the hemorrhage, the vesical irritability, or the impossibility of erecting the watershed. It is in these very conditions, however, that catheterization of the ureter is most difficult, and in any one case the choice of instrument will depend on the habit of the operator. Either may fail at one time and succeed the next; indeed, it is a rule that positive evidence derived from either procedure is valuable, while negative evidence—i. e., the absence of urine—is not to be regarded as final. The inconsistencies and imperfections of ureteral catheterization with its 20% to 40% of failures and its danger of infecting the kidneys are graphically set forth in Harris's latest article.[1] Unfortunately segregation gives little better results.

In examining the urine, whether obtained from the segregator or the catheter, the presence of blood and of the albumin due to it must always be discounted, for either instrument is likely to cause hemorrhage, the one in the bladder, the other in the ureter.

The indications for the use of these instruments are best laid down with the description of each particular disease, and no attempt will be made to discriminate between them. The surgeon will use whichever he sees fit. I may confess that I am not particularly enthusiastic about any form of urine segregation. I have employed the procedure in order to determine the presence of both kidneys, I recognise its applicability to the diagnosis of unilateral renal tuberculosis, and I have employed the ureteral catheter to diagnose a suspected ureteral stone. But I am absolutely opposed to the free use of the cystoscope or the ureteral catheter as a familiar means of diagnosis. The clinician should do as well without them; the patient much better. The therapeutic uses of the ureteral catheter are not important, and their description may be brief.

[1] How great this danger of infection may be it is impossible to estimate. The advocates of the segregator make a great to-do about it while expert catheterizers do not take it into account at all. I can only say that I have several times catheterized the healthy ureter through an inflamed bladder and have seen no bad result.

Therapeutic Uses.—The ureteral catheter may be employed for three purposes:

1. To wash out the pelvis of the kidney.
2. To cure hydronephrosis or fistula.
3. To dislodge ureteral stone and to dilate stricture.

1. Kelly, Pawlick, Albarran,[1] and Casper[2] have done pioneer work in washing out the pelvis of the kidney through the ureteral catheter for the cure of pyelitis. The solutions employed have usually been boric acid and nitrate of silver, 1:1,000; 10 to 30 c. c. may be injected at a time. Casper once employed 10 c. c. of 2% nitrate-of-silver solution in a case of acute pyelitis. Its effect was as magical as that produced at the neck of the bladder in acute gonorrheal cystitis!

It has been my experience that simple pyelitis—and this treatment is avowedly only applicable to the simplest cases—is readily controlled by internal medication; while complicated cases may be held in check by medication and often cured by operation. In view of the further fact that irrigation of the renal pelvis has been followed by chills and death, I shall not perform the operation.

2. Albarran[3] has been particularly successful in curing hydronephrosis and renal fistula by means of the ureteral catheter. He leaves the instrument in place a week or two and in some cases changes from a smaller to a larger catheter every few days, going from a No. 6 or 7 French to a No. 12 or 14 French. He claims to have achieved admirable results, but one cannot help fearing that they may prove only temporary.

3. Stones have been successfully washed from the ureter by injections of olive oil, a procedure which is alleged to alleviate and shorten attacks of renal colic. Kelly and Albarran have dilated ureteral strictures by the use of bougies. Here, again, the permanence of the cure may be doubted. Before using the instrument in these or in any other conditions, the possibility of infecting the kidney must be seriously considered and guarded against.

---

[1] Revue de gyn. et de chir. abdom., 1897, i, 457.
[2] Handbuch der Cystoskopie, 1898, p. 186. Berl. klin. Wochenschr., 1899, xxxvi, 27.
[3] Guyon's Annales, 1900, xviii, 790, 799.

CHAPTER XXXI

DISEASES OF THE URETER

URETERAL ANOMALIES

Anomalies of Number.—Variations in the number of the ureters are attributable to anomalies in the kidneys. Thus, when one kidney is absent its ureter is missing as well. A fused kidney, however, commonly has two distinct pelves and ureters. When a kidney has two or more separate pelves the ureters are correspondingly increased in number. These multiple ureters run side by side and usually become fused in the upper part of their courses, or else open into the bladder by two distinct orifices placed close together.[1]

Anomalous Point of Origin.—When a ureter rises from any but the most dependent point in the renal pelvis it may so interfere with the outflow of urine as to cause hydronephrosis (p. 545).

Anomalous Implantation.—The ureter may empty into the urethra, the rectum, or the seminal passages (or the vagina in the female). Such cases are rare. The subject is discussed by Beuckhiser [2] and Olshausen.[3]

Dilatation of the Lower End of the Ureter (*Intravesical Ureteral Cyst*).—This rare condition is due to constriction of the vesical orifice of the ureter. Stricture at this point causes a back pressure that is chiefly felt in that part of the ureter which underlies the vesical mucous membrane. The ureteral wall gradually stretches at this point until there is a large cyst projecting into the bladder. There is often hydronephrosis as well. The cyst may grow large enough to obstruct the urethra, or even, in the female, to protrude from the meatus (prolapse of the vesical mucous membrane). On the other hand, the pouch may become inverted into the ureter (De-

---

[1] *Cf.* Spaletta, Bull. de la soc. anat., 1895, lx, 616.
[2] Zeitschr. f. Geb. u. Gyn., 1899, xli, 413.
[3] *Ibid.*, 1899, xli, 423.

lore[1]). Englisch[2] has collected 23 cases of such cysts, in 7 of which the ureter terminated in an abnormal locality.

Congenital stricture occurs at the lower end of the ureter. It causes the condition just described.

Kinking of the ureter over a branch of the renal artery or vein probably occurs only as the result of nephroptosis (p. 521).

RUPTURE AND WOUNDS

Rupture.—Subcutaneous rupture of the ureter is very rare. Morris[3] finds 24 reported cases, of which he rejects 12 and classifies the others as verified (3), probable (4), and possible (5). Macdonald, of Minneapolis, has added an authentic case.[4] The small size, loose attachments, and protected position of the ureter render it peculiarly likely to escape injury except from a penetrating wound.

It is quite impossible to distinguish rupture of the ureter from rupture of the renal pelvis except by operation (p. 637).

Wounds.—Accidental wounds of the ureter are even more uncommon. Morris has found only 5 reported cases (2 bullet wounds), and quotes Otis's conjecture that these injuries do not come to the surgeon's notice because the trunk vessels are likely to be punctured.

Operative Wounds.—The ureter, in most instances so safe from the onslaught of the surgeon, is frequently wounded during the course of a hysterectomy. "To-day there are few surgeons who have done many major operations upon the pelvic and abdominal organs who have not had the misfortune, once or oftener, to divide, or even excise, a portion of a ureter, either through necessity or by accident" (Morris). So common is this occurrence, indeed, that Howard Kelly advises catheterization of the ureters (that they may be readily recognised) as a preliminary to every hysterectomy. Discussion of these preventive measures we leave to the gynecologist, with the assurance that a maturing experience will serve to reduce the number of accidental wounds of the ureter, which thus far has seemed to wax rather than to wane.

Symptoms.—1. If the ureter is tied off or otherwise occluded the kidney, after going through a preliminary period of congestion, atrophies without dilatation (p. 586). In such a case if the patient survives the uremia the accident may never be recognised. On the other hand, unless both ureters are tied off so that there is complete

[1] Gaz. hebdom., 1899, iv, 325.
[2] Centralbl. f. d. Krank. d. Harn. u. Sex. Org., 1898, ix, 373.
[3] Surg. Dis. of the Kidney and Ureter, Lond., 1900, ii, 332.
[4] Med. Record, 1901.

anuria (p. 544), the symptoms, however severe, are merely characteristic of the partial suppression of urine so usual after capital operations, and are indistinguishable from it (except possibly by ureteral catheterization).

2. If the ureter is divided and the accident passes unrecognised, the position of the wound is usually such that the urine discharges into the vagina and a utero-vaginal fistula remains to be dealt with.

3. If the wound is so situated that the urine is extravasated within the peritoneal cavity, it sets up peritonitis, immediate and general if the urine is bacterial, remote and localized if the urine is clean. The source of the infection is suspected only when urine is discovered in the discharge.

Treatment.—In the early days of pelvic surgery nephrectomy was the only alternative offered to those women who were left with uretero-vaginal fistulæ after hysterectomy. But in 1886 Schopf, Fritsch, and Tauffer (twice) each recognised at the time of operation that he had divided the ureter and proceeded to sew the ends together. Thus began the conservative surgery of the ureter, and thus from the mishaps of gynecology has arisen the most brilliant conservative achievement of urinary surgery, the preservation of the healthy kidney whose duct has been severed.

Yet it was fully seven years later before any general notice was taken of the operation. Since 1893 the rapid development of the technic of uretero-ureteral anastomosis has been almost exclusively American. E. W. Cushing (1893) performed a successful end-to-end anastomosis, supposing the operation to be original. In the same year Van Hook suggested lateral implantation,[1] and Howard Kelly performed it successfully. Bache Emmet then suggested a modification of Van Hook's operation,[2] and Wesley Bovée performed oblique end-to-end anastomosis.[3] The only other notable modification is Poggi's end-to-end invagination.[4] Uretero-cystoneostomy was a later development, and all the while futile attempts have been made at anastomosis with the bowel and implantation in the skin—futile because of the high mortality and the ultimate renal infection.

A review of these various operations and their relative merits and demerits is reserved for a subsequent chapter.

Ureteral Calculus.—(See *Renal Calculus.*)

Ureteritis.—(See *Pyelo-nephritis.*)

Ureteral Tuberculosis.—(See *Renal Tuberculosis.*)

---

[1] J. of the Am. Med. Ass'n, 1893, xx, 225.

[2] Am. J. of Obstet., 1895, xxxi, 449.

[3] Ann. of Surg., 1897, xxv, 25; xxxvi, 314.

[4] Riforma medica, 1887, i, 314.

Ureteral Stricture results from one or other of the above conditions, and is not clinically separable from them.

URETERAL NEOPLASMS

Cysts of the ureter are extremely rare. Mucous cysts may occur, and there are some half-dozen reported cases of multiple small cysts of the ureter and pelvis of parasitic origin (psorosperms) (Morris [1]).

Epithelial Growths.—The solid neoplasms of the ureter are almost as rare as the cysts. They are all epithelial formations, papilloma, carcinoma, and epithelioma.[2] These tumours have been studied by Albarran,[3] who has collected 32 cases. Their histogenesis is quite the same as that of vesical tumours. They usually begin as benign growths and become malignant secondarily, arising in the renal pelvis and being propagated downward by direct extension or by implantation. In the kidney they may produce secondary deposits or give rise to hydronephrosis, hematonephrosis, or pyonephrosis. The kidney, bladder, retro-peritoneal glands, and less often the liver or the pleura, may be involved secondarily. The youngest patient was thirty-two years old, the oldest eighty-nine. In 7 cases there was stone in the kidney.

Symptoms.—The symptoms are those of renal stone or tumour. Bleeding is usually noted (72%) and is often the first symptom. Tumour was noted in one third of the cases, pain in one fourth. The diagnosis has been made only by the observation (through a cystoscope) of a villous tumour protruding from the ureteral orifice. The tumour has otherwise been either unrecognised or mistaken for a renal growth. Albarran suggests the possibility of diagnosis by the urine obtained from a ureteral catheter. If the urine is bloody, not purulent, and yet contains cylindrical or pavimentous epithelium, there must be an epithelial neoplasm. In the presence of pus, however, this sign is of no value, since such cells occur abundantly in chronic pyelitis. As a matter of fact, however, the diagnosis is commonly made only when nephrectomy is undertaken for supposed renal growth.

Treatment.—The treatment is wholly operative. Nephrectomy has been performed 13 times, with 3 deaths and 1 known recurrence. One case of papilloma was known to be well fourteen months, and 1 of carcinoma twenty-six months after operation.

Of 2 nephrotomies, with curettage, for a supposedly benign papil-

---

[1] Surgical Diseases of the Kidney and Ureter, ii, 480.

[2] Morris has, however, collected 3 reported cases of sarcoma.

[3] Guyon's Annales, 1900, xviii, 701, 918.

loma, 1 relapsed and died, the other relapsed and underwent successful nephrectomy.

Complete nephro-ureterectomy is, therefore, the only appropriate treatment. The cystoscope will determine whether or not the disease has reached the ureteral orifice. If not, the kidney and ureter may be removed by the lumbo-inguinal incision (p. 637). If so, the nephrectomy must be combined with complete removal of the ureter and perhaps a portion of the adjoining bladder wall (p. 500). Above all things it is essential not to be misled by gross appearances. The ureter must always be removed well down into the pelvis, for the growth may be propagated by implantation, forming a secondary tumour in the ureter at a distance from the original growth.

URETERAL FISTULÆ

Ureteral fistulæ have many causes. Congenital uretero-rectal and uretero-vaginal fistulæ are extremely rare. In these cases it is usually possible to make an opening into the bladder through a suprapubic wound. The termination of the ureter is then obliterated by extirpation or cauterization. Acquired fistulæ, on the contrary, occur in any portion of the ureter: at the upper end after nephrectomy, especially if the ureter is actively tuberculous. In other parts of its course cutaneous fistulæ form after the duct has been inadvertently divided during an abdominal operation or after rupture from stone, stricture, or other disease, such as tuberculosis and neoplasm, or from trauma or pressure of some intra-abdominal growth usually of the uterus or ovary, or from injuries inflicted during labour.

The discharge from the ureteral fistula is usually uro-purulent, sometimes simply purulent, and rarely simply urinary. The presence of urine in the discharge may be taken as presumptive evidence that the fistulous ureter leads up to a functionating kidney. Yet the absence of urine does not necessarily prove that the kidney is past all usefulness, nor does its presence prove a connection with the kidney; for it has been observed by Hartman and Desnos (Morris) that the urine may regurgitate from the bladder through a ureteral fistula.

Treatment.—The treatment of cutaneous fistula is ureterectomy if the kidney has ceased to functionate, ureteral anastomosis or some allied procedure if the kidney is worth saving.

The treatment of uretero-vaginal and uretero-uterine fistula is no simple matter. The great variety of operations employed for its cure, the great proportion of failures after most of these, and the total absence of concerted surgical opinion upon the subject, attest the complexity of the problem. While the number of operations is legion and the choice among them lies rather with the gynecologist than with the genito-urinary surgeon, a few simple principles may here be laid down.

When practicable Tuffier's[1] operation should be employed, as it combines the attributes of simplicity and perfect safety. The steps of the operation are as follows: (1) Introduce a director into the fistulous opening, and, using this as a guide, dissect free the lower 2 or 3 cm. of the duct. (2) Split up the orifice for 1 cm. in order to insure an ample opening. (3) Make a triangular opening in the most accessible point of the bladder wall (pushed down by a sound). (4) Suture the ureteral and vesical mucous membranes with catgut and the muscular layers with silk. Finally, close the wound in the anterior vaginal wall. A ureteral catheter, or at least a permanent vesical catheter, is necessary for the first week after operation.

If this operation fails or is impracticable, abdominal uretero-cysto-neostomy should be tried and should succeed. Hysterocleisis and colpocleisis are operations of last resort. The functional result of including the uterus or the vagina in the urinary reservoir is anything but satisfactory. If all attempts at uretero-vesical anastomosis fail and the opposite kidney is healthy, nephrectomy would be preferable to colpocleisis. Let it not be forgotten, however, that at least once the wrong kidney has been removed. This deplorable accident may, for a certainty, be avoided by catheterization of the fistulous ureter at the time of operation and palpation of the catheter within the pelvis of the organ to be removed.

---

[1] Bull. de la soc. de chir., 1895, xxi, 270.

CHAPTER XXXII

OPERATIONS UPON THE URETER

Excluding the special operations for uretero-vaginal fistula (p. 484), the operative surgery of the ureter may be considered under two heads: Plastic Operations and Extirpation.

Plastic Operations.

1. For kinks, valves, and strictures. (See *Hydronephrosis.*)
    - Ureterotomy.
    - Pyelo-ureterotresis (uretero-pyelo-neostomy).
    - Pyeloplication (or nephropexy).
    - (Any operation in the list below.)
2. For wounds, strictures, necrosis, disease or fistula entailing loss of continuity of the duct.
    - Uretero-ureteral anastomosis.
    - Cysto-ureterotresis (uretero-cysto-neostomy).
    - Closure of the ureter or nephrectomy.
3. For exstrophy of the bladder (p. 337).
    - Cutaneous fistulization.
    - Entero-ureterotresis.
    - Maydl's operation.
    - Recto-vesical fistulization (Frank).

Extirpation.

- Partial ureterectomy.
- Complete ureterectomy.

OPERATIONS FOR KINKS, VALVES, AND SIMPLE STRICTURES

Kinks, valves, and strictures of the ureter manifest themselves by causing hydronephrosis (or pyonephrosis or atrophy of the kidney), and are accordingly discussed in that connection (p. 545). These obstructions may occur at the upper or the lower extremity of the ureter or somewhere in its course (usually at the point where it crosses the brim of the pelvis). Their only treatment is operative. Cures have been reported through dilatation with ureteral catheters; but our experience with strictures of the urethra, the rectum, and the esophagus produces the conviction that dilatation must prove inadequate in the majority of cases. Catheterization can scarcely be relied upon to affect a valve or a kink. The knife only remains.

Now these obstructions may be divided arbitrarily into two classes: Obstructions which may be relieved by operation upon the ureter only, and obstructions which cannot be relieved without operation upon the kidney or its pelvis.

Obstructions Remediable by Ureterotomy.—Such obstructions are commonly strictures, congenital or due to the presence of ureteral stone or disease of the ureter or of the adjacent viscera. These strictures occur at the lower orifice of the ureter, where they cause intravesical ureteral cyst (p. 480), (the treatment of which is transvesical incision), or at or above the pelvic brim. Strictures in this latter location are reached after evacuation of the hydronephrosis by inguinal prolongation of the oblique lumbar incision (p. 637).

A probe introduced into the ureter from the renal pelvis will at once detect the site of stricture (some surgeons prefer a preliminary ureteral catheterization for this purpose). The peritoneum is lifted forward and the ureter followed down until the strictured point is reached. It will here be found adherent to the peritoneum, which may be torn before the ureter can be freed. Such a tear should be immediately sutured. The ureter is then brought up into the wound and an attempt made to perform ureteroplasty on the principle of the Heinecke-Mikulicz operation for pyloric stenosis. The accompanying figures show the method by which a longitudinal incision is sutured transversely (Figs. 127, 128, 129). The sutures enter the lumen of the duct and must therefore be of catgut. They may be re-enforced by suture of the peritoneal tissues.

If, for any reason, this operation cannot be performed: if the ureter cannot be freed, if it is accidentally torn across, if the stricture is too wide or the wall of the ureter above it too friable to permit the sutures to be satisfactorily applied, the ureter must be divided, resected, and some form of ureteral anastomosis employed.

Obstructions requiring Operation upon the Pelvis or the Kidney.—Such obstructions, usually due to nephroptosis, and often the cause of intermittent hydronephrosis, are relatively common. The obstruction is at or near the junction of ureter and pelvis, and usually consists of a kink closely surrounded by adhesions and perhaps associated with a valve or a stricture.

In attempting the operative relief of such an obstruction it is well to remember that the object of the operation is simply to insure a free outflow of urine. To this end kinks must be straightened, stenosis relieved, and the ureteral orifice placed at the most dependent point of the pelvis. In order to accomplish this threefold purpose the simplest operation—viz., reposition of the prolapsed kidney, after the liberation of adhesions—is usually all-sufficient. The pelvis having been emptied of its contents and adhesions having been freed as far as necessary, the internal ureteral orifice is palpated and inspected through the incision in the pelvis. If it is not constricted and a probe passes freely down the ureter, the kidney is replaced high up under the ribs, and it will probably be found that, with the organ in this position, the dilated pelvis falls into a funnel shape with the ureter leading directly from its apex. In such a case nephropexy (p. 527) is all that is required.

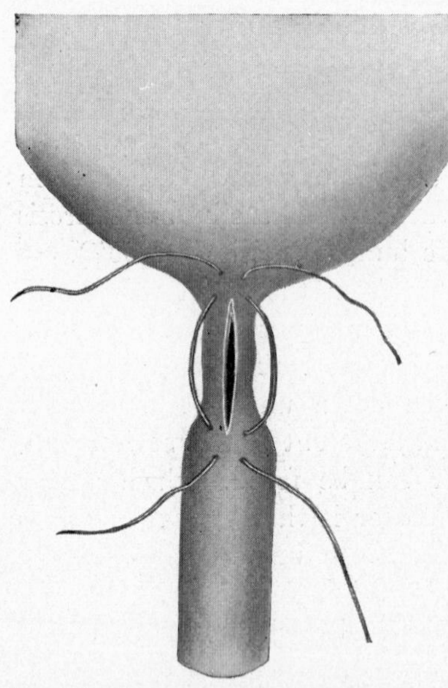

FIG. 127.—URETEROPLASTY OR PYELO-URETEROTRESIS (after Morris).
The stricture is incised longitudinally and two sutures are inserted.

But conditions may be complicated in three ways:

1. *It may be Difficult to find the Orifice of the Ureter.*—The search may be facilitated if the hydronephrosis is large by everting the sac (Fenger) and subjecting its internal surface to a careful scrutiny, or by identifying the ureter below the constriction and pulling upon it in order to dimple its orifice, or by introducing a probe (through a longitudinal incision) upward along the ureter, or by ureteral catheterization.

2. *There may be Stricture of Valve.*—This may be relieved by ureteroplasty or by pyelo-ureterotresis (Figs. 127, 128, 129).

3. *The Pelvic Dilatation may have occurred irregularly, so that when the Kidney is replaced high up in the Loin there is still a Pouch hanging below the Ureteral Orifice, calculated to invite Infection of the Retained Urine and to lead to Renewed Nephrectasis.*—This condition is unusual, and its treatment depends upon whether or not it is associated with valve or stricture. When there is a simple pouching of the pelvis which cannot be remedied by nephropexy

it may be obliterated by suturing the two walls of the pouch together (pyeloplication) after scarification of the mucous membrane (Israel, Albarran). Albarran even went so far in one case as to resect the

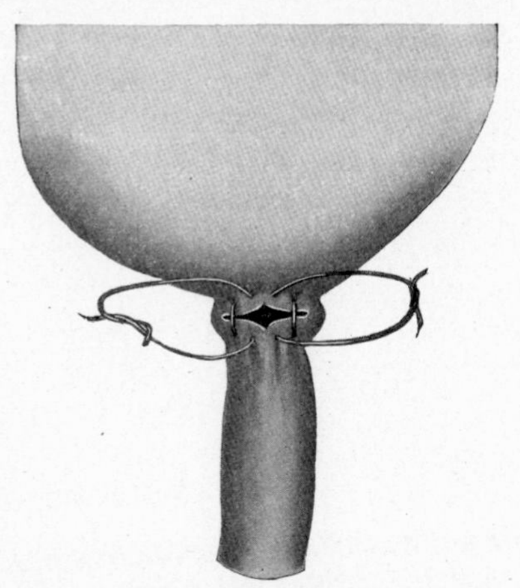

Fig. 128.—Ureteroplasty or Pyelo-ureterotresis (after Morris).

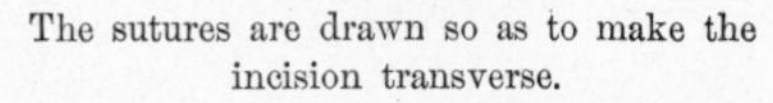

The sutures are drawn so as to make the incision transverse.

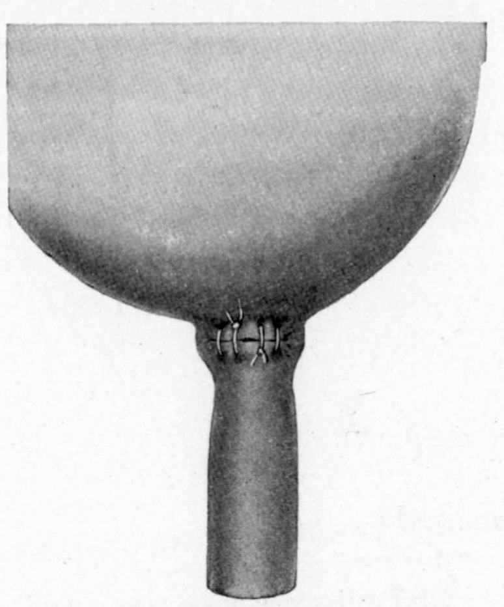

Fig. 129.—Ureteroplasty or Pyelo-ureterotresis (after Morris).

The result.

lower pole of the dilated kidney with the adjoining portion of the pelvis.

When ureteral stricture and pelvic pouching coexist the best operation is lateral anastomosis of the ureter with the pelvis (pyeloureterotresis). A longitudinal incision in the ureter below the stricture is sutured with fine catgut to a corresponding incision at the most dependent point of the pelvis. This operation has been performed unsuccessfully by Helferich, successfully by Delbet and Albarran.

Yet, in spite of the success that has attended almost every plastic operation proposed for the relief of renal retention, it is a suggestive fact that Tuffier has cured 17 consecutive cases by nephropexy, and that Guyon, as recently as 1898, maintained that simple nephrotomy with drainage is superior to every other operation for the relief of this condition. Certainly the great majority of hydronephroses were cured by these methods before the days of plastic ureteral surgery, and, while our wider knowledge of the subject makes it the surgeon's duty not to be satisfied until he has identified the source of obstruction, he may rest assured that fixation of the kidney in its proper place and removal of calculi—if any be present—will almost always suffice to relieve the obstruction and to prevent its recurrence.

URETERAL ANASTOMOSIS

Under this caption may be grouped all operations for the purpose of re-establishing the flow of urine through a ureter divided by accident or design, together with an estimation of the obstacles to the success of such an operation and a consideration of the proper procedure to elect in case anastomosis is impossible. Thus we shall review the technic and merits of, 1, anastomosis of the ureter with itself and with the bladder; 2, anastomosis with the intestine and cutaneous fistulization; 3, closure of the ureter and nephrectomy.

Uretero-ureteral Anastomosis

A rough history of the development of this operation has already been given. Since the end-to-end anastomosis of the earlier operators is now generally condemned as predisposing to stricture, there remain but three operations to be considered—viz.:

1. End-in-end anastomosis.
2. Oblique end-to-end anastomosis.
3. Lateral anastomosis (end-in-side).

End-in-end Anastomosis.—This operation was first suggested by Poggi, and has been modified by Mayo Robson [1] and Gubaroff.[2] The upper end of the ureter is cut obliquely (to prevent stricture) and the lower end dilated (Poggi) (Fig. 130) or incised longitudinally (Robson). The upper end is then drawn into the lower by a single suture, as in Van Hook's operation, the longitudinal incision closed by Lembert sutures of fine silk, and the union strengthened, if the operator deems it necessary, by a circle of fine silk Lembert sutures around the external line of union.

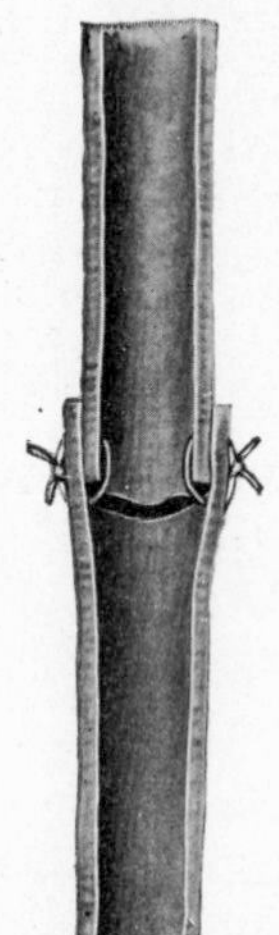

Fig. 130.—End-in-End Anastomosis (Poggi).

Oblique End-to-end Anastomosis (Wesley Bovée).—Both ends are cut obliquely, dilated,[3] and sutured with rectangular and simple interrupted sutures of silk traversing only the outer coats of the duct and re-enforced by a few Lembert sutures (Fig. 131).

It is convenient in this, as in most of the other plastic operations upon the ureter, to suture the tube after the introduction (from the bladder) of a ureteral catheter, or, as Howard Kelly [4] has sug-

[1] Internat. Med. Ann., 1896, p. 602.

[2] Centralbl. f. Chir., 1901.

[3] It has been observed by various writers that the ureter could be dilated with ease to twice its normal size.

[4] J. of the Am. Med. Ass'n, 1900, xxxv, 860.

gested, a guide introduced through a longitudinal incision in the wall of the duct.

Lateral Anastomosis (Van Hook).—To quote the author's lucid description:

"*a.* Ligate the lower portion of the tube $\frac{1}{8}$ or $\frac{1}{4}$ inch from the free end. Make with fine sharp-pointed scissors a longitudinal incision twice as long as the diameter of the ureter in the wall of the lower end, $\frac{1}{4}$ inch below the ligature.

"*b.* Make an incision with the scissors in the upper portion of the ureter, beginning at the open end of the duct and carrying it up $\frac{1}{4}$ inch. This incision insures the patency of the tube (Fig. 132, *A*).

"*c.* Pass two very small cambric needles armed with one thread of sterilized catgut through the wall of the upper end of the ureter $\frac{1}{8}$ inch from the extremity, from within outward, the needles being from $\frac{1}{16}$ to $\frac{1}{8}$ inch apart, and equidistant from the end of the duct. It will be seen that the loop of catgut between the needles firmly grasps the end of the ureter.

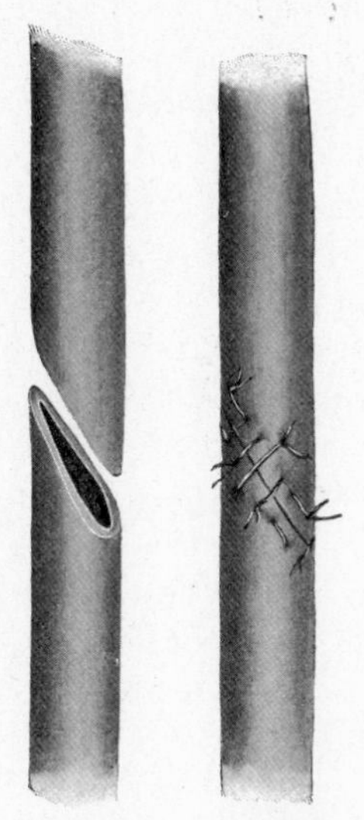

Fig. 131.—Oblique End-to-End Anastomosis (Bovée).

"*d.* These needles are now carried through the slit in the side of the lower end of the ureter into and down the tube for $\frac{1}{2}$ inch, where they are pushed through the wall of the duct side by side (Fig. 132, *B*).

"*e.* It will now be seen that the traction upon this catgut loop passing through the wall of the ureter will draw the upper fragment of the duct into the lower portion. This done, the ends of the loop are tied together securely, and, as the catgut will be absorbed in a few days, calculi do not form to obstruct the passage of urine (Fig. 132, *C*).

"*f.* The ureter is now enveloped carefully with peritoneum. This may be done by lifting the duct gently into the cavity of the peritoneum, drawing down the serous membrane carefully behind the ureter, and after pulling the peritoneum around it, stitching it in a position to permanently inclose and protect the tube." [1]

---

[1] Van Hook is here speaking of an intraperitoneal operation, which ureteral anastomosis almost always is. If, however, the duct has been approached from behind the peritoneum, the risk of opening that structure into a cavity over which urine of at least doubtful cleanliness has been poured would scarcely be compensated for by the advantage of a peritoneal investment. It would seem much more to the

Bache Emmet employs three sutures to drag the upper segment into the lower one. This for the purpose of puckering the upper segment, if it is considerably dilated (Fig. 133).

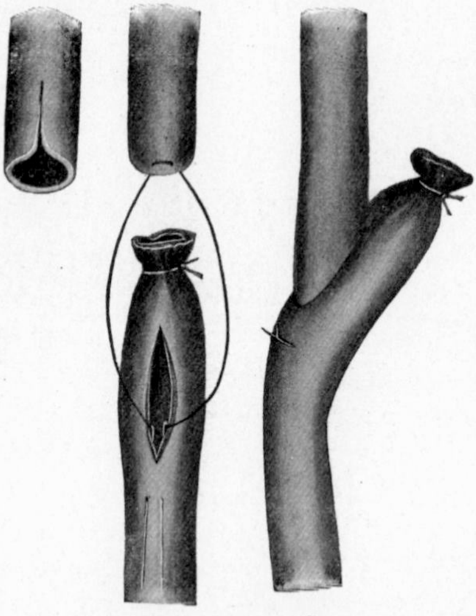

A B C

Fig. 132.—Lateral Anastomosis (Van Hook).

We may justly disregard the discussion of the relative methods of the three procedures, but the following observations seem apposite:

1. All of the operations have been equally successful.

2. Invagination, whether end-in-end or end-in-side, may be performed more easily and rapidly than Bovée's operation.

3. End-in-side anastomosis wastes more of the length of the duct than either of the other two. Bovée claims that his operation may be performed even though as much as 3 inches of the duct have been cut away.[1] He has also suggested that in case of need the kidney may be loosened and stitched low in the loin.

4. Whatever method is employed it is customary to use catgut for all sutures that enter the lumen of the duct, and silk for the others: this in order to avoid calculous incrustation. (Yet it is known that silk sutures in the kidney do not become incrusted, and it is at least possible that ureteral sutures might escape.)

5. When the lower end of the ureter is

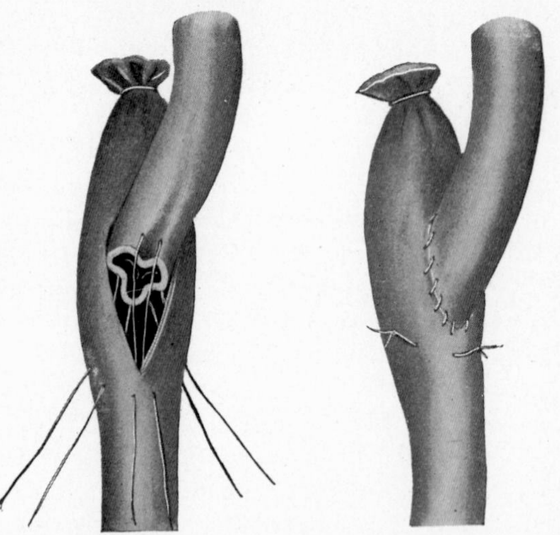

Fig. 133.—Lateral Anastomosis (Bache Emmet).

point to scarify the mucous membrane of the lower segment in order to make it adhere to the upper.

[1] J. of the Am. Med. Ass'n, 1901, xxxvii, 254.

lost or useless for any reason, cysto-ureterotresis is the operation of choice. When this is impracticable the choice lies between entero-ureterotresis and nephrectomy (or shutting off the ureter with the object of causing atrophy of the kidney—a dangerous though simple procedure), with a preference for the latter, if the opposite kidney is able to support life.

CYSTO-URETEROTRESIS

Cysto-ureterotresis (uretero-cysto-neostomy) has been employed usually for the relief of uretero-vaginal fistula, rarely for other conditions when ureteral anastomosis proved impracticable.

Poggi in 1887 made the first experiments in reference to this operation. Novaro and Bazy were the first to perform it.

Three routes have been chosen—viz., vaginal, sacral, and abdominal. The best of the vaginal operations has already been described. The sacral route has nothing to recommend it.

Almost every surgeon who has performed the abdominal operation has devised his own technic. The various methods have been enumerated by Boari [1] and Morris.[2] To avoid confusion, it is best to describe only a type operation. The peculiarities of each case will suggest the necessary modifications.

Whether the ureter is to be attached intraperitoneally or extraperitoneally is often decided by the features of the case. It is safer to operate extraperitoneally through the lumbo-inguinal incision when possible, elevating the peritoneum until the bladder (distended with boric-acid solution) is entirely exposed, freeing the ureter from the peritoneum and drawing it down.

The bladder is then emptied by catheter and incised on the point of a sound at the most convenient point, as near as possible to the trigone. The ureteral orifice is then split to prevent stenosis, and attached to the bladder by means of a catgut traction suture (as in the Van Hook anastomosis). It is convenient at this juncture to introduce a ureteral catheter and upon it to suture the outer layers of ureter and bladder. When the operation is performed within the peritoneum the line of union should be protected by a peritoneal or an omental fold.

While the Boari button has twice been employed successfully, it has the obvious disadvantages of its prototype, the Murphy button—viz., possibility of stricture and difficulty of extraction (it cannot be used in the male for this reason), and these more than counterbalance the advantage of time-saving.

---

[1] Guyon's Annales, 1899, xvii, 1059, 1141. [2] *Op. cit.*, ii, 563.

After operation it is customary to leave the ureteral catheter in place for four or five days.

In several instances the ureter has seemed too short. An inch or more may be gained by loosening the pubic attachments of the bladder (Witzel, Kelly, Penrose) and suturing its fundus to the lateral pelvic wall. Boari has succeeded experimentally in bridging a greater gap. He dissected up as a flap the whole thickness of the anterior bladder wall an inch wide with its base at the fundus. This he turned back and sutured as a sleeve about a ureteral catheter and the extremity of the ureter. He then closed the wound in the bladder. Such an extensive line of suture would require protection by drainage for fear of leakage. Dislocation of the kidney to gain slack has not been performed in connection with cysto-ureterotresis. An isolated loop of intestine has been employed experimentally to bridge the gap between ureter and bladder.[1]

STATISTICS

Having discussed the chief operations of ureteral surgery, a brief review of the clinical statistics will fitly impress the brilliant practical results of these procedures in marked contrast with those which we have yet to note.

Plastic Operations at the Upper End of the Ureter.—Christian Fenger,[2] who has himself performed 10 out of the 30 operations for renal retention which he is able to collect, clearly and succinctly sets forth the brilliant results of these operations.

One case of division of pelvic partitions and transpelvic section of spur was successful.

Nine cases of valve were operated upon transpelvically by incision of the valve and transverse closure.

Of these, 1 died of uremia, 1 of ileus.

Five were completely successful.

Two relapsed.

Eleven cases of valve and stricture were subjected to extrapelvic incision and transverse suture.

Of these, 10 were successful, 1 unsuccessful.

Six cases were subjected to resection and reimplantation of the ureter (uretero-pyelo-neostomy).

Of these, one died of sepsis or iodoform poisoning. Three proved successful, and 2 failed; 1 because of an extensive stricture

---

[1] J. of the Am. Med. Ass'n, 1901, xxxvii, 323.

[2] Ann. of Surgery, 1901, xxxiii, 369.

lower down the ureter, the other because of the friability of the tissues.

While 3 cases were subjected to pyeloplication and capitonnage, and all 3 were successful, in 2 a valve was incised as well.

We may disregard 1 case of unkinking the ureter.

In 2 cases a ureteral stricture was successfully divided and sutured transversely. These may be grouped with the 12 extrapelvic incisions:

To summarize:

Ten intrapelvic operations—
- Two deaths.
- Six successes.
- Two relapses.

Thirteen extrapelvic operations—
- No deaths.
- Twelve successes.
- One failure.

Six uretero-pyelo-neostomies—
- One death.
- Three successes.
- Two failures.
- One simple pyeloplication successful.

With no deaths directly attributable to the operation, and only 25% of failures among these first attempts, we may well look forward to a brilliant future for this class of work.

Ureteral Anastomosis.—Bovée[1] has collected 12 cases of transverse end-to-end anastomosis with 2 deaths not directly attributable to the operation, 1 oblique end-to-end successful, 9 end-in-end with 1 death, and 5 end-in-side with 1 death. In all 27 cases with 7.5% mortality. That no case of obstruction by contracture of the scar is reported possibly illustrates the inaccuracy of statistics. Yet even this negative evidence has some weight, and certainly the enthusiasm of surgeons over the brilliant series of successes in these cases is not unwarranted.

Cysto-ureterotresis.—Bovée records 79 operations, 42 for the cure of fistula (1 death) and 37 for operative accidents (2 deaths). While the attempts at vaginal operation have been remarkably unsuccessful, the worst complication of the abdominal procedures has been a temporary leakage of urine, and even this has been extremely rare. The theoretical objections to the operation are stenosis of the ureteral orifice and ascending pyelo-nephritis in case cystitis occurs,

[1] Ann. of Surgery, 1900, xxxii, 165.

since the ureter is not guarded by its natural muscular orifice. The former danger need not be feared if the end of the ureter is enlarged by splitting it, and the latter is probably a theoretical rather than a real objection, for no case of renal infection attributable to this cause has been recorded.

On the whole, then, the results already obtained in plastic ureteral surgery are excellent. They preserve the healthy kidney and permit it to remain sound, and are not attended by any notable difficulty in technic nor any considerable mortality. In direct contrast are the operative methods employed to divert the course of the urine, which, by the difficulty of their technic, their high mortality, and small percentage of actual cures, may well deter the most experienced. In the table at the beginning of this chapter they have been listed "for exstrophy of the bladder" because this unfortunate deformity is almost the only warrant for their performance.

Closure of the Ureter and Nephrectomy.—When all attempts at re-establishing the continuity of the ureter fail, nephrectomy may be contemplated as preferable to cutaneous fistulization or entero-ureterotresis. Indeed, if the opposite organ is known to be sound the removal of one kidney may be perfectly compatible with the maintenance of life. Under these circumstances the operation is quite free from danger.

In a few instances surgeons have been satisfied to tie off the ends of a divided ureter and so to leave the kidney to atrophy. As far as I know the result has always been happy; yet to leave the kidney thus as a possible focus for suppuration is no small risk, for numerous experiments have shown that with the ureter thus tied off the kidney falls a victim to bacteria which, under ordinary circumstances, it could transmit without harm to itself. Hence of the two operations nephrectomy is to be preferred.

OPERATIONS TO DIVERT THE URINARY STREAM

Cutaneous Fistulization.—Although this operation has been performed several times, and with some success, it leaves the patient in a deplorable condition of constant wetness, is followed within a few months by infection of the kidney, and has no feature other than its simplicity to recommend it. To quote Morris:[1] "Surface grafting the ureter, with its resultant fistula, is only less objectionable than nephrectomy; indeed, some patients have undergone nephrectomy to get rid of the fistula, as Poggi's patient did. It is only in

[1] Surg. Dis. of the Kidney and Ureter, 1901, ii, 596.

cases of ectopia vesicæ and in those where the ureter of a *single kidney* is blocked that such an expedient can be willingly resorted to; and in my opinion it ought not to be done at all in the case of ectopia vesicæ, since uretero-colic grafting (i. e., Maydl's operation) has become, during the last few years, a comparatively safe procedure."

Entero-ureterotresis.—The implantation of one or both ureters into the bowel (the rectum or the sigmoid flexure is usually selected) is followed, when successful, by results which, at first sight, are encouraging. The rectum becomes accustomed to retain the urine perfectly for a space of from three to six hours, and the immediate result is by that much better than cutaneous fistulization. This fact has led many surgeons to advocate the operation. But recent researches tend to prove that the conclusion was precipitate. Animal experiments from the time of Glück and Zoller (1881) down to Peterson,[1] Zeit,[2] and Frank[3] have been extremely discouraging. The immediate mortality runs from 60% to 90%, while those dogs that survive show interesting lesions. "Dogs which had fully recovered from the operation and the resulting pyelo-nephritis,[4] and were, to all appearances, in perfect health and vigour again, *all* had granular, contracted kidneys, due to induration and cicatrization of diseased areas. . . . Dogs which had fully recovered after unilateral implantation were living by the other kidney. The kidney of the side operated on was atrophic and granular, the result of an early pyelo-nephritis. The functionally active kidney was from 2 to 8 times the size of the atrophic one" (Zeit).

The results of the operation upon man have been but little better. According to Peterson, double implantation has been performed 18 times with 8 deaths (44%) immediately due to the operation, and 3 deaths from a subsequent pyelo-nephritis (total mortality 61%). Unilateral implantation fared somewhat better with 3 primary deaths among 15 cases and 2 secondary deaths. Of those followed for more than a month after operation Peterson has compiled the following table:[5]

1 ureter implanted, well after	6	months.
1 ureter implanted, well after	18	months.
1 ureter implanted, well after	2	years.
1 ureter implanted, well after	8	years.
2 ureters implanted, well after	5	weeks.

[1] J. of the Am. Med. Ass'n, 1901, xxxvi, 444, 506, 569, 632, 735.

[2] N. Y. Med. J., 1901, lxxiii, 756, 839.

[3] J. of the Am. Med. Ass'n, 1901, xxxvi, 1466.

[4] Which seems always to occur.

[5] I have advisedly omitted the cases of Beck and Evans, since both have died of pyelo-nephritis, though reported well at the end, respectively, of 7 and 13 months.

2 ureters implanted, well after...............................	3½ months.
2 ureters implanted, well after...............................	10 months.
2 ureters implanted, well after...............................	1 year.
2 ureters implanted, well after...............................	3½ years.

It is obvious, then, that about 1 out of every 3 cases upon whom unilateral implantation is done may be expected to live (whether with an atrophied kidney or not, we need not decide), while one in four bilateral implantations should recover. The evidence is, I agree, ample to condemn either procedure, even without the strong probability that the survivors all have damaged kidneys.[1] But fortunately, we have, in Maydl's and Frank's operations, procedures which, while not by any means bereft of danger, allow such a chance of recovery as to bring them well within the scope of practical surgery.

Maydl's Operation.—In 1894 Maydl[2] reported his first cases of uretero-trigonal anastomosis. This operation consists of the implantation into the colon, not of the ureter itself but of the bladder wall surrounding the mouth of the ureter. The operation has only been employed for exstrophy of the bladder and allied conditions, and is performed as follows: A probe or a ureteral catheter is introduced into each ureter after the operative field has been cleansed as well as may be, and an elliptical section surrounding the mouths of both ureters is then cut from the bladder wall, great care being taken not to injure the ureters. Next, the peritoneal cavity is opened. A convenient loop of the sigmoid flexure or the rectum is selected and brought out of the abdominal wound. The ureters, with their attached portion of trigone, are then freed, a longitudinal incision is made in the wall of the gut, with the necessary precautions, and into this the section of trigone is sutured. The remainder of the bladder is now stripped of its mucous membrane and the abdominal wound closed as tightly as possible, with splitting and transposition of the recti, if necessary. As a final precaution the sphincter ani is stretched and a tube inserted and left in for several days to establish drainage and so to minimize the danger of leakage and renal retention.

This operation avoids several of the dangers associated with simple uretero-intestinal anastomosis. For the cicatricial ureteral orifice, which has proved so liable to contracture with disastrous results to the kidney, it substitutes the normal muscular orifice of the ureter,

[1] J. of the Am. Med. Ass'n, 1901, xxxvi, 1263.

[2] Wien. med. Wochenschr., 1894, xliv, 1113, 1169, 1209, 1256, 1297. *Ibid.*, 1896, xlvi, 1241, 1333, 1373. *Ibid.*, 1899, xlix, 249, 304, 360.

and, while this is not an absolute protection, it has proved very effectual clinically. Among 36 cases collected by Peterson there was a primary mortality of 14% (5 cases) and a secondary mortality of 5% (2 cases). Sphincteric control proved good in 27 cases, fair in 4, and poor in 1. The convalescence of 6 cases was delayed by temporary urinary fistulæ. These figures proclaim the practical advantage of Maydl's operation. Yet even this procedure cannot be considered ideal. A capital operation in the course of which a foul bladder and the peritoneal cavity are simultaneously invaded must always retain an appreciable mortality, and diverting the urine from the bladder into the rectum can never be accepted except as a makeshift to avoid greater evils. Yet as surgery stands to-day no plastic operation has had a success to compare with Maydl's operation in the treatment of exstrophy of the bladder. In resection or extirpation of that organ for malignant growths Maydl's operation is ruled out by the fact that the growth almost always involves one ureteral orifice or both; yet the other forms of uretero-intestinal anastomosis offer so uninviting a prospect that, until something better presents itself, the prudent surgeon must be inclined not to extirpate these tumours unless a cysto-ureterotresis is possible.

Frank's Operation.—Frank[1] has applied the methods of modern surgery to vesico-rectal fistulization in dogs with such good results as to suggest that his procedure is as satisfactory as Maydl's. It is certainly far simpler. He opens the abdominal cavity and unites the bladder to the rectum by a bone coupler of his own devising—a Murphy button would doubtless do as well. The obvious objections to the operation are: first, the necessity of closing the (exstrophied) bladder—no simple matter; and, second, the possibility of continuous severe cystitis. Halstead performed this operation on one patient who died of shock. Among the advantages of his operation Frank claims that there is no danger that the trigone will slough, yet statistics do not show that this has been an important element in the prognosis of Maydl's operation.

URETERECTOMY

Ureterectomy has been repeatedly performed for tuberculosis, less often for neoplasm, stone, and stricture. In these last conditions ureterectomy is only indicated when it is deemed inadvisable or impossible to preserve the kidney. Indeed, the operation commonly passes by the name of nephro-ureterectomy, for, excluding the cases

---

[1] Med. Record, 1896, l, 469. J. of the Am. Med. Ass'n, 1900, xxxiv, 1174, 1237.

of resection already alluded to, excision of the ureter implies a previous or a simultaneous nephrectomy.

"As to whether primary or secondary ureterectomy is better, the following considerations will guide us. If, during the course of nephrectomy, the ureter for some inches from the renal pelvis is seen to be in a dilated and suppurating condition, or affected with tuberculous disease, the rule ought to be to excise the affected portion of the ureter together with the kidney; but if there is no evidence from the history and symptoms and from the conditions found at the time of the operation that the greater part or the whole of the ureter is in a similar state, the surgeon must be guided by the condition of the patient. If this is not good, it will be best to remove the kidney and wait until the patient has recovered from the nephrectomy before excising the ureter. If the condition of the patient warrants it, the ureter should be at once removed—i. e., primary ureterectomy should be performed" (Morris).

As a matter of fact, a tubercular ureter left fixed at the lower angle of the wound may cease to be fistulous after a few weeks, just as tubercular lesions of the bladder are known to heal after the primary renal focus has been removed. At any rate, the patient's condition usually improves greatly after nephrectomy, and so ureterectomy—total ureterectomy certainly—may be always safely and often preferably deferred.

The Operation.—The ureter has been extirpated transperitoneally by Howard Kelly through an incision to the outer side of and parallel with the semilunar line. But as all other operators have found the extraperitoneal route adequate, that only need be described.

With the patient lying upon his side the oblique lumbo-ilio-inguinal incision is made (p. 637) and carried down as far as need be, even to the external abdominal ring. When the peritoneum is reached it is carefully elevated and the ureter sought for. If the operation is being performed with nephrectomy the ureter is usually readily traced down; but if the ureterectomy is secondary it is preferable to disregard the fistula and to search for the duct where it crosses the brim of the pelvis. The peritoneum is carefully elevated until the finger feels and recognises by their pulsations the internal and external iliac arteries. Opposite the junction of these, closely confined to the peritoneum by its fibrous sheath, the ureter will be found. The sheath is nicked, an aneurysm needle passed under the ureter, and after that the dissection is easy unless there are adhesions, in which case great care must be exercised not to tear the peritoneum. The ureter may be followed down into the pelvis to its vesical orifice, where it is to be divided between ligatures. The external wound is then sutured in layers after such irrigation and with such drainage as the surgeon deems advisable.

Several surgeons have employed the combined abdominal (extraperitoneal) and vaginal method devised by Kelly, but it has not proved as satisfactory as the method described above.

The excision of that part of the bladder wall adjoining the mouth of the ureter is difficult and unnecessary except in those rare cases of ureteral neoplasm which extend into the bladder. The operation is best performed by extraperitoneal abdominal section combined with suprapubic cystotomy, the wound in the bladder being sutured according to the usual method (p. 462).

CHAPTER XXXIII

SURGICAL ANATOMY AND PHYSIOLOGY OF THE KIDNEY —EXAMINATION OF THE KIDNEY—ABNORMALITIES OF THE KIDNEY

ANATOMY

Gross Anatomy.—Although familiarity with the minute anatomy of the kidney is an essential part in the equipment of every practitioner, be he physician or surgeon, it is quite impracticable to enter upon this intricate subject here. A brief survey of the gross anatomy of the organ must suffice. The rest we leave to the histologist.

The kidney is ovoidal in shape, flattened antero-posteriorly, and with a deep notch, the *hilum*, in its inner border. The renal vessels and nerves enter the organ through the hilum, the vein lying in front of the artery, while behind these is the *conical pelvis*,[1] terminating below in the ureter. The *sinus* of the kidney is the irregular cavity of which the hilum is the orifice.

The normal kidney is 11 cm. long, 6 cm. wide, and 4 cm. thick. It weighs from 125 to 200 grammes.

The kidney is closely surrounded by a fibrous capsule sending fine processes between the secreting tubules. A thin irregular layer of unstriped muscle lies between the capsule and the kidney. When the organ is healthy its capsule may be stripped from it, but inflammation causes the capsule to become adherent.

A vertical section through the kidney (Fig. 134) shows its secreting structure to consist of two parts: an outer (cortical) portion and an inner (medullary) portion, the latter made up of rounded cones (pyramids) whose apices (papillæ, mammillæ) project into the sinus of the kidney; while between the medullary pyramids the lighter coloured cortical portion of the organ also abuts on the sinus.

---

[1] Although, strictly speaking, the pelvis is the dilated upper extremity of the ureter, it is customary and convenient to speak of the renal pelvis rather than the ureteral pelvis.

Vessels and Nerves.—The *renal arteries* are given off one from each side of the abdominal aorta, and proceed directly outward to the kidney, lying behind the veins (the right renal artery runs behind the inferior vena cava). As the artery enters the hilum of the kidney it divides into several branches, which enter the cortical substance and are thence distributed throughout the organ.

The *renal veins* accompany the arteries, lying in front of them, and empty into the inferior cava. On the left side, the spermatic, inferior phrenic, and suprarenal veins are tributaries of the renal.

The *nerves* of the kidney are derived through the renal plexus from the solar plexus, the semilunar ganglion, and the lesser and smallest splanchnic nerves. The spermatic plexus is derived from the renal plexus.

The *lymphatics* accompany the blood-vessels and empty into the lumbar glands.

Position. — The kidneys lie on each side of the spine in the upper lumbar region, behind the other viscera and outside of the peritoneal cavity (Fig. 135). They rest on the diaphragm and the psoas magnus and quadratus lumborum muscles between the twelfth dorsal and the third lumbar vertebræ. Their upper extremities lie nearer to each other than the lower, and the internal borders face a little downward and forward, the outer borders upward and backward. The right kidney lies rather lower than the left on account of the position of the liver above it (Fig. 136).

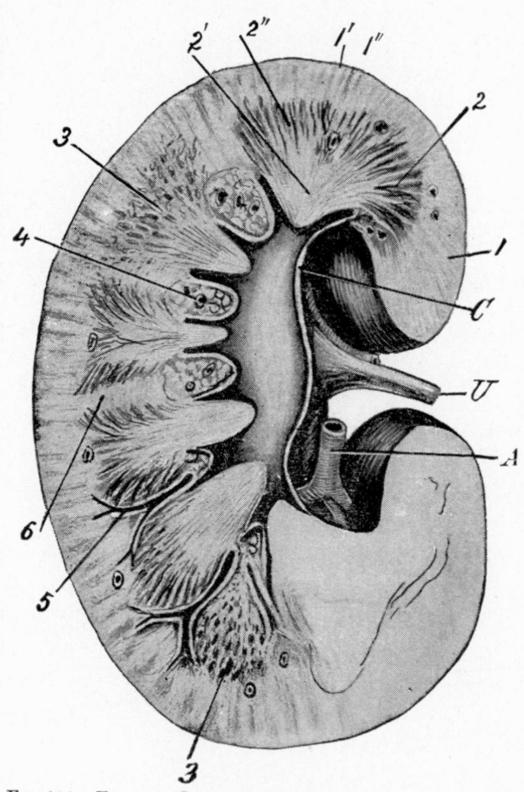

Fig. 134.—Frontal Section through the Kidney, Pelvis, and Calices (Henle).

A, branch of the renal artery; *U*, ureter; *C*, calyx; *1*, cortex; *2'*, medulla; *2"*, boundary zone; *4*, fat of sinus of kidney; *5*, arterial branches.

The average normal variation in the position of the kidneys is well expressed by Brewer's[1] statistics obtained in the dissecting-room. He found the upper end of the right kidney opposite the eleventh rib in 78 cases, opposite the twelfth rib in 62 cases, and lower still in 9 cases. The upper end of the left kidney was opposite the tenth rib in 1 case, opposite the eleventh in 100 cases, opposite the twelfth in 43 cases, and below the ribs in 6 cases. Yet it must be borne in mind that during life the kidneys move up and down with every respiration, and are peculiarly susceptible to downward displacement.

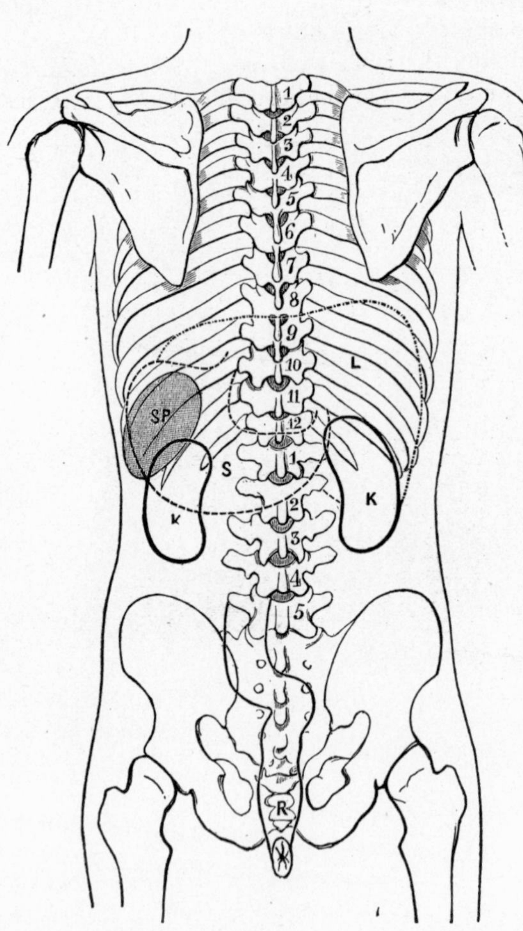

Fig. 135.—Diagram showing Relation of the Viscera to the Parietes, Posterior View (Treves).

S, stomach; *L*, liver; *K*, kidney; *SP*, spleen; *R*, rectum.

Fatty and Fascial Envelope.—The kidney, surrounded by its fibrous capsule and topped by the adrenal, lies embedded in a mass of loose cellular tissue, usually containing a considerable amount of fat, and calculated to permit slight changes in its size and position. This fatty envelope (perirenal fat) quite fills the hollow of the loin, and is surrounded and held in place by a distinct fascia. This fascia has been studied by Zückerkandl, Gerota, and Glantenay and Gosset.[2] It completely surrounds the kidney, the suprarenal capsule, and the peri-

[1] Med. News, 1897, lxxi, 129.

[2] Guyon's Annales, 1898, xvi, 113.

renal fat. In front it blends with the subperitoneal fascia, internally it adheres to the vertebral column, and above to the dia-

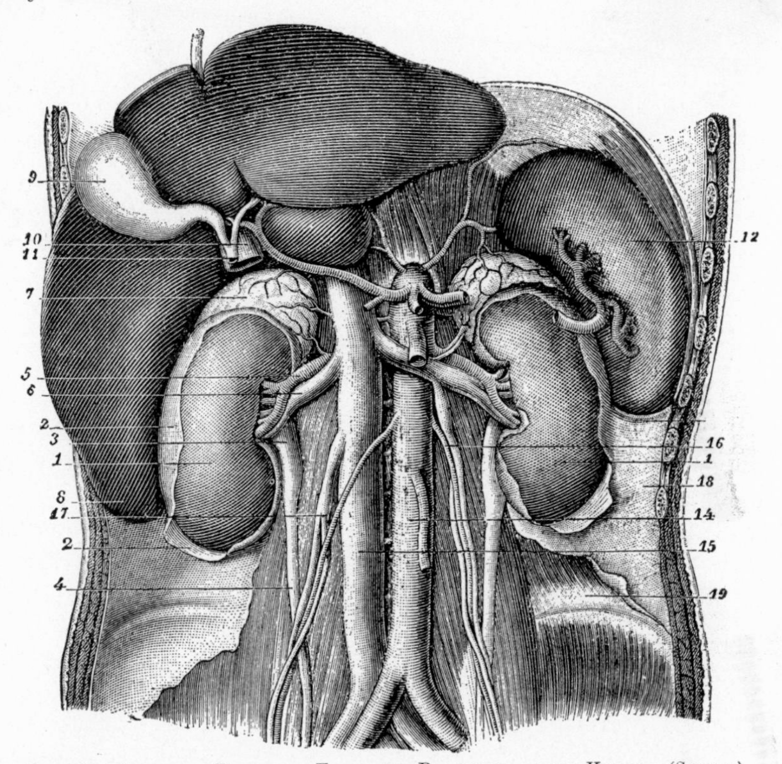

Fig. 136.—Situation, Direction, Form, and Relations of the Kidneys (Sappey).

1, *1*, the two kidneys; *2*, *2*, fibrous capsule; *3*, pelvis; *4*, ureter; *5*, renal artery; *6*, renal vein; *7*, suprarenal capsule; *8*, the liver lifted up; *9*, gall-bladder; *12*, spleen; *14*, abdominal aorta; *15*, inferior vena cava; *16*, left spermatic artery and vein.

phragm. It sends a few fibres to the aponeurosis of the quadratus lumborum which lies immediately behind it. It thus forms a distinct sac firmly anchored to the diaphragm and the spine. It is everywhere closed, except at its lower extremity, where the posterior layer thins out and sends only a few fibres across to the subperitoneal fascia. (Were it not for this hiatus floating kidney would be impossible.) Below and behind this fascial envelope lies another mass of fat, practically continuous with the perirenal fat, but distinguished by the Germans as the " pararenal " fat.

Relations.—Behind, the kidney is in relation with the diaphragm and the psoas and quadratus muscles. The last dorsal nerve runs transversely between the muscles and the perirenal fascia, and the pleura usually descends between the ribs and the diaphragm low enough to cover the upper third of the organ.

In front of the right kidney lie the duodenum and the ascending colon. A fold of peritoneum separates kidney and liver above the colon, while lower down a peritoneal fold separates colon and duodenum.

The left kidney is crossed by the tail of the pancreas and lower down by the descending colon, while its upper portion is separated from the stomach by the lesser sac of peritoneum.

The upper extremity of each kidney is capped by the adrenal. In fetal life this is closely adherent to the kidney and almost completely envelops it, but after birth the adherence becomes slight.

The Pelvis of the Kidney.—The pelvis belongs anatomically to the ureter, of which it is the dilated upper extremity, but surgically to the kidney, of whose secretion it is the reservoir and in whose surgical diseases it participates.

At the bases of the renal pyramids the epithelium of the uriniferous tubules joins with the fibrous covering of the cortex, the one to form the inner, the other the outer, coat of a tube surrounding one or more papillæ, and called a *calix* (infundibulum). The calices unite to form the pelvis, an irregularly funnel-shaped pouch which protrudes from the lower and back part of the hilum, whence it runs downward, narrowing rapidly to become the ureter proper at a level with the lower end of the kidney.

The structure of the pelvis resembles that of the ureter (p. 469).

PHYSIOLOGY

The physiology of the kidney, in so far as it interests the surgeon, may be studied under three divisions:

I. Estimation of the Renal Function.

II. Renal Reflexes.

III. The Effect of Anesthetics upon the Kidney.

Estimation of the Renal Function

The surgery of the urinary organs would be an exact science were we able accurately to estimate the functional capacity of the kidneys. Renal insufficiency, be it in the form of an acute suppression of urine or of a slowly progressing uremia, is the most elusive, the most threatening element of post-operative prognosis. In every operation from urethrotomy to nephrectomy we are taught by bitter experience that however careful the preparation, however minute the asepsis and antisepsis, however brilliant the execution, however promising the outlook, suppression or uremia may claim the victim. We are becoming expert in urinary bacteriology and antisepsis. Our ideas grow more incisive, our fingers more adept, but now and again the kidneys trick us still. Wherein does our knowledge fail? We can estimate accurately the quantity and quality of the renal secretion. We can recognise the clinical picture of urinary toxemia and septicemia. We can even delve into urinary toxicity, cryoscopy, and the phloridzin and pyoktanin tests. By these means we can learn with considerable accuracy what the kidneys *are doing*, and hence we may make certain fairly correct inferences. But what the kidneys *will do*, how they will bear the shock of anesthesia and operation, how much reserve energy they have, we are far from comprehending. I make no attempt to discredit the present trend of scientific investigation in this department: on the contrary, I hope as fervently as any one that we are on the right track. But as yet the experimental stage has not been passed. While all are agreed that the estimation of specific gravity, urea, etc., affords very inadequate evidence of functional activity of the kidneys, the newer methods have yet to show that they are much better for the surgeon's purposes.

Methylene Blue and Phloridzin.—In 1897 Achard and Castaigne proposed to test the permeability of the kidneys by means of subcutaneous injections of methylene blue. After the injection of 1 c. c. of a 5% solution, they found that if the kidneys are normal the blue appears in the urine within a half hour, reaches its maximum concentration in about two hours, and gradually diminishes, disappearing at the end of twenty-four to forty-eight hours. The elimination of the methylene blue is accompanied, sometimes preceded, sometimes followed, by the elimination of a colourless chromogen, which is detected by acidulating with acetic acid and boiling.

It was at first believed that the elimination of both the blue and its chromogen was retarded by any disease which interfered with the excretory power of the kidneys (producing the so-called renal insufficiency). But further experience has shown that while, as a rule, the excretion of methylene blue is retarded by interstitial nephritis, it is accelerated by parenchymatous nephritis; while in a fair proportion of cases the opposite is true, interstitial change hastens and parenchymatous change retards elimination. Albarran and Bernard [1] have studied, by the aid of ureteral catheterism, the elimination of methylene blue in surgical diseases of the kidney.

On the other hand, it has long been known that the subcutaneous injection of phloridzin would cause a temporary glycosuria. This fact has been utilized as a test of renal permeability. If 5 mgm. of phloridzin are injected subcutaneously, sugar should appear in the

[1] Guyon's Annales, 1899, xvii, 336, 465.

urine within an hour and disappear within four hours, the total amount of sugar excreted varying from 0.5 to 2.5 grammes. Disease, especially interstitial disease, retards and decreases the glycosuria or even prevents it completely. In other cases the glycosuria is excessive.

Cryoscopy.[1]—Cryoscopy is the determination of the freezing point of fluids containing certain substances in solution. Urinary cryoscopy consists in determining the relation of the freezing point of the urine to that of the blood. The most important studies in these relations have been made by Koranyi. Urinary cryoscopy has been applied to the study of renal permeability, cardiac disease, and physiological metabolism. It is currently stated that with the reduced elimination of urinary insufficiency the urinary freezing point falls. But the case is by no means so simple. The theory is based upon a series of chemical formulæ and hypotheses that cannot be familiarly handled by any but a trained physiological chemist; while as an evidence of the delicacy of the technic we may adduce the testimony which Huddleston [2] offers in his able review of this subject —viz., that his earlier experiments were rendered useless by instrumental inaccuracy, in spite of the great care which he evidently bestowed upon every detail.

Comparison of Methods.—When one endeavours to compare the relative values of the different tests of renal permeability, one is confronted by a remarkable discrepancy of authorities. We learn that the results of the methylene blue and the phloridzin tests are neither consistent with nor conformable to each other. A happy, though possibly incorrect, elucidation of these discrepancies appears in the theory that either test measures only the renal permeability to a single substance, not to all substances—a selective, not a general permeability. Again, while all award to cryoscopy a pre-eminent precision, Casper [3] claims that the phloridzin test always accords with the findings of cryoscopy, while Achard [4] proclaims the supremacy of the methylene-blue test. And finally, Bernard [5] confesses that there is no stable relation between uremia and impermeability, and Vaquez adds that the absence of any sign of reduced permeability or of reduced freezing point does not preclude the possibility of uremia.

From these diverse opinions several conclusions may be drawn. In the first place, it is evident that none of these new methods is infallible, while, unhappily, the most promising of the lot—viz., cry-

---

[1] *Cf.* La Cryoscopie des urines. H. Claude et V. Balthazard, Paris, 1901.

[2] Phila. Med. J., 1901, vii, 1246.

[3] Berlin. klin. Wochenschr., 1900, xxxvii, 643.

[4] Semaine méd., 1900, xx, 247.

[5] Guyon's Annales, 1901, xix, 206 *et seq.*

oscopy—is the most difficult to carry out accurately, and can only be performed by a trained chemist with special apparatus. It is also obvious that any one of the methods may hint at an important renal insufficiency, which other methods of diagnosis might fail to show; and yet that very insufficiency need not necessarily indicate an impending uremia. Finally, it is an open question whether the routine observance of the daily excretion of urea, the presence or absence of polyuria or anuria, and above all a broad-minded estimate of the patient's general condition, of the presence or absence of urinary toxemia or septicemia, do not give surer results than a too close technical examination by methods whose value is as yet only vaguely determined. I confess a greater confidence in the older familiar methods until such time as we can apply the newer elimination tests with greater precision than is as yet attainable.

Renal Reflexes

Here, again, we enter a field that merits further exploration. So vague is our knowledge of renal reflexes that the description of them resolves itself into the enumeration of a series of disconnected facts and opinions. We may consider reflexes concerning the secretion of urine and painful reflexes.

Reflexes concerning the Secretion of Urine.—The function of the kidneys is regulated by the nervous system. Roughly speaking, the excretion of solid matter (in solution) by the kidney depends upon the amount of such matter in the blood and the health or the disease of the renal cells. But the amount of water excreted varies widely with the nervous condition of the individual, as is best exemplified by the phenomena of hysterical polyuria, and nocturnal polyuria.

Hysterical Polyuria.—Hysterical polyuria occurs almost exclusively in young adults. By day the attacks occur as follows: the subject urinates naturally, emptying his bladder completely. Within a short time, perhaps within fifteen or twenty minutes, he is surprised by a desire to urinate—often an imperious desire. In relieving himself he notices a scalding in the perineum and along the urethra, which is the more remarkable since the urine is almost clear water. But the most startling feature of the case is the amount of urine passed. More than a pint of this clear limpid fluid may be secreted by the kidneys within a half hour. These attacks are purely neurotic, of short duration, and irregular in recurrence. They are indicative either of an acute nervous strain or of a chronic state of nervous tension and weakness. Beyond this they have no significance.

Nocturnal Polyuria.—Nocturnal polyuria might be termed the neurasthenic polyuria of the decline of life. As such it has a far more serious import than hysterical polyuria. When a man beyond his prime complains of passing great quantities of urine at night, while his output by day is about normal, it invariably means that he is suffering from some form of nervous debility. He may be suffering from chronic nephritis or hypertrophy of the prostate as well, and the former may cause a polyuria both diurnal and nocturnal, the latter a nocturnal pollakiuria; but unless the man's nervous energy—his power of resistance, his vital force—is impaired, the nocturnal polyuria will not assume notable proportions. In such a condition surgical operation of any sort is a grave risk. Treatment of any existing prostatic retention or renal disease is not to the point. What the man needs is hygiene and tonics, and, more than anything else, relief of mind from the troubles that oppress him.

Hysterical Anuria.—Anuria the result of nervous conditions may be a benign or a grave condition. Complete anuria is one of the manifestations of true hysteria (p. 634). It may last for hours, even days, during which time the kidneys secrete not one drop of urine. This anuria (or it may be only an oliguria) may be alarming, but I do not know that it has ever proved fatal. It is habitually succeeded by an extreme polyuria, as though the kidneys were striving to make up for lost time.

Reflex Anuria.—A more serious type of anuria is that which sometimes follows traumatism to the urethra, the passage of a sound, or the performance of urethrotomy. The kidney secretion is immediately inhibited. There may or may not be urethral chill; there may or may not be evidence of renal disease. The clinical features of this anuria, so often fatal, have already been discussed (p. 43). In most cases it is associated with infection and disease, but by its very clinical features it is evidently reflex in origin, due to the irritation of the nerves of the deep urethra.

Of no less importance is the reno-renal reflex anuria. This is not a purely nervous anuria, for it occurs only under such circumstances of anesthesia or of bilateral kidney disease as make it in great part evidently referable to an irritative and compensatory congestion. But the fact remains that when one kidney is cut down upon, the other is very likely to cease functionating for a time. The details of this condition may best be discussed elsewhere (p. 644).

Pain Reflexes.—The pain reflexes of the kidneys are threefold: pain referred from the prostatic urethra to the kidney; pain referred from the kidney to the prostatic urethra; pain referred from one kidney to the other.

As a rule pain referred from the prostatic urethra to the kidney is of no great importance. Patients with posterior urethritis, especially at its onset or during an exacerbation, may complain of a dull ache in the loins (not due to sandal-wood oil). I have not known this ache to prove unbearable nor to portend any serious consequences. Again, the sufferer from prostatic neuralgia may complain bitterly of pains radiating up the ureter to one or both kidneys. Such pains merit no especial attention.

Pain referred from the kidney to the prostatic urethra will be referred to later (p. 584).

Pain referred from one kidney to the other is alleged to be a misleading feature of some cases of renal calculus, but it must be rare. Morris has never met with it nor have I.

The Effects of Anesthetics upon the Kidneys

It is generally admitted that whatever the anesthetic employed, anesthesia has no permanent or serious ill effects upon the kidneys. The lists, published from to time, of urinary analyses taken before and after operations upon individuals whose kidneys are presumably sound, show the appearance of albumin and casts after operation where none existed before, and it is familiarly recognised that after any serious operation, whether on account of operative shock or anesthesia, the urinary output is markedly decreased during the first twenty-four to forty-eight hours. Beyond this there is no universally accepted rule. Some maintain that if the kidneys are seriously diseased and unequal to withstand a severe shock it is safer to use ether, while others cling to chloroform. I believe, however, that the majority of clinicians prefer chloroform to ether in such cases. Such has always been my preference, and the researches of Thompson and Kemp [1] add scientific support to this belief.

These observers state:

"As regards ether, it would appear that this agent produces a special contraction of the renal arterioles, with a consequent damaging effect upon the renal secretory cells, similar to that which follows clamping the renal artery. The kidney shrinks in bulk, with consequent fall of the oncometric tracing, and accompanied by diminution of secretion, marked albuminuria, and, finally, suppression. As remarked before, this condition of the kidney is not due to any change in the general arterial circulation.

"These facts would seem to contra-indicate the use of ether as

---

[1] Med. Record, 1898, liv, 325.

an anesthetic when renal disease is present, and particularly when with albuminuria there is a tendency to pulmonary edema.

"The effect of chloroform upon the kidney seems to be nil. The oncometric curves are nearly normal and are affected only through sharing in general circulatory changes. The secretion of urine continues up to the last moment of life, and the albuminuria is so slight that its presence at all is apparently due only to respiratory interference. Meantime the action of chloroform on the heart, as shown by the carotid tracings, is directly depressing. Ether, on the other hand, shows evidence of cardiac stimulation throughout.

"The A. C. E. mixture shows the special effects both of ether on the kidneys and of chloroform on the heart, either being predominant according to the mode of the administration. . . . These objections appear to be still more applicable to Schleich's anesthetic."

In this connection, however, the depressing effect of chloroform upon the heart must not be forgotten. A myocarditis often accompanies advanced renal disease, and it may be a delicate question whether it is wiser to imperil the kidneys by administering ether, or the heart by chloroform. When this question arises it is safe to hold to the rule (other things being equal): in nephrotomy spare the heart, the incision and drainage of the kidney will stimulate it to secretion sufficiently to make up for the added risk; in nephrectomy spare the remaining kidney, which will have strain enough put upon it. In any case spare the patient; make the anesthesia as short and as light as possible.

EXAMINATION OF THE KIDNEY

Inspection.—Inspection of the patient's abdomen or loin reveals nothing in reference to the kidney, unless it be greatly enlarged. The thick spinal muscles prevent tumours of the kidney from projecting backward. Hence they protrude first in the loin and thence push forward the antero-lateral portion of the upper abdomen. No definite information can be gained, however, without palpation.

Palpation.—The kidney, normal in size and situation, cannot be palpated. Indeed, it may be distinctly enlarged, especially in a stout subject, and still be impalpable.

For a proper palpation of the kidney the patient should be flat on his back with the head and shoulders elevated on a small pillow and the lower extremities flexed. In this position the abdominal wall is entirely relaxed, unless the patient voluntarily stiffens his muscles, either by lifting his head for the purpose of seeing what the surgeon is doing, or his side in a futile endeavour to help in the manipulations, or by tightening up the abdominal muscles in instinctive resistance. A few words and a gentle touch will overcome these difficulties.

The simplest and most efficacious method of examination is Guyon's *ballottement rénal.* To examine the right kidney the patient lies, as above described, at the edge of a couch, beside which, and to the right side of the patient, the surgeon sits. With the index and middle fingers of the left hand the surgeon now identifies and makes pressure upon the triangular depressible spot between the last rib and the vertebral column. The right hand is then placed close under the free border of the ribs, and firmly pressed upward and inward, while the patient is required to breathe deeply. Then, at the moment of deepest inspiration, the fingers of the left hand are suddenly and sharply pressed forward. If the kidney is tender this blow upon it will evoke pain. If it is enlarged or movable it will be thrown forward against the fingers of the right hand, which recognises the impact, the ballottement of a solid body. This examination should be repeated several times to preclude the possibility of error, positive or negative.

If an enlarged or a movable kidney is thus identified, further information may be gained by making the patient take long deep breaths, and endeavouring, at the beginning of expiration, just as the abdominal wall relaxes, to catch the kidney between the two hands. If the kidney is freely movable deep inspiration may send it wholly below the surgeon's hands, and he may feel its size, shape, and tenderness by gentle pressure as it slides back again during inspiration. Similarly if it is merely enlarged or only slightly movable, the examining fingers can detect the contour and tenderness of more or less of the organ. Many surgeons claim that by this method it is sometimes possible to feel even the normal kidney.

When the kidney is notably enlarged it may be examined by simple abdominal palpation and percussion. A movable kidney may usually be satisfactorily examined by the method above described, though Israel and Morris prefer that the patient lie on his side with the loin to be examined uppermost. Occasionally a kidney is displaced downward so far that it never returns to its place in the loin. The patient complains of a tumour or of a tender spot in the iliac or the lateral umbilical region, and the movable kidney, which can be returned towards or into the loin, is recognised by deep palpation with the flat of the fingers.

I have not found palpation advantageous with the patient in the erect, sitting, stooping, or knee-elbow position. Exploration by means of the ureteral catheter and the X-ray need not be dwelt upon here. Exploratory laparotomy has been almost entirely abandoned in favour of lumbar nephrotomy. This operation will be described elsewhere (p. 637).

ABNORMALITIES OF THE KIDNEY

The abnormalities of the kidney are either—

1. Abnormalities of Form (Congenital Malformations).
2. Abnormalities of Number, or
3. Abnormalities of Position (Misplaced Kidney).

Since operations upon the kidney have become so frequent each variety has assumed a practical importance.

Frequency.—Abnormalities of the kidney are very rare. Morris[1] has collected the records of 11,168 post-mortem examinations at the Middlesex Hospital and Guy's. Excluding floating kidneys, 16 cases of double ureter, and 53 cases of acquired atrophy and small cirrhotic kidneys, his cases may be tabulated thus:

Congenital atrophy (unilateral)	11 cases.
Fused kidney	1 case.
Horse-shoe kidney	16 cases.
Lobulated kidney (4 bilateral)	9 cases.
Malformed kidneys (1 bilateral)	6 cases.
Misplaced kidneys	10 cases.

About 1 case in 211.

Congenital Malformations

Variations in the size of the kidney are interesting only when they amount to atrophy. Apart from these malformations, we may consider malformations without union and malformations associated with fusion or union of the two kidneys.

Simple Malformation.—Slight irregularity in the shape of the kidney, a greater or less persistence of fetal lobulations, is not uncommon and has no surgical interest. Considerable malformation of the kidney is usually associated with displacement, and is of interest in the latter connection. Bergmann[2] states that malformed kidneys are peculiarly subject to tuberculosis.

Fusion.—(See Abnormalities in Number.)

Abnormalities in Number

Morris recognises five subvarieties—viz.:

A. Single, or unsymmetrical kidney, where one is entirely absent.

---

[1] Surgical Diseases of the Kidney and Ureter, 1901, i, 32.

[2] Deutsch. Chir. von Billroth u. Lücke, 1896, lii, i, 113.

B. Solitary or fused kidney, where the two kidneys are massed together.

C. Imperfect development, or atrophy of the kidney.

D. Absence of both kidneys (no clinical significance).

E. Supernumerary kidneys.

In each of the first three subvarieties there is but one kidney, yet embryologically the conditions differ widely. In class *A* one kidney is entirely absent; in class *B* both kidneys are more or less fully developed and united; in class *C* one kidney is never sufficiently developed to perform its functions.

Single Kidney.—Single kidney is very rare. Morris has collected records of 10 instances among 24,542 autopsies. The kidney is hypertrophied and may be situated normally or displaced downward. The ureter is wanting on the opposite side. The absence of one kidney is not necessarily a great evil, for Newman has recorded 17 cases of patients with this abnormality living beyond the sixtieth year. But it is of paramount importance should the question of nephrectomy arise.

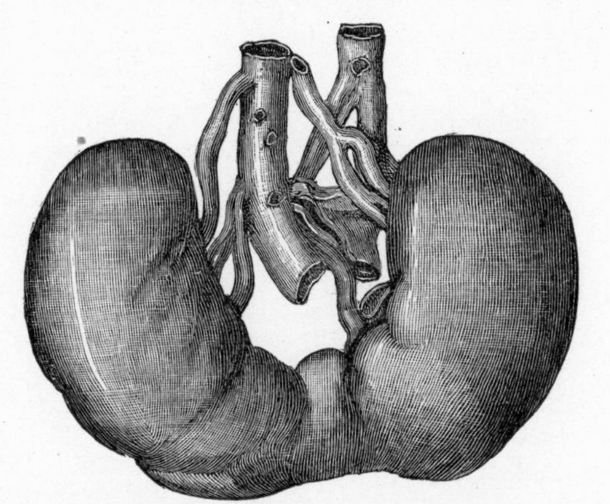

Fig. 137.—Horse-shoe Kidney (Morris).

Fused Kidney.—Fused kidney may be horse-shoe-shaped, completely fused, or irregular in shape. The two latter forms are extremely rare. In each the kidney has two ureters running from it into opposite sides of the bladder, and may be situated normally, displaced downward, or lying in the median line.

The horse-shoe kidney (Fig. 137) is the most common of all renal abnormalities. Morris noted it 19 times among 18,244 autopsies; Preindlsberger [1] 6 times among 1,344 autopsies; and Socin [2] 5 times among 1,630 autopsies—in all, 30 cases among 21,218 autopsies (1 in 707). The fused organ is made up of two fairly normal kidneys lying low in the loin, and more or less intimately united by a band of renal tissue running across the median line and connecting the lower poles of the two organs. (In one of Socin's and one of

---

[1] Wien. klin. Rundschau, 1901, xv, 197, 215.

[2] Quoted by Bergmann, *op. cit.*, p. 117

Preindlsberger's cases the upper poles are united instead of the lower ones.) The great vessels habitually lie behind the central mass, while, as a rule, the ureters descend in front of it. There are usually two separate and normal pelves and ureters, but ureteral and vascular abnormalities often occur. Since the possibility of partial nephrectomy has become generally recognised, the horse-shoe kidney has lost its terrors. A contemplated nephrectomy need not be abandoned if this condition is encountered. Resection of the affected half of the organ may be performed, although, of course, the other half must be spared.

Atrophy of the Kidney.—Atrophy of one kidney may be congenital or acquired. Congenital atrophy is infrequent, while acquired atrophy, the result of interstitial nephritis or of ureteral obstruction, is common. The existence of this condition enforces the rule, *Never perform nephrectomy unless you are sure that the opposite kidney is present and functionating* (p. 640).

Supernumerary Kidney.—Supernumerary kidneys are most uncommon. Morris records 3 cases, of which 2 were examples of small accessory organs lying near one of the kidneys. The third case, reported by Watson Cheyne,[1] is unique in that the supernumerary kidney lay at the pelvic brim and was found during a laparotomy.

Misplaced Kidney

A misplaced kidney is by no means a movable or floating kidney, though the two conditions may coexist. A fused kidney is usually misplaced, a misplaced kidney often misshapen. Usually only one kidney is affected. The misplaced organ commonly lies near the sacro-iliac synchondrosis, exceptionally in the true pelvis or the opposite loin. The condition is usually congenital, though a movable kidney may become fixed in an abnormal position.

The clinical features of misplaced kidneys are: (*a*) the danger of mistaking them for abdominal tumours, and (*b*) the painful and pathological effects of pressure upon the misplaced organ itself as well as upon the adjoining organs. Hochenegg [2] records 9 nephrectomies for this condition. Buss [3] reports an additional nephrectomy, and Dewis [4] a nephrotomy.

---

[1] Lancet, 1899, i, 215.
[2] Wien. klin. Wochenschr., 1900, xiii, 4.
[3] Zeitschr. f. klin. Med., 1900, xxxix, 439.
[4] Boston Med. and Surg. J., 1901, cxlv, 35.

CHAPTER XXXIV

MOVABLE OR FLOATING KIDNEY—NEPHROPTOSIS

The kidney is naturally endowed with a certain degree of mobility. Like the other abdominal viscera it moves with respiration and its position is influenced by the attitude of the subject. Yet this condition is entirely normal. Such a kidney is not distinctly palpable. A movable kidney, on the other hand, is one that is subject to downward displacement to such an extent that it may be distinctly palpated by the usual methods of examination. English authors distinguish between movable kidney and floating kidney. The former is subject to downward displacement only behind the peritoneum; the latter may also be displaced forward towards the anterior abdominal wall, and often possesses a mesonephron. Continental writers distinguish mobility of the first degree (the fingers can grasp the kidney), the second degree (the fingers can be brought together above the organ), and the third degree (the kidney can be depressed into the iliac fossa).

Frequency

The recorded frequency of movable kidney varies with the point of view of the author and the delicacy of his sense of touch. The widely divergent opinions of various writers may be tabulated thus:

	Women.		Per cent.	Men.		Per cent.
	Cases examined.	Movable kidney.		Cases examined.	Movable kidney.	
Bergmann[1]	905	40	4.41	828	4	0.48
Einhorn[2]	543	112	20	772	14	1.81
Idem[3]	832	240	28	1,080	42	3.88
Mathieu[4]	306	85	25	...	..	....
Godard-Danhieux[5]	603	212	35	268	6	2.33
Suckling[6]	100	42	42	100	6	6
Harris[7]	126	71	56	...	..	....

[1] *Op. cit.*, p. 134.
[2] Med. Record, 1898, liv, 220.
[3] *Ibid.*, 1901, lix, 561.
[4] Le bull. méd., 1893, vii, 1113.
[5] Guyon's Annales, 1901, xix, 197.
[6] Edinb. Med. J., 1898, iv, 228.
[7] J. of the Am. Med. Ass'n, 1901, xxxvi, 1527.

Many of these statistics are obviously compiled *in camera*, and represent only the physician's interpretation of the term "movable kidney" without any reference to the patient's symptoms. The average observer will probably recognise a movable kidney in 20% of women and 2% of men; yet the cases which have symptoms and require treatment are far fewer than this.

There is a general agreement that in 8 cases out of 10 the right kidney only is movable; of the remainder the majority are bilateral, unilateral left-sided nephroptosis being most unusual. When both kidneys are movable, the right kidney is usually more movable than the left.

Although movable kidneys have been discovered in patients of all ages, as a rule the symptoms of the disease appear in the third decade of life and disappear between the fortieth and fiftieth years.

Pathogenesis

Our conceptions of how the kidney becomes movable are only just emerging from an overwhelming mass of contradictory assertions. Without pausing to confuse the issue by reporting every shade of opinion, it is safer to plunge at once into the subject, guiding ourselves by a symptom rather than by any man's views, placing our credence only in facts that are proved, and leaving open questions open still. To be satisfactory, a theory must explain (*a*) the predominance of movable kidney in woman, (*b*) the frequency with which it occurs on the right side, and (*c*) its importance between the ages of twenty and forty.

We shall consider:

a. Causes of Congenital Nephroptosis.
b. Causes of Acquired Nephroptosis.
- Primary Predisposing Cause.—Shape of the lumbar recess.
- Secondary Predisposing Causes { Enteroptosis. Pregnancy. Emaciation.
- Exciting Causes { Corsets. Trauma.

a. **Causes of Congenital Nephroptosis.**—The existence of congenital nephroptosis has been doubted, but the possibility of such a condition is proved by such cases as Dr. W. R. Stewart's. In this case an exploratory operation performed for intestinal obstruction on an infant eight months old disclosed a floating kidney. Abt [1] and Morris have collected similar cases. Yet the discovery of a movable

[1] J. of the Am. Med. Ass'n, 1901, xxxvi, 1166.

kidney in a child is undoubtedly exceptional, and the presence of any symptoms before puberty is rarer still.

With our present knowledge it is impossible to say what may be the cause of this condition. It has not been determined how far the factors that operate in later life are at work, and how great a part actual abnormal development plays.

b. **Causes of Acquired Nephroptosis.—Primary Predisposing Cause.**—Wolkow and Delitzen[1] have shown by an extensive series of pathological investigations that there is quite a wide variation in the size of the niche in the loin occupied by the kidney. The paravertebral niche, as they call it, is shallower in women than in men, shallower on the right side[2] than on the left. The feminine peculiarity appears with the broadening of the pelvis at the advent of puberty; and it is this feminine, right-sided shallowness of the bed in which the kidney lies that is the chief predisposing cause of nephroptosis. Harris has gone even further, and maintains that the chief characteristics of the body form that predispose to nephroptosis "are a marked contraction of the middle zone of the body with a diminution in the capacity of this portion of the body cavity. This diminution in the capacity of the middle zone depresses the kidney, so that the constricted outlet of the zone comes above the centre of the organ, and all acts, such as coughing, straining, lifting, flexions of the body, etc., which tend to adduct the lower ribs, press on the upper pole of the kidney and crowd it still farther downward. It is the long-continued repetition, in a suitable body form, of these influences, which collectively may be called internal traumata, that gradually produces a movable kidney." Not every one is willing to lay so much stress on the predisposing cause, though Wolkow and Delitzen have proved that its influence has been much underrated.[3]

Secondary Predisposing Causes.—The internal traumata just mentioned, and many others, such as intermittent renal congestion during menstruation, prolapse, and inflammation of the pelvic organs, etc., may be included here; but we need discuss only four alleged causes—viz., enteroptosis, weakness of the abdominal wall, pregnancy, and emaciation.

Enteroptosis is a general condition, of which nephroptosis is often one of the features. Glenard[4] considers that nephroptosis never exists without a general enteroptosis, but he stands alone in this

[1] Die Wanderniere, 1899, Berlin.

[2] Chiefly because the liver fills the upper segment of the niche on this side.

[3] The theory that enteroptosis is an evidence of degeneracy has been propounded by Stiller, Tuffier, and Albarran, but this theory has not met with general acceptance.

[4] Les Ptoses viscérales, Paris, 1899. Lyon méd., 1885, xliv, 8.

opinion. Einhorn [1] has seen 27 cases of enteroptosis without nephroptosis, and 213 cases in which both conditions existed; hepatoptosis occurred with nephroptosis only 30 times, 54 times without it; while in 57 cases only the kidney was movable. Similarly Godard-Danhieux [2] records 131 cases of nephroptosis without enteroptosis, and 81 cases with it; while in 97 instances there was enteroptosis without nephroptosis. Obviously, then, enteroptosis plays only a secondary rôle. When the two coexist it is quite as possible they are due to similar causes as that the one depends upon the other. I can comprehend how a loose liver should depress the kidney below it and favour its mobility; but a general enteroptosis can influence the position of the kidney only by leaving room for its displacement.

Pregnancy introduces another dispute. It is an accepted fact that repeated pregnancies favour relaxation of the abdominal wall and enteroptosis, yet there is an absolute disagreement in the statistics on nephroptosis. Landau, Senator, Moulin, Morris, and others maintain that movable kidney is more frequent in women who have borne children, while Küttner, Godard-Danhieux, and Lindner defend the opposite theory. It would certainly seem probable that tendency to mobility in a kidney would be increased by the abdominal strain of parturition, and the resultant abdominal flaccidity.

Weakness of the abdominal wall, Wolkow and Delitzen insist, is a strong predisposing factor in enteroptosis and nephroptosis. The abdominal viscera are deprived of their necessary support, and therefore sag downward, carrying the kidneys with them, in case the shallowness of the paravertebral niches makes these organs liable to prolapse. Many authors agree in this theory, which has the merits of lucidity and appositeness.

Emaciation, it is stated, causes nephroptosis by absorption of the perirenal fat. Morris has often noted the small quantity of fat that surrounds kidneys requiring nephrorrhaphy. Yet one can scarcely believe that the absorption of fat could be so sudden as to leave a space into which the kidney would sag. On the other hand, it is quite conceivable that the excursions of a movable kidney should discourage the deposition of fat within its fascial envelope.

Exciting Causes.—*Corsets* have been alternately praised and condemned. A corset that brings pressure to bear below the kidney region will, if applied while the kidney is in place, help to retain

---

[1] Med. Record, 1898, liv, 220; 1899, lvi, 397; and 1901, lix, 561.

[2] Gaz. hebd., 1900, v, 159.

a movable organ; while a long-waisted corset that compresses the ribs is equally likely to encourage renal mobility. The fact that Egyptians suffer from movable kidney is evidence that the corset does not deserve all the blame which has been heaped upon it. Yet it does weaken the abdominal wall and so increases the liability to nephroptosis.

Trauma of one sort or another is certainly the exciting cause of all cases of movable kidney. But it is equally certain that the trauma in question is usually of a mild type. Suckling mentions the influence of constant stooping. The internal traumata recognised by Harris have been enumerated. The influence of pregnancy and corsets has already been mentioned. Bergmann insists upon the evil effect of horseback riding.

The effect of acute trauma, such as falls, kicks, and blows, is an open question. Harris absolutely denies its influence, and though many acute cases from this cause have been enumerated, I believe that in most instances the trauma has been only the cause of symptoms in an organ already movable.

Morbid Anatomy

Congenital Mobility.—" A floating kidney with a mesonephron is, of course, always congenital " (Morris). Such cases are rare; but it is also possible that the kidney may be congenitally movable behind the peritoneum.

Acquired Mobility.—The kidney may be movable within its fatty capsule, or fat and kidney may move together within the fascia. The adrenal does not habitually move with the kidney. The kidney, however great its acquired mobility, does not come to have a mesonephron. It moves about behind the peritoneum, rarely making its way between mesenteric layers.

Secondary Changes.—As a result of long-continued mobility the *renal vessels* may become considerably lengthened. They are the radii of the circle in which the kidney moves; as they lengthen mobility increases.

The *ureter* may become kinked, and in this event, which is by no means uncommon, the free outflow of urine is obstructed and the kidney becomes hydronephrotic. Kinking of the ureter is due to the fact that it is held fast to the peritoneum, and therefore cannot partake in the renal excursion.

Adhesions may form as a result of repeated attacks of hydronephrosis or of other inflammation of the kidney itself or of the surrounding tissues. Such adhesions increase the ureteral obstruction and may give rise to considerable pain.

The secondary changes in the kidney are referred to in connection with hydronephrosis.

Exceptionally *gangrene of the kidney* has occurred from torsion of the pedicle.

Symptoms

So as to bring order out of the contradictory opinions concerning the symptoms of movable kidney, we may take as the basis of our description a few commonly accepted facts. In the first place, any surgeon familiar with abdominal palpation appreciates that, in examining a patient, one occasionally finds a movable kidney—perhaps even a floating kidney—which has never given any symptoms, and of whose existence the patient will not become aware unless the surgeon announces his discovery. Then there is a second class of cases who, while having a movable kidney and suffering from various symptoms—digestive, neurotic, or pelvic—have no symptoms directly referable to the kidney itself. The organ is neither tender, adherent, nor enlarged. There is no history of hydronephrosis, no evidence of either urinary infection or renal sclerosis. Finally, there are other cases with symptoms directly referable to the kidney itself. Thus nephroptosis is encountered clinically under three aspects:

1. Nephroptosis without symptoms.
2. Nephroptosis without symptoms directly referable to the kidney.
3. Nephroptosis with symptoms directly referable to the kidney.

Nephroptosis without Symptoms directly Referable to the Kidney.—The greater number of cases commonly classed as movable kidney come under this head, and it is the infinite variety of symptoms which such cases present, the doubtful origin of these symptoms, and the uncertainty of their cure that has obscured the whole subject and given rise to opinions so divergent and to discussions so virulent. And so long as man retains his individuality opinions upon this subject must continue to differ. Therefore I shall not attempt the futile task of reconciliation, but shall rest satisfied with expressing a point of view which may afford a basis for discrimination in the surgical treatment of this malady which, after all, is the main point at issue.

The class of cases under discussion has but two common features: (1) The subjective symptoms are referable to any one of several diseases of organs other than the kidneys, and (2) one or both kidneys are movable, but present no signs, either subjective (pain) or objective, of disease. Such patients may present nervous symptoms, digestive disorders, or painful symptoms. These symptoms are exhibited in greater or less degree and in various combinations.

Nervous Symptoms.—It is quite impracticable to detail here the various symptoms of neurasthenia with abdominal manifestations that have been attributed to renal mobility. Their name is legion. But the question that always arises is, Does the neurasthenia depend upon the movable kidney? Two answers may be suggested. If temporary reposition of the affected organ brings temporary relief from the symptoms, and if with renewal of the kidney prolapse the symptoms recur, there is, clinically speaking, an established connection between the mobility of the kidney and the nervous symptoms. In the second place, it may be found that, perhaps as a result of slight retention from kinking of the ureter, there is interstitial nephritis. In this case the nervous symptoms may possibly be attributed to renal auto-intoxication.

Digestive Disorders.—The flatulent dyspepsia and constipation that figure so prominently among the symptoms of nephroptosis are but rarely referable to the kidney. Einhorn's opinion upon this subject deserves quotation:

"Most of the gastric and intestinal symptoms, such as pains, eructations, nausea, occasional vomiting, irregularity of the bowels (chiefly constipation, sometimes diarrhea), which are present in persons with movable kidney, occur usually independently of the latter, and require therapeutic measures appropriate to such conditions. Gastric neuroses, which originate by reflex action from a movable kidney, are met with but rarely; among them I would place nervous vomiting and nausea. Whether cases of periodic attacks of continued gastro-succorrhea can be regarded as reflex symptoms of a movable kidney appears to me doubtful. Of course these conditions are found in patients suffering from movable kidney, yet I have observed cases in which neither the wearing of an abdominal bandage nor the performance of nephrorrhaphy caused the disappearance of the periodic gastro-succorrhea."

Here, again, the tests applied to the neurotic cases are of service. If reposition of the kidney relieves the symptoms, or if there is renal insufficiency, some connection between the renal condition and the digestive disturbance may be suspected.

We may mention here the theory maintained by Edebohls[1] that movable kidney on the right side may cause chronic appendicitis by pressure upon the superior mesenteric vein. The relative infrequency of appendicitis in women discourages this belief.

---

[1] Post-Graduate, 1899, xiv, 85.

Painful Symptoms.—The pains most often caused by movable kidney are: (1) Pain and tenderness in the kidney itself. (2) Pain of a dull, dragging character low down in the back, a pain comparable to that commonly attributed to uterine retrodisplacement. (3) Frequent and painful urination. It is characteristic that these pains should be increased by exercise, and should be more severe during the menstrual period. It is evident that any or all (except the first) may be attributable to conditions other than nephroptosis. Therefore it is essential that they should be known to disappear with reposition of the kidney, and to reappear with its prolapse before we can be sure of any connection between the pain and the renal mobility.

Nephroptosis, with Symptoms directly Referable to the Kidney.—Here we enter upon a more definite field of investigation. If the kidney is tender and painful, if the tenderness is relieved by reposition of the organ, if there is renal colic, or if the tender kidney is enlarged or adherent in an abnormal position, we have direct physical evidence that the symptom is due to the nephroptosis. Even more characteristic is the *intermittent hydronephrosis* due to movable kidney. This condition in its fully developed form is unmistakable. The patient comes with history of a tumour in the flank. This tumour gradually grows larger during a few days or weeks and then suddenly disappears. There is an interval of a few days and then the tumour once more begins to grow. It is usually very painful and tender, and its growth is often attended by renal colic, while its disappearance is signalled by relief of the pain and accompanied by the discharge of an excessive quantity of urine. In other cases the kidney does not fill sufficiently to give a perceptible tumour, but there are repeated attacks of renal colic without passage of stones or evidences of pyelo-nephritis. Examination then reveals a movable kidney, swollen and tender during paroxysms.

Intermittent *pyonephrosis* may also occur.

The outcome of these obstructive cases is that of hydronephrosis.

Diagnosis

If the kidney is only slightly movable this may be detected by ballottement and the other methods already described (p. 512). A floating organ may be discovered almost anywhere in the abdomen. As a rule, it is not difficult to distinguish a floating kidney from other abdominal tumours. The very mobility of the organ, the fact that it may be replaced in the loin, together with its general contour, and the sickening sensation, similar to and yet not the same as the ovarian sensation, caused by pressure upon it, are sufficiently characteristic. Tumours arising from the ovaries or uterus may be distinguished by their pelvic attachments. To distinguish a movable kidney from a distended gall-bladder, Morris proposes the following criteria: (1) The enlarged gall-bladder as well as the kidney is a frequent cause of *movable* abdominal tumour. (2) History of jaundice. (3) The tumour caused by an enlarged gall-bladder can, in almost every case, at all times be felt, whereas a movable kidney (unless also enlarged) cannot. (4) Variability in the size of the tumour goes for nothing unless associated with sudden diuresis. (5) A calculous gall-bladder feels much harder than a movable kidney. (6) The radius of mobility of the gall-bladder differs from that of the kidney. Morris also mentions the fact that the two conditions often coexist, and that inflation of the colon for the purpose of pushing the kidney outward and the gall-bladder upward is a most unreliable means of diagnosis, since the hepatic flexure of the colon may be displaced downward and inward when either affection exists. The ultimate method of diagnosis in a doubtful case is exploratory incision. Exploratory aspiration cannot be too strongly condemned.

But the discovery of a movable kidney by no means completes the diagnosis. It is equally important to ascertain whether the symptoms are due to the nephroptosis or to something else. In some cases there can be no doubt that the kidney is at fault. If a hydronephrosis, a pyonephrosis, or an adherent organ is discovered, here is a pathological condition demanding treatment. Then there are the tender kidneys and those cases whose symptoms are temporarily relieved by rest and reposition of the displaced organ. These form a doubtful class, and merit the most minute examination and the closest watching, of which the palliative treatment of the disease forms an important part. The majority of them are complicated by some neurotic tendency, enteroptosis, or gastro-intestinal or pelvic disease. Their judicious treatment is peculiarly difficult. Finally, there are the cases in which no test can show a direct connection between the renal ptosis and the symptoms.

Treatment

In deciding upon the proper course of treatment for any individual case of movable kidney, the surgeon must bear in mind the following facts:

1. In many cases nephroptosis produces no symptoms.

2. In many instances nephropexy, while it retains the kidney in place (which it does not always do), either fails to relieve or aggravates the neurotic or dyspeptic symptoms attributed to the renal mobility.

In view of these facts we must hesitate to elect nephropexy, a treatment which, though surgically a success, may prove clinically a failure, or worse than a failure. Mechanical treatment—supporting the kidney by a suitable belt—may always be experimentally employed in doubtful cases. But to have recourse to surgery is a grave matter. Not because of the danger or discomfort connected with the operation, for the former is almost nil, the latter inconsiderable, but because in most instances the patient is distinctly neurotic, and, while the influence of the operation *per se* may be beneficial, it may also be injurious. In short, the knife is no proper instrument for a faith cure. Its brilliant successes should not blind us to its failures. Yet where palliative measures fail, and the symptoms are apparently dependent upon the renal mobility and require relief, there is no choice. An operation is then surely the lesser evil. So we may conclude that *the treatment of subjective symptoms due to renal mobility is palliative; surgical measures should be reserved for the treatment of hydronephrosis and other similar pathological conditions that cannot be relieved without them, and for those cases that do not respond to persistent, intelligent palliative treatment.*

Palliative Treatment.—The broad lines of palliative treatment are:

1. To remedy digestive and menstrual derangements.
2. To regulate exercise so as to avoid overfatigue.
3. To improve the general vitality and combat neurasthenia by overfeeding, massage, hygiene, electricity, and tonics, and
4. To apply an abdominal supporter.

Much emphasis is placed upon the kind of belt or corset employed to support the abdomen. Edebohls [1] reviews the opinions of various writers upon this subject, even to that of Gurtzburg, who "administers a yeast ferment with the object of producing meteorism, and thus sustaining the prolapsed kidney." This is an extreme example of the fallacious impression that a support must be worn solely for the purpose of retaining the kidney in place, and that, this accomplished, the cure is assured. Nothing could be further from the truth. As a matter of fact, it is the patient's general condition that should be attacked primarily, the local condition only secondarily. Many a case of movable kidney is cured by hygiene, diet, and exercise, while the kidney remains as loose as ever. Moreover, in applying a belt or a corset the effort must be made to support all the abdominal viscera, not the kidney only. It is not conceivable that any form of pad should hold the kidney in place, and

---

[1] Med. Record, 1901, lix, 690.

therefore it is wiser to dispense entirely with pads and to support the abdominal contents *en masse.* For this purpose the modern straight front corset may be employed. Some women find that this article, if applied in the recumbent position, acts as an admirable supporter. If this fails a snug elastic abdominal belt should be tried. And all the while the systemic treatment must be attended to.

Surgical Treatment—Nephropexy.—Nephropexy or nephrorrhaphy is the operation of fixing the prolapsed kidney against the abdominal wall. With abdominal or transperitoneal nephropexy we need not concern ourselves. The operative treatment of hydronephrosis and adherent kidney will interest us in another chapter. Here we need dwell only upon the operation of lumbar nephropexy and its consequences.

The preparation of the patient and the incision in the abdominal wall are made according to the usual rules (p. 637). When the fascial capsule of the kidney is reached it is incised and the kidney laid bare by blunt dissection. The kidney must now be fixed in its proper position. Harris states that the persistence of pain after operation is often due to squeezing of the kidney, which has been replaced by the surgeon in a paravertebral niche too small to contain it. If replacement is not easy, it is certainly legitimate to fix the organ in any available position; but in most cases it is quite possible and eminently proper to replace the kidney well up under the ribs with only its lower half protruding below them. Then arises the question of fixation. Quite a variety of methods have been employed, which may be classified as follows:

1. Suture............ { *a.* Without decortication.
   b. With decortication.
2. Support........... { *a.* By means of the fascia.
   b. By means of cicatricial tissue.

Suture without Decortication.—The obvious way to fix a loose kidney is to remove the greater part of its fatty envelope, and then to attach the organ by 2 or 3 sutures passed through the fibrous capsule, the parenchyma and the parietal muscles. The sutures may be slowly absorbable (chromicized catgut or kangaroo tendon) or silk.

In transfixing the kidney the sutures may be applied along the convex border (Hahn, Bassini, Albarran) or in the posterior surface (Morris). They may be made to transfix the fibrous capsule only (Hahn, Bassini) or the kidney substance as well (Albarran, Morris). The sutures should not be tightly tied lest they cause necrosis of the kidney substance within their grasp. It is useful to scarify the fibrous capsule in order to promote adhesions (Albarran).

Suture with Decortication.—On account of the frequent relapses following nephropexy, as performed in the early days, it seemed doubtful whether simple suture suffices to hold the kidney in place. Accordingly Tuffier suggested that the fibrous capsule be split and turned back along the convex border of the organ, and the sutures be passed through the parenchyma itself. His example has been widely imitated. In some cases the sutures were found to cut through the kidney, and therefore the majority of those who employ decortication apply the sutures to the reflected edges of the fibrous capsule. Dr. J. F. Baldwin [1] carries the capsule flaps into the belly wall between bundles of muscle fibres.

Fascial Support.—Hahn, who was the first to perform nephropexy (in 1881), endeavoured to hold the kidney in place by suturing the fatty and fibrous capsule below the organ. Seven of his 27 cases relapsed, and the operation has been thereby discredited; but Harris [2] has recently suggested a similar operation which he claims has given perfect results. He excises the perirenal fat and sutures the two layers of the fascial capsule together, so as to obliterate the cavity in which the kidney moves, while still permitting the organ a mobility comparable to that of the normal kidney. He counsels opening the peritoneal cavity to the outer side of the colon in case the suturing cannot otherwise be carried out. Andrews [3] counsels carrying the fascial layers out through the parietal incision.

Cicatricial Support.—Every nephropexy by suture is performed with the expectation that firm adhesions will form between the kidney and the abdominal wall, and so prevent any further prolapse of the kidney. But in view of the nervous hyperesthesia of most of these patients many surgeons, of whom I am one, object to suturing the kidney or stripping back its capsule, or in any way injuring it unless something is to be gained thereby. Hence the attempts at obtaining a fascial support, and hence also the advantage of obtaining a cicatricial support without sutures. Jaboulay was the first to employ gauze packing to support the kidney. Senn [4] scarifies the posterior surface of the kidney, applies a sling of iodoform gauze about its lower pole, and stuffs a strip of the same material below the kidney between it and the perirenal fat, thus forming a gauze platform upon which the kidney rests. Since 1892 I have employed a similar method and have found it eminently satisfactory.

Results of Nephropexy.—The earlier nephropexies were so uniformly followed by relapse that many physicians opposed the opera-

---

[1] J. of the Am. Med. Ass'n, 1899, xxxiv, 177.
[2] *Op. cit.*
[3] *Ibid.*, 1900, xxxv, 877.
[4] *Ibid.*, 1897, xxix, 1190.

tion on the ground that a permanent cure was *never* accomplished by operation; but recent statistics tell an entirely different story. Morris has performed 98 nephropexies with one death ("cardiac thrombosis in a stout female whose kidney was incised and explored before being fixed"), and only "a few" relapses after operations performed according to "a plan different from the present methods." Edebohls [1] reports 193 cases (68 bilateral) with 3 deaths and 2 known relapses. All of my own cases have been successful.

But nephropexy may be regarded from another point of view. In a very considerable proportion of cases the patients have complained of more pain after the operation than before. This may be due to one of several factors; perhaps the pain did not commence in the kidney, and therefore was not relieved by operation, but was rather intensified by the shock and disappointment; or perhaps it was due to adhesions or kinks of the ureter which were not relieved by the surgeon; or perhaps the kidney was replaced high up in the loin in a niche from which it had descended because there was not sufficient room for it (Harris), and where it is continually compressed. However this may be, I have had only one patient complain of a recurrence of pain. Nephropexy was performed upon her as a lesser evil than exploratory abdominal section with which she was threatened by another surgeon. Her various neurotic symptoms, which had existed for years, immediately disappeared. Five years later they returned, and she underwent at the hands of various surgeons the extraction of several teeth, drainage of the antrum of Highmore, excision of the inferior dental nerve, nephrectomy (the kidney was found firmly adherent), vesico-vaginal fistulization, an infinite variety of other treatments, all to no avail. It has been interesting to find two reports of her cure, the one by a dentist, the other by a physician. Finally, exploratory laparotomy was performed a year ago. A normal appendix was removed—and she has remained better ever since, though far from well. She has recently been poisoned by a rectal injection of boric acid, but survived!

Choice of Method.—An ideal nephropexy should be free from mortality, should fix the kidney in place, and should incur the least possible risk of subsequent pain. In the matter of mortality there is no preference among the various methods. None of them is dangerous if performed by a competent surgeon upon a patient free from grave organic disease. Relapse is not to be expected after any operation, provided the fatty capsule is removed so as to allow direct adhesion of the kidney to the muscle. There is no need to split the

[1] Med. Record, 1901, lx, 635.

fibrous capsule. Experience has proved that nephropexy is quite as successful without decortication as with it. But pain is the surgeon's bugbear. In these neurotic patients it is quite conceivable that pain may be due to forcing the kidney too high in the loin, to attaching it too firmly (as by decortication or numerous sutures) in any position, or to the presence of silk sutures. Therefore the ideal operation is to reef the fascial capsule, after removal of the perirenal fat, so that the kidney is left relatively free in a confined space. But the capsule-reefing operations lack the confirmation of time, and, therefore, I prefer to support the kidney by packing gauze beneath it, a procedure certain to hold the kidney in place and likely to leave it surrounded by less adhesions than any of the suture methods. On the other hand, if the kidney has to be incised for hydronephrosis or stone, it is obviously appropriate to retain it in place by suture through the reflected capsule.

CHAPTER XXXV

INJURIES TO THE KIDNEY—ANEURYSM OF THE RENAL ARTERY

SUBPARIETAL INJURIES—RUPTURE

THE subparietal injuries of the kidney are often classified as contusions and ruptures; but inasmuch as with every rupture there is contusion, and with almost every contusion at least a partial rupture, while clinically contusion and rupture exhibit the same symptoms and demand the same treatment, they need not be distinguished.

Subparietal injury of the kidney, though more frequent than any other form of renal trauma, is rare. Among 13,455 autopsies there occurred only 31 instances of ruptured kidney (Morris and Herzog[1]). Güterbock,[2] however, encountered 36 ruptured kidneys among 925 autopsies, and 9 such cases among 9,500 patients admitted to St. George's Hospital. Among 198 cases collected by Tuffier, 136 occurred in adult men, and in only two were both kidneys injured. Two hundred and eighty-one of Küster's 306 cases were males. Of 272 in which the particulars are stated, 142 occurred on the right and 118 on the left side, 12 being bilateral (Morris).

The kidneys may be contused by a variety of accidents, such as kicks, buffer accidents, falls, and even simple muscular effort. The lower ribs may be broken and driven into the organ, and many of the accidents are explicable only on the theory that the kidney is burst by the impact of the floating ribs compressing it against the spine.

MORBID ANATOMY

Subcapsular Hemorrhage.—Morris relates two instances of extravasation of blood under the fibrous capsule of the kidney, caused by slight muscular exertion and producing severe pain. Calculus was suspected, but nephrotomy revealed only a subcapsular hematoma,

---

[1] Morris, *op. cit.*

[2] Die chirurgischen Krankheiten der Harnorgane, Leipzig u. Wien, 1898, iv, 900.

the evacuation of which effected a cure. He believes that this form of rupture is not uncommon, and that the compression of the parenchyma, perhaps increased by repeated small hemorrhages, explains the irregular and protracted course of the symptoms in some cases, until ultimately the capsule gives way, the blood and disorganized parenchyma escape into the perirenal space, and this late hematoma demands operation which reveals a disorganized kidney. Such cases are usually classified as *subcapsular lacerations of the kidney substance.*

Laceration of the Parenchyma.—The kidney substance may be lacerated in any direction and to any extent (Fig. 138). Portions of the organ may be lopped off, or the whole kidney may be reduced to a pulp or torn away from its vessels and ureter. If the capsule and ureter remain intact the primary reaction is often slight; but usually one or both are torn, and as a result blood and urine are immediately poured into the perirenal space, at first distending it and forming a tumour in the loin, and later escaping from the orifice at the lower part of the perirenal fascia (or through any tear in it) to form a more or less generalized subperitoneal infiltration. This extravasation of blood and urine is more or less rapid in proportion to the size of the ruptured vessels.

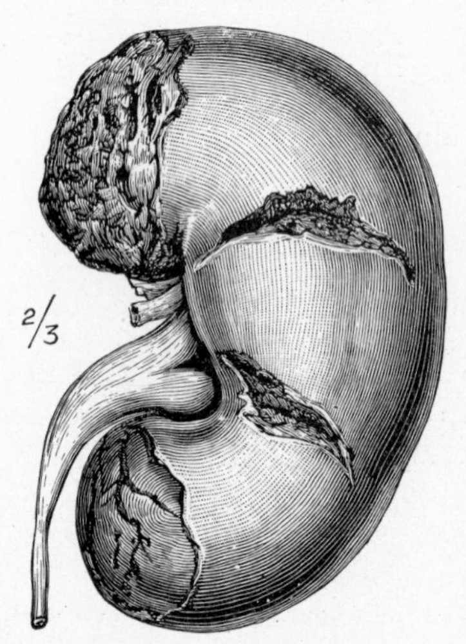

Fig. 138.—Ruptured Kidney (Morris).

The blood also pours down the ureter into the bladder and is expelled therefrom (hematuria).

Associated Lesions.—Laceration of the perirenal fat may occur alone or in connection with rupture of the kidney. It is unimportant. Fortunately laceration of the peritoneum is rare. In the adult there is a distinct layer of fat between the kidney and the peritoneum, which permits complete disintegration of the former without any injury to the latter; but in children this layer of fat is not developed, and, therefore, rupture of the peritoneum permitting rapidly fatal hemorrhage is more frequent in them than in the adult. Rupture of the renal artery and vein is also rare. Rupture of the liver occurred in 10 out of Morris's 12 cases (an unduly large proportion). Rupture of the spleen is a less frequent complication, though, in either case, the free hemorrhage from the intraperitoneal organ is likely to make the renal lesion a secondary consideration. Fracture of the lower ribs and puncture of the diaphragm, the pleura, and the lung are among the less frequent associated lesions.

The Process of Repair.—Slight injuries of the renal parenchyma may heal promptly with but slight associated inflammation,[1] and perirenal hematoma of some size may disappear within a few weeks by diffusion and absorption. Yet the usual outcome of rupture of the kidney—if the patient survives the immediate results of the injury—is infection of the urohematoma, suppuration throughout the wound in the kidney, and gangrene of such portions of the organ as have been partially or completely torn away. The urinous, purulent collection burrows in various directions until the patient succumbs or the surgeon intervenes.

Symptoms

Apart from the systemic shock and the local pain and ecchymosis due to the bruising of the abdominal wall, there are four cardinal symptoms of rupture of the kidney directly referable to the organ itself. These are, hematuria, variations in the quantity of urine excreted, tumour, and pain.

Hematuria.—The passage of bloody urine after a contusion of the loin is the most characteristic symptom of ruptured kidney. Yet the hematuria may occur when the kidney is not ruptured,[2] and, on the contrary, there may be no hematuria, even though the kidney is ruptured. Thus the blood cannot reach the bladder if there is (1) subcapsular rupture, (2) occlusion of the ureter by clot, or (3) avulsion of the kidney from the ureter. Yet hematuria was a feature in 65 of the 71 cases collected by Maas.

The course of the bleeding is very irregular. The blood usually flows freely for several days, and then ceases, either because the hemorrhage has stopped, or because the ureter becomes obstructed by clots. Blood cells and albumin may persist in the urine for many days, and recurrence of bleeding is not uncommon. Exceptionally there is no hematuria for the first few days. The blood passed has the characteristics of kidney blood (p. 419), and is usually eliminated in sufficient quantity to dye the urine a deep red. Yet, as a rule, the actual amount of blood passed is not alarming.

---

[1] *Cf.* Yarrow, N. Y. Med. J., 1900, lxxi, 1.

[2] Morris gives a long list of exceptional causes of hematuria after contusion of the loin, such as slight contusion of the kidney, renal congestion, thrombosis of the renal vessels, stone, malaria, villous tumour of the bladder. But the only feature of clinical importance is the persistence of bleeding. Uncontrollable bleeding, from whatever cause, demands operation.

Variations in the Quantity of Urine.—During the first day after the injury there is oliguria, perhaps anuria, from shock. Continued anuria indicates rupture of both kidneys, or else the incapacity of the opposite kidney (if there be one) to act, and is therefore an indication for immediate nephrotomy (p. 593). But usually a polyuria replaces the primary oliguria, and lasts two or three days or longer. There may be reflex dysuria or retention.

Tumour.—The extravasation of blood and urine about the kidney develops a tumour in the loin. This swelling may appear immediately, or its advent may be delayed several days, or no tumour may ever appear. The tumour is usually quite diffuse, filling the whole loin and perhaps extending even to the groin. The swelling is elastic, but fluctuation cannot be made out. A general abdominal tension from the accumulation of flatus and from the tenderness of the bruised parietes may obscure a large perirenal hematoma.

Pain.—The pain of a ruptured kidney is an inconstant symptom. The superficial contusion produces local pain and tenderness; the passage of clots through the ureter may evoke renal colic, and the distention of the kidney, or its compression by effused blood, may produce an active pain radiating chiefly to the groin and testicle, and perhaps causing retraction of the latter.

Course of the Disease.—1. *The injury is slight.* There is some shock, a temporary oliguria, and hematuria. After a few days the urine becomes quantitatively and qualitatively normal. No notable tumour appears in the loin, and the patient is well within ten days or so.

2. *The injury is apparently slight*, but the symptoms, instead of growing less, or perhaps after an apparent remission, become more severe. The lumbar tumour grows larger, pulse and temperature run high, the digestive functions are not properly established, the abdomen remains distended and tympanitic, there is constipation, anorexia, perhaps vomiting, the tongue is dry, the patient listless and irritable. This clinical picture indicates progressive urinary toxemia and sepsis, and calls for prompt nephrotomy if the patient is to be saved. The presence of pleurisy, pneumothorax, or edema of the lung must not be overlooked.

3. *The injury is severe.* At first the patient is dazed, unconscious, or in a state of collapse. Hematuria and hematoma develop rapidly. He may fail rapidly and die of shock, of internal hemorrhage, of suppression, or later, of septic complications. Or the hematoma may be gradually absorbed, and recovery may occur after a prolonged and severe illness.

4. In the most serious cases *the renal rupture is only one among*

several visceral injuries. Rapidly fatal intraperitoneal hemorrhage may occur from the kidney, liver, or spleen. The triple infliction of shock, hemorrhage, and peritonitis can be combated only by immediate abdominal section with slight hope of success.

Diagnosis

While slight injuries to the kidneys may be overlooked, especially if overshadowed by more important lesions of the other viscera, a kidney rupture of any great significance always manifests itself by loin tumour, usually associated with hematuria and oliguria or anuria.

The use of instruments of precision, such as the cystoscope or ureteral catheter, in the diagnosis of these injuries must be deprecated, for any renal rupture that cannot be diagnosed by the symptoms above narrated is either mild enough to deserve expectant treatment or severe enough to require immediate exploratory section.

Treatment

The treatment of shock is of the first importance. The patient is put to bed, surrounded by hot-water bottles and stimulated with alcohol, strychnin, and nitroglycerin, according to his needs. In extreme cases an intravenous saline infusion is admirably efficacious. Opium must be sparingly employed for fear of masking the symptoms. To check hemorrhage cold may be applied locally, and ergot or gelatin injected subcutaneously by those who put faith in them. Food should be of the lightest description, and the bowels should be moved by mild laxatives if possible, since active peristalsis is said to encourage hemorrhage from the kidney. The catheter should be employed with the most minute antiseptic precautions, for the bloody vesical pool is more than usually receptive of infection, and infection is—after the primary shock and hemorrhage have passed—the only noteworthy danger to the patient.

But all the measures detailed above are palliative at best. By them the symptoms are modified, but the essential features of the case—the hemorrhage, the function of the opposite kidney, the infection of the perirenal hematoma—are, to all intents, unaffected. Only by the knife can the surgeon reach these, and thus the momentous questions in the treatment of rupture of the kidney are, Whether to operate? and when to operate?

Immediate operation is required only when the patient fails to rally from his shock, and becomes weaker and weaker in spite of the surgeon's ingenuity. The possibility of intraperitoneal hemorrhage or rupture of some of the other viscera will lead the surgeon to fortify the patient by a large intravenous infusion, and then to operate, in the desperate hope of averting the fatal issue.

The only other cases that may be subjected to immediate operation are those whose evidence of grave internal injury is associated with so little shock as to encourage the hope that immediate exploration may prevent other and worse evils.

After the first shock is over expectant treatment may be continued on condition that the patient grows progressively stronger. Yet the surgeon must be ready to operate, and the patient and his friends prepared to submit, as soon as any unfavourable symptom manifests itself. The usual indication for operation at this juncture is continued hemorrhage, as evinced by the growing tumour in the loin, for "it is not the visible loss of blood by the bladder, but the easily overlooked but far more dangerous bleeding into the perinephritic tissues, or into the peritoneal cavity, that should receive the chief attention" (Keen[1]). Anuria persisting for twenty-four hours is an indication for immediate operation (p. 593). Finally, beginning sepsis, suggested by an unfavourable temperature and pulse, must be prevented by operative drainage.

Although severe wounds in the kidney have been known to heal, the prospects of cases treated expectantly are not good. Thus among Küster's 222 uncomplicated cases there were 67 deaths (30% mortality), while among 84 cases complicated by grave lesions of other viscera, 77 died. Of the former class 30 died of hemorrhage, 27 of suppuration, 5 of shock, 3 of chronic nephritis, 2 of calculus and edema of the lungs. Keen's figures tell the same story. Among 100 uncomplicated cases there were 34 deaths—14 from hemorrhage and shock, 16 from suppuration or peritonitis, the other 4 from coma, anuria, and nephritis. Thus almost one half the cases die of suppuration, which should be preventable, and fully one half die of hemorrhage which can usually be checked by nephrotomy. Yet up to 1896 the mortality after operation was relatively high (Keen), there being 8 deaths attributed to 22 nephrectomies (36.4% mortality), whereas among 78 uncomplicated cases treated expectantly there were 27 deaths (34.5%). Undoubtedly the operative mortality has decreased since then. I have operated on but 3 cases, and they all recovered.

The Operation.—The surgeon employs the incision with which he is most familiar, as speed is all-important. The choice between the abdominal and the lumbar route depends upon whether any other visceral lesions are suspected. Though the abdominal route affords

[1] Annals of Surgery, 1896, xxiv, 138.

quicker control of the renal artery, the lumbar incision is habitually employed. Upon incision of the fascial envelope clots, blood, bloody urine, or pus exudes, and should be quickly washed away. If copious bleeding is encountered, the renal artery must be clamped or tied (p. 642) immediately, though, as a general rule, the hemorrhage may be controlled by suture of the kidney and packing. The earlier operators performed nephrectomy for rupture of the kidney as they did for every other surgical affection of the kidney, but this grave operation is rarely, if ever, necessary. Generous drainage will allow for the expulsion of such detached fragments of kidney tissue as the surgeon overlooks. A final irrigation and plentiful gauze drainage complete the operation. Secondary nephrectomy may be required if prolonged suppuration ensues.

WOUNDS OF THE KIDNEY

Wounds of the kidney (other than ruptures) are extremely rare. Even in military practice they are unusual. Of *incised and punctured wounds* (excluding bullet wounds) there are no instances recorded in the Medical History of the War of the Rebellion. Küster [1] collected 43 cases. In 10 there were severe injuries to other organs, and of these 6 died (60%), while among the 31 uncomplicated cases, there were only 4 deaths (12.9%). Keen records 8 cases with 2 deaths. Among Küster's cases 10 were operated upon (2 primary and 6 secondary nephrectomies) with no deaths; Keen records 4 nephrectomies without a death.

Morris sums up the diagnostic features of the condition as follows: "It may be stated (1) that a wound in the renal region succeeded by the escape of urine through the wound is conclusive of injury to the kidney; (2) that such a wound quickly succeeded by the discharge *per urethram* of urine heavily mixed with blood, or of pure blood, is almost conclusive, if not quite so; (3) that such a wound succeeded by retention of urine, or lumbar or abdominal pain and dysuria, even without hematuria, is highly suggestive of a superficial wound of the kidney, or of a deeper wound and the blockage of the ureter; (4) that hematuria succeeded by traumatic peritonitis is strong evidence of an injured kidney."

The chief clinical features of a penetrating wound of the kidney, other than the symptoms of rupture of that organ, are: (1) External hemorrhage, (2) greater likelihood of infection from particles of clothing and dirt carried into the wound, (3) frequent involvement

[1] Deutsch. Klinik, 1896, lii, 1, 221.

of the peritoneum and of the other abdominal viscera, (4) prolapse of the kidney, if the wound is extensive.

Treatment.—The treatment is much the same as that of rupture, except that exploration of the wound for the purpose of cleansing it, and exploratory abdominal section to insure the safety of the other viscera are more often necessary.

Gunshot Wounds.—Although the recorded cases of gunshot wounds of the kidney show a very high mortality—viz., 59 deaths among 85 cases in the War of the Rebellion, and 8 deaths among 15 cases in the Franco-Prussian War—it is evident that this death-rate is due to associated injuries. (Thus Edler [1] collected 20 uncomplicated cases with 5 deaths, and 18 complicated cases with 15 deaths.) Hence, as Küster remarks, "the danger of a gunshot wound of the kidney increases with the velocity of the bullet."

The only special features of these wounds are (1) the explosive effect of high-velocity projectiles—similar to that observed in the other semisolid viscera—(2) the advantage of employing the X-rays to locate the bullet in case its extraction is desirable.

ANEURYSM OF THE RENAL ARTERY

Morris has collected 19 instances of aneurysm of the renal artery, of which 12 were traumatic in origin. He calls attention to this very rare condition because, apparently, it is always fatal (if of any size) unless the patient submits to operation.

The *symptoms* are tumour, pain, and hematuria. It is remarkable that pulsation is rarely detected. Morris detected a loud systolic bruit in his case, but no thrill. The *diagnosis* is made by nephrotomy.

The *treatment* is operative. The aneurysmal sac should be disturbed as little as possible until the pedicle is secured. Albert, Hahn, and Keen have operated successfully; Morris unsuccessfully. A transperitoneal operation presents a better field for securing the renal vessels than does the lumbar route.

---

[1] Arch. f. klin. Chir., 1887, xxxiv, 379.

CHAPTER XXXVI

PERINEPHRITIC EXTRAVASATIONS AND INFLAMMATIONS

EXTRAVASATION

THE extravasation of feces from the intestine or of air from the lung or bowel into the perirenal tissues is an unimportant phenomenon sometimes associated with grave visceral lesions.

Effusions of urine and blood are more frequent, and, since the source of the blood is usually the kidney, they often occur together.

The extravasation consists of blood alone if it results from an injury to the renal artery or to the renal parenchyma without affecting the pelvis or the ureter. (Bilateral retroperitoneal hematoma may also result from rupture of an aortic aneurysm.) If both the kidney and its pelvis are torn a *urohematoma* results, the blood preponderating at first (unless the kidney is hydronephrotic), the urine later; or rather, a lumbar tumour appearing immediately after an injury to the loin and rapidly increasing in size during the first twenty-four hours is a hematoma; while urinary extravasation (unless preceded by hematoma) produces a slowly growing tumour, which may not be noticed until some weeks after the infliction of the injury. Occasionally the lesion in the pelvis or ureter is so small, and the escape of urine so gradual, that the cellular tissue forms a tense sac about the fluid. The name *traumatic hydronephrosis* has been given to this condition, in spite of the fact that there is no true dilatation of the renal pelvis. True traumatic hydronephrosis results from cicatricial stricture of an injured ureter, and is excessively rare. Sollers (Rattier[1]) and Pye Smith (Morris) have reported authentic cases. In Mannasse's case (Rattier, Obs. XXIV) a pseudo-hydronephrosis appeared eighteen months after injury.

Course.—The effusion spreads as long as hemorrhage or urinary leakage continues. As the perineal fascia is usually uninjured,

---

[1] Des épanchements urineux d'origine rénale, Paris, 1899, p. 17.

the extravasation forms an elastic swelling filling the loin. Thence it may extend downward to the inguinal region, the pelvis and thigh; but this is exceptional.

If the extravasation is hemorrhagic, it is likely to remain aseptic and to become a blood cyst, with grumous or serous contents if it is too large to be absorbed. But when the tumour is a urohematoma, as is usually the case, the danger of infection is great, not so much from the urine itself—since this fluid is habitually aseptic—but by the bacteria habitually passed through the urinary channels without finding any lodgment, but which find ideal conditions for their proliferation in so excellent a culture medium as is formed by the mixed blood and urine. Suppuration with secondary perinephritic abscess is the usual outcome.

Treatment.—The proper treatment of perinephritic extravasation, be it hematoma or urohematoma, is incision, exploration, and drainage, for the purpose of (*a*) preventing suppuration, (*b*) suturing large rents in the kidney or its pelvis, and (*c*) removing any ureteral kink, valve, obstruction, or stricture in order to re-establish the urinary flow through the natural passages. Therefore it is especially important to investigate the condition of the pelvis and ureter (p. 640).

PERINEPHRITIS AND PERINEPHRITIC ABSCESS

Perinephritis is an inflammation of the fatty fibrous envelope of the kidney. It is encountered under three forms: (1) Suppurating perinephritis, (2) fibro-lipomatous perinephritis, and (3) sclerotic perinephritis. The two latter varieties may be dismissed with a word.

Fibro-lipomatous and Sclerotic Perinephritis

Each of these allied processes is a protective inflammation of the perirenal fat secondary to suppurative inflammation of the kidney itself. When the fatty capsule is found contracted and condensed, as it were, into a solid mass of firm fat bound to the kidney by dense bands of fibrous tissue, the inflammation is termed fibro-lipomatous; when the fat is entirely replaced by fibrous tissue the term sclerotic is used. In each instance the reaction in the perinephritic tissue is a chronic fibrosis aroused by long-continued suppuration within the kidney. If the renal inflammation is chiefly confined to the pelvis, the perirenal reaction manifests itself by the accumulation of dense masses of fat and fibrous tissue about that part of the organ. If there is a considerable inflammation of the renal parenchyma, the whole kidney is enveloped in the fibro-lipomatous mass, which may be sufficiently thick to produce a considerable tumour (Fig. 139).

Suppurating Perinephritis—Perinephritic Abscess

Perinephritic abscess may be primary or secondary, simple or tubercular.

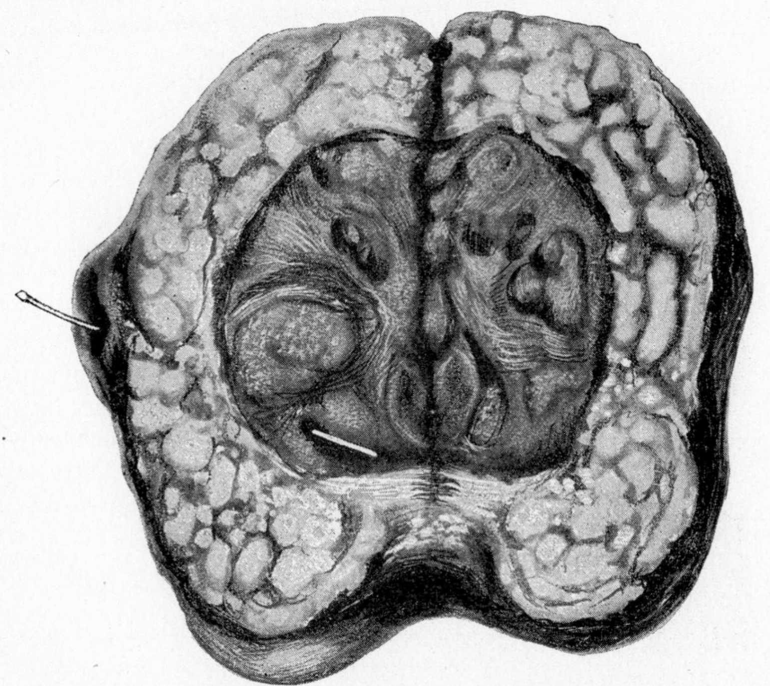

Fig. 139.—Perinephritis (Morris).
Dense fibro-lipomatous perinephritis due to intrarenal suppuration. The probe shows a fistula, through which the suppuration has extended to the perirenal tissue in spite of the protective inflammation.

Etiology.—The causes of perirenal abscess may be tabulated as follows:

Primary abscess—
- Traumatic—
  - Infection from the kidney.
  - Infection from the wound.
- Spontaneous—
  - Attributed to a sprain, a chill, or to general debility.

Secondary abscess—
- Of renal origin—
  - Calculous or tubercular pyelo-nephritis.
  - Pyonephrosis.
  - Suppurative nephritis.

From other viscera—
Appendix.
Liver.
Gall-bladder.
Pelvic organs.
Vertebræ (often tubercular).

I have encountered traumatic abscess, abscess due to calculous and to tubercular pyelo-nephritis, abscess arising from an acute appendicitis, abscess secondary to cystotomy, and spontaneous tubercular abscess without evident connection with any bone or viscus.

Symptoms.—The *onset* of suppuration is usually insidious, marked by irregular fever (rarely by a chill), tenderness over the kidney, a stiffness and tendency to favour the affected side in walking or sitting, and restricted extension of the thigh, without obstruction to flexion. Gibney has indicated the possibility of mistaking beginning perinephritis for hip disease. Even when perinephritis succeeds injury the history may be so obscure as to be misleading. A careful physical examination, however, will show that the seat of inflammation is the loin, and not the spine or hip.

The *course* of the disease is that of a retroperitoneal lumbar abscess. Resolution without the formation of an abscess is rare. The irregular fever usually continues (it is often mistaken for typhoid), the pain and tenderness in the loin, the forced flexion of the thigh grow more marked, and a tumour appears in the loin.

This tumour is quite characteristic. The whole loin is perceptibly bulged outward and backward, with less protuberance in front than is the case when the tumour is intrarenal. Moreover, the tumour formed by perirenal abscess is quite immobile. When large, fluctuation can be elicited, and edema of the overlying skin may appear.

The *termination* of the disease, unless subjected to operation, is death by septicemia or by rupture. Küster records 34 cases of rupture distributed as follows:

Pleura and bronchi	18 cases.
Intestine (colon)	11 "
Peritoneum	2 "
Bladder, or bladder and vagina	3 "

Morris says: "Compared with the frequency with which perinephritic abscesses perforate the colon, the pleura, or the lung, the other forms of spontaneous opening are rare. Probably it is not an exaggeration to say that of every 12 cases which pursue their own course, 4 or 5 open into the pleural cavity or the lung." External rupture through the loin is rare.

Diagnosis.—While the diagnosis may be difficult in the early stages the presence of leukocytosis, the absence of malarial organisms from the blood, and a negative Widal reaction, will show that the fever is due to suppuration somewhere; and tenderness in the loin suggests the site of suppuration. There are no urinary signs essentially connected with this malady.

In the later stages the tumour is pathognomonic. The one tubercular case I have seen was unmistakable, although the only subjective symptom was an inability to cross the corresponding leg over the other without lifting it with the hand. Yet a mere inspection of the flank showed the presence of the abscess, which, when incised, yielded a litre of pus.

Prognosis.—Spontaneous cure by resolution, encapsulation, or rupture is very rare, and is never to be expected.

Early operation gives good results. The longer the operation is delayed the worse the prognosis.

Treatment.—The only treatment for suppurating perinephritis is incision and drainage. Even when the case is diagnosed so early that the presence of pus is doubtful, an exploratory incision—although nothing be found—offers a better prospect of cure than any expectant treatment. Rupture of the abscess into the intestine is no contra-indication to operation; it is rather an incentive, since the abscess drains but poorly and the admixture of feces with its contents is calculated to add fuel to the inflammation.

In operating, the primary object is to secure free drainage. The usual oblique incision insures this and permits thorough exploration. As soon as the abscess is opened, and while it is being copiously irrigated with salt solution, the finger is introduced, and with it the cavity is carefully explored for the purpose of discovering whether the abscess arises fom the kidney, the appendix, or some other organ. Bimanual palpation may reveal a diseased kidney; but the question as to whether, in such event, nephrotomy should be performed immediately, or delayed until the perirenal suppuration is reduced, is one that must be decided upon the merits of the case, especially in reference to the condition of the patient, the severity of the infection, the amount of intrarenal suppuration, and the condition of the opposite kidney. The possibility of associated empyema should not be forgotten. After-treatment consists in prolonged drainage.

CHAPTER XXXVII

HYDRONEPHROSIS

Obstruction to the outflow of urine from the kidney is of two kinds: 1. Sudden complete obstruction. 2. Gradual or incomplete obstruction.

Sudden complete obstruction occurs clinically under two forms —viz., by a calculus, and by the surgeon's ligation. In either event the result is the same. The urine is dammed back upon the kidney, causing an acute renal congestion (Fig. 146) and a diminished secretion of urine; but even this increases the intrarenal pressure. The congestion is exchanged for atrophy, thus terminating the usefulness of the organ. The details of these changes do not interest us at present. They are fully described under Calculous Anuria.

Gradual, incomplete, or intermittent urinary obstruction sets up a very different train of events. Some urine escapes past the obstruction, continuously or from time to time, and affords partial relief to the renal tension, while still keeping up a very considerable pressure. Thus the organ does not atrophy. It continues to excrete an amount of urine equivalent to what can pass the obstruction, while the continued high pressure within the kidney causes a gradual dilatation of its cavity. Pelvis and calices gradually dilate—and there is hydronephrosis (cystonephrosis, nephrectasis, renal distention).

The above-described pathogenesis of renal atrophy and hydronephrosis has been experimentally worked out by Guyon,[1] Byron Robinson,[2] and others, and confirmed by observations in clinic and dead-house.

Etiology

The cause of hydronephrosis is gradual, incomplete, or intermittent urinary obstruction. The obstruction may be urethral or ureteral.

---

[1] Guyon's Annales, 1892, x, 161.

[2] Annals of Surgery, 1893, xviii, 402.

Urethral Obstruction.—The common urethral obstructions are stricture of the canal and hypertrophy of the prostate. But the former always and the latter usually damages the kidneys more by infection than by dilatation. The bladder bears the brunt of the distention, and, although the kidneys and ureters become dilated by chronic urethral obstruction (Fig. 38), this dilatation is clinically subordinate to the inflammatory features of the disease.

Ureteral Obstruction.—Ureteral obstruction acts differently. No distensible bladder intervenes to distribute the pressure, and infection is often entirely absent; so that the aseptic dilatation of kidney and ureter progresses rapidly and unobscured.

The ureteral obstructions are:

1. Obstruction from within by stone, tumour, or foreign body (Fig. 147).

2. Pressure from without by aberrant renal vessel (common) (Fig. 140) or by pelvic growth (uncommon).

3. Kinking of the ureter from nephroptosis.

4. Strictures and valves of the ureter, especially those caused by anomalous origin of the duct or by stricture at its termination (p. 480).

Roberts[1] has examined 52 cases in reference to their etiology. Twenty were bilateral and 32 unilateral. The cause was congenital in 20 cases. In 2 of these a supernumerary renal artery crossed and compressed the ureter near its origin; in 4 the ureter was congenitally imperforate; in 4 the ureter entered obliquely into the pelvis of the kidney; in 1 the ureter was kinked and adherent; in 1 there was stricture at the vesical extremity. Thirteen of these congenital cases were bilateral. Of these, 2 were still-born, 5 died within six months (3 within forty-eight hours) after birth. Four lived from five and a half to twenty years. One[2] survived to the age of thirty-eight.

Of the 32 cases of acquired hydronephrosis, 11 were due to impacted ureteral calculi (3 others were attributed to the same cause); 5 showed inflammatory or ulcerative stricture; 9 were occluded by external pressure—by peritoneal adhesions (3 cases), gravid uterus, ovarian cyst, cancerous growth.

Among Roberts's cases 25 were male, 23 female.

Morris has analyzed 142 cases, of which 128 were due to obstruction of the ureter, by cancer of the pelvic organs (118), cancer of the abdominal organs (3), ovarian cysts (4), and "constriction of the

---

[1] Urinary and Renal Diseases. Second American Edit., Phila., 1872, p. 482.

[2] Kinked and adherent ureters, doubtless not congenital.

ureter" (3). Yet hydronephrosis due to cancerous obstruction is rarely noted except post-mortem.

The so-called traumatic hydronephrosis is almost always an encysted perinephritic extravasation.

A special cause of hydronephrosis, a cause that figures but rarely in statistics and yet is commonly encountered in practice, is nephroptosis. Since so few movable kidneys become hydronephrotic it is an open question which is the antecedent condition. Certainly renal mobility is associated with practically every case of intermittent hydronephrosis, and I believe that in a great majority of hydronephroses due to kinked and adherent ureters, whether over an aberrant renal vessel or not, and to oblique implantation of the ureter in the kidney pelvis, the first kinking of the ureter or pouching of the pelvis is attributable to a nephroptosis (Fig. 140). Why so small a proportion of movable kidneys becomes hydronephrotic is not clear.

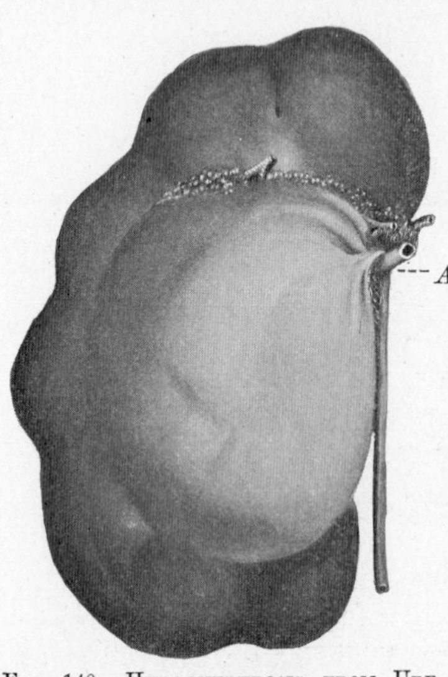

FIG. 140.—HYDRONEPHROSIS FROM URETERAL COMPRESSION (AT *A*) BY A BRANCH OF THE RENAL VEIN.

This obstruction caused an intermittent hydronephrosis, which was permanently cured by the liberation of adhesions and nephropexy.

MORBID ANATOMY

The morbid ureteral conditions at the point of obstruction require no detailed description. The strictures, adhesions, etc., present no peculiar features.

The Hydronephrotic Sac.—The tumour may consist of only a part of the kidney, whether because the kidney possesses two ureters only one of which is blocked, or because a single calyx becomes occluded by a stone. Either condition is very rare; as a rule, the sac consists of the entire kidney and its pelvis. The ureter may also be dilated.

The size of the tumour varies from that of a normal kidney to that of a child's head.

The sac wall consists of the renal pelvis and capsule. The kidney caps the tumour. The outer surface of the mass is irregularly ovoidal, the inner surface is irregular. If the hydronephrosis is small its interior consists of the dilated pelvis and calices (Fig. 141). If large, it is a great, smooth-walled cavity crossed by fibrous septa representing the remains of the columns of Bertini (Fig. 142). The sac wall may be thin, but is usually tough and fibrous. Cartilaginous nodules have been observed in it.

Renal Changes.—The changes in the kidney substance are interesting. At first the kidney is congested, the canaliculi dilated, and the cells flattened. This process soon manifests itself macroscopically by the thinning out of the kidney tissue. Thus the kidney becomes more and more spread out on the surface of the sac with a great portion of its secreting substance atrophied.[1] But this is not the only change. The remaining parenchyma cells — for the kidney is never completely atrophied— undergo a compensatory hypertrophy. They grow to 3 or 4 times their normal size and their secretory capacity increases accordingly. It is for this reason that every hydronephrotic kidney should be recognised as a useful, though an impaired organ, and should not be sacrificed unnecessarily.

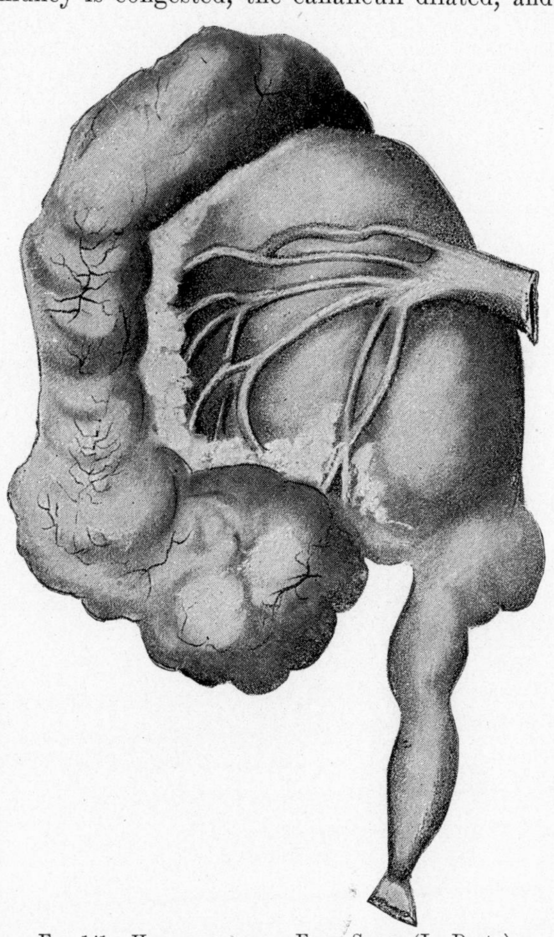

Fig. 141.—Hydronephrosis; First Stage (Le Dentu).

The hydronephrotic sac may be open or closed. If the ureter is merely kinked, the hydronephrosis is usually intermittent. If contractured or obstructed, the hydronephrosis is fixed or con-

[1] There is no interstitial sclerosis, no production of fibrous tissue, in simple uninflamed hydronephrosis.

stant, and the orifice of the sac may finally become absolutely sealed.

The Fluid.—The quantity of fluid in a hydronephrotic sac often reaches 5 or 6 gallons. One case is reported (Glass) containing 30 gallons.

The quality of the fluid varies. It is usually a simple solution of sodium chlorid, though it may contain urea, albumin, urinary

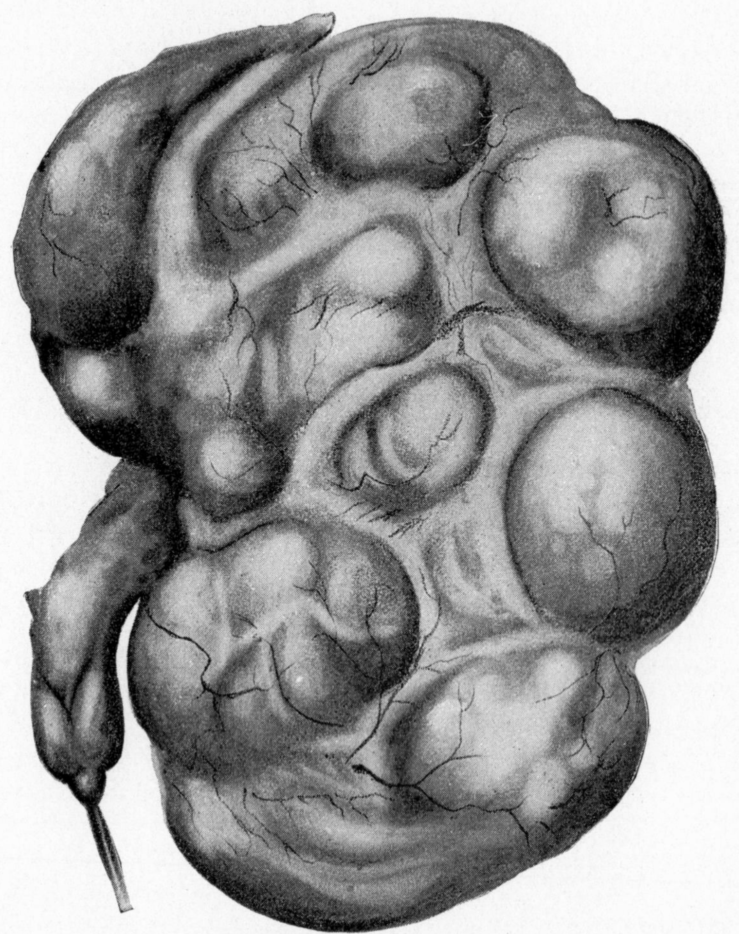

Fig. 142.—Hydronephrosis; Second Stage, the Kidney Substance being completely Atrophied (Le Dentu).

crystals, epithelial cells, and leukocytes, and less often blood, cholesterin, or bacteria, and flakes of pus, indicating an impending suppuration. There may be a catarrhal pyelo-nephritis, with slight infection of the contents of the sac (uropyonephrosis), but this light infection does not materially influence the clinical aspect of the case.

Physiology.—It has long been the generally accepted belief that the hydronephrotic kidney secretes a urine less rich in solids than that of a normal organ, but the functional activity of such an organ has never been accurately tested in man, except by Guyon and Albarran.[1] They have shown that even the kidney whose ureter has been occluded for a great while will begin to secrete when the obstruction is removed. Urea appears in the secretion, though it may have been entirely absent from the fluid in the sac; while the quantity of fluid secreted by the diseased organ may exceed that secreted on the sound side. In one case (uropyonephrosis) in which the renal tissue was so compressed that it was only 2 or 3 millimetres thick, the kidney excreted a litre a day after the pressure had been removed.

The kidney whose outlet has not been entirely closed acts in a similar manner. While a normal quantity of urine may be excreted by the diseased organ, it is poorer in urea and salts. It usually contains one quarter to one third of the total urea. A curious fact is that, while the total excretion of urea may vary widely from day to day, this variation takes place almost entirely in the sound kidney, the diseased organ excreting an approximately constant amount.

Symptoms

The majority of kidneys found hydronephrotic post-mortem give no symptoms during life. The one characteristic symptom by which attention is called to the kidney is the presence of a tumour. There are clinically two varieties of hydronephrosis. When the tumour is constant the hydronephrosis is spoken of as fixed; when the tumour varies in size the hydronephrosis is said to be intermittent.

Fixed Hydronephrosis.—When the hydronephrosis is fixed the patient usually gives a history of a slowly growing *tumour* in his side. Or soreness and *pain* may first call attention to the kidney; but, as a rule, unless the kidney is misplaced and adherent, fixed hydronephrosis is uncomfortable rather than painful. The tumour grows very slowly. It may burst either into the peritoneal cavity, or into the perirenal space; either event is rare.

On examination a smooth, elastic, fairly movable, and, as a rule, insensitive tumour is found filling the side. The absence of systemic disturbance is remarkable. There is no fever, and, unless both kidneys are affected, no evidence of renal insufficiency.

---

[1] Guyon's Annales, 1897, xv, 1200.

Intermittent Hydronephrosis.—This condition presents an entirely different picture. The trouble begins with irregular attacks of severe pain in the side. These pains are habitually attributed to the intestines, to hysteria, or to renal colic. When the patient is examined between attacks the discovery of a movable and tender kidney only confirms the diagnosis of hysteria, and if the patient becomes thin and anemic and has flushes of watery urine, this only adds colour to the picture.

But affairs go from bad to worse. The attacks of pain become more and more severe, they recur every few days. During the attack the distended kidney may be felt filling the entire loin. The pain, after lasting several hours or days, is suddenly relieved by the passage of a large quantity of urine; but the relief is only temporary. At the end of the usual interval the pain recurs. In a personal case the pains began twenty years before the tumour was found, while in another the tumour reached enormous dimensions after less than ten years' growth.

Morris justly remarks that not all these cases are due to renal mobility, and cites instances attributed to stone and to vesical papilloma. Yet Terrier and Baudouin,[1] who collected 83 reported cases, showed that the condition was almost always associated with nephroptosis.

The usual outcome of an intermittent hydronephrosis is that it becomes fixed. The variations in size decrease and the pain becomes less constant and more severe.

Diagnosis

It is scarcely possible to mistake a fully developed intermittent hydronephrosis. The large recurrent lumbar tumour is characteristic.

A fixed hydronephrosis may be distinguished as a chronic noninflammatory renal tumour (p. 624). When large the cystic nature of the growth is obvious. It may then be mistaken for ovarian cyst. When small it is not always possible to distinguish a hydronephrosis from other tumours of the kidney. The occurrence of hematuria may obscure the diagnosis.

Rarely a pyonephrosis pursues so chronic a course and causes so little constitutional disturbance as to be mistaken for hydronephrosis.

Prognosis

Unless both kidneys are affected hydronephrosis does not threaten life. The development of the tumour is very slow, and

[1] Revue de chir, 1891, xi, 719, 833, 1055.

treatment is usually demanded for the relief of pain or on account of the size and discomfort of the tumour. Although secondary suppuration may occur, transforming the hydronephrosis into a pyonephrosis, this is singularly rare. Rupture of the sac into the peritoneum—an accident usually fatal—is most exceptional. Rupture into the perirenal space, with the formation there of a false hydronephrosis, may occur. Morris noted the spontaneous and permanent disappearance of 6 or 7 out of 47 hydronephroses observed by him.

Treatment

Just as hydronephrosis has been known to disappear spontaneously, so massage and repeated aspirations of the cyst can boast their cures. I can see no advantage in massage, and if the dangers of aspiration are not great neither are its chances of success. Albarran has achieved some cures by the use of the ureteral catheter (p. 479). This has at least the advantage of pretending to straighten out the ureter. But in the majority of cases these palliative measures must fail; there is a definite ureteral obstruction, and until that obstruction is removed the hydronephrosis must persist. Hence the sole treatment in which confidence may be placed is operation.

Operative Measures.—Although a number of plastic operations upon the ureter for the relief of renal retention are described in another chapter (p. 486), and although some surgeons proclaim that they cure all their cases by this or that operation—by nephrotomy, by nephropexy, or even by nephrectomy—yet the only intelligent way to undertake the surgical cure of hydronephrosis is to recognise that the procedure is exploratory, the object sought being the discovery and relief of the ureteral obstruction.

When the hydronephrosis is intermittent, it may be fairly presumed that its cause is a nephroptosis, and that nephropexy, preceded by the loosening of adhesions, will effect a cure. The usual lumbar incision reveals the distended kidney. If the tumour is so large as to encumber the operative field, its contents are allowed to drain away through a small incision, preferably in the pelvis.[1] Then the kidney is forced upward under the ribs and its pelvis carefully freed of adhesions by blunt dissection until the ureter is reached; here the kink will usually be found. The adhesions must be carefully separated. When the obstruction is apparently relieved, the patency of the duct should be tested by passing a ureteral catheter from the pelvis of the kidney into the bladder.

In other cases, an impacted stone, a ureteral stricture, or exter-

[1] The line of incision should radiate from the neck of the pelvis.

nal pressure will be found to cause the obstruction (p. 486). While the operative technic must differ with each case, it may be said in general that—

1. The discovery and removal of the obstruction is the first object of the operation.

2. Until the ureteral catheter has been passed from the pelvis of the kidney down and into the bladder one cannot feel sure that the obstacle has been removed.

3. No matter how dilated the kidney, it is still of some service to the patient, and should not be extirpated unless nephrectomy is considered a less formidable procedure than the removal of the obstruction.

4. Operating to preserve the kidney does not imply the performance of any of the so-called conservative plastic operations for renal retention. Simple nephropexy, or even nephrotomy, is a far safer and, in all but the exceptional cases of ureteral valves and strictures, an equally certain procedure.

5. Yet to return to the original point, the ease with which certain cases may be cured is no excuse for overlooking the obstructive cause of the retention, since, unless this cause is known, we have no means of judging how much relief may be expected from the operation.

I have purposely consigned the description of the plastic operations upon the ureter to another chapter (p. 486) in order to emphasize the fact that they are rarely needed here. After what has been said it is scarcely necessary to repeat that nephrectomy for the relief of hydronephrosis is a last resort.

CHAPTER XXXVIII

ETIOLOGY, MORBID ANATOMY, AND GENERAL SYMPTOMATOLOGY OF SURGICAL INFLAMMATIONS OF THE KIDNEY

No common disease is so persistently and so comprehensively misunderstood as is pyelo-nephritis. The physician, encountering mild chronic cases, is contented with the diagnosis and treatment of chronic interstitial nephritis; while the surgeon is too apt only to see in the pyuria characterizing the severer inflammations an evidence of cystitis. Yet the only way to appreciate the frequency of the disease is *to suspect of pyelo-nephritis every case of bacteriuria or pyuria that is not a urethritis.* Investigation will show that almost every case of long-standing stricture or hypertrophied prostate, and many cases of stone and tumour of the bladder, show some pyelo-nephritis, while occasionally a case will be encountered in which the characteristic symptoms of cystitis—viz., frequent and painful passage of purulent urine—are the sole obvious indications of a suppurating kidney uncomplicated by cystitis.

Varieties.—The four varieties of pyelo-nephritis are—

Catarrhal pyelo-nephritis (pyelitis).

Suppurative pyelo-nephritis.

Pyonephrosis.

Abscess of the kidney.

These four conditions constitute the surgical inflammations of the kidney. They represent the various degrees and varieties of suppuration in the kidney and its pelvis. Hence it is convenient to group their etiology, morbid anatomy, and general symptoms all together, leaving the consideration of special symptoms, diagnosis, prognosis, and treatment for the next chapter.

The terms explain themselves. Catarrhal pyelo-nephritis is a light inflammation of the kidney and its pelvis productive of little pus. Suppurative pyelo-nephritis is a similar condition more severe in type, with much pus collected in the pelvis of the kidney and passed off with the urine. Pyonephrosis is suppurative pyelo-nephritis in a dilated kidney. Abscess of the kidney is suppuration within the organ uncomplicated by pyelitis.

Etiology

The surgical inflammations of the kidney are microbic in origin, and may be caused by any pyogenic bacteria. It is to be remarked, however, that the milder forms of pyelo-nephritis are habitually caused by the bacillus coli, and are characterized by an acid urine.

The route of bacterial invasion has been noticed in a previous chapter (p. 357). An ascending invasion is accepted as the cause of the inflammation when it is secondary to some disorder of the bladder, prostate, or urethra. But when the renal inflammation is primary it is attributed to infection by microbes excreted through the kidneys—the so-called descending invasion.

Predisposing Causes.—The predisposing causes of pyelo-nephritis are all-important. Bacteria are always present. Every attack of constipation doubtless sends myriads of colon bacilli through the kidneys, and from every infected wound a sufficient number of staphylococci and streptococci doubtless enter the circulation and pass through the kidneys to cause suppuration ten times over in those organs, if only they are vulnerable; but they are not. Unless there is some trauma, irritant, or congestion, the bacteria are passed off without so much as multiplying in the urine. Thus the predisposing cause literally produces the inflammation—more than this, it often determines the quality of inflammation.

The chief predisposing causes are—

1. *Retention.*—Urethral retention, whether by stricture or prostate, is a common cause of catarrhal pyelo-nephritis, and may cause suppuration. Ureteral retention, which usually causes hydronephrosis, may cause pyonephrosis.

2. *Stone.*—Renal calculus is the most common cause of suppurative pyelonephritis, and may, by obstructing the ureter, cause pyonephrosis.

3. *Tuberculosis or Neoplasm.*—Malignant or tubercular disease may occasion suppuration in the kidney by producing a tissue ill fitted to repel bacterial invasion, or by blocking the ureter.

4. *Trauma.*—If a contused or ruptured kidney becomes infected there results a suppurative pyelo-nephritis or abscess of the kidney, or both (Fig. 144).

5. *Other Causes.*—A number of exceptional causes of renal suppuration are occasionally encountered. Among these may be mentioned the pressure of pelvic growths, pregnancy (see Acute Pyelonephritis), decrease in the power of resistance, such as occurs in wasting diseases, and especially in tabetics and paralytics, and such

septicemias as overwhelm the kidneys by the multitude of microbes these organs are called upon to transmit.

Morbid Anatomy

It is customary to describe suppurative pyelitis and nephritis as though they were quite independent conditions, or at least often met with separately. Such is not the case. While doubtless the inflammation has its first beginning in the one or the other, it is impossible clinically to distinguish pyelitis without nephritis or nephritis without pyelitis, excepting only those rare cases of renal abscess which begin within the parenchyma of the kidney and do not implicate the pelvis. With this one exception, then, suppurative nephritis does not occur without pyelitis, nor does pyelitis, whether catarrhal or suppurative, occur without nephritis.

The Renal Pelvis.—**Catarrhal Pyelitis.**—When the pelvis of the kidney is acutely inflamed it is congested and may be covered with a layer of pus or false membrane. There may be petechiæ and spots of epithelial desquamation.

In chronic conditions the pelvis is thickened and its mucous membrane rough and bereft of its normal polish.

Suppurative Pyelitis.—Suppurative pyelitis is characterized by more important changes. Besides a considerable inflammatory thickening of its walls, and more or less ulceration of its surface, the very shape of the pelvis may be distorted. There is often sufficient pouching of its sides to allow the accumulation of pus and calculi in a sort of pocket which, like the *bas fond* of the bladder, is the microbic breeding-place—the source of the pus.

The ureter is usually inflamed throughout its length in severe or acute cases. Its congested vesical orifice may be observed through the cystoscope.

Pyonephrosis.—In pyonephrosis the pouching and dilatation of the kidney pelvis reach their limit. The pelvis is usually greatly thickened and dilated, and is often irregularly pouched, ulcerated, and filled with pus, calculi, or a magma of lime salts (Fig. 143). The ureteral orifice is usually stenosed or completely obstructed.

The Kidney.[1]—**Catarrhal Nephritis.**—A light bacterial infection does not necessarily provoke suppuration in the kidney. The bacteria (usually the bacillus coli) obtain a foothold, probably in the mucous membrane of the calices, and thence attack the whole kidney, not by suppuration, but by chronic interstitial sclerosis.

The kidneys become small and dense, slightly lobulated on the

---

[1] *Cf.* Albarran.

surface, with adherent capsule, and perhaps a few small cysts with serous or sero-purulent contents. On section the cortex is found chiefly affected. While the pyramids retain a normal appearance the cortex may be quite converted into a mass of fibrous tissue containing lobules of fat. The microscope reveals infiltration of the stroma with fibrous and fatty tissue compressing and obliterating tubules and glomeruli alike. The areas of sclerosis are unevenly distributed about the organ, and wherever there is no sclerosis the secreting epithelium undergoes hypertrophy.

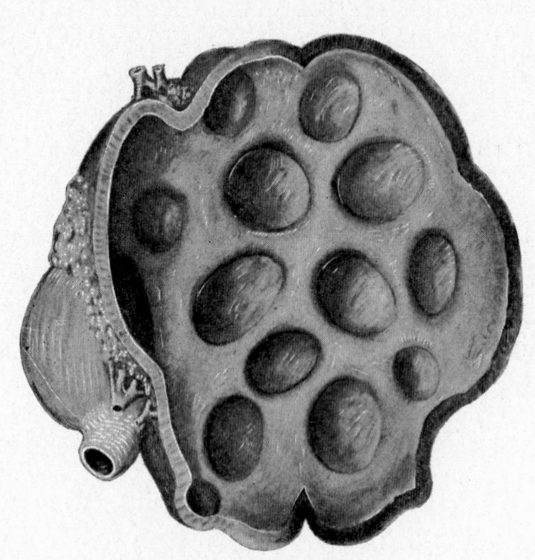

Fig. 143.—Pyonephrosis.
The kidney is reduced to a multilocular suppurating cavity.

The difference between the lesions just described and those of renal retention (*cf.* Hydronephrosis) must not be forgotten. *Retention alone causes* congestion and edema first, later epithelial *atrophy without any production of new interstitial tissue; while inflammation*, whether catarrhal or suppurative, whether associated with retention or not, *causes chronic interstitial nephritis* with a temporary acute congestion if the onset of the nephritis is acute.

Suppurative Nephritis.—Inasmuch as no two suppurating kidneys present exactly the same lesions it is quite impracticable to give a detailed picture fitting the requirements of every case. In general it may be said that—

1. There is always more or less of the chronic interstitial change described above.

2. In chronic suppurative pyelo-nephritis the kidney is habitually enlarged and congested, while the sclerosis is marked and the suppuration may be confined to the surfaces of calices; or there may be one or more foci of suppuration within the kidney substance, or dense globular scars showing where abscesses have been.

In the more acute cases the whole kidney may be infiltrated with pus. The bacteria, and with them the suppuration, follow the tubules, so that the pyramids are traversed by radiating yellow streaks surrounded by zones of congestion (*néphrite rayonnante* of

Albarran). In other cases the purulent infiltration follows no defined lines, the kidney is simply riddled with small foci of suppuration. If the patient survives, these foci coalesce to form one or more large abscesses, which ultimately burst into the pelvis of the kidney or reach the perinephritic tissue by rupture or by lymphatic invasion.

3. In pyonephrosis the kidney is commonly reduced to a dense multilocular abscess cavity (Fig. 143) containing pus, perhaps urinous or cheesy, and usually calculi. The loculi may intercommunicate widely or may be quite shut off, forming separate abscesses. Albarran mentions the occurrence of large subcapsular abscesses. Yet, in spite of all this sclerosis and chronic suppuration, the pyonephrotic, like the hydronephrotic, kidney almost always retains some epithelial elements and some power of secretion. Yet, in discussing the treatment of this condition, we shall see that the conservatism with which this should inspire the surgeon is often more than outweighed by the dangers of leaving a suppurating kidney and the inconvenience of secondary nephrectomy.

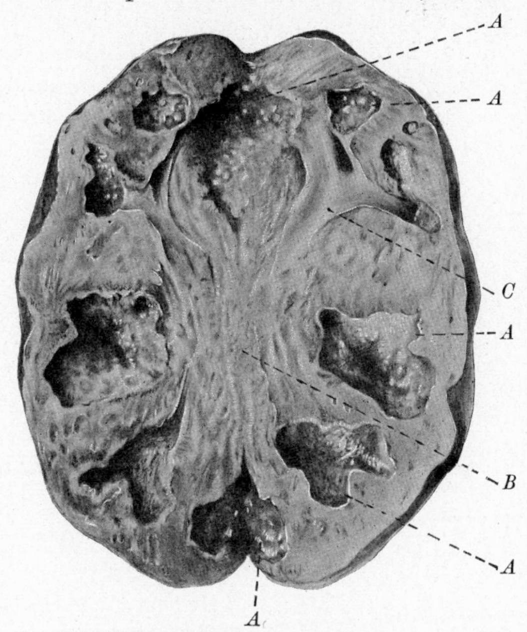

FIG. 144.—MULTIPLE ABSCESS OF THE KIDNEY DUE TO RUPTURE AND CICATRICIAL OBLITERATION OF THE PELVIS (Nephrectomy, by Dr. Chetwood).

A, abscesses; *B*, pelvis replaced by scar; *C*, sole remaining calyx.

4. True abscess of the kidney of hematogenous origin usually begins with one or more foci of suppuration in the cortex that grow and coalesce to form large abscesses (Fig. 144). These terminate by invading the pelvis or the perinephritic tissue, thus setting up pyelo-nephritis, pyonephrosis, or perinephritis, unless the patient dies before this stage is reached.

5. Albarran has described two hyperacute fatal forms of renal infection characterized only by an accumulation of bacteria and the evidences of an acute congestion of the kidneys.

The Urine.—The urine excreted by an inflamed kidney is absolutely pathognomonic; and if there is any clinical confusion in determining the urinary signs of the surgical inflammations of the kidney, it is for one of three reasons:

1. Because the urine from the inflamed area (abscess of the kidney, closed pyonephrosis) is not passed off;

2. Because the products of vesical and prostatic inflammation (the vaginal mucus in the female) habitually mingle in the urine and obscure the products of renal inflammation; or

3. Because there is a superficial resemblance between the urinary signs of inflammation in any portion of the urinary tract.

In view of these confusing elements it will be useful to consider consecutively how to obtain the kidney urine uncontaminated by vesical, prostatic, or vaginal pus, what the characteristics of such a urine are, and how renal inflammation may be diagnosed therefrom.

To obtain the urine uncontaminated from the kidneys, it is not necessary—current opinion to the contrary, notwithstanding—to employ the ureteral catheter or the urine segregator. Any one who depends entirely upon these instruments will certainly blunt his diagnostic acumen by his inability to discover renal inflammation in that very large class of every-day patients upon whom their use is impracticable or impossible. But there are many other methods that serve for all practical purposes. To be satisfactory the method employed must always obtain the renal urine uncontaminated by bladder pus, and it must sometimes determine from which kidney such urine is derived.

When a patient comes complaining of any inflammation of the urinary tract, it is customary to have him urinate into two glasses (p. 83). This test may suffice. The second flow of urine may show the characteristics of kidney urine plainly enough. But the diagnosis is often not so easy. If there is still a doubt this may usually be solved by washing the bladder gently and repeatedly with boric-acid solution until the wash returns clear. The urine previously passed is preserved for comparison, and the patient dismissed for an hour. At the end of that time he returns and passes the urine meanwhile accumulated in his bladder. If this is as cloudy as the second flow before washing, the diagnosis of pyelo-nephritis may at once be made and will be confirmed by testing the urine last passed.

But another question may arise. If the kidney urine thus obtained shows evidences of pyelo-nephritis, it may still be necessary to determine—especially if an operation is contemplated—which kidney is inflamed, or whether both are implicated. If, on the other hand, the kidney urine is clear, the surgeon may still suspect renal suppuration—e. g., closed pyonephrosis or abscess of the kidney, the evidences of which do not escape down the ureter. To decide these questions it is rarely necessary to appeal to the ureteral catheter. A closed pyonephrosis or a parenchymatous abscess declares itself plainly by the local signs and general symptoms; while to determine from which kidney the pus comes there are four criteria: (1) The lumbar tumour and tenderness, (2) observation by the cystoscope of the congested ureteral orifice, (3) segregation or ureter-catheterism, and (4) exploratory nephrotomy. I confess that, except in tuberculosis, I prefer double nephrotomy to ureteral catheterization.

The Urinary Signs of Pyelo-nephritis.[1]—Since the lesions of pyelo-nephritis are catarrhal or suppurative inflammation of the kidney and its pelvis, combined with a chronic interstitial nephritis, *we always find in the urine excreted from such a kidney pus, bacteria, albumin, and renal casts.* Each of these has its special characteristics.

The *pus* may be present in great quantity, or it may be possible to obtain only a slight deposit by the centrifuge. Yet some pus is always present, varying in quantity from time to time. If the case is closely watched it will often be found that the urine remains for days almost clear of pus, during which period the patient's general and local symptoms become progressively more marked. Then, suddenly, and without any assignable cause, the urine becomes loaded with thick creamy pus and immediately the symptoms are relieved—only to recur gradually as the pus pocket in the renal pelvis refills. This symptom-complex, of *markedly remittent pyuria with increasing symptoms while the pus collects and relief when it is poured out,* is almost pathognomonic of pyelo-nephritis. The seminal vesicle may give similar gushes, but the symptoms and the local and urinary signs of the two conditions differ so widely that an error of diagnosis is hardly possible.

But these gushes of pus are not constant, and to distinguish them may require long and careful observation. Yet if there is at any time a quantity of renal pus in a given specimen its characteristics are usually quite distinctive. If the urine is allowed to stand an hour or so in a glass vessel, it will be found that *the pus sinks to the bottom of the glass and lies flat and solid like a bed of sand, while the supernatant fluid remains hazy with bacteria* (Plate IX). The pus has often a sallow greenish hue, or it may be creamy; but these signs are of little moment. It is the flatness and solidity of the de-

---

[1] I advisedly employ the term pyelo-nephritis, since the urinary signs in pyonephrosis or abscess of the kidney are not to be depended upon.

posit that are characteristic. Bladder pus never settles in this way. However intense the cystitis, however deep the layer of pus at the bottom of the glass, it is always capped by a fluffy, rolling muco-cloud (like the thunderheads on the horizon of a summer sunset) if the pus comes from any part of the urinary tract except the kidney (Plates V, VI).

But this distinctive pyuria is only encountered in the suppurative forms of pyelo-nephritis. When the lesion is mild and catarrhal we must look further for our diagnosis.

Bacteria appear in the pyelo-nephritic urine in a characteristic manner. When there is a notable pyuria the bacteria need not be especially noted. They befog the supernatant urine, but that is all. Yet there are many phases of mild catarrhal pyelitis, acute as well as chronic, in which pus is present in so small a quantity that the urine is clouded by the bacterial swarm rather than by pus—i. e., there is *bacteriuria* with all its characteristics, already studied at length (p. 363). We need not repeat them here.

Albumin is always present in the urine of pyelo-nephritis. In the catarrhal (bacteriuria) cases there is habitually not enough albumin present to give Heller's ring; but careful acidulation and boiling after filtration will produce the characteristic light albuminous cloud. In the graver or more acute cases albumin may be present in great quantities, whether from renal exudation or from the presence of blood.

The *casts* are characteristic of the grade of kidney lesion. They often contain blood, pus, and epithelial cells.

Certain other characteristics of the urine of pyelo-nephritis are its *light colour and low specific gravity*, attributable to the deficient excretion of solids, and its *acidity*. The urine is always acid in catarrhal and almost always so in suppurative cases, and this is the more striking when the urine is so malodorous and purulent as to suggest ammoniacal cystitis.

To sum up: A characteristic pyelo-nephritic urine is light in colour and acid in reaction. It is hazy with bacteria, and if it contains pus in any quantity, this deposits in a solid flat mass, green or yellow. (Compare Plates V, VI, and IX.) Albumin may be discovered in the filtered urine, and the microscope reveals casts unless their presence is obscured by pus.

The Perinephritic Tissue.—Fibro-lipomatous perinephritis (p. 540), characterized by condensation of the perirenal fat into a dense fibro-lipomatous envelope, is constantly met with in severe cases of long standing, while some fibro-lipomatous masses are found about the pelvis in almost all cases.

PLATE IX

THE URINE OF ACID, SUPPURATING PYELO-NEPHRITIS

The urine is acid and milky when passed. On standing it becomes almost clear, retaining only a bacterial haze, while the pus accumulates in a flat, cohesive, yellow or greenish mass at the bottom. The specific gravity of this urine is always low, and the amount of pus varies from day to day.

PLATE IX

THE URINE OF ACID, SUPPURATING PYELO-NEPHRITIS

The urine is acid and milky when passed. On standing it becomes almost clear, retaining only a bacterial haze, while the pus accumulates in a flat, cohesive, yellow or greenish mass at the bottom. The specific gravity of this urine is always low, and the amount of pus varies from day to day.

PLATE IX

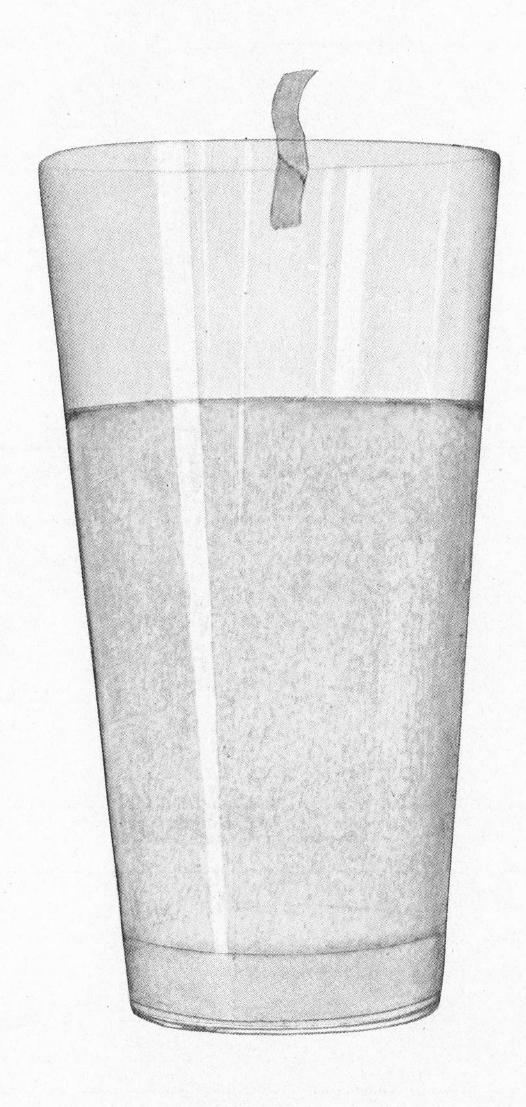

Suppurative Perinephritis.—The result of irruption or extension of a renal abscess into the perinephritic tissue has already been described (p. 541).

The Opposite Kidney.—Catarrhal pyelo-nephritis is habitually bilateral, and it is common for a catarrhal pyelo-nephritis to occur in the fellow of a kidney affected by any extensive suppuration.

But whether the opposite kidney is catarrhal or sound, it tends to undergo a compensatory hypertrophy to make amends for the deficient excretion of the diseased organ. Indeed, the catarrhal nephritis which so often affects it is doubtless due to the congestion of overwork.

Other Organs.—**Urinary Organs.**—When the kidney is primarily inflamed the infection is spoken of as descending, though, as a matter of fact, it is not common for the inflammation to descend to the bladder. Indeed, the patient often seems singularly immune from the consequences that might be anticipated from the zealous soundings and washings to which he is so often subjected. In spite of purulent urine and surgical trauma Nature for once is kind, and tries to spare the prostate and bladder. On the other hand, when the prostate and bladder are primarily infected, the additional renal lesion does them no harm, except inasmuch as it deteriorates the patient's powers of resistance.

Other Organs.—That the bacterial sclerosis of the kidney now under consideration has any relation to general arterio-capillary fibrosis, I do not know. The two may be met with in one patient. The cardiac hypertrophy of renal sclerosis is encountered here. The digestive disorders are apparently toxemic and functional. Septicemia and pyemia are possible complications.

General Symptomatology

The general symptoms of surgical renal infection may be due to auto-intoxication from renal insufficiency (urinary toxemia) or to actual septicemia or pyemia. We need not here concern ourselves with that special and peculiar form of urinary toxemia occurring when both ureters are suddenly and completely obstructed (see Calculous Anuria).

Urinary Toxemia

Urinary toxemia is a chronic auto-intoxication due to renal insufficiency—i. e., to the inability of the diseased kidneys properly to perform their function of eliminating certain excrementitious substances from the circulation. This condition is common to all the diseases of the renal parenchyma, whether medical or surgical. It is usually called uremia, a misleading term, for which I prefer to substitute the more accurate title, urinary toxemia, which serves to distinguish it clearly from urinary septicemia; while at the same time it does not hint, as uremia does, that the retention of urea (itself a diuretic) plays any part in causing the symptoms.

Etiology.—The causes of urinary toxemia are all reducible to one condition—viz., inability of the renal epithelium to perform its function. This the surgeon encounters in an acute and a chronic form.

Acute urinary toxemia occurs as (*a*) acute post-operative renal congestion, and (*b*) acute reflex renal congestion after operations, etc., upon the urethra and bladder (see Urinary Fever). Calculous anuria will interest us elsewhere.

Chronic urinary toxemia may occur from the chronic congestion of urinary retention—be it urethral, prostatic, or ureteral—or from chronic interstitial nephritis. In practice the two causes act together. The congestion of retention permits infection; that, in turn, causes interstitial nephritis, and the congestion continuing hastens the functional dissolution of the diseased organs.

Symptoms.—The symptoms of urinary toxemia, whether acute or chronic, are those commonly described in text-books on the practice of medicine as the symptoms of chronic interstitial nephritis and uremia. The picture in acute cases is anuria (or oliguria), auto-intoxication, and death—unless, perchance, the attack subsides spontaneously or the surgeon intervenes. In chronic cases, when the surgeon sees them, the symptoms of chronic urinary toxemia are commonly intermingled with and obscured by those of urinary septicemia.

Treatment.—1. For the acute forms, *diuresis* by mineral waters, or, in emergencies, by saline infusion, *diaphoresis* by the hot pack, by pilocarpin, etc., the administration of urotropin (p. 373), cupping the loin, even venesection, if the patient is plethoric, to *reduce renal congestion*, and such mechanical or operative measures as may be appropriate *to remove the cause of the renal congestion*—among these last nephrotomy may figure, if the future justifies the confidence Harrison and Edebohls place in it (p. iv).

2. For the chronic forms the diuretic waters are useful, as are the various diuretic drugs employed by the physician, among which I especially favour the sodio-salicylate of theobromin, the bichlorid of mercury, and the tincture of the chlorid of iron. Appropriate diet, regulation of the bowels, such hygienic measures as exercise, climate, etc., and avoidance of mental strain, are important accessories to the treatment. But best of all, when this chronic urinary toxemia arises from a surgical cause, is the surgical relief—

whether by drugs, manipulation, or operation—of the cause (retention, infection, etc.) of the toxemia. If this can be removed the progress of the renal sclerosis may be checked, and, to all appearances, even cured, an outcome to which no medical or hygienic measures aspire.

Urinary Septicemia

Urinary septicemia is septicemia arising from the absorption through the kidneys of bacterial products in the urine. It is due to the retention of infected urine. Therefore it always includes urinary toxemia, and to this are due some of its peculiar features.

Many forms of septicemia and pyemia result from diseases of the genito-urinary organs. A prostatic abscess, a periurethritis, an infiltration of urine, a suppurating testicle (to mention only a few of the more notable causes), may and do set up a generalized infection. But this is not *urinary* septicemia.

Occurrence.—Urinary septicemia results from retention of purulent urine. It is most commonly encountered in cases of prostatic hypertrophy. Old, tight strictures evoke it, and it always occurs with pyonephrosis and suppurative pyelo-nephritis.

Pathogenesis.—It will be observed that urinary septicemia is always due to changes in the kidneys. Any renal suppuration in which there is accumulation of pus in the kidney inevitably gives rise to urinary septicemia. On the other hand, urethral stricture and prostatic hypertrophy cause urinary fever only by producing renal retention and suppuration.

Symptoms.—The symptoms of this condition may be grouped under several heads—viz.:

Fever.—The fever of urinary septicemia is as irregular as that of any septicemia. When acute it may be interrupted by successive chills, or it may merely run high in the afternoon and low in the morning. In mild chronic cases there may be but a slight afternoon rise, with perhaps a subnormal temperature at night, while occasionally the temperature may remain subnormal for days at a time.

Circulation.—The circulatory conditions vary through an equally wide range. The heart may show the feebleness of age or the hypertrophy of chronic nephritis. If the patient is robust the pulse is rapid and tense, and as he fails it may grow more so, or it may become weak and thready. Arterial sclerosis is a common complication in long-standing cases.

Digestive Organs.—The condition of the digestive organs is usually characteristic. The bowels are constipated, the appetite poor, and, while any acute indigestion is unlikely, that general digestive discomfort common to every form of auto-intoxication is met with here. Nausea, vomiting, and hiccough are symptoms of grave uremia. A foul diarrhea may bespeak intense poisoning. *In severe cases the condition of the tongue, mouth, and fauces is pathognomonic. The tongue is bright red*[1] on its tip and sides, while the dorsum is coated and brown or grayish (Plate X). The entire organ, indeed *the entire mouth and fauces are dry and parched.* The saliva is diminished in quantity, viscid in consistence, and acid in reaction. In the last stages of the disease the foul breath, the sordes, the cracked, parched tongue brown in the centre and bright red all about, form a characteristic and repulsive picture.

The result of this condition of the mouth and tongue is the *buccal dysphagia,* first described by Guyon. On account of the dryness of his mouth the patient accepts with avidity all fluids, but has an aversion to solids, which he can masticate and swallow only with considerable discomfort.

Uremic Symptoms.—Drowsiness and torpor are often the earliest uremic symptoms. Later the drowsiness may deepen, or may alternate with or give place to a mental restlessness with wanderings and hallucinations, whence the patient may at first be recalled, though later he goes into a permanent maniacal or comatose condition. At the same time hiccough and persistent vomiting are likely to occur, with absolute constipation or severe diarrhea—and then the end.

The Urine.—The urine is albuminous, purulent, perhaps bloody, often ammoniacal and fetid. It contains casts, but these may be obscured by the pus. These qualities are not peculiar, but the striking and ominous characteristic is the polyuria. The gravity of the patient's condition may often be fairly well estimated by this symptom alone. For as he loses ground his kidneys, instead of ceasing to secrete, as might be expected, habitually pour out a torrent of dilute urine. The patient passes from 4 to 6 litres (quarts) during the twenty-four hours, two thirds of it by night. This polyuria is a warning sign. It indicates a collapsed nerve force and threatens the worst.

The Patient's Aspect.—When a patient comes complaining of his bladder or kidneys a glance will reveal the presence of urinary septicemia to the experienced eye. His face is usually thin, drawn, and sallow, or, if fat, flabby and pasty. There is a history of failing digestion and lost weight. The skin is dry, perhaps feverish. There may be a slight edema of the extremities, but this symptom is often

[1] The *redness* and dryness of the tongue are directly due to the renal condition and are therefore constant, while the *coat* is attributable to the digestive disturbance and is therefore variable, or may even be entirely absent.

PLATE X

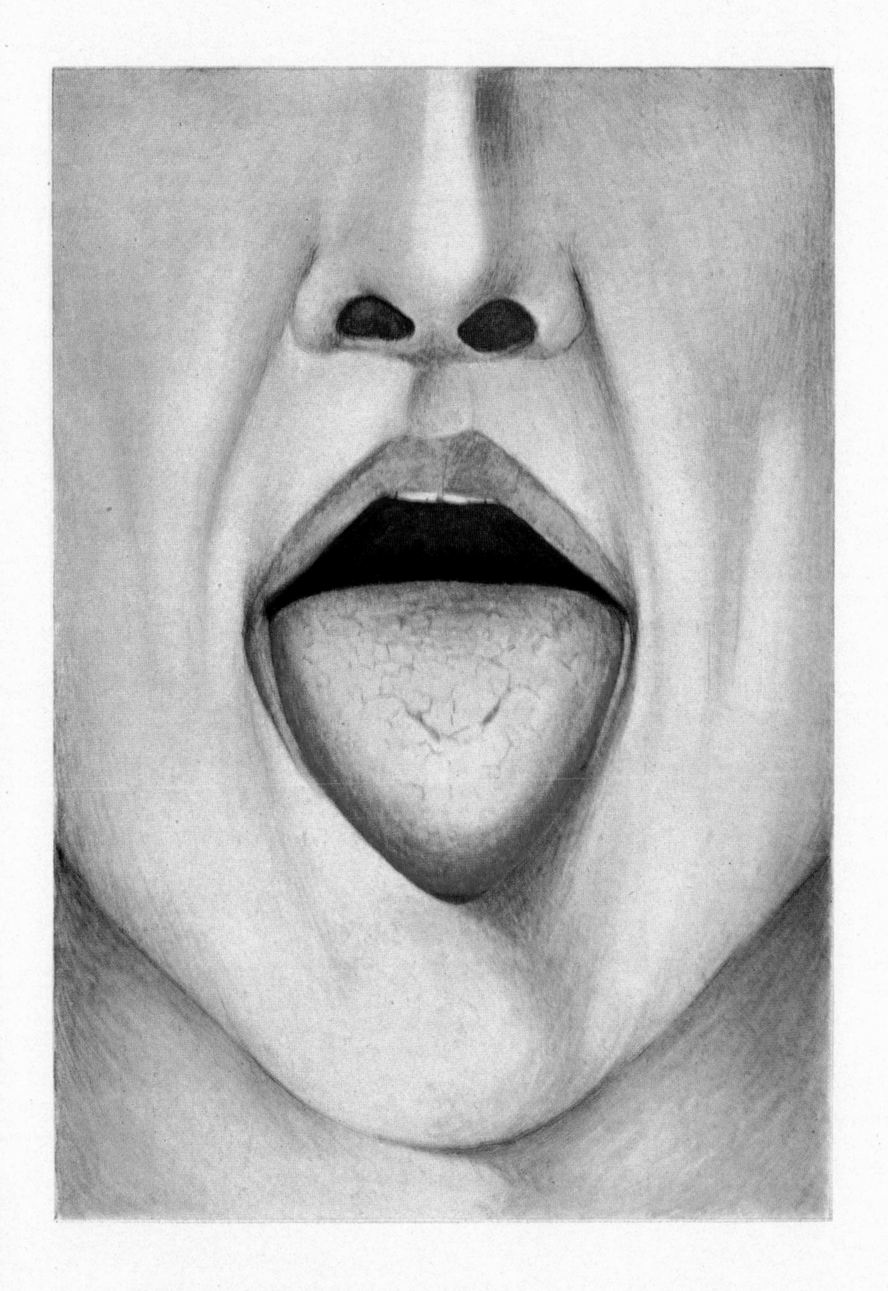

THE DRY, SCARLET TONGUE OF URINARY SEPTICEMIA.

notable by its absence. The actions of the man betoken lassitude, even stupidity.

Types of the Infection.—Urinary septicemia manifests itself in one of four types—viz.:

Urethral Chill.—This condition, which has already been described (p. 43), may be defined as an acute form of urinary septicemia that may occur in a relatively sound individual as the result of urethral instrumentation.[1] This short, sharp chill usually passes off promptly, exceptionally kills the patient, and rarely ushers in the second type of urinary septicemia.

Acute Septicemia or Pyemia.—This type is characterized by repeated chills. The infection usually begins with a chill following urethral instrumentation. This rigor, instead of appearing suddenly, comes on slowly, is not intense, and instead of being succeeded by defervescence, initiates a febrile state, which continues interrupted by chills at irregular intervals of a few hours to a few days. The urine is often dense with urates. Desnos[2] asserts that the urine is not albuminous, but that the kidneys are sensitive to pressure in one half the cases. Among the complications may be mentioned toxic erythema, hypostatic pneumonia, and pyemic abscesses. As a rule, the chills may be controlled by the end of a week, and the patient gradually recovers, or he dies or passes into chronic urinary septicemia.

Chronic Urinary Septicemia.—This is urinary septicemia as encountered in every-day practice. It rarely begins as an acute septicemia. Its onset is habitually gradual, even obscure. The various symptoms that combine to make up the picture of this disease have been described above. Two classes of cases are encountered—viz.:

Dyspeptic cases, in which the patient complains solely or chiefly of his digestive disturbance. Such are the old men who suffer from prostatic retention, with little inflammation and little irritability. They recognise only that they are failing, losing weight and strength, becoming more and more drowsy, and utterly dyspeptic. They present the characteristic tongue, and show slight irregularities of temperature and some polyuria. Relief of the prostatic retention will cure the symptoms, unless, perchance, the surgeon's efforts, catheteral or operative, result in provoking the septic type of chronic urinary septicemia. If let alone these patients deteriorate slowly, and, if not carried off by intercurrent disease, pass finally into the septic type.

---

[1] The exceptional cases in which the kidneys are sound and there is no infection do not concern us here.

[2] Traité élémentaire des maladies des voies urinaires, 1898; 2de éd., p. 909.

The septic type of chronic urinary septicemia is the grave condition that precedes the fatal termination of any chronic retention and suppuration in the bladder or kidneys. It may last for years, or death may close the scene within a few weeks of its onset. While the mildness of its symptoms may at first contrast vividly with those of urethral chill or acute urethral septicemia, it is in still more marked contrast to them, in that it always terminates fatally if left to itself. The approach of the fatal issue is betokened by accentuation of the polyuria and buccal dysphagia, and by the appearance of vomiting, hiccough, and diarrhea.

Treatment.—The treatment of urethral chill has already been described. The *prophylaxis* of urinary septicemia consists in the relief of retention and the prevention of inflammation.

The *curative treatment* of urinary septicemia, in whatever form, is conducted along the same general lines. Retention and suppuration are to be relieved by drainage (catheterization, urethrotomy, cystotomy, or nephrotomy), irrigation, and the administration of urinary antiseptics (pp. 371, 373), while the patient's vitality is reenforced by rest in bed and stimulants, his toxemia combated by diuresis, catharsis, and diaphoresis, and his symptoms appropriately relieved. Urotropin (or salol), diuretic waters, saline infusion, saline cathartics, nitroglycerin, and strychnin form the basis of treatment, while drainage is afforded according to the requirements of the case.

It is impossible to particularize beyond this. The treatment is reviewed in general elsewhere (p. 367), and the particular methods by which drainage should be obtained are discussed under the various appropriate sections. This much may be said, however, that, while the existence of urinary septicemia is evidence of retention and absorption of bacterial toxins through the kidneys, the retention to which the infection is attributable often occurs in the urethra or prostate, and hence, to relieve renal retention and suppuration in such cases, it is the bladder, and not the kidney, that must be drained.

CHAPTER XXXIX

SPECIAL SYMPTOMS, DIAGNOSIS, AND TREATMENT OF SURGICAL INFLAMMATIONS OF THE KIDNEY

SYMPTOMS AND DIAGNOSIS

Acute Catarrhal Pyelo-nephritis.—This inflammation is characterized by total bacteriuria, fever, and a few local symptoms. It seems to be caused solely by the bacillus coli communis and the typhoid bacillus. It occurs during pregnancy or in the course of a typhoid fever. It may also be the first stage of many ascending renal infections.

It is an ephemeral inflammation. I have known it to begin with repeated chills and a sharp rise of temperature, though it may commence less acutely. In the few cases I have seen the temperature ran a septic course, low in the morning, high in the evening, and was associated with little prostration and no evidence of urinary toxemia or septicemia. After a few days the temperature runs lower, and becomes normal between the fourth and the fourteenth day.

Meanwhile the local symptoms amount to nothing more than a slight ache and tenderness in the loins. The urine, however, shows a characteristic acid total bacteriuria (p. 363) and contains albumin and casts.

As the acute inflammation subsides, it is possible for the infection to be overcome spontaneously and for the kidneys to return to their normal state. Otherwise chronic catarrhal or suppurative pyelo-nephritis supervenes.

Diagnosis.—Acute catarrhal pyelo-nephritis is not an uncommon inflammation, but practically it is always overlooked. When it occurs in the course of a pregnancy the obstetrician recognises the albuminuria, but pays no attention to the bacteriuria. If the fever is low it is overlooked, if high it is misinterpreted. The inflammation soon becomes chronic, and so continues indefinitely, or disappears without any diagnosis or treatment other than that of puerperal nephritis.

The acute catarrhal pyelo-nephritis of typhoid fever is also misinterpreted. Whatever rise of temperature or albuminuria it causes is attributed to the enteric inflammation, and the bacteriuria is treated and cured without any clear recognition of the nature of the lesion.

Acute catarrhal pyelo-nephritis occurring in the course of a cystitis is still more obscure. The urinary evidences of cystitis overshadow the renal bacteriuria, and the general and local symptoms are not sufficiently definite for a diagnosis. Hence the renal inflammation is overlooked until the cystitis is controlled and the pyelo-nephritis has become chronic.

To diagnose acute pyelo-nephritis it is only necessary to distinguish the symptom-complex of bacteriuria, albuminuria, and fever. This can often be done in the puerperal cases, sometimes in the typhoidal cases, and rarely in the cases of ascending infection.

Chronic Catarrhal Pyelo-nephritis.—The symptoms of chronic catarrhal pyelo-nephritis are acid renal bacteriuria (p. 363) and urinary toxemia. In the earlier stages of the disease bacteriuria is the only symptom, but as the renal sclerosis alvances the evidences of kidney insufficiency gradually appear. There are no local symptoms.

I suspect that chronic catarrhal pyelitis always begins acutely or remains as the last trace of a suppurative inflammation of the kidneys. Yet I have encountered many cases that gave no history of either origin. The inflammation is habitually encountered as the result of stricture or of prostatic hypertrophy. In many such cases the cystitis may be conquered, leaving the patient with no evidence of disease other than the passage of acid bacterial urine containing casts, a mere trace of albumin, and a few pus, blood, or epithelial cells. Less frequently a chronic catarrhal pyelitis persists after pregnancy or typhoid fever. In other cases the catarrhal pyelitis originates as a suppurative inflammation. After the kidneys have been thoroughly emptied of pus, an acid renal bacteriuria still persists.

The course of the inflammation is much the same whatever its origin. It may resolve spontaneously or under treatment during the first months. The typhoid cases usually resolve, while those originating from a retention cystitis or from suppurative pyelo-nephritis very rarely do. More often it continues indefinitely. At first it gives no subjective symptoms. Unless the patient's attention is called to his urine by its haziness or its odour, he is quite unconscious that there is anything wrong with him. But the interstitial sclerosis progresses slowly as the months and years go by and the renal parenchyma is slowly destroyed, so that the patient passes into a condition of chronic interstitial nephritis.

As the vital forces weaken nocturnal polyuria occurs, while the quantity of albumin in the urine remains slight. There may be occasional hematuria. The heart undergoes compensatory hypertrophy, and general arterio-sclerosis is likely to ensue. The digestion is not good. Constipation is the rule. Edema does not often appear. In short, there is renal insufficiency and the patient suffers from urinary toxemia. While he would not style himself actually ill, he is obviously not well. He has an unhealthy look, an impaired digestion, a poor circulation, and damaged kidneys. He may still be able to endure hard work and severe mental strain, but sooner or later he is smitten down. A slight cold brings on pneumonia, edema of the lungs or acute congestion of the kidneys, with suppression of urine; an excessive exertion or emotion induces apoplexy. Or, if he is more fortunate, his eyesight fails, and the ophthalmoscope reveals the origin of his troubles, or a chance examination for life insurance discloses the urinary conditions. Such is one side of the picture—what might be termed its medical aspect. It is that of chronic interstitial nephritis from whatever cause.

In many instances, however, the surgical conditions overshadow the interstitial nephritis. Perhaps the retention of prostate or stricture has never been relieved, or perhaps it recurs; perhaps the suppurative nephritis has left pockets in the pelvis of the kidney that invite a local retention; perhaps stone forms. From one or other of these causes there is an ever-present possibility that suppurative pyelo-nephritis may ensue. Hence the treatment is directed almost as much against this mishap as towards curing the disease.

Diagnosis.—The diagnosis of chronic catarrhal pyelo-nephritis is the diagnosis of bacteriuria and of chronic interstitial nephritis. Both diagnoses are essential to appreciate and treat the case. If it has originated in a chronic cystitis, the surgeon is peculiarly prone to neglect the kidneys and to torture the bladder with syringes, cystoscopes, sounds, and section in vain efforts to check an inflammation that is in the pelvis of the kidney. A careful urinary examination (p. 365) will set him right, and on this alone he must depend.

On the other hand, the general practitioner will be quick enough to appreciate the renal aspect of the case, but, through neglect to note the obvious haze in the urine, he overlooks the bacterial cause, and all his medical treatment avails nothing. The diagnosis of chronic catarrhal pyelo-nephritis is simple enough, if one only suspects its existence.

Suppurative Pyelo-nephritis.—Suppurative pyelo-nephritis is caused by stone, tubercle, injury or abscess of the kidney, or by ascending infection from the bladder. Suppuration from the first three causes is usually confined at first to one kidney; but ascending infection attacks the two kidneys simultaneously, and it is this form of the inflammation that concerns us here.

Ascending suppurative pyelo-nephritis has been termed *the surgical kidney*, and such it is in every sense. It is a surgical disease; it demands surgical treatment; it is caused, often enough, by the careless surgical treatment of retention cystitis.

The *lesions* of surgical kidney are commonly bilateral, but the suppuration is almost always more severe in one kidney than in the other.

The course of the disease may be acute or chronic.

Acute Cases.—The symptoms of *acute suppurative pyelo-nephritis* are urinary septicemia, pyuria, and local evidences of abscess. The infection of the kidney is announced by a chill, perhaps by a succession of chills. The temperature rises abruptly and runs a septic course. Already worn out by a severe cystitis, the patient is greatly prostrated. At this time there may be no urinary evidences of the renal infection, for the pus may be pent up in the kidney or its pelvis. But there pain and tenderness to pressure over the kidney exist —a tenderness best elicited by Guyon's ballottement—though bimanual examination reveals little or no enlargement of the organ. The tumour and septicemia increase day by day, and the patient may succumb to the infection or pass into what might be termed the second stage of the disease. The abscess bursts. Exceptionally it bursts into the perirenal tissue and gives only temporary relief; habitually it bursts or overflows into the pelvis of the kidney and down the ureter. The aspect of the case is immediately altered. The urine is loaded with renal pus; pain, tenderness, and tumour disappear from the loin, or at least perceptibly diminish, and the septicemia abates. If the patient is able to rally, his condition greatly improves and the inflammation becomes catarrhal, or the abscess refills and the suppuration becomes chronic.

Chronic Cases.—The symptoms of *chronic suppurative pyelonephritis* are general, local, and urinary. There is urinary septicemia, renal pyuria, intermittent or continuous, pain, tenderness, and tumour of the affected organ. The symptoms habitually run a remittent course. While the pus is draining well the fever is low, the local signs obscure, the urine full of pus. As the abscess fills up the general and local symptoms become more marked, while the pus disappears from the urine. So definite may be this association of symptoms that the patient himself learns that when his urine is foul and muddy he feels far better than when it is comparatively clear.

In other cases the course of the disease is more steady. The collection of pus in the kidney drains badly. There is little variation in the general, local, and urinary symptoms. Such cases may pursue one of several courses.

1. *The symptoms are all referable to the bladder.* It may be that a severe cystitis obscures the symptoms of pyelo-nephritis; but more often it is the symptoms of the pyelo-nephritis itself that are referred to the bladder. It is a singular fact that suppuration in the kidney—and this is especially true of calculous pyelo-nephritis—may cause the most torturing tenesmus in the bladder without any pain in the loin. The association of pyuria and dysuria encourages the surgeon in his treatment of the bladder, while he neglects a suppurating kidney that may fill the whole loin. The records of innumerable futile cystotomies attest this fact, and the only way to avoid such a mistake is by a careful urinary examination. Renal pus will be found in quantity, or else there will be a suggestive bacteriuria, albuminuria, and cylindruria. Following up this suggestion, the surgeon will obtain unmistakable confirmatory evidence from the tongue, the temperature, and an examination of the loin.

2. In other cases the *local symptoms in the loin* attract the patient's notice. The *tumour* may not be so large as to compel his attention; but the *pain* may be marked. It varies from a slight soreness and tenderness to the excruciating agony of renal colic. These painful types of the disease commonly occur in calculous cases (p. 589).

3. *Dyspeptic and septic cases,* in which the symptoms of urinary septicemia (p. 563) predominate, are often obscure, especially if the kidney is not notably enlarged or tender. Yet here again a careful urinary examination will disclose evidences of renal inflammation.

The inflammation runs one or other of the above courses for weeks, months, or years before it *terminates.* It may end in resolution. The foci of renal suppuration are effectively drained, and there is no further accumulation of pus. In the process of cure the inflammation passes through a catarrhal stage that may be prolonged indefinitely. The kidney does not recover from its sclerosis unless by hypertrophy of its remaining parenchyma cells.

On the other hand, the patient may die of sepsis or of suppression of urine. The fatal event may be hastened by extension of the inflammation to the perinephritic tissue, or by recurrent pyonephrosis from ureteral obstruction.

Diagnosis.—The most important suggestions as to diagnosis have been made in the preceding paragraphs. Whether the symptoms assume a vesical, dyspeptic, or septic type, the urine affords ample evidence of the involvement of the kidney. But, given a suppuration in the kidney, it may be extremely difficult to distinguish between the simple, the calculous, and the tubercular forms of suppurative pyelo-nephritis. The history is of some value in this regard, and so are the X-rays (p. 590), while exploratory nephrotomy is a perfectly legitimate means of determining the question and treating the condition found. I have on several occasions been able to discover which kidney was the source of pus by cystoscopy, which revealed a congested ureteral orifice emitting cloudy urine.

Pyonephrosis.—Pyonephrosis is not a primary condition. It may develop from suppurative pyelo-nephritis (whether simple, calculous, or tubercular) by occlusion of the ureter, or from hydronephrosis by infection of the contents of the sac. Like hydronephrosis, pyonephrosis may be fixed or intermittent. It is usually the former; yet, however intermittent the pyonephrosis, it does not (with the rarest exceptions) empty itself completely.

The symptoms of pyonephrosis may best be expressed by comparison with those of pyelo-nephritis. They are more severe in almost every respect. The symptoms of pyonephrosis are habitually constant, not remittent. There is grave chronic urinary septicemia with considerable fever. The pains, vesical or renal, like those of pyelo-nephritis, may be of any intensity; but the tumour is marked. The kidney is much enlarged; it may be enormously dilated. If the ureter is entirely shut off the urine offers no indication of the renal condition. If not entirely occluded, pus and bacteria appear as in pyelo-nephritis.

The striking features of pyonephrosis are the lumbar tumour and the septic condition of the patient. The lumbar tumour may be felt by almost any method of palpation; indeed, it may often be seen. The urinary septicemia is always marked.

The outcome of the disease is death by sepsis or suppression, or rupture into the ureter, into a neighbouring viscus, or into the perinephritic fat. Exceptionally the contents of a pyonephrotic sac undergo a sort of caseation and become aseptic, so that the urinary septicemia disappears while the renal tumour remains. A cure may result if the sac empties into the ureter.

Diagnosis.—Pyonephrosis is diagnosed from hydronephrosis by the presence of urinary septicemia. It is not always possible nor is it necessary to distinguish between a small pyonephrosis and a pyelo-nephritis. The distinctions between the pyonephrotic tumour and other abdominal growths are discussed elsewhere (p. 624).

Abscess of the Kidney.—Many cases that we clinically classify as pyelo-nephritis and pyonephrosis the pathologist might justly term abscess of the kidney. But there is a marked clinical distinction between suppuration of kidney and pelvis together and suppuration confined—for the time, at least—to the substance of the kidney.

Suppurative nephritis without pyelitis is rare. It is usually unilateral, and due to a descending infection. It occurs most commonly in the course of a pyemia, less frequently as the result of embolism, or as a complication of any severe constitutional infection. It may result from wounds or contusions of the kidney.

The course of the disease may be either acute or chronic. Abscess of the kidney occurring during any severe infectious disease may not add any definite symptoms to those already existing, and may only be discovered post mortem. Indeed, it may be difficult to make a diagnosis even when there are no overshadowing symptoms. There is hectic fever and evidence of suppuration somewhere in the body, *but there is neither renal tumour nor any urinary evidence of renal suppuration.* The disease runs its course as an obscure internal suppuration. There may chance to be tenderness to ballottement, or a history of injury to the loin to guide the surgeon. But in the absence of these signs he may remain in complete ignorance, unless enlightened by the appearance of lumbar pain, tenderness or tumour, or by the rupture of the abscess into the pelvis of the kidney or into the perinephritic tisuse.

The prognosis is bad. Renal suppuration lessens the prospects of recovery from pyemia. If the abscess bursts into the perirenal tissues, perinephritis ensues; if it opens into the pelvis of the kidney the suppuration becomes pyelo-nephritic. Morris believes that " in some cases it is pretty certain that the contents of the abscess, instead of escaping in any of the directions mentioned, become inspissated and remain quiescent for the rest of life."

Diagnostic Table

I have classified the chief distinguishing features of chronic cystitis and the various forms of surgical renal inflammations in the appended diagnostic table.

	Chronic cystitis.	Catarrhal pyelo-nephritis.	Suppurative pyelo-nephritis.	Pyonephrosis.	Kidney abscess.
Appearance of urine	Bladder pus.	Bacteriuria.	Renal pus.	Usually no pus.	No pus.
Reaction of urine ..	Usually alkaline.	Acid.	Usually acid.	....	....
Albumin	From pus or blood.	Present.	Present.	Usually.	Usually.
Casts..............	Absent.	Present.	Present.	Usually.	Usually.
Bladder symptoms .	Present.	Absent.	Sometimes.	Sometimes.	....
Renal symptoms...	Absent.	Usually none.	Pain, tenderness, tumour.	Large tumour, pain, tenderness.	Indefinite.
Urinary toxemia...	Absent.	In later stages.	Present.	Present.	....
Urinary septicemia.	Absent.	Absent, unless acute.	Present.	Present.	Present.

PROGNOSIS

As to prognosis, the various surgical inflammations of the kidney have been dealt with separately. Dealing with them collectively we may say that the prognosis depends upon the damage done to the kidney tissue (*a*) by the bacterial inflammation, and (*b*) by the interstitial nephritis. When an acute catarrhal pyelo-nephritis is cured, the casts and albumin disappear from the urine after a few months, and no sign of the inflammation remains. With chronic catarrhal pyelo-nephritis the case is different. While this inflammation does not directly threaten life, and while the bacteria may usually be driven from the kidney by a prolonged course of suitable treatment, the interstitial sclerosis remains, and the kidneys never return to a normal state. Whether this sclerosis continues stationary after its bacterial cause has been eliminated, or whether it progresses slowly after the fashion of the medical chronic interstitial nephritis, I cannot say.

When there is actual suppuration in the kidney substance, whether the condition be a suppurating pyelo-nephritis, a pyonephrosis, or an abscess of the kidney substance, the prospect is still less encouraging. The patient often escapes with his life, and the suppuration may be controlled by appropriate measures, but in many instances the resultant catarrhal pyelo-nephritis cannot be entirely conquered; and even if it is, the kidney is always left badly scarred. But one of the most striking features of renal pathology is compensatory hypertrophy of the kidney. Not only will one kidney do the work of two after nephrectomy, but the merest shell of a kidney, the dense fibrous sac of a pyonephrosis in which the naked eye detects no secreting structure whatever, is still a functionating organ. Its power of excreting solids may be much diminished, but its capacity for transmitting water is practically unimpaired; and it is still a useful organ, one that should be spared to the patient if the inflammation in it can be cured.

The prognosis as regards life and death depends chiefly upon the treatment.

TREATMENT

Prophylaxis.—All ascending infection of the kidney may be prevented by prompt and efficient treatment of the cause of retention, be it stricture, prostate, or what not. Descending infections do not so readily lend themselves to prophylaxis; yet it is often possible to nip acute puerperal or typhoid pyelo-nephritis in the bud, if the possibility of this renal infection is borne in mind. The operative prevention of calculous pyelo-nephritis does not concern us here.

The condition of the bowels is of the utmost importance in the prevention of infection of the kidneys. The bacillus coli is the infective agent in almost every case of descending renal infection. This bacillus reaches the general circulation from the intestine only when the bowels are constipated or otherwise diseased, and is excreted from the general circulation through the kidneys. Hence as long as the regular daily movements of the bowels are uninterrupted there appears to be little danger of spontaneous infection. It is intestinal stagnation that applies the spark.

Hence renal inflammations are preventable in two ways: The retention that prepares the kidney for infection and the intestinal stagnation that supplies the infectious agent may both be prevented.

Curative Treatment.—The inflamed kidney may be considered an abscess cavity. What it requires is drainage and irrigation with an antiseptic fluid.

Drainage.—The kidney affected by *catarrhal pyelo-nephritis* is habitually normal in shape and size. There is no abscess cavity in its parenchyma, no pouch in its pelvis; yet as a rule it is not properly drained. The outflow of urine is impeded by stricture, hypertrophied prostate, pelvic tumour, peritoneal adhesions, or pregnant uterus. In order to establish proper drainage this retention, whatever its nature, must be relieved. Without this it is quite impossible to relieve the renal inflammation (p. 380).

Suppurative pyelo-nephritis (not calculous or tubercular) may sometimes be relieved by the same indirect method of drainage that applies to catarrhal inflammations. Thus a surgical kidney due to cystitis from prostatic retention may usually be cured by draining the bladder. In such cases the restored equilibrium of urinary pressure permits the pus to drain freely. But often enough vesical drainage does not suffice. The pelvis is so pouched or the renal substance so riddled with abscesses that the kidney itself must be drained by nephrotomy. If the kidney is palpably dilated at the time cystotomy is performed, it is proper forthwith to establish drainage through the loin. The patient's condition may render the procedure a desperate one, yet the alternative of leaving a poorly drained abscess is even more desperate than a rapid nephrotomy.

In other cases the cystotomy does not relieve the patient. In spite of efficient bladder drainage the sepsis continues, the patient does not gain in strength, perhaps one or both kidneys become tender or enlarged. The proper treatment of such a case requires the ablest prognostic acumen. Nephrotomy may prove fatal. The patient may recover without it. When performed soon enough it will cure if it does not kill; when performed too late it can only kill, it cannot save. Yet who shall say too late! The best technical judgment and skill may err. One can only say that a septic patient is a better risk than a uremic one, and that proper drainage should at all risks be afforded before the kidneys give out. Perhaps in the future cryoscopy or the elimination tests will aid us to decide.

Nephrotomy is the Treatment for Pyonephrosis.—Cystotomy, ureterotomy, or some other operation may be required as well, for the urinary right of way must be cleared from top to bottom; but nephrotomy is the essence of a cure. The operation is not a severe one. Perhaps my experience has led me to be too optimistic; but certain it is that when death has followed nephrotomy at my hands, the cause has been urinary septicemia, which could be relieved by no means other than nephrotomy. Yet I have not escaped the accidents that befall other surgeons. I have opened the peritoneal cavity. I have encountered severe secondary hemorrhage. And still I assert confidently that properly performed nephrotomy is an operation simple for the surgeon, safe for the patient, and brilliant in its results.

The object of nephrotomy is drainage. The surgeon wishes to obtain (*a*) thorough drainage through the wound for a few weeks, and then (*b*) thorough drainage through the ureter. To get satisfactory wound drainage it is only necessary thoroughly to open up the suppurating foci and to drain from a dependent point (p. 640). But to establish drainage through the ureter is no such simple matter. In speaking of hydronephrosis some space was devoted to the consideration of operations for the relief of the various ureteral obstructions. Such operations are feasible in hydronephrosis, but the suppurating kidney, whether dilated (pyonephrotic) or not, is so surrounded by dense adhesions as to make plastic procedures difficult or impossible. The patient is in no condition for a protracted operation; while the inner surface of the suppurating organ is often so subdivided, so pocketed that the establishment of permanent perfect drainage is impracticable. No two cases are alike. In one a small central abscess requires incision and drainage. In another the removal of a calculus effects a cure. A third requires some plastic work about the ureter. A fourth demands urethrotomy or prostatotomy. A fifth calls for nephrectomy. A sixth is so debilitated that it is deemed unwise to attempt anything more than simple drainage: if lucky he will recover and his lumbar fistula will heal. If the lumbar fistula persists a secondary operation is called for.

One hears much discussion on the comparative merits of *nephrotomy and nephrectomy* in the treatment of suppurating kidney. Inasmuch as the question can never be decided one way or the other for all cases, the discussion will doubtless continue. But the essence of the matter is this: if adequate ureteral drainage can be established nephrotomy suffices. Nephrectomy is required when the kidney is so pouched that the urine and pus cannot be made to drain efficiently through the ureter, or when its suppuration will do the patient more harm than its secretion will do him good.

Nephrectomy may be primary or secondary. There are advantages on each side. For secondary nephrectomy it is claimed that it exposes the patient to a severe shock—which nephrectomy always does—only when he has been given the opportunity to rally from his septicemia by a palliative nephrotomy. On the other hand, it is urged that secondary nephrectomy, on account of the adhesions formed after nephrotomy, is far more difficult and dangerous than primary nephrectomy. Both contentions are just, and, in order to reconcile the opposing views, it has been suggested that secondary nephrectomy be performed after the patient has somewhat recovered from his sepsis, but before dense adhesions can form. So long as any mortality remains to either operation, there will be a difference of opinion in this matter. But it is generally conceded that:

1. If the patient is gravely septic or uremic, it is safest to perform rapid nephrotomy with no thought of the ultimate result.

2. If the general condition is good, every effort should be made to re-establish ureteral drainage, and the kidney should be removed only (*a*) when it is obvious that ureteral drainage can never be re-established, or (*b*) when the suppurating cavity is so large and the remaining renal tissue so slight that it does not appear possible for the cavity to close down without subjecting the patient to a pro-

longed course of suppuration, for which the possession of an extremely disabled kidney would never compensate.

3. If, for any reason, ureteral drainage is doubtful, the patient should be given the benefit of this doubt, and nephrectomy postponed until the persistent lumbar sinus has shown that the re-establishment of ureteral drainage is not to be expected.

4. Nephrectomy, primary or secondary, should not be thought of until it is proved that the opposite kidney is capable of supporting life.

Such are the general and more or less defined rules that must guide the surgeon. Their practical application, the technic, and the results of operation, are described in another chapter.

Abscess of the kidney requires nephrotomy or nephrectomy, if it is possible to save the patient by these means. When the renal lesion is only one phase of a pyemia, it is needless to add to the patient's discomfort by cutting holes in his back. Yet an acute case, especially if it occurs in a comparatively young person, may perhaps be saved from otherwise certain death by prompt nephrotomy.

Irrigation and Antisepsis.—This—the medical and palliative part of the treatment—is accorded a secondary place because, while it may be the only treatment required for a given case of surgical renal disease, yet the essence of all treatment must be drainage. Drainage without medicine may cure; medicine without drainage cannot cure. Drainage we must have, whether afforded by Nature or by the surgeon. Yet our medical treatment is most important. It is employed for three purposes:

1. To prevent infection. (*Cf.* Prophylaxis.)

2. To control inflammation when perfect drainage cannot be obtained, and

3. To cure inflammation.

The routine medical treatment is twofold: irrigation and antisepsis. The principles upon which this treatment is founded have been laid down in another chapter (p. 373).

Acute catarrhal pyelo-nephritis yields promptly to urotropin and diuresis. The administration of urotropin should be continued for several weeks after the bacteriuria has ceased. It may be necessary to increase the dose to 3 or 4 grammes a day, in order to conquer the bacteriuria, but as soon as this is controlled, it may be reduced to 1.5 grammes. Even when the higher doses are intolerable, I look for better results from a prolonged course of diuresis and urotropin, at the highest dose possible, than from salol or benzoic acid.

Chronic catarrhal pyelo-nephritis demands the same treatment. There is usually a prostatic retention to be corrected and constipation to be overcome. Urotropin and diuresis should be continued for months. There is no advantage in pushing them. If perfect drainage is not obtainable (because the patient will not submit to systematic catheterism or to operation) the medical treatment is still useful as a palliative, to prevent exacerbations of inflammation. Hygiene and climate are often very beneficial in these cases.

Suppurative pyelo-nephritis demands medical treatment chiefly for the urinary septicemia. Persons suffering from mild chronic suppuration in the kidneys are often unwilling or unable to undergo the operation required to establish perfect drainage. Moreover, it is just such cases that are least amenable to operation. There may be no very definite obstruction, but only a slight renal dilatation. I have cured such cases by nephrotomy; but I have cured them—or they have cured themselves—equally well without it. When the X-rays demonstrate the absence of stone (p. 590), and there is no renal enlargement nor any evidence of vesical retention, a cure may be expected from purely medical treatment. A climate and water cure at almost any mineral spring, and the long-continued use of urotropin or salol, will always benefit the patient, and will often cure.

The more acute or severe cases demand perfect drainage and vigorous treatment of the septicemia, followed by a prolonged course of mild diuresis and urotropin or salol.

Pyonephrosis requires purely surgical treatment. Drainage is almost the sole essential. Diuresis and urinary antisepsis are important but secondary features.

Abscess of the kidney calls for the knife.

Other Methods of Treatment.—Some surgeons employ the knife, others the ureteral catheter for the cure of almost every form of renal inflammation. I confess that the knife can almost always be employed with advantage; but I believe that the comfort and safety of the patient may be best insured by some such plan of surgical conservatism as outlined in the preceding paragraphs.

As for the ureteral catheter and lavage of the kidney pelvis, I cannot see that their vaunted cures atone for their manifest inconveniences, dangers, and uncertainties.

CHAPTER XL

RENAL AND URETERAL CALCULUS

The general description of urinary calculi, their macroscopic and microscopic characteristics, pathogenesis, etc., are discussed in Chapter XXVIII. Only a few words need be added here.

Renal calculi are usually single. Exceptionally a great number of stones are found. Thus Morris removed 200 stones from 1 case and Dessirier and Legrand [1] found 400 calculi in the left kidney and 60 in the right at the autopsy of a young soldier who during life had shown no symptoms referable to the kidneys. Renal calculi run up to about 100 grammes (3 ounces) in weight, the large stones being irregularly branched to fit into the distorted and dilated pelvis and calices (Fig. 145). In operating upon a suppurating kidney one occasionally meets with very small stones, scarcely more than phosphatic dust.

Kraft [2] found renal calculi 40 times in 2,953 autopsies; both kidneys were affected 15 times. Legueu and Albarran agree that in about half the cases both kidneys contain calculi, yet recent X-ray investigations go to show that in the living the proportion of bilateral cases is not very great.

Renal calculi occur more frequently in men than in women. They are oftenest encountered in middle life.

Morbid Anatomy

The changes that a calculus may undergo, such as phosphatic incrustation, spontaneous fracture, etc., have been described (p. 434).

The changes that occur in the kidneys and ureters from the presence of calculi may be considered under three heads—viz., retention, ulceration, and inflammation.

Retention.—A calculus formed in the renal pelvis may at any moment slip down and be caught at the orifice of the ureter, or at any physiological or pathological narrowing in that duct. This usu-

[1] Méd. mod., 1901.

[2] Hospitals Tidende, 1900, No. 29.

ally occurs at or near the upper end of the ureter (Fig. 147), less frequently at the vesical orifice of the canal (Fig. 104) or at the point where it crosses the brim of the pelvis. Such an impaction may be partial or complete. It is usually partial, and as the urine dammed up behind this sudden obstacle brings pressure upon it, the stone is forcibly driven into the ureter, setting up a *renal colic*. This is relieved by the passage of the stone into the bladder, by its slipping back into the pelvis, or by the gradual accommodation of the parts to the new conditions. If the stone remains impacted it causes either partial retention resulting in *hydronephrosis*, or complete obstruction resulting in an acute congestion and subsequent atrophy of the kidney (unless the obstruction is relieved). This complete retention is evinced by *anuria*—calculous anuria it is called—which is temporary if the opposite kidney is able to continue its functions, permanent and fatal if the opposite kidney stops secreting, whether on account of reflex congestion or of bilateral calculous obstruction.

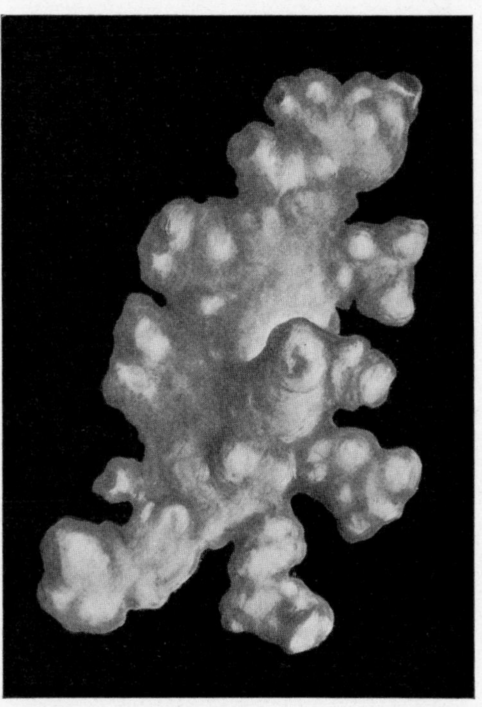

Fig. 145.—Large Branched Renal Calculus.

Ulceration.—Ulceration occurs at whatever point in the kidney, the pelvis, or the ureter a stone may rest. If the stone is small and movable the ulceration may be insignificant. If it is large or impacted the ulceration may be so deep and extensive that actual *perforation* occurs, permitting the stone to escape from the kidney (the pelvis or the ureter) into the surrounding tissues. This complication, associated as it is with urinary extravasation, is as unusual as it is grave. *Ureteral stricture* may result from prolonged calculous impaction.

Inflammation.—A more common—in fact, *the* most common—effect of ulceration is infection. The congested ulcerated spot and the stone itself, coated with the muco-serous exudate, form admirable breeding-places for bacteria, and if there is retention to cause a general congestion, so much the more likely is it that infection will occur. The infection is habitually descending and spontaneous. While the resulting pyelo-nephritis may assume a catarrhal form, and perhaps is usually of that nature at first, the surgeon sees it only after the suppurative stage is reached: *suppurative pyelo-nephritis* or *pyonephrosis*. It is futile to attempt the enumeration of the various lesions that may be caused by one or more stones in the various portions of the upper urinary tract. The lesions of retention, ulceration, and inflammation are combined in endless variety. There may be only localized suppuration about a small pelvic calculus, or there may be numerous calculous pockets throughout the kidney; the entire organ may be reduced to a multilocular abscess cavity filled by a great branching stone (Fig. 145). The kidney may be found atrophied, and closely contracted around a stone that had caused complete obstruction years before. Pyonephrosis results from obstruction of the ureter by stone or stricture when there is infection. Suppuration within the organ may be associated with *peri-nephritis* from extension of the inflammation or from rupture of the sac. The longer the disease continues the more extensive the destruction of renal tissue and the greater the likelihood of bilateral calculous disease.

Symptoms

Any general discussion of the symptoms of renal calculus must be prefaced by the statement that the condition may exist for years without causing any symptoms whatever. The influence that this fact must have upon diagnosis and therapeusis will be considered later.

Morris mentions the notable symptoms caused by renal calculus in 103 cases of his own. These he tabulates as follows:

Pain occurred in	71 cases	(69%).
Pyuria " "	50 "	(48%).
Renal colic occurred in	44 "	(43%).
Hematuria " "	41 "	(40%).
Tumour " "	27 "	(26%).
Troubles of micturition occurred in	24 "	(23%).
Tenderness occurred in	17 "	(16%).

Pain.—Of calculous diseases, Morris writes: "They are the most frequent and most painful of surgical diseases of the kidney. Probably no disease, except acute tetanus, is capable of causing worse suffering." The various pains due to renal and ureteral calculi are renal colic, pressure pains, and reflex pains.

Renal Colic.—This is the most characteristic symptom of stone in the kidney. It is due to the impaction of a stone in the ureter.[1] The pain is paroxysmal in character. It commences suddenly at any time when the patient is seemingly in the best of health, perhaps most frequently shortly after rising in the morning. It shoots down the ureter into the scrotum and to the end of the penis. The testicle of the affected side is often strongly retracted. Indeed, the entire scrotum and penis may be drawn up into a hard knot, as it were. The pain may also extend down the thigh on the affected side. There is usually an incessant desire to pass water, although there is almost absolute suppression. What little urine is voided comes away high-coloured and in small quantities at a time, often tinged with blood and mixed with epithelium from the kidney. Pain attends urination, chiefly towards its close, running down to the end of the penis. If the paroxysm is severe, faintness, nausea, and vomiting occur, the skin is covered with a cold sweat, the patient tosses restlessly about, seeking relief, but finding none. In the intervals between paroxysms there is a sense of soreness and discomfort perhaps amounting to continued pain, or the relief may be absolute. After one or more paroxysms, lasting from a few hours to many days, all pain suddenly ceases. This sudden cessation indicates that the stone has been liberated. It may have fallen back into the pelvis of the kidney, have passed down into the bladder, or have reached some dilated portion of the ureter, where it rests without interrupting the urinary outflow.

The nature of the *termination* of an attack may usually be diagnosed from the symptoms. If the calculus remains in the ureter some pain and tenderness usually persist at the point where it rests. If the impaction has occurred at the upper end of the ureter and is relieved by the stone slipping back into the pelvis, the pain during the attack is usually most intense in the loin and radiates across the back as much as down the ureter. On the other hand, if the stone travels down the ureter to the bladder, its descent is often marked by a progression of the pain from the loin to the pelvis—a progression which may be interrupted by periods of relative or absolute ease—with a corresponding increase in the vesical irritability and the pain and retraction of the testicle.

It may be here remarked that the period of calm following an attack of renal colic should be a time of utmost vigilance on the part of the surgeon (p. 592).

---

[1] Renal colic caused by the passage of gravel or by kinking of the ureter is discussed elsewhere (p. 631).

Pressure Pains.—When the stone is in such a position or of such a size as to fill the cavity in which it lies, it commonly causes a dull continuous ache associated with tenderness. This ache is not necessarily severe, indeed, some persons will endure it for years without attaching any great importance to it, but to the surgeon it is of the utmost importance. The history of such an ache, whether past or present, especially if associated with a point of local tenderness, may be the chief symptom determining the location of the stone.

Reflex Pains.—The two most notable renal reflex pains excited by stone are: (1) Pain following the course of the ureter into the pelvis and thence radiating to the testicle and thigh, and (2) painful and frequent urination. Both reflexes originate from distention or irritation of the pelvis or the ureter rather than from the kidney proper,[1] and may rarely occur from any irritation other than stone.

The painful and frequent urination that so often misleads the surgeon into the belief that the bladder is diseased can only be distinguished by a careful examination of the patient and the urine. This symptom occurred in 23% of Morris's cases.

It is questionable whether stone in one kidney may give pain referred only to the opposite organ. Morris, who has had more experience in this malady than any other surgeon, says: "There is not, so far as I know, any case on record in which there is completely satisfactory evidence of symptoms on one side only being caused by a stone in the kidney of the opposite side. The presence of a stone on one [2] side is not proof that the opposite and painful side is not also affected. That the attacks referred to one side have ceased after operating upon the opposite and painless side is not conclusive; this may be a coincidence due either to the accidental shifting of a calculus in the painful kidney or to the calculus becoming lodged in some immovable manner. There may be very advanced disease of the kidney on the painful side and a symptomless calculus in the opposite kidney." And again: "It is important to know that a stone in one kidney will sometimes excite sympathetic pain and irritation in the other; but this transferred or sympathetic pain is of an aching character, not of a spasmodic or colicky description, is only occasional, and never occurs except as an accompaniment of more severe pain on the affected side."

Hematuria.—As shown by the table, considerable hematuria is a fairly constant symptom of stone. Yet it is variable to the last

[1] I cannot accept Bryson's theory that vesical pains are always due to irritation at the lower end of the ureter.

[2] Painless.

degree. Some hematuria usually accompanies and follows a renal colic, and in most cases there is a fairly constant oozing of blood, showing itself only by the presence of a few red cells and a trace of albumin in the urine. Blood casts and long ureteral clots rarely occur. The bleeding is usually made worse by exercise (though the pain is not), and hence the presence of a great number of red cells in the sediment centrifuged from the urine passed after exercise is suggestive of stone. But after all, the hemorrhage caused by renal stone is an inconstant symptom.

The remaining symptoms on the list require no notice here.

Course of the Disease

The course of the disease is entirely irregular. The character of the symptoms bears no relation to the size or position of the stone; and the progress of the disease varies from the cases that have only a single fatal attack of calculous anuria to those that drag on for years with chronic renal suppuration, or that die of some intercurrent disease without ever having manifested any symptom referable to the calculi with which their kidneys are filled. Yet we may agree with Morris that "no disease gives rise to such a variety of morbid changes in the kidney as calculus, and none is more certainly fatal when allowed to progress without surgical interference."

Several types of the disease may be mentioned, due allowance being made for the fact that the clinical aspect of any given case is often a compound of several types. The surgeon encounters: (1) Cases without symptoms, (2) cases of renal colic, (3) cases of calculous anuria, (4) cases of renal distention, and (5) cases of renal suppuration.

Cases without Symptoms.—Morris distinguishes cases without symptoms from quiescent cases that have shown symptoms (e. g., renal colic) at some previous time. Clinically the conditions are much the same. After several years have intervened it may be impossible to obtain a convincing history of even so impressive an attack as a renal colic. Moreover, a stone may certainly remain for many years unsuspected in the kidney, and at the end of that time set up calculous anuria or perinephritic abscess (Morris), or any other form of calculous trouble. The clinical warning impressed by these cases is that after a renal colic or after any other manifestation of stone in the kidney, the subsidence of symptoms is no evidence that the stone has passed. In such a case it is the surgeon's duty to *find out* that the stone has passed. (*Cf.* Diagnosis.)

Renal Colic and Other Pains.—When the calculus does begin to give symptoms, pain of one sort or another becomes a feature of the disease. A renal colic is often the initial symptom of stone. A single colic may result in the passage of the offending stone; or the stone may remain quiescent for years thereafter, or give rise to repeated attacks of colic, or to a continuous dull pain. The attacks of colic may be singularly regular in their recurrence. I have encountered a case in which the paroxysms recurred every Sunday afternoon for several weeks; but this systematic recurrence is always suggestive of a neurosis rather than of a straightforward calculous colic (p. 631). Other cases run their course with no other notable symptom than a constant ache in the loin. There may or may not be intercurrent attacks of colic or other pains.

Other cases again give only reflex symptoms. One of my earliest professional recollections is of an old man who for years suffered only from painful and frequent urination. His bladder was washed, searched, sounded, and even cut—all to no avail. New York's best surgeons of those days could do nothing for him. Finally, his protracted agony was terminated by a fatal attack of suppression of urine, as it was called. Autopsy revealed a normal bladder and one kidney atrophied and tightly contracted about a calculus, the other somewhat dilated and with a stone plugging the ureteral orifice. Yet he had never complained of a symptom referable to either kidney.

Calculous Anuria.—Calculous anuria is a cessation of the urinary flow, caused by the plugging of one or both ureters with calculi. It is part suppression, part retention. The terminal anuria in the case mentioned above was a pure retention. One kidney had been out of commission for years; the flow of urine from the other was stopped by the obstructing stone. In other cases the blockage of one ureter throws such a burden of excretion upon the opposite kidney that it becomes acutely congested, and suppression ensues. Thus anuria may ensue (1) when both ureters are completely obstructed, or (2) when one ureter is obstructed and the opposite kidney absent, hypertrophied, or sufficiently diseased to be incapable of enduring the congestion forced upon it. The acute obstruction is clinically unilateral, but unless both kidneys are diseased anuria—prolonged anuria, at least—does not occur.

Morbid Anatomy.—The morbid anatomy of calculous anuria is striking and characteristic. The affected kidney, which may be hydronephrotic or suppurating, is intensely congested (Fig. 146). It is enlarged to twice or thrice its normal size, dark in colour, and mottled. On section its tissues are found friable and edematous. Such a large, soft, purple organ once seen is never forgotten.

The opposite kidney (Fig. 147)—if there is one—may undergo

like changes in a less degree, but the absence of congestion in it may be in striking contrast to its fellow. In all but 3 of the 58 cases collected by Morris, the opposite kidney was absent or completely disorganized.

Symptoms.—The symptoms of calculous anuria may be divided into three stages: 1. The Premonitory Stage. 2. The Tolerant Stage. 3. The Uremic Stage.

1. In the *premonitory stage* there is more or less pain, perhaps an actual colic, referred to the kidney. Happily this pain always occurs, for it is the chief sign by which the surgeon is able to decide which kidney most requires operation. It persists from a few hours to a few days.

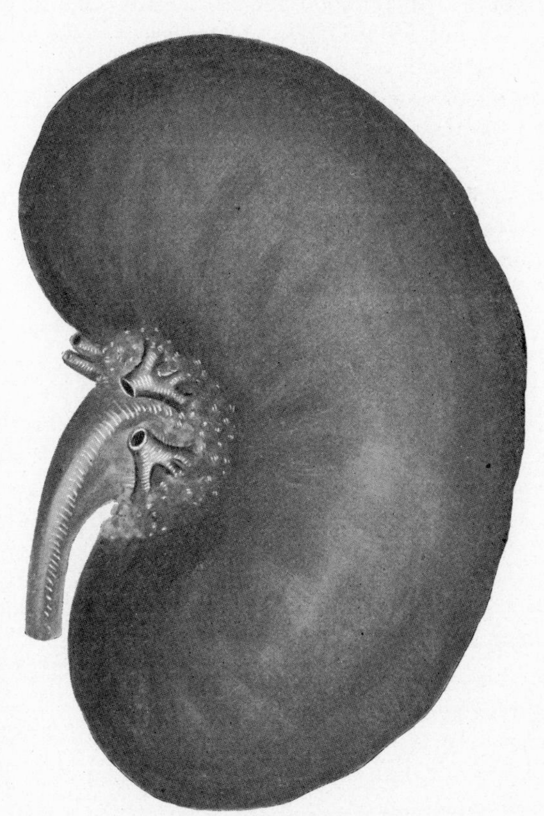

FIG. 146.—CALCULOUS ANURIA: THE CONGESTED KIDNEY. The stone was impacted lower down the ureter. (Compare Fig. 147.)

2. The *tolerant stage* is characterized by but one symptom—viz., anuria. The patient does not pass water. This anuria is rarely absolute. A few grammes of urine tinged with blood are passed every day, or perhaps the anuria runs a remittent course. At one time or another 2 or 3 litres of urine may gush forth, a misleading promise of relief, for the flow is but temporary. This state of affairs lasts from three days to a week. *Not a drop of urine may be passed during several days and yet the patient may, apparently, remain in the best of health.* No more striking contrast could well be imagined than that presented by calculous anuria: on the one hand, the grave renal lesion, the absolute retention, the swift fulminating character of the uremic period soon to follow; and,

on the other hand, this entire absence of symptoms, local or general. The patient goes about well content. He eats, sleeps, and works pretty much as usual. Whatever pain he has had in the loin is past, and his present discomforts are insignificant. And yet all the while there is brewing within him a crisis swift and terrible.

Spontaneous recovery may occur. The obstruction is relieved; the urine gushes out, 3 or 4 litres a day, and all is well. This may occur in 20.8% (Morris) to 28.5% (Legueu) of all cases. In Legueu's[1] cases the spontaneous cure took place on the third day once, between the fifth and the tenth day twice; later still in five instances. Yet it is obvious (*Cf.* Treatment) that no time should be lost in the expectation of a spontaneous cure; for even if this occurs, unless the calculus is actually passed, the patient thereafter goes about in imminent danger of a recurrence of his attack.

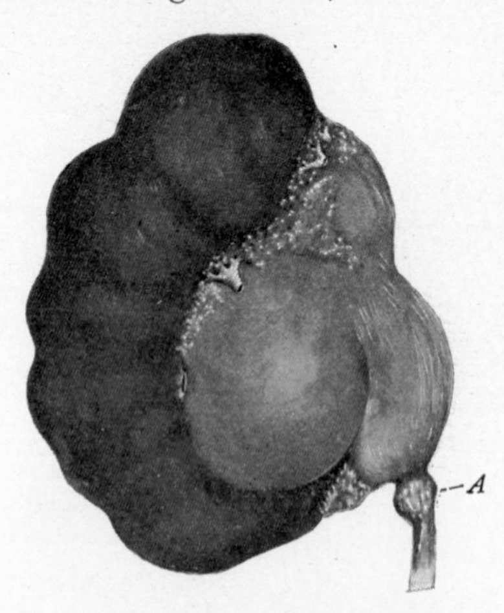

Fig. 147.—Calculous Hydronephrosis. A small stone was found lodged at *A*. This kidney is the fellow of the one shown in Fig. 146. They were obtained from a patient who died of calculous anuria.

When spontaneous recovery does not occur the patient passes into the third stage of the disease at the end of a week or ten days.

3. The *uremic stage* is usually ushered in by hiccough or vomiting. This is the first warning. It may continue for a day or two without additional symptoms. The pulse is tense, the temperature usually subnormal. Constipation becomes absolute and the intestines are distended with gas. The vomiting grows more severe, the intellect becomes dulled and stuporous. The patient's mind may wander a little, and he may even have maniacal attacks. There is often a restlessness of both mind and body. And thus he sinks away and dies, often within two or three days of the first hiccough or vomiting.

Such is the clinical picture of what Morris has aptly termed the gravest and most fatal of the many serious complications of urinary lithiasis. Of course there are atypical cases, the obstruction may be intermittent or partial; but such cases require no special notice.

Calculous Hydronephrosis.—Calculous hydronephrosis is due to the impaction of a stone in the ureter (Fig 147), or rarely

[1] Guyon's Annales, 1895, xiii, 865.

to a stricture secondary to a calculous ulceration. The development of the hydronephrosis is habitually marked by a series of renal colics, and hydronephrosis may be one of the features of calculous anuria. The symptoms and signs of hydronephrosis are detailed elsewhere.

Renal Suppuration.—Stone in the kidney is probably the most common cause of suppurating pyelo-nephritis. It also causes pyonephrosis (Fig. 148); while secondary phosphatic calculus or phosphatic deposit upon a pre-existing calculus results from the inflammation. Catarrhal inflammation is not encountered with calculus. The irritation caused by the stone is such that when inflammation occurs it promptly assumes a suppurative type.

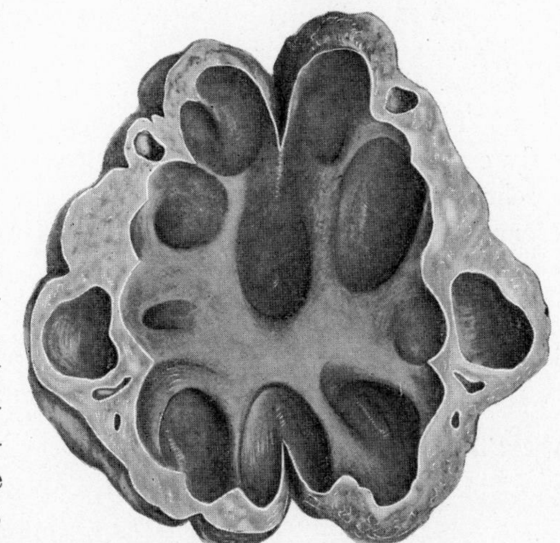

FIG. 148.—CALCULOUS PYONEPHROSIS.
This kidney contained the stone shown in Fig. 145.

The variations imprinted upon the classical picture of suppurative pyelo-nephritis by the presence of stone are few. There is the same urinary septicemia, the same absence of any great enlargement of the kidney. There may be colic, and there is usually a constant ache in the side. Hemorrhages occur from time to time. The inflammation is rarely acute or virulent, but progresses slowly, involving the whole organ and terminating finally in pyonephrosis or perinephritic abscess.

DIAGNOSIS

Not one of the symptoms of renal calculus is absolutely pathognomonic. In another chapter I have collected cases illustrative of anuria, hematuria, and renal colic caused by something other than a calculus. Even the passage of a stone may be misleading. Not long ago a patient came to me with a history of having passed several calculi, and complaining of pain in her right loin. The urine showed evidence of mild suppurative pyelo-nephritis; there was local tenderness but no tumour. I performed nephrotomy, and found nothing but a dense spherical scar 2 cm. in diameter in the kidney substance and some thickening of the pelvis: no obstruction, no pouching, no stone. She was drained for several weeks, sent to a mineral spring, kept on a long course of urotropin, and in six months the pus disappeared from her urine; she gained many pounds in weight and remains well now after three years. To be brief, there is no one subjective symptom of calculus that can be depended upon. The cessation of symptoms after a stone has been passed no more indicates the absence of another stone than their continuation indicates its presence. That a stone is present in the ureter or kidney cannot be absolutely affirmed unless it is seen or felt. Palpation, ureteral catheterism, skiagraphy, and exploratory nephrotomy constitute our diagnostic measures.

Palpation.—Palpation of the loin has been known to elicit a distinct grating of two or more renal calculi upon one another. In a few cases it has been possible to distinguish a large stone by palpation. These are most exceptional signs, and, as a rule, palpation is only employed to distinguish such renal enlargement or tenderness as characterizes hydronephrosis, or pyelo-nephritis, without any reference to the calculous nature of the disease. Abdominal palpation along the course of the ureter, and rectal (or vaginal) palpation of its lower extremity are useful to determine the presence of stone in these localities (p. 472).

Ureteral Catheterization. — Ureteral catheterization with wax-tipped bougies has been successfully employed by Howard Kelly for the diagnosis of pelvic or ureteral calculi. The stone leaves scratches upon the wax. This device will commend itself to those who frequently employ the ureteral catheter, but can never afford the satisfactory evidence obtainable from the X-rays.

Radiography.—Radiography will some day solve our diagnostic difficulties. It has not done so yet.[1] The possibility of X-ray burns has not been entirely eliminated, nor has sufficient experience accumulated to justify the belief that the skiagraph is an infallible index both of the presence and absence of a stone.[2] Yet experienced manipulators have already attained such perfection of technic that radiography stands first as a means of diagnosing ureteral and renal stones. The density of the shadow thrown by a stone seems to depend upon the amount of lime it contains. Hence oxalate and phosphate stones show well, while a pure uric-acid stone would be quite indistinguishable. Yet, clinically speaking, uric-acid calculi usu-

---

[1] J. of Cut. and G. U. Dis., 1901, xix, 341 and 368.

[2] Dr. C. L. Leonard (Annals of Surgery, 1900, xxxi, 163, and 1901, xxxiii, 435) has so perfected the technic that the examination of 136 cases, in 100 of which he made a negative diagnosis, has netted him only one known error. But there are numerous instances, especially in fat persons, in which most authorities are liable to err.

ally contain enough urate or phosphate of lime to produce a faint shadow (Williams[1]).

I have employed radiography 7 times. In 3 cases the result was unsatisfactory—one of these probably has a stone. In 2 it was negative and correct. In 2 it was positive and correct; but I am strongly inclined to believe that in one of these the stone was bilateral, though the plate showed only one stone.

Radiography is useful in all cases, even when the presence of stone can be determined without it, for it shows every detail of position with the greatest accuracy. A good radiograph is therefore invaluable to the surgeon, since it tells him just where to look for the stone and relieves him of any responsibility as to the presence in ureter or kidney of other calculi that might be difficult to locate in the course of an operation.

Nephrotomy.—Exploratory nephrotomy until recent years has been the only accurate method of diagnosis. There has been keen discussion as to the relative merits of needling, pyelotomy, and nephrotomy for the discovery of calculi. Stones have been overlooked, no matter what the method employed; and since exploratory nephrotomy bids fair to be superseded by the X-ray, it need only be noted that palpation of the exterior of the kidney and the process known as needling—i. e., the insertion of needles into the kidney substance—may disclose the stone, but are peculiarly fallacious. In order to make an adequate examination the kidney must be laid open, every portion of its pelvis carefully palpated, and a probe inserted down the ureter into the bladder. The renal incision may pass through the pelvis or through the cortex (p. 639). I have not found it necessary to bisect the kidney. An incision in the lower pole large enough to admit the finger suffices for adequate examination of the entire organ.

Suggestive Symptoms.—Many renal conditions secondary to calculus require nephrotomy for their relief without reference to the presence or absence of stone. Such cases (e. g., anuria, pyonephrosis, hydronephrosis, pyelo-nephritis, persistent pain or hematuria) may be suspected to be calculous from the nature of their pain and hemorrhage and from the absence of the positive signs of tubercle or of neoplasm. Yet before operating, I repeat, it is convenient to have radiographic evidence of the exact position of any stones that may be present, in order to spare the patient a tedious and uncertain digital exploration.

---

[1] The Roentgen Rays in Medicine and Surgery, 1901.

Treatment

The *prophylactic treatment* has been discussed elsewhere (p. 439).

Palliative and Symptomatic Treatment.—Many of the morbid conditions caused by renal stone require palliative treatment, either in the hope that the stone will pass or for the purpose of alleviating symptoms until operation may be performed. These conditions are reducible to three—viz., colic, anuria, and suppuration.

The Treatment of Renal Colic.—The first thing demanded by a renal colic is relief from pain. A gramme of antipyrin may suffice—if not morphin should be injected hypodermically with a generous hand. Muscular relaxation should be encouraged by means of hot baths and by the local application of heat to the loins. Beer and gin are useful adjuvants to produce free diuresis. If the pain is not relieved by morphin administered to the limit of endurance, it is customary to administer chloroform, keeping the patient anesthetized to the obstetrical degree for as long as an hour. In such an emergency it is proper to introduce a ureteral catheter for the purpose of pushing the stone back into the pelvis of the kidney, or, if all else fails, to perform nephrotomy at once; this will afford immediate relief.

As the pain passes, the patient and his attendants should be warned to watch for the stone. If the point of maximum tenderness remains in one place, it may be inferred that the stone is immobile; but if the pain and tenderness pass down the course of the ureter, and cease after causing an attack of frequent and painful urination, the assumption is that the stone has passed into the bladder. For a week or ten days thereafter the closest watch should be kept for the stone. It may be ejected by the bladder without a symptom or with a sharp urethral spasm. It is not likely to become impacted in the urethra unless there is a pin-hole meatus. If the stone does not soon appear the bladder should be searched with a large litholapaxy tube (p. 452).

Whether the stone passes or not, the surgeon should explain to his patient that other stones may be present, and should insist that a radiograph be taken by an expert in order to clear up this point. Unless this is done the patient is blindly exposed to all the complications of renal stone, and is deprived of his safest opportunity of avoiding them. With a satisfactory radiograph before him the surgeon is in a position to declare that there are or are not any more stones present. If so, and they are very small and lie in the ureter or free in the pelvis, an attempt may be made to wash them through by sharp diuresis. But if the stones are of such size or in such a position that the surgeon deems their spontaneous passage impossible, the patient should be so informed, and he should be enlightened upon the propriety and prospects of operation, to which he should be urged to submit.

The Treatment of Anuria.—Until within the last few years the treatment of calculous anuria has been expectant. It has been the custom, and still is the practice of many physicians, to stand by and watch the case, deluded by the absence of uremic symptoms and misguided by an occasional spontaneous recovery, until the sudden intense uremia closes the scene or summons the surgeon too late. Such a course of action cannot be too heartily condemned. Morris states that "so useless is medicinal and expectant treatment that I have refused to attend consultations in cases of calculous anuria unless I have permission beforehand to operate at once if I think the case suitable." Such should be the attitude of every surgeon. Though the patient, his family, or his physician may see fit to trifle with this swift and mortal condition the surgeon cannot afford to countenance any delay.

So much for what should not be done. The positive aspect of the situation is not so clear. It is true the majority of cases require nephrotomy; but there is a proportion of recoveries—one quarter of the recorded cases—that must be respected. In view of this, during the first forty-eight hours of the attack diuresis may be pushed to the utmost in the hope of dislodging the stone, and the opportunity of obtaining a radiograph should be seized; but if the anuria is not relieved on the third day, or if the patient is not seen until that time, no palliative measures may be considered; immediate operation must be insisted upon. The date of operation is recorded in 37 cases of Morris's list: 21 of these were operated upon on or before the fifth day, with 8 deaths, a mortality of 38%; 16 after the fifth day, with a mortality of 50%. Append the 75% mortality of the non-operative treatment of anuria and the inference is complete. No matter how well the patient may appear, the operation should not be postponed after the second day of anuria; in some cases it may be wiser to resort even sooner to the knife.

The Treatment of Calculous Pyelo-nephritis.—Renal suppuration due to stone may be only one degree less benign in appearance and less malignant in reality than anuria. Suppuration caused by calculus cannot be overcome by any medical or hygienic treatment. Unless the stone can be passed off spontaneously—an outcome to the last degree improbable in suppurating cases—its growth is fostered by secondary phosphatic deposit, while the irritation it provokes in turn feeds the renal suppuration. Palliative treatment is futile except as a preparation for the knife.

Pyonephrosis and perinephritic abscess, whether calculous or not, require radical surgery.

Radical Treatment.—The radical treatment of renal and ureteral calculus consists of three operative procedures: nephrolithotomy, nephrotomy, and nephrectomy. Nephrolithotomy (pyelolithotomy or ureterolithotomy) is incision of the kidney (pelvis or ureter) for the purpose of extracting a stone. The term has been restricted by Morris to operations performed upon the aseptic kidney, to distinguish them from nephrotomy performed upon the suppurating kidney. This distinction is valuable from a surgical point of view. The term nephrolithotomy, therefore, will be employed to designate extraction of a stone from a non-suppurating kidney, while nephrotomy, in this connection, will imply lithotomy of a suppurating organ.

Indication for Operation.—The general indication for operation upon a calculous kidney is the presence of a stone too large to pass down the ureter. Leonard[1] has suggested that by means of the X-rays it is possible to estimate with great accuracy the size of small calculi. He mentions the recognition of 3 ureteral calculi weighing a grain or less, all of which were passed spontaneously. In such cases the surgeon may adopt expectant treatment and endeavour to expel the calculus by free diuresis. But if the calculus is too large to pass of itself it must be removed by the surgeon. Such then is the indication for operation—a stone that will not pass. In the preceding paragraphs the modifying circumstances have been discussed—the delusive nature of the calm succeeding a renal colic, the imperative necessity for operation during anuria, the futility of delay whether the kidney is suppurating or not.

Yet there is another point of view, one most frequently assumed by the patient—viz., What are the risks and inconveniences of operation? For to the patient the immediate horror of the knife is a far more potent incentive than the "ifs" and "ands" with which a conscientious surgeon must mitigate the non-operative prognosis. For calculous disease, though swift and fatal in anuria, torturing in colic, and slowly, grimly progressive in suppuration, also presents possible vistas of years of comparative health and comfort, a delusive prospect with which the timorous sufferer would fain brace his refusal of the knife. But the surgeon can offer a prognosis whose brilliancy eclipses anything the patient may expect from Nature's

---

[1] J. Am. Med. Ass'n, 1901, xxxvii, 1451.

unaided efforts. The general mortality from nephrolithotomy and ureterolithotomy does not run above 3% or 4%. That is to say, it is lower than the mortality of Bottini's operation, and almost equals that of litholapaxy. In fact, an experienced surgeon may assure the average patient that this operation is perfectly safe. Its discomforts are minimal. The distress so frequent after vesical, pelvic, and intestinal operations need not be anticipated, and the discomfort of lying in bed for about two weeks is almost the sum of the convalescence. Such a prospect with its assurance of future safety, its lack of present danger, and its unimportant discomforts, outweighs a single renal colic, and is not for a moment to be compared with the progressive unsafety and discomfort to which the patient subjects himself by refusing operation.

The advantage of early operation, before the kidney becomes infected, is still further enforced by the relative mortality of nephrolithotomy, nephrotomy, and nephrectomy. Nephrolithotomy—the removal of a stone from an uninflamed kidney or ureter—has, as remarked above, a mortality of 3% to 4%. Nephrotomy—the incision of a septic kidney—has a mortality of 20% to 25%, while the mortality of nephrectomy in like conditions runs from 30% upward. Add to this the mortality of nephrotomy for calculous anuria, 50%, and the conclusion is obvious that the patient who refuses surgical relief while the kidney is yet uninflamed spurns a comparatively safe and sure cure and subjects himself to a disease which, apart from its other dangers and discomforts, may at any moment bring him to a critical condition of renal obstruction or suppuration, from which he can only escape by submitting to an operation many times more dangerous and distressing than the one he seeks to avoid.

Nephrolithotomy.—No operation is more exact and straightforward than nephrolithotomy if a good skiagraph of the kidneys and ureters has been obtained. No operation is more indefinite in its possibilities nor more dependent for success upon the surgeon's experience and skill than is nephrolithotomy without a skiagraph. Therefore any amount of time and trouble may be deemed well spent if only it ends in the acquisition of an exact skiagraph. With this at hand the surgeon has but to cut boldly down upon the kidney and to extract the stone by pyelotomy or nephrotomy, as is most convenient. Without the skiagraph nephrolithotomy is a purely exploratory operation. Even if the surgeon feels sure that there is stone, he cannot ascertain to a certainty whether it is single or multiple, whether renal, pelvic, or ureteral; or, perchance, all three. The methods employed in this tedious and comparatively uncertain search have already been alluded to.

Ureterolithotomy.—A calculus may lodge at either end of the ureter or at the point where it crosses the brim of the pelvis. Several calculi may be found in different portions of the ureter. The seat of impaction is stated in 56 cases collected by Morris. Seven times the calculus lay in the renal pelvis blocking the upper end of the ureter (4 bilateral). Thirty times the stone occupied the upper extremity of the ureter (5 bilateral, 3 multiple). Seven times the stone lay at or near the brim of the pelvis (1 bilateral, 2 multiple). Ten times the stone lay within the bladder wall or just outside of it (3 bilateral, 1 multiple). Twice both ureters were obstructed by the pressure of a large vesical calculus.

The X-rays may be depended upon to locate a stone in any of these positions. Without their aid the surgeon needs all the information afforded by history and physical examination in order to decide upon what operation he should undertake, for different procedures are required to meet different conditions.

Calculus at the upper extremity of the ureter should be reached by the usual lumbar incision, and extracted by ureterotomy or pyelotomy.

Calculus at the brim of the pelvis may be attacked extraperitoneally through the lumbo-vaginal incision, or intraperitoneally through an incision in the linea semilunaris. In some measure the choice of route depends upon the surgeon's prejudices, though the extraperitoneal incision is usually preferred if there is infection.

Calculus at or near the vesical orifice of the ureter may be reached in a variety of ways. If the stone is within the bladder wall, bulging the mucous membrane or projecting into the vesical cavity, it may be extracted by a transvesical route. Dilatation of the urethra in the female, suprapubic cystotomy (Morris prefers perineal section) in the male, permits the removal of the stone by divulsion or incision of the ureteral orifice, perhaps aided by the lithotrite or scoop. I have performed this operation once successfully.

When the stone lies outside of the bladder, low down in the pelvis, it is singularly inaccessible. Sometimes it may be reached by an incision in the vault of the vagina—risking a uretero-vaginal fistula. Such a stone has been reached through a transverse perineal incision (Hurry Fenwick). The rectal route presents obvious objections. Morris has successfully operated by the sacral route. But usually the line of attack has been intraperitoneal or inguinal. These last two routes are probably preferable.

Technic.—Four technical points must be remembered in every ureterolithotomy:

1. The incision in the ureter should be longitudinal—i. e., parallel with its long axis.

2. Before making the incision the stone should be pushed up from the pouch in which it lies, in order that the incision made upon it may pass through a portion of the ureteral wall unaffected by pressure or ulceration.

3. Before closing the incision a long probe should be passed upward and downward in search of other stones, and the ureter should be minutely examined for stricture at the point where the stone has rested. If found the stricture is to be treated *secundum artem* (p. 486).

4. The ureteral incision may be closed by fine silk sutures not piercing the mucous membrane, or by catgut sutures through and through. Drainage is always appropriate to avoid a possible infiltration of urine.

Nephrotomy, Pyelotomy.—These operations are performed with the double purpose of removing the stone and of providing adequate drainage for pus. The incision in the kidney should preferably pass through renal tissue, but the main object to be kept in view is speed —without haste—in order to spare the patient the shock of a prolonged operation. The ureteral exploration must not be forgotten. The operative details are described elsewhere (p. 637).

Nephrectomy, Nephro-ureterectomy.—The indications for nephrectomy are those rehearsed in the preceding chapter (p. 577). When sacculated and full of calculi the ureter should be removed with the kidney.

CHAPTER XLI

TUBERCULOSIS OF THE KIDNEY

Etiology

Tubercular inflammation of the kidney occurs with tuberculosis of the genital tract or of the lungs. It also occurs as a primary lesion. The theory that the primary tubercular deposit may occur in the kidney was first developed by Vigneron.[1] It has been confirmed by but few autopsies. Whatever the original seat of the disease, death does not often occur until the tubercular inflammation has spread to several organs. But the strongest support of the theory of primary renal tuberculosis lies in the results of nephrectomy. The remarkably large percentage of cases that remain free from evidences of the disease for a number of years after this operation is sufficient evidence that in these cases, at least, the primary inflammation is in the kidney (p. 610).

Renal tuberculosis is a disease of youth. Its more acute forms occur during adolescence, while its chronic caseating forms are usually encountered between the ages of twenty and forty. Thus Israel [2] states that 80% of his operations were performed upon persons between these ages. Exceptionally the tubercular kidney is encountered in later life.

French and German authors are agreed that women suffer from renal tuberculosis twice as often as do men, though the smaller statistics of English and American authors (Morris,[3] Tilden Brown,[4] Watson [5]) show a preponderance in the opposite direction.

Pathogenesis.—The tubercle bacillus may reach the kidney by direct extension of a tubercular process from an adjoining organ, or by invasion from the lymphatics, or from the blood current.

---

[1] Thèse de Paris, 1892.

[2] Chir. Klin. d. Nierenkrankh., Berlin, 1901, p. 180.

[3] *Op. cit.*, p. 484.

[4] N. Y. Med. J., 1897, lxv, 377, 447, 479.

[5] Boston Med. and Surg. J., 1895, xxxii, 121, 135.

The extension of a tubercular inflammation to the kidney through its capsule is most exceptional. Tilden Brown justly remarks that tuberculosis of the suprarenal capsule does not involve the kidney, and I have known a kidney to remain normal, although it lay for several months surrounded by a tubercular perinephritic abscess.

The constant association post mortem of vesical, ureteral, and renal tuberculosis long misled pathologists to believe that the kidney is always attacked by a tuberculosis mounting the ureter from a primary lesion in the bladder. Hence extension of the disease along this route is still generally regarded as an established fact, although we are learning to recognise that this method of invasion is by no means so frequent as has been believed. Yet the documentary evidence in favour of this view is singularly slight. It is known that the disease travels down the ureter from the kidney, and that extirpation of the kidney is often succeeded by a cure of the ureteral and vesical inflammation; but, so far as I know, there is no recorded case of a vesical tuberculosis extending up the ureter without reaching the kidney. The discovery of tubercular lesions in the kidney, ureter, and bladder may be explained in several ways. The infection may work its way up along the ureteral mucous membrane; it may proceed by a lymphatic infection along the ureteral wall; or it may reach the kidney from the circulation, and thence pass down the ureter to the bladder. This last explanation seems the most plausible, and, according to it, every renal tuberculosis, whether primary or secondary, is hematogenous in origin. Such a theory has at least the merit of explaining the occurrence of tuberculosis in the kidney and genitalia—a not uncommon phenomenon—without any lesion whatever of the bladder.

Infection from the blood stream is the usual source of primary renal tuberculosis. Why the kidney should be able sometimes to transmit tubercle bacilli and at other times fall victim to them, why so many cases show involvement of one kidney years before that of its fellow—in other words, what the predisposing causes of renal tuberculosis may be, the future must decide. Our ideas upon this subject are not yet sufficiently clear to merit debate here.

Morbid Anatomy

Primary Tuberculosis.—There are four varieties of primary renal tuberculosis—viz.:

1. Acute miliary tuberculosis.
2. Subacute diffuse tuberculosis.
3. Chronic papillary ulceration.
4. Chronic caseous tuberculosis.

1. Acute miliary tuberculosis of the kidney is a phase of acute general miliary tuberculosis interesting only to the pathologist.

2. Subacute diffuse renal tuberculosis holds a middle place in point of virulence between acute miliary tuberculosis and chronic caseation. It usually attacks both kidneys simultaneously and is habitually associated with tubercular lesions in other parts of the body. The kidneys are riddled with tubercles, which are found chiefly in the cortex, in the glomeruli, and along the vessels. As they break down they form caseous and purulent foci radiating from the pelvis, itself inflamed, simulating the purulent collections seen post mortem in the acuter forms of surgical kidney—a condition for which this variety of tuberculosis is often mistaken.

The course of the disease under this form is rapid and fatal. It occurs in children, and only interests the surgeon from the fact that it is likely to be mistaken for chronic renal tuberculosis. If so diagnosed and operated upon the surgical intervention only hastens the fatal issue.

3. Tuberculous ulceration of a papilla is a very rare form of primary tuberculosis. A tubercular deposit occurs in the tip of one or more of the papillæ, ulcerates, and gives rise to considerable hemorrhage with but few other symptoms. Such an ulcer appears to have little tendency towards dissemination. Hurry Fenwick and Israel have operated successfully upon such cases.

4. Caseous renal tuberculosis is the *surgical* tuberculosis of the kidney. The tubercular process usually begins in one or other extremity of a single kidney. The usual stages of tuberculization, ulceration, and caseation occur, so that, as seen by the surgeon, the disease presents itself under the form of multiple tubercular nodules and caseous areas. The kidney may be affected in whole or in part. Section reveals a number of tubercular nodules in various stages of development, some solid, others caseous. As the inflammation progresses new tubercular deposits appear, and the old nodules break down and coalesce. Secondary pyogenic infection occurs, and finally the kidney becomes more or less of a shell surrounding one or more large caseous foci (Fig. 149). The pelvis and ureter become thickened and studded with tubercles. In extreme cases the ureter may be obliterated and the dilated pelvis filled with the solid caseous mass.

Secondary Tuberculosis.— Secondary or ascending renal tuberculosis may be either miliary or caseous. Exceptionally a hydronephrotic kidney becomes tubercular, so that, while it retains the macroscopic appearance of an aseptic hydronephrosis, microscopic examination reveals tubercular lesions in it and tubercle bacilli in its fluid contents.

Secondary Pyogenic Changes.—The tubercular kidney, like the tubercular lung, is liable to secondary infection by pyogenic micro-organisms. Such a double infection adds to the virulence of the case. Mixed infection in subacute, diffuse tuberculosis hastens

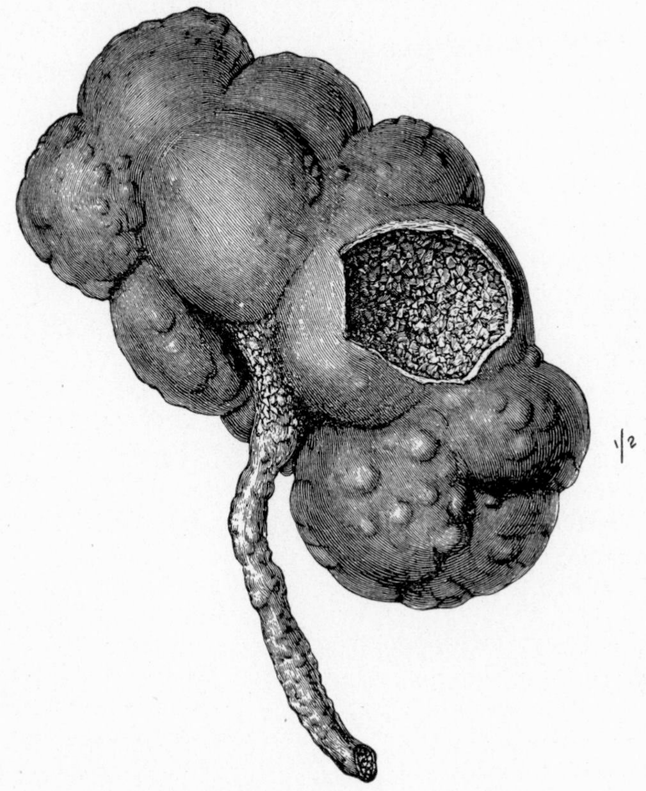

FIG. 149.—TUBERCULAR KIDNEY (Morris).

the fatal issue; mixed infection in caseous tuberculosis causes tubercular pyelonephritis. The sacculated kidney suppurates throughout, and the tubercular and pyogenic inflammations spread rapidly to the bladder and soon affect the opposite kidney. In fact, nothing stimulates the progress of a chronic caseating tuberculosis so much as secondary infection by pyogenic microbes.

Accessory Lesions.—Fatty and fibrous *perinephritis* results from chronic renal tuberculosis as well as from chronic suppuration (p. 540). Perinephritic phlegmon and abscess are rare, and are usually due to mixed infection. *The ureter* is involved by the extension of the tubercular inflammation downward (or upward); its walls are much thickened and ulcerated, its lumen is pouched and usually constricted, sometimes entirely obstructed. As the tubercular inflammation extends downward it reaches the *bladder* and extends to *that portion of the vesical wall surrounding the orifice of the ureter.* Even before the tubercular process has reached thus far some congestion or simple inflammation of this region often occurs as the result of mixed infection in the kidney. The presence of this congestion or tubercular inflammation in the bladder around the orifice of the ureter is of great importance. If tuberculosis of the kidney is suspected and cystoscopy reveals congestion, tuberculization, or ulceration about the orifice of one ureter, it may be concluded that the kidney to which that ureter leads is certainly tubercular, although it is by no means fair to infer that the opposite kidney is free from involvement. Israel estimates the frequency of this descending bladder tuberculosis at 59%.

The Opposite Kidney.—From a prognostic point of view the condition of the opposite kidney is of the greatest importance. Statistics derived from the dead-house are of no value here, for what the surgeon must know is not whether the second kidney was involved at the time of the patient's death, but whether the second kidney is involved at the time the patient presents himself for treatment. Vigneron [1] collected the records of 205 cases subjected to operation, of which only 106 were known to have bilateral renal tuberculosis. Israel records 21 cases of primary renal tuberculosis operated upon, of which only 2 (9.5%) were bilateral. The statistics of all other surgeons agree on this capital point: that *in chronic renal tuberculosis the two organs are not inflamed simultaneously; the second kidney becomes diseased many months after the first;* and, in about one half the cases, the disease is unilateral at the time the patient presents himself for treatment.

It is not to be forgotten, however, that amyloid degeneration and chronic inflammation may attack the opposite kidney even though it be not tubercular. This fact has a particular bearing upon the postoperative prognosis of nephrectomy for renal tuberculosis. Thus 3 of Israel's 9 deaths are attributed to this condition.

Symptoms

Tubercle of the kidney, like stone in the kidney, may run its whole course and lead to the patient's death without ever giving any recognisable symptom referable to the urinary organs. Yet this is rare. Usually there are symptoms, but these symptoms are most misleading. The ordinary evidences of renal surgical disease, such

[1] *Op. cit.*

as pain and tumour in the loin, are inconspicuous in all but the most advanced stages of the disease. The characteristic early symptoms are painful and frequent urination and hematuria, a symptom-complex which directs attention to the bladder, where the discovery of a tuberculous ulceration may well lead the surgeon to overlook the primary focus of the disease in the kidney.

Painful and Frequent Urination.—The first symptom of tuberculosis of the kidney usually is a frequency of urination. This is the case whether there is any tuberculosis of the bladder or not. This frequency is spontaneous, and may be quite inexplicable if the urine contains no pus or blood. There is usually some polyuria even in the early stages. After a time urination becomes painful. The pain occurs during the urinary act, or at its termination if there is ulceration about the bladder neck. Needless to relate, pain and frequency are uninfluenced by any local treatment of the bladder. They continue, varying in intensity, and even disappear at times. As a rule they are not extreme unless the bladder is tubercular.

Hematuria.—Sometimes the first evidence of renal tuberculosis is hematuria. The bleeding is not particularly characteristic. It has not the severity of a hemorrhage from a neoplasm, nor is it so continuous or so constantly associated with pain as that from stone. The primary bleeding is likely to last for a short time, to be followed by a protracted period during which there is little or no blood in the urine. Although most authorities incline to the belief that hematuria is a fairly constant sign of tuberculosis of the kidney, Israel only noted it 4 times among 18 primary cases, and I believe that its frequency is generally overestimated. In the later stages of the disease, if there is mixed infection the purulent urine is very likely to show some traces of blood. Violent hemorrhage rarely occurs, though the bleeding from an ulcerated papilla may be so severe as to endanger life.

Renal Pain and Tumour.—There is usually a dull soreness in the loin, but little active pain. Renal colic from the passage of clots of blood or shreds of caseous matter is exceptional. The kidney enlarges sufficiently to form a notable tumour only when such a complication as pyelonephritis or perinephritis occurs. The tuberculous ureter may sometimes be felt by rectal or vaginal palpation or through a thin abdominal wall. A tubercular thickening in the ureter has been mistaken for stone.

Urinary Signs.—The urine usually is of low specific gravity and from the beginning somewhat increased in quantity, and this polyuria accounts in some degree for the frequency of urination. Hematuria may occur, and pyuria appears with the occurrence of ulceration and mixed infection, whether in the kidney, in the bladder, or in both. The purulent urine of the later stages of renal tuberculosis is acid, always acid; it is albuminous, perhaps tinged with blood, and contains casts of various qualities.

General Characteristics.—The patient presents the usual tubercular characteristics: a history of tuberculosis in other members of the family and evidence of the disease elsewhere in his body, either in the lungs, the epididymis, the bladder, or the cervical lymphatics. He is usually under forty, and is pale, thin, and lymphatic in appearance. Israel states that there was the usual tubercular evening rise of temperature in only 22% of his cases of uncomplicated renal tuberculosis, while 80% of those patients whose bladders were involved had fever. The loss of weight so characteristic of tubercular disease is usually noted, and it has been my experience that the pulse is habitually rapid.

Diagnosis

It is the commonly accepted belief that diagnosis of tubercular kidney is extremely difficult. In many senses this is true. It is difficult even for an expert to diagnose a tubercular kidney in its earliest stages; it may be impossible for him to distinguish between chronic caseous renal tuberculosis and subacute diffuse tuberculosis. It is often quite impossible for the practitioner who is unaccustomed to use the cystoscope and the ureteral catheter to diagnose the disease in any but its most advanced stages, and it requires the greatest diagnostic acumen to decide in many cases whether or not the disease is of such a nature as to merit treatment by hygienic and climatic agencies or by the knife.

In order to simplify the matter as much as possible we may first enumerate the forms of the disease that can be readily distinguished. In its advanced stages the disease can almost always be recognised either by examination of the urine or by palpation of the loin.

The gross urinary aspects often suggest the existence of an inflammation of the kidney or of the bladder. The urine may be purulent; it may contain blood, albumin, and casts. It is habitually acid. If the bladder is involved the signs of bladder tuberculosis may be detected (p. 401), and *if the bladder is found to be tubercular it is the rule always to suspect a similar condition in the kidneys.* If, however, the bladder is not inflamed, the only urinary sign to distinguish a tubercular pyelo-nephritis from a suppurating one may be the presence in the urine of the tubercle bacillus. Unhappily, in a large proportion of cases, it is quite impossible to discover this bacterium in the urine (p. 403). Thus it was identified microscopically in only 15 of the 67 cases reported by Küster, König, and Czerny. It is in such cases that injection of the suspected urine into guinea-pigs affords a positive and conclusive physiological test. Morris relates a convincing case in which tubercle bacilli could not be distinguished by a most careful examination until, after the success of guinea-pig inoculation, a second microscopical investigation disclosed the incriminated microbe. The tubercle bacillus should be thus sought by microscopic and physiological tests in every case of pyelo-nephritis of obscure origin.

The presence of a tumour or a markedly tender point in the loin may be the first thing to draw attention to the kidney. Here again obscure cases merit a searching investigation for Koch's microbe.

In other cases an unexplained dysuria is the most marked symptom. The urine may be clear and disclose no evidences of the renal condition beyond an insignificant polyuria, with perhaps a slight albuminuria. The tubercle bacillus may not be discovered in the urine and the cystoscope may not reveal the pathognomonic inflammation about the ureteral orifice. Such cases represent the earlier stages of the disease in which it may be impossible to make an absolute diagnosis. The patient's history and physical type, the presence of lesions elsewhere in the body, an unexplained loss of flesh, an afternoon temperature—all these are suggestive elements to the experienced diagnostician. But any or all of them may be lacking, so that the diagnosis cannot be made until the disease has reached a more advanced stage. And even if the presence of tuberculosis in the kidney is suspected, one cannot feel sure of it unless (1) tubercle bacilli are disclosed by the microscope or the guinea-pig, or (2) unless the cystoscope shows a tubercular process about the mouth of the ureter.[1]

Having diagnosed the presence of renal tuberculosis, the next point is to discover the condition of the two kidneys. Is the disease bilateral, or, if it be unilateral, is the opposite kidney present and functionating properly? This is the finest point of diagnosis, it has no interest for those who are committed to a purely medical treatment of the disease. But if there is question of nephrectomy it is absolutely essential to know which kidney is tubercular and what is the condition of its fellow. These points can be determined only by examining the urine obtained separately from each kidney; which is to say that the urine segregator or the ureteral catheter

---

[1] I formerly employed tuberculin injections for the diagnosis of these cases, but gave them up because I found them to contain an element of danger as well as an element of uncertainty.

must be employed.[1] Of the two, I rather prefer the ureteral catheter for most cases. This is especially true if there is any tubercular lesion of the bladder, for in such cases contact of the segregator with the ulcerated bladder wall is likely to provoke a hemorrhage sufficiently profuse to nullify the result of the examination. It is scarcely necessary to say that the insertion of a ureteral catheter into a ureter whose mouth is tuberculous is quite uncalled for. The duct undoubtedly leads to a tubercular kidney. It is the opposite and apparently healthy kidney that requires catheterization.

The examination of the urine obtained by the ureteral catheter should be both bacteriological and chemical. The pathologist should seek for tubercle bacilli, for the evidences of surgical inflammation, and for evidence of the renal function. The surgeon is not justified in assuming that this kidney is in a satisfactory condition unless the urine obtained from it shows (1) no tubercle bacilli, (2) no pus, (3) no more than a trace of albumin and a few casts, and no marked decrease in the excreted solids. It is worthy of note that a very considerable proportion of those persons who die at a greater or less length of time after a successful nephrectomy for tuberculosis lose their lives on account of amyloid degeneration or chronic nephritis of the opposite kidney. Another point that must be determined is the presence of tuberculosis elsewhere in the body. I need only enumerate the lungs, the testicles, the vesicles, and the prostate as probable seats of tubercular deposit.

The nature of the lesion in the kidney can be determined only by a just appreciation of all these data. The surgeon is not justified in assuming that he has to deal with chronic caseous tuberculosis (the only form of the disease for which a radical surgical cure can be expected) unless he knows that the tubercular lesion is confined to one kidney; and he cannot justly expect to achieve such a radical cure unless he knows that the disease exists only in a mild or latent condition elsewhere in the body. Thus tuberculosis of the ureter and of the adjoining portion of the bladder is no contra-indication to nephrectomy, nor is a slight lesion of the lung. But the presence of active pulmonary or genital tuberculosis will usually nullify the effect of the most successful nephrectomy.

Prognosis

The prognosis of tuberculosis of the kidney depends upon the nature of the lesion, the age of the patient, and the presence of le-

[1] If the case is known to be tubercular, the cystoscope or the segregator should never be employed academically for the mere purpose of distinguishing the extent of the bladder disease, but only as a preliminary to nephrectomy.

sions elsewhere in the body. The prognosis of the acute and subacute forms of renal tuberculosis is extremely bad. Usually the patient rapidly loses ground, the disease spreads from one organ to another, and runs its course within a year or two. On the other hand, the caseous form of tuberculosis, if not complicated by a secondary mixed infection and if associated with few lesions elsewhere in the body, is very slow to progress and may last for many years. Apparently the course of the papillary tubercular ulcer is equally chronic. The age of the patient has an indirect bearing upon the prognosis, for tuberculosis of the kidneys, like that of other organs, assumes its more malignant forms in the young and advances more slowly in later years. Finally, the distribution of the disease among the other organs of the body has a marked influence. For, even though the renal lesion be caseating and chronic, the patient may die of some more acute process in the lung or in some other portion of the genito-urinary tract. Tuberculosis of the kidney may progress to a spontaneous cure. Such an event is most unusual, and yet it may occur. Moreover, appropriate hygienic treatment will in many cases delay the fatal issue for years, and sometimes effect a cure.

Treatment

We are now on the crest of a wave of operative success in the treatment of renal tuberculosis. We look backward into the depths of the pre-operative period and appreciate—fairly, I think—that a great advance has been made; but looking forward there is another depth which can only be dimly outlined. A cursory review of current therapeutic reports would lead one to suppose that the treatment of renal tuberculosis is purely surgical. A few isolated voices are raised in protest; but it is impossible to deny the great success of modern surgery in eradicating tuberculosis of the kidney, and in our first flush of appreciation of this success it is quite impossible sanely to appreciate how much evil there may be intermingled with the good. Perusal of the works of Tuffier, Israel, Simon, Küster, and Morris is calculated to enforce the conviction that surgery is the ideal treatment—the only treatment deserving of the name. Yet I believe that the future will modify this view. I believe we shall learn that the operative successes are not so permanent as the figures now before us would seem to indicate, and that, lasting as they may be, in the majority of cases hygienic and tonic treatment will prove more effective still. In short, tuberculosis of the kidney, like tuberculosis of any other organ, is not a local disease. I doubt if the surgeon is ever able to diagnosticate tuberculosis of the kidney at a time when there are no other tubercular lesions in the body. Certainly he can never feel sure, so long as the patient lives, that the tubercular kidney is not complicated by some other lesion. The gravity of this doubt is impressed upon us by the unexpected failure of some of the most promising cases. For tuberculosis of the urinary tract is a no less treacherous disease than that of the respiratory tract. In some cases it is chronic and advances but slowly, in others it is frightfully malignant; and we have as yet no absolute criterion by which to distinguish the two classes.

Such being the case, the operative treatment of tuberculosis of the kidney must be recognised as palliative only—that is to say, the surgeon may chance to control the disease by extirpating the kidney, but the probabilities are against him; and, inasmuch as he cannot feel sure that the procedure is radical, I think it only just to class the operation as a palliative measure to be employed when hygienic treatment fails, and when employed to be followed by a further course of hygienic treatment in order to complete the cure. Nephrectomy for tuberculosis should hold the same place in reference to hygienic treatment as urethrotomy for stricture does to the employment of sounds. I have nowhere seen a set of cases more beautifully illustrating this relative uncertainty of operative treatment than that recently published by Dr. Tilden Brown,[1] of this city.

Operative Treatment.—In spite of the fact discussed in the preceding paragraphs that, strictly speaking, all operative treatment for renal tuberculosis is palliative, it is convenient to distinguish between those operations employed for the avowed purpose of eradicating the disease and those employed to relieve symptoms or to prolong the patient's life. The so-called radical operations are nephrectomy, nephro-ureterectomy, and partial nephrectomy. The operative technic of these various procedures is described in a subsequent chapter. The indication for nephrectomy is the existence of advanced localized chronic tuberculosis of one kidney. When the kidney is known to be seriously damaged by the disease and the opposite kidney known to be sound, and no active tuberculosis can be discovered in the genital tract or in the lungs, it is proper to extirpate the tubercular portion of the kidney or the whole kidney and the ureter as well, if necessary, in the hope of relieving the patient of his main foci of disease. The presence of tubercular cystitis about the mouth of the ureter, or of a chronic circumscribed tuberculosis in the lung, is no contra-indication to nephrectomy. The statistics published by various surgeons show that patients do about as well after operation whether the bladder is involved or not. In-

[1] Boston Med. and Surg. J., 1901, cxliv, 513.

deed, Israel's detailed descriptions in most cases show a spontaneous cure of the vesical lesion within a year after nephrectomy.

For the same reason there is no absolute need for total ureterectomy unless the duct is very seriously diseased. A moderately inflamed ureter will atrophy spontaneously after nephrectomy in 9 cases out of 10. For the same reason again, it is proper to perform partial nephrectomy upon cases showing macroscopical lesions of only one end of the kidney. It is true, as some authorities contend, that the opposite pole of the kidney probably contains some tubercles; but just as the ureter and bladder will heal spontaneously after the main focus of disease has been removed, so, I believe, may the lesser renal lesions be expected to disappear after extirpation of the disorganized tissue.

To pursue the argument still further—further, indeed, than most surgeons are willing to pursue it—I cannot indorse nephrectomy for tuberculosis in its earliest stages. I believe that the beginning of the disease in the kidney may be checked and cured as promptly and effectively by hygienic treatment as can its beginnings in the lung, and I therefore *restrict nephrectomy to those cases which do not respond to hygienic measures.* The knife is called for if the patient progressively loses weight or if in spite of palliative measures the kidney fills with pus.

Nephrotomy is the recognised palliative surgical treatment for tubercular kidney, and it is a very unsatisfactory measure. Nephrectomy has a fair chance of controlling the disease, but nephrotomy seems only to hasten the patient's downward course. Yet in some cases when both kidneys are so involved that nephrectomy cannot be undertaken, and one of them is suppurating freely, nephrotomy must be performed to open the abscess and afford a temporary relief, however unpromising may be the ultimate outlook. Curiously enough, it would seem that in some of these cases nephrectomy gives better results than nephrotomy, even though the opposite kidney is somewhat diseased. Secondary nephrectomy, after an unsuccessful nephrotomy, does not show so great a proportion of cures as primary nephrectomy. Yet, in the presence of pyonephrosis or perinephritis it is sometimes wiser first to incise, and then to remove the kidney when the patient is somewhat relieved of his septicemia. Yet even in these cases nephrectomy (if done at all) should be done within a few weeks of the nephrotomy, for after nephrotomy the tubercular kidney is peculiarly prone to form dense adhesions with the surrounding tissue.

Statistics.—I append the operative statistics of those surgeons who have had the widest experience in this field. I allow the figures to speak for themselves.

	Primary Nephrectomy.							Secondary Nephrectomy.						Partial Nephrectomy.			Nephrotomy.							
	Cases.	Operative mortality.	Unrelieved; died.	Died later of the disease.	Fistulous or improved.	Recent.	Cured.	Cases.	Operative mortality.	Unrelieved; died.	Died later of the disease.	Recent.	Cured.	Cases.	Secondary nephrectomy.	Cured.	Cases.	Operative mortality.	Unrelieved; died.	Died later of the disease.	Fistulous.	Secondary nephrectomy.	Recent.	Cured.
Israel[1]......	27	3	3	2	2	..	17	1	..	..	..	..	1	1	1	..	2	1	..	..	..	..	1	..
Morris[2].....	17	3	2	1	1	..	10	5	1	..	1	..	3	7	3	4	8	2	1	..	..	2	..	3[7]
Tuffier[3].....	6	..	..	..	..	..	6	2	..	..	..	..	2	..	..	..	21	..	1	3	..	15	1	1
Czerny[4].....	11	2	..	1	..	1	7[8]	16	1	1	4	1	9[8]	1	..	1	7	2	..	..	3	..	..	2
Albarran[5]...	19	1	..	..	1	..	17	..	..	..	..	..	..	..	..	..	12	1	..	9	..	..	1	1
König[6]......	18	3	3	3	1	1	7	..	..	..	..	..	..	..	..	..	..	..	..	..	..	..	..	..
	98	12	8	7	5	2	64	24	2	1	5	1	15	9	4	5	50[7]	6	2	12	3	17	3	7

[1] *Op. cit.*, p. 218.

[2] *Op. cit.*, p. 510. Renal Surgery, London, 1898.

[3] Tuberculose rénale, Paris, 1898.

[4] Brüns. Beiträge, 1901, xxx, 1.

[5] Traité de chir., par Le Dentu and Delbet, 1899, viii, 865. Trans. Fr. Cong. of Surgery, 1897.

[6] Deutsch. med. Wochenschr., 1900, xxvi, 109.

[7] One bilateral.

[8] Including those that died of intercurrent disease after an interval of a few years.

Thus 159 patients were operated upon; 61.63% of them were deemed fit subjects for primary nephrectomy: of these, 12% died as a result of the operation; 8% were unrelieved and died soon after (total immediate mortality, 20%); 7% died later of the disease, and 64% were apparently cured.

Nephrotomy was performed upon 38.81%. The total immediate mortality was 16%; 24% died later of the disease, 34% underwent secondary nephrectomy, and only 12% were apparently cured.

Only 5.66% were deemed fit subjects for partial nephrectomy, and 44% of these relapsed and underwent secondary nephrectomy, while 55% were cured.

Secondary nephrectomy was necessary in 15.09% and netted an operative mortality of 8%, a total immediate mortality of 12% (considerably less than that of primary nephrectomy), a secondary mortality of 20% (considerably greater), while 62% were cured (about the same).

Cures from nephrectomy are known to persist twenty-one years, twelve years, eleven years (3 cases), ten years; in 13 cases from five to ten years; in 13 cases (2 partial nephrectomies) from three to five years, and in 15 cases (1 partial nephrectomy) one or two years.

Nephrotomy cures are known to persist two, four, and five years.

In short, of 159 cases 31 (19%) died shortly after the operation; 24 (15%) were temporarily relieved, but died later of the disease, and 90 (56.6%) are believed to be cured; though in only 34 of these (20%) is the cure known to have persisted for three years or more.

After-treatment.—The after-treatment of operative cases is the same as the preliminary treatment. It consists in antitubercular hygienic measures. The special complications of the various operations do not concern us in this place.

Medical Treatment.—A critical survey of the original surgical reports quoted above leaves the impression of uncertainty fixed in the reader's mind. While many of the operative successes are brilliant to the last degree, and while the knife saves some cases that have sunk to a depth where recovery seems impossible, yet the element of uncertainty prevails and the most promising case may go entirely wrong. Therefore it is that while the disease is purely tubercular and uncomplicated by any mixed infection, pyonephrosis or perinephritis, hygiene and medical treatment are more likely to succeed than the knife with its associated shock and a more or less prolonged after-treatment in unhygienic surroundings.

I find no satisfactory statistics showing the results of medical treatment upon renal tuberculosis; indeed, from the very facts of the case, the surgeon who makes the diagnosis must send the patient to some health resort in order to do him justice, and thus, in the majority of instances he loses sight of the case.

Yet in every discussion of surgical reports upon this subject some few men will be found who record their belief in the satisfactory results of hygiene. The absolute diagnosis of tubercular kidney, except in its advanced and obviously surgical conditions, is such a recent refinement of science that few of us can feel sure of spontaneous cures, and only in a few instances has the dead-house disclosed healed lesions of renal tuberculosis. Yet I have seen several cases, most of them obviously inoperable on account of the extent of tubercular involvement, go on for many years, better or worse, in accordance with the amount of care they took of their physical condition. I believe appropriate hygiene will almost always check the disease and in many cases will prolong life indefinitely, while I look forward to the time when we can say with certainty that medical measures promptly undertaken and thoroughly carried out will be probably curative. There are no specific drugs for this form of the disease: creosote has a record of cures and so has ichthyol, but climate and hygiene are our chief dependence.

one of the 68 cases seen by Israel occurred between the fiftieth and the seventieth year. The majority of the tumours of childhood are sarcomata, while those of later years are carcinomata. Of 138 cases of sarcoma collected by Walker,[1] 116 occurred before the fifth year. Trauma and heredity have not been shown to influence tumours of the kidney, while nephritis, suppuration, and stone are accidental and secondary rather than primary.

Morbid Anatomy.—Benign and malignant adenoma, carcinoma, and sarcoma of many varieties have been described. They are alleged to arise from adrenal rests or inclusions, or from the normal or diseased renal parenchyma, or from encapsulated portions of that tissue (Albarran). To enter into a brief discussion of these varieties is only to complicate confusion. Ample discussion of the facts may be found in the writings of Kelynack, Morris, and Albarran.[2] Suffice it to say that tumours are encountered involving the whole kidney (Fig. 151) or only a part of it; and that without exploratory

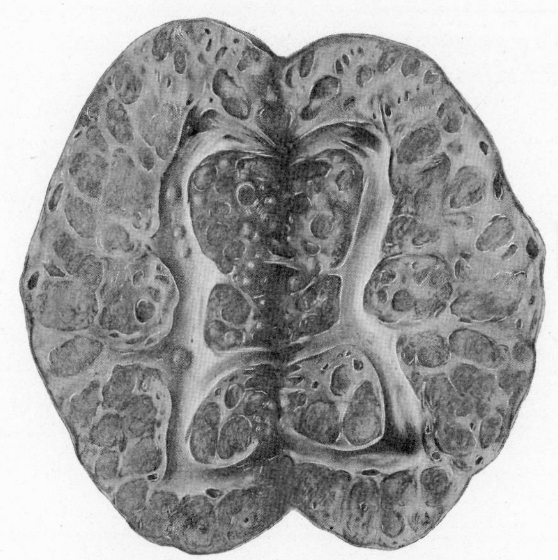

Fig. 151.—Malignant Adenoma of the Kidney.

incision it is impossible to distinguish clinically between tumours of the kidney itself, tumours of the suprarenal gland, and tumours of the perirenal tissue. The sarcomata of childhood grow far more rapidly and to a far larger size than do the malignant growths of later years. Thus Morris mentions a 31-pound tumour removed post mortem from a child, who without the tumour weighed only 100

[1] Annals of Surgery, 1897, xxvi, 529.
[2] Guyon's Annales, 1897, xv, 243, 387.

pounds. In one of Abbé's cases the tumour weighed $7\frac{1}{2}$ pounds and the child 15 pounds. In Mackenzie's case the tumour weighed 22 pounds, the child 39 pounds.

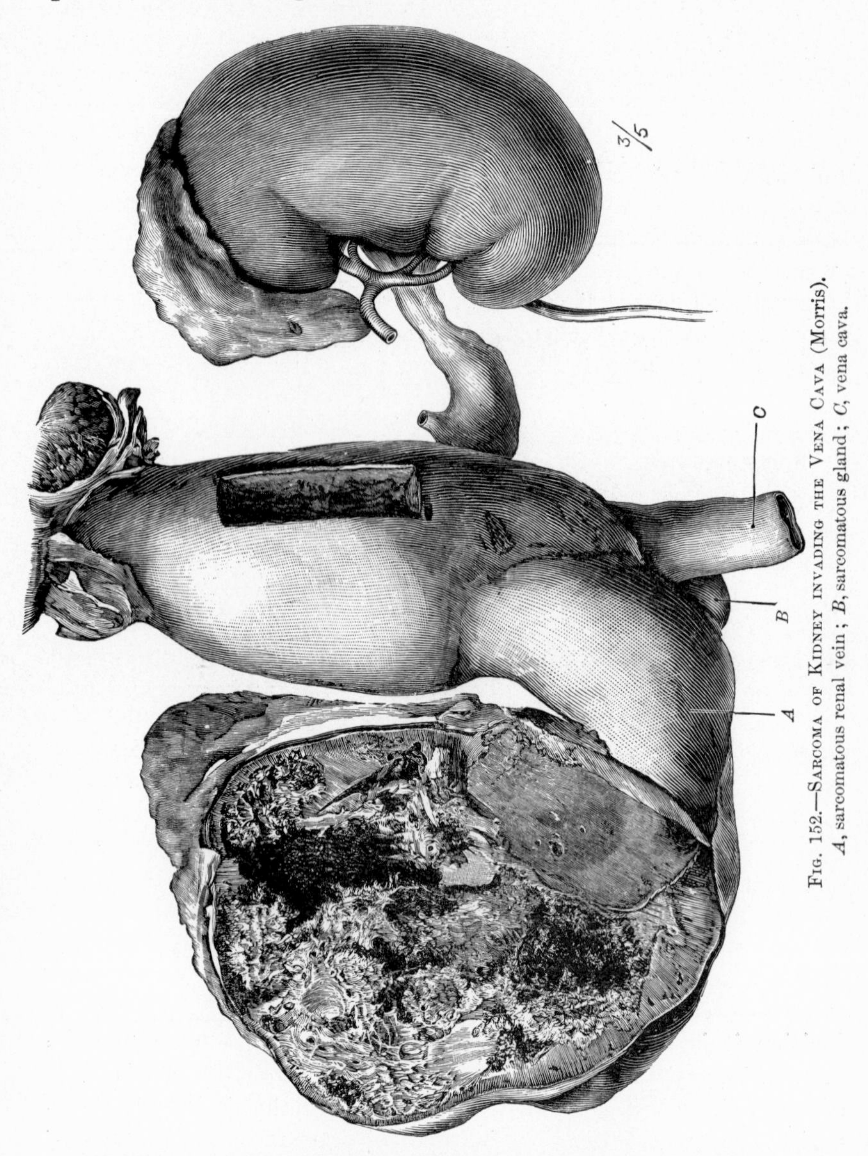

Fig. 152.—Sarcoma of Kidney invading the Vena Cava (Morris).
A, sarcomatous renal vein; *B*, sarcomatous gland; *C*, vena cava.

Extension of the Disease.—Primary malignant disease of the kidney may extend directly through the capsule, along the renal vein (Fig. 152), through the lymphatics, down the ureter, or by metastasis. Extension through the capsule or down the ureter is most exceptional. In a certain percentage of cases the renal vein is involved by the disease. Thus Israel encountered this complication 7 times in 43 operations. As may be imagined, involvement of the wall of the vein or its occlusion by clots forms one of the greatest operative complications, for the vein may be torn by manipulations of the kidney, clamps may tear through it and ligatures may slip from it; while the disturbance of the vessels incident to the various stages of the operation may break off a large clot and instantly kill the patient from cardiac or pulmonary embolism. All of these accidents have been encountered. Extension along the lymph channels is singularly slow, although it occurs in the majority of cases; but circulatory metastases are common. The occurrence of metastases cannot be foreseen, nor can their probability at any stage of the disease be denied. Israel cites several cases in which metastatic tumours gave the first evidence of the primary renal disease. In other cases, however, the renal tumour may grow to an enormous size without any metastasis or other extension.

Symptoms.—*In childhood* the symptom that overshadows all others is the lumbar tumour. Generally speaking, the only symptoms of a renal growth in childhood is the appearance of a rapidly growing lateral abdominal tumour associated with progressive cachexia. Early hematuria, so characteristic of this disease in the adult, is but rare in children, the striking condition being the wasting away of the child coincident with the enormously rapid growth of the abdominal tumour. *The characteristics of the renal tumour*, whether occurring in childhood or in adult life, are the following: At first the growth retains the rounded shape of the kidney itself, so that a small tumour, whether growing in the upper pole and pushing the kidney downward or itself protruding from the lower pole, is difficult to distinguish from a movable kidney, for adhesions to the surrounding tissue are unusual, and the tumour is readily mistaken for the lower end of a normal kidney and slips up and down between the examining fingers in a similar manner. As it grows larger the tumour still retains its rounded outline, so that, although so large as no longer to be mistaken for a normal kidney, it may still be distinguished from a tumour of the spleen or of the liver by the fact that at no place do its rounded sides present the sharp edges usually to be detected in a growth arising from one of the two latter organs.

The position of the renal growth or enlargement, be it hydronephrosis, pyonephrosis, or tumour, is quite characteristic. As it enlarges it first projects laterally, effacing the natural curve of the loin, although there is never any marked protrusion of the growth directly backward unless from edema and circulatory disturbance in the parietes. As the tumour grows it extends forward into the outer segment of the umbilical region, and finally it may come to occupy the whole half of the abdomen, extending down into the false pelvis and up into the epigastrium. In a few instances a renal tumour has been known even to encroach upon the opposite half of the belly. Given a tumour so large as to be visible, the characteristics that mark its renal origin are its rounded outline and its mobility with respiration, which latter, though not so great as the mobility of a hepatic or a splenic tumour, is more marked than that of a pelvic growth. Another characteristic usually to be determined is the presence of the large intestine in front of the tumour. It is a rule—not without numerous exceptions—that as the kidney enlarges it pushes the colon forward between it and the anterior abdominal wall. If the abdominal wall is thin and relaxed, the position of the colon when empty can be determined by rolling it beneath the fingers, while percussion reveals a resonant note over the large intestine inflated either by its own gases or by carbonic-acid gas injected by the surgeon.[1] The characteristic line of resonant large intestine running upward in front of the tumour is found in the majority of renal tumours, never in splenic tumours, and only rarely in tumours of pelvic or hepatic origin; while, on the other hand, tumours growing from any organ other than the kidney habitually have a line of resonance behind instead of in front of them. The surface of the renal growth may be smooth or irregular, hard or elastic, yet the rounded outline without any edge is usually maintained.

In children the disease runs a rapid course, and, according to Kelynack, the expectation of life lies between eight months and two years from the time the diagnosis is made.

In Adults.—In adults the course of the disease is usually slower than in the child and the development of the symptoms distinctly different.

Hematuria.—The first symptom usually is hematuria. The *hematuria* of renal tumour has the characteristics of being *spontaneous, profuse, and uninfluenced by exercise or jolting.* It is often preceded by or associated with pain when by its very profuseness it obstructs the ureter with clots. These clots are passed with more or less soreness or actual renal colic, and when passed they

---

[1] This injection of carbonic-acid gas may be readily made through a long rectal tube by means of an inverted siphon of any carbonated water. The only necessary precaution is to allow the escape of gas into the tube very slowly and regularly.

are often to be found in the voided urine as elongated narrow bits roughly moulded to the shape of the ureter. It is characteristic of this bleeding, as of every other hemorrhage from the kidney, that the blood is habitually intimately mixed with the urine, so that at no time during the hemorrhage is any blood passed without urine in it or any urine without blood. However, Israel relates a few exceptional instances in which this intermingling did not occur. The same author reports 66 cases, most of them in adults, of which 61 had hemorrhages at one time or another during the disease, while 70% of them noticed a hematuria as the initial symptom. He notes, however, that the bleeding may occur before the tumour has attained palpable dimensions; or it may not be noticed at all until the tumour has attained such a size as to produce a distinct fulness in the loin. While the blood from a renal tumour has not always the characteristics of spontaneity and profuseness these suggestive attributes are usually noted.

Tumour.—The second striking symptom of renal growth in the adult is the presence of tumour. Morris states that tumour is the first symptom in 23% of cases in the adult. Yet if the kidney region is carefully examined by ballottement and by deep bimanual pressure the presence of a tumour can be discovered in a far larger proportion of cases. Thus Israel was able to recognise the enlargement in 62 out of 68 cases; and he especially notes that in 5 of these the growth was extremely small, and could be distinguished only by palpation at the moment when the abdominal wall is relaxed immediately after full inspiration.

Varicocele.—The importance of varicocele as a symptom of renal tumour has been somewhat overestimated on account of the insistence of Legueu that the spermatic vein dilates only when the renal vein becomes compressed by enlarged glands. If this were the case, the presence of an acute varicocele due to tumour of the kidney would be an absolute contra-indication to operation; but several cases cited by Heresco, Israel, and Morris show that acute varicocele may occur without any involvement of vein or glands. Be this as it may, the characteristics of the acute renal varicocele are that it appears suddenly on the right or the left side, dependent upon the situation of the renal tumour, and occurs at a time of life when primary varicocele is never encountered.

Pain.—Pain is not a notable symptom of renal tumour, except in connection with bleeding; yet when a sharp hemorrhage occurs from the kidney in 50% of the cases there will be a sufficiently distinct localized pain or colic to identify the organ from which the bleeding proceeds.

Other Symptoms.—Cancerous cachexia makes its appearance as the disease progresses. Uremia and jaundice, ascites, or anasarca may occur, but they are not often prominent symptoms until the disease is far advanced. *Urinary examination* is only negatively important. The absence of any pus from the urine is particularly suggestive of cancerous hemorrhage. The *disorders of micturition*, so common with other surgical diseases of the kidney, do not seem to occur with tumour, a fact which lends weight to the supposition that they are due rather to involvement of the pelvis and the ureter than to disease of the kidney proper.

It has been observed that generalization of the disease occurs especially late in the rapidly growing sarcomata of childhood.

Diagnosis.—The existence of a malignant growth in the kidney is not suspected unless there is hematuria or tumour in the loin. *When there is tumour* one must first be sure that the tumour is renal in origin. The characteristics of a renal growth which have been detailed above usually are adequate to solve this difficulty. Exceptionally the tumour is so small that it is mistaken for the lower end of a slightly movable kidney, or so large that it has formed connections with the liver or spleen which so modify its shape and position as to mislead the surgeon. In the latter case the tumour is usually inoperable, while in the former the youth or advanced age of the patient will speak against the diagnosis of nephroptosis. A malignant tumour on the posterior wall of the colon is often especially difficult to distinguish from a renal growth. However, such a tumour is never associated with hematuria, and usually causes digestive disturbances.

Having determined that the enlargement belongs to the kidney, the nature of the growth may be inferred from the absence of inflammation. Except in those rare instances of renal growth complicated by stone or by perinephritis, the patient has absolutely clear urine, and shows no signs of urinary septicemia. These facts rule out pyonephrosis and stone. In a few cases gummatous enlargement of the kidney has been mistaken for tumour and thus an unnecessary nephrectomy has been performed. The clinical evidences of syphilitic disease of the kidneys are, however, not sufficiently distinctive to permit of generalization. When the tumour is small and the patient gives a syphilitic history it is proper to put him through a short and sharp course of iodids and mercurial injections in order by this therapeutic test to eliminate the possibility of syphilis.

Another and larger class of renal tumours is that in which *hematuria is the most marked symptom.* When hematuria occurs before the tenth year suspicion naturally points to tumour; when it occurs between the tenth and the thirty-fifth year the probabilities favour tubercle; while later than this the presumption again refers to tumour. At any age such a hemorrhage may be due to stone, whether vesical or renal; but the associated symptoms, and especially the examination by searcher and X-ray, should distinctly determine this point. Given a hematuria, its renal origin may be determined by the nature of the bleeding (p. 623), by the fact that vesical instrumentation has no effect upon the hemorrhage, and by cystoscopic examination, which will usually demonstrate the flow of blood from one or the other ureter. Renal blood has usually a darker colour than vesical blood.

The side from which the hemorrhage comes is determined by renal colic—if there is any—by the presence of tumour, or, in the absence of these, by the use of the cystoscope, the segregator, and the ureteral catheter. Having determined that there is renal hemorrhage from one kidney, the absence of pus from the urine narrows down the diagnosis to tubercle, cancer, and the so-called idiopathic hematuria, although, exceptionally, stone may enter into consideration. The age of the patient and the size of the tumour will often make the existence of neoplasm morally certain. In doubtful cases investigation of the urine for the tubercle bacillus, the X-ray, and all the aids that physical examination and history afford, should be employed to arrive at a definite conclusion. But in a certain number of instances it will be found impossible to achieve this without an exploratory operation, which is always a proper and usually a safe procedure. The only special preliminary precaution required is that the presence and integrity of the other kidney be insured and that the patient's permission be obtained for removal of the kidney if this seems called for by the conditions described.

Prognosis.—The prognosis of malignant tumours of the kidney is always absolutely bad unless the kidney is removed. In the infant the expectation of life is usually but a few months, always less than two years. In the adult a tumour progresses more slowly, and the expectation of life varies from two to five years. Death usually results from cachexia, hemorrhage, or uremia.

Treatment.—*The treatment of tumour of the kidney is wholly operative.* Unless the whole growth and the whole kidney be removed it is useless to employ any measures other than the desperate alternative of narcotics. Until within the last decade the immediate mortality of nephrectomy for cancer has been so great as to be almost deterrent. Thus Guillet collected the operations up to 1889, and found a mortality of from 60% to 70%. The statistics of Rovsing and Küster, published in 1895, showed that the operative mortality had fallen to 25%, while more recent figures show even better results. Thus Heresco[1] collected 165 nephrectomies for tumour performed since 1890 with only 32 deaths within a month of the operation—a mortality just under 20%; while Israel lost 9 cases out of 43, a mortality of 20.9%. The statistics of individual operators show the same improvement. Morris lost 2 cases, and has since operated 10 times without a death. Tuffier's mortality has fallen from 65% to 5%. Czerny lost 7 of his first 9 cases, and since then has operated 9 times successfully. The late results of this operation have not kept pace with the decrease in operative mortality. Thus of the 89 survivors in Heresco's table, 62 were followed, and of these 22 died of recurrence within three and a half years, 4 of intercurrent disease, while 36 were known to survive from two months to seven years after the operation. Israel records 29 cases operated upon three years before, of whom 7 died as the result of operation or of intercurrent disease. Of the remaining 22, 14 died of recurrence and 8 (36%) remained cured after more than three years, the longest records extending to ten, twelve, and fourteen years. Yet of Morris's 8 cases all died of recurrence except 1, who was well three months after nephrectomy. Until statistics grow larger they will not yield any accurate results. Yet it is obvious that with increasing accuracy of diagnosis operations will in future be performed earlier in the disease, and the successful extirpation of cancerous kidneys will be more frequent.

Contra-indications.—The only absolute contra-indication to operation is extension of the disease along the renal vein, along the lymphatics, or by metastasis of other organs. The opposite kidney can almost always be depended upon, unless there is diabetes (Israel). Chronic myocarditis has been the cause of the majority of the operative deaths. Five of Israel's 8 deaths resulted from heart failure, while 13 of the 39 deaths reported by Heresco were due to the same cause. Other causes of death are embolism, hemorrhage primarily from rupture of the renal vein or the cava, and secondarily from slipping of ligatures or clamps on a diseased vessel.

---

[1] Thèse de Paris, 1899.

CHAPTER XLIII

IDIOPATHIC RENAL HEMATURIA AND NEPHRALGIA

IDIOPATHIC OR ESSENTIAL RENAL HEMATURIA

WHEN a hemorrhage occurs in the kidneys its outward sign is hematuria. The only condition in which a serious hemorrhage can occur without hematuria is rupture of the kidney, when, as has already been remarked, the blood effused into the lumbar recess or into the perirenal cavity is of far more importance than the relatively small amount that escapes down the ureter. Apart from this condition, renal hemorrhage is expressed by hematuria. The characteristics of renal hematuria have been described in the preceding chapter, for the hematuria that occurs with tumour of the kidney is at once the most important and the most profuse spontaneous hemorrhage from that organ. Bleeding is also a common symptom of renal stone and renal tuberculosis; and when the kidney bleeds, one of these three conditions—stone, tubercle, or tumour—is usually suspected. But there are a great many other diseases, a few of them surgical in their aspects and most of them medical, in which renal hemorrhage—even profuse renal hemorrhage—may occur. To such profuse hemorrhage from an obscure cause has been given the name of essential or idiopathic renal hematuria.

Etiology.—The causes to which this essential renal hematuria has been attributed may be classified as follows:

1. Hematuria, scurvy, purpura.
2. Drug-poisoning (turpentine, cantharides, etc.).
3. Parasites (e. g., distoma, hematobium—Sondern[1]).
4. Acute or chronic febrile diseases (scarlet fever, malaria).
5. Surgical diseases (hydronephrosis, renal mobility).
6. The passage of urinary crystals.
7. Angioneurosis.
8. Chronic nephritis.

It is not necessary to consider all these conditions in detail. Distoma, for instance, is practically never heard of in these latitudes.

[1] Medical News, 1897.

Renal hemorrhage caused by drugs or occurring in the course of one of the bleeding diseases has no surgical interest. There remain the hematuria due to surgical causes, that due to angioneurosis, and that due to chronic nephritis. It is possible that any of these three causes may produce a profuse renal hemorrhage. Physical examination of the loins should eliminate hydronephrosis and movable kidney, and there are left for our consideration only angioneurosis and chronic nephritis.

When it was first recognised that an apparently normal kidney might bleed spontaneously and profusely, it was believed that the cause of this hemorrhage was probably some idiopathic dilatation or rupture of the renal capillaries, hence the name of idiopathic or essential renal hematuria was bestowed upon this condition. Without stopping to review the various opinions upon this subject, let it suffice to say that modern investigations have shown that in almost all, if not in all such cases, there is organic disease of the kidney. The disease may be slight, it may be obscure, but some abnormal condition has been found to exist in every case that has been carefully examined in the light of modern pathology.

According to the older theories the bleeding was an angioneurosis, an oozing from the spontaneously dilated renal vessels. According to the theory now generally accepted, the bleeding occurs in a kidney which is chronically inflamed, and is usually a congestion aroused by some form of toxemia. Exceptionally, it is a bleeding from an ulcerated papilla.[1] Thus, the bleeding that occurs in acute nephritis, the bleeding of scurvy and of malaria, the bleeding that sometimes occurs in the course of a chronic nephritis, the bleeding due to drugs, and the idiopathic renal hematuria, are all much the same in origin. Each and every one of them originates in a congestion caused by the endeavour of the kidney to eliminate a poison. If the poison is sufficiently irritant (e. g., cantharides) it may cause the normal kidney to bleed; but in most cases the kidney itself must be diseased before it will react in this way.

Symptoms.—The brief narration of a characteristic case may suffice for a description of the symptoms of this disease:

Mr. C. D., single, aged thirty, has been treated by me for several attacks of non-specific urethritis, terminating in 1872 in a soft stricture at the bulbo-membranous junction, admitting only a No. 13 F. blunt steel sound. After many relapses and irregularities, in

[1] Hurry Fenwick has described two successful operations for renal hemorrhage in which nephrotomy disclosed the existence of a bleeding point upon the tip of a papilla. It is possible that these ulcerations were tubercular or malignant.

1880 this was dilated to 27 F., and has remained well. The patient is nervous; the urine overacid, overheavy, and containing oxalate-of-lime crystals in abundance.

August, 1887.—A spontaneous attack of left nephralgia and hematuria lasting eighteen hours.

April, 1890.—Pyuria and hematuria. A little blood in the urine all the time until

July 29.—An attack similar to that of August, 1887. The blood is bright red; the bleeding ceases spontaneously; the pain is not very severe.

September.—Similar attack.

December 18th.—Similar attack. The left kidney is sensitive. Except under orders he has not been confined to bed during any of these attacks.

February, 1891.—An attack of hematuria lasting five weeks, with pain and tenderness in the left kidney. This continues until

March.—Nephrotomy; left kidney exposed. It appears normal; no stone felt. Needling discloses several areas of tissue so dense that a distinct creaking sound is produced by the needle as it passes through them. Bleeding ceased.

The patient has been occasionally seen since the operation, and in the summer of 1899 I operated upon him for acute appendicitis. He has never had any further hematuria, although from time to time the urine contains oxalate-of-lime crystals, and once (1896) he has had some aching in the left kidney. No stone or gravel has passed at any time, nor has there ever been any real attack of renal colic.

Diagnosis.—The bleeding may last a few hours or it may continue for days; having once occurred it may never appear again; or it may return time after time, and be so profuse as to threaten the patient's life. In the presence of a condition so various in its manifestations, so comparable in its only symptom to the most serious affections of the kidney, so dangerous sometimes in its continuance, a diagnosis is of the utmost importance, and a diagnosis is difficult to obtain. If the hemorrhage ceases, the presence of a trace of albumin and a few casts lends weight to the probability that it was not due to surgical disease. But an appreciation of the fact that the bleeding, which is so often the first symptom of malignant growth in the kidney, may occur two, three, or even five years before any other symptom, cannot fail to impress upon the surgeon the necessity for the utmost caution in deciding the nature of the malady. It is not sufficient that the hemorrhage cease. This it may do spontaneously or as the result of the administration of some drug. But the patient should be warned that this bleeding may be the first symptom of some serious renal disease and should be instructed to watch for further developments, and even to report occasionally for examination.

In view of the frequency of idiopathic renal hemorrhage such a course may seem extreme, and in certain cases it may be best to withhold from the patient any knowledge of the real possibilities of the case in order to spare his own nerves as well as those of the surgeon. But the surgeon at least should recognise that the more spontaneous the bleeding and the more entirely free the patient from any other symptom, the greater is the probability of malignant disease. It is for this reason that I am not inclined to discourage exploratory nephrotomy for the purpose of clearing up the diagnosis. This operation has no mortality and few discomforts; and although the hemorrhage may often be checked without it, the assurance that there is no beginning cancer in the kidney is worth having at this cost.

Treatment.—Idiopathic renal hemorrhage may usually be checked by the administration of 0.5 gramme of turpentine in capsules 3 times a day. By this treatment, sometimes adding a fluid diet and diuresis by mineral waters, I have been able to cure some 5 or 6 cases. In one striking case the patient had been bleeding profusely for a month. Every drop of urine passed was stained dark red by the contained blood. One week on turpentine sufficed to check the bleeding absolutely and permanently. Yet in another case the bleeding was checked by turpentine, recurred several years later, and was then not amenable to that drug, nor would the patient accept the suggestion of operative exploration.

Cantharides in small doses has been serviceable in the hands of some, and the fluid extract of senecio aureus has its supporters, though it has not proved as useful in my hands as turpentine.

Most surgeons have submitted these cases to nephrotomy, and so often has a cure followed exploration of the kidney that, in order to explain the fact, the theory has been devised that incision of the organ relieves the congestion and so checks the bleeding. This theory fits well with that of Harrison and Edebohls concerning nephrotomy for chronic nephritis. Yet in this connection it is noteworthy that in several instances the bleeding has stopped after such efforts as my own related above, in which the kidney was neither incised nor split; while other kidneys continued to bleed in spite of the exploration. In this desperate extremity nephrectomy may be considered if the patient's life is threatened by the continued hemorrhage. Ordinarily speaking, nephrotomy may properly be performed not so much to check the bleeding as to prove the innocence of its cause.

IDIOPATHIC NEPHRALGIA

Although the occurrence of renal pain without renal lesion has not attracted so much attention as has essential renal hematuria, this is due to the relative insignificance rather than to the rarity of the pain as compared to the bleeding. Renal pain and even renal colic are often due to hysteria or to the passage of crystals of uric acid or of oxalate of lime without the presence of any actual calculus. Such pain may assume the proportions of renal colic, and may be associated with the most characteristic symptoms of stone, especially in overworked men and in hysterical women. The narration of two characteristic cases will throw more light upon this subject than pages of discussion.

Case I.—The patient is a short, thick-set muscular individual, the president of a large corporation, and has been engaged in the manufacturing business for many years without any vacation. He had never been ill a day in his life until his present troubles began, and believes himself to be organically sound. But his pulse is rapid; in comparison with that of his brother who accompanied him his complexion is sallow and his air dejected and spiritless. His present complaint began in the summer of 1897, with an attack of sharp colicky pain in the right loin. This pain having recurred on several occasions, he comes with the diagnosis of renal stone expecting operation. The pains are typical attacks of renal colic, beginning in the right loin, running down into the groin and testicle with retraction of that organ. They last for several hours and terminate as suddenly as they begin. No stone has ever been passed. Recent attacks have occurred as follows:

November 17th.—Pain from 2 to 4 A. M.
November 23d.—Pain from 8 to 10.30 A. M.
November 25th.—Pain from 2 to 9 A. M.
November 29th.—Pain from 2 to 5 A. M.
December 1st.—Pain at 2 A. M.

He passes 32 ounces of urine a day. Examination of that fluid shows it to be acid, of a specific gravity of 1.030, containing a trace of albumin and a few blood cells to account for it; no sugar; loaded with oxalates, urates, and phosphates.

Patient eats too much, exercises too little; is constipated; weighs 203 pounds; has been married five years, and has no children. Neither kidney is tender or enlarged.

The following treatment was instituted:

1. Low diet, meat only once a day.
2. Rest from business.
3. Walk six miles a day.
4. Suwannee water, 4 quarts daily.
5. Citrate of potash, 4 grammes 3 times a day.
6. Calomel, rhubarb, and soda.

Since beginning treatment he has never had another colic. Occasionally the loin is sore. He was several times awakened at 2 A. M. by a profuse night-sweat. The exercise and diet were indefinitely continued. During the following six months he gained 21 pounds, impregnated his wife, and was operated upon for appendicitis (!) in another city. The specific gravity of the urine dropped to about 1.020, the crystals, albumin, and blood disappeared, and in April, 1900, he reports himself perfectly vigorous, weighing 172 pounds (a proper reaction from his first excessive gain in weight), and free from all trouble so long as he continues to eat lightly, to exercise freely, and to take a reasonable vacation from business.

Case II.—Female domestic, thirty-nine years old, comes May 7, 1900, complaining of a stone in the left ureter. Six years ago she had some pain in her pelvis, especially during the menstrual period. This was attributed to uterine retrodisplacement, and was treated mechanically without much relief. Since then she has continued to have considerable pain during menstruation and some soreness between times. The pains are pelvic and confined to the left side. On April 12, 1900, she was seized with a sudden sharp pain in the left loin, the pain lasting a few hours and being accompanied with nausea. The attack recurred on April 16th and was relieved by morphin. It was followed by a profuse flow of blood, although menstruation was not due. Since then she has not passed more than a pint of urine during any day. There has been continual pain in the loin, interrupted by four attacks of renal colic, during which she had complete anuria for as long as twelve hours. No stone has ever been passed. The left kidney is just palpable, but not tender. There is one markedly tender spot where the ureter crosses the brim of the pelvis. Vaginal examination is negative. The urine has a specific gravity of 1.010 and contains blood cells and albumin.

Under the impression that a stone was impacted in the ureter, the patient was ordered to drink 6 pints of beer a day. On the following day there was a slight colic, followed by a copious flow of urine, and on May 14th the kidney was no longer palpable, the ureteral tender point had disappeared, and she felt perfectly well.

In July a number of left renal colics were succeeded by tenderness on the left side of the pelvis low down. Supposing that the stone had reached the lower end of the ureter, I examined her under general anesthesia and found an elastic, movable mass behind the uterus, while cystoscopy and ureteral catheterization revealed nothing. I subsequently removed a cyst the size of a billiard-ball from the right ovary and several smaller ones from the left. Her kidney pains were thereby checked for two years. The colics then returned, and she put herself under the care of another surgeon, who, after obtaining a negative X-ray picture, split the left kidney and passed a probe down into the bladder, finding nothing. During her convalescence the colics returned.

Case I is a good example of renal colic caused by the passage of crystals. The diagnosis depends upon a satisfactory X-ray picture, and must be confirmed by the effects of over-exercise, under-feeding, and general mental and physical hygiene. Such cases may also be relieved by exploratory nephrotomy.

Case II is chiefly hysterical. The pains were doubtless primarily due to the ovarian cyst, and their return after this had been removed is explicable only by the persistence of an impression upon a weak nervous system.

RENAL DECAPSULATION

The disappearance of albuminuria after an operation performed for surgical disease of the kidney has been noted by various authors, and is not a very uncommon experience. I have encountered several such cases in which the operations of nephro-lithotomy, nephropexy, and nephrotomy for suppurative pyelonephritis have resulted not only in the cure of the surgical condition, but also in the apparent *restitutio ad integrum* of the affected organ. In 1901, Dr. Edebohls,[1] having observed these facts in a number of nephropexies, conceived the idea of aiding the return to normal of the kidney by stripping from it its fibrous capsule, on the theory that tension would thus be relieved and that the new capsule formed from the cellular tissue about the kidney might prove more vascular than the old, and thus supply more blood to the kidney.

Following out this theory, at first chiefly upon cases of albuminuria due to nephroptosis, later upon all kinds of albuminurics, Edebohls [2] reported, in 1903, 51 cases, of which 14% died, 44% improved, and 14% were definitely cured. But in the meanwhile, Rovsing,[3] by a series of careful investigations, demonstrated that bac-

[1] Med. Record, 1901, lx, 690. [2] Med. Record, 1903, lxiii, 481.
[3] Mitteil. aus d. Grenzebiet. d. Med. u. Chir., 1902, x, 288.

terial nephritis (i. e., catarrhal pyelonephritis), or nephritis causing renal pain or hematuria, could be cured by nephrotomy with decapsulation, but that true Bright's disease, non-surgical nephritis, could not be so cured.

Experiments upon dogs, rabbits, and cats have shown that the capsule of scar tissue formed after decapsulation, although more vascular at first, soon develops into a fibrous layer closely resembling the original capsule, and is, if anything, more closely adherent to the kidney. Autopsy reports are few and conflicting, but in the main confirm this view. At present the clinical findings, which have accumulated to a considerable number, form a safer guide. Suker [1] investigated 19 decapsulations for chronic interstitial (17) and diffuse (2) nephritis with ocular complications. Of these (excluding 2 cases) 6 died in a few days, 10 more died within the year (94% total mortality), and 1 is alive, "improved," at the end of a year. Elliott [2] collected 112 reported decapsulations, among which 29 cases of nephroptosis, with albuminuria, operated upon by nephropexy with or without decapsulation, almost all did well. His 79 cases of medical nephritis may be grouped as follows:

	No. of cases.	Died within one month.	Died later.	Made worse.	Unimproved.	Improved.	Cured.
Glomerulo-nephritis (*subacute*).....	2	—	—	—	—	2	0
Arterio-sclerotic (*renal atrophy*)...	1	—	1	—	—	—	0
Interstitial nephritis (*early*).......	14	1	—	1	2	10	0
Nephritis (*advanced*)..............	29	12	10	1	2	4	0
Parenchymatous nephritis.........	33	7	6	—	8	12	0
Total chronic nephritis...........	76	20	16	2	12	26	0

In other words, only 34% of the cases of true Bright's are alleged to have improved after decapsulation. Unfortunately, most of these were reported less than six months after operation, and, inasmuch as relief of symptoms often occurs (8 of Suker's cases that died within the year showed improvement after operation), even these figures can not be accepted as wholly accurate. Thus the present status of decapsulation is failure to improve most cases of Bright's disease and failure to establish anastomotic circulation for the kidney, against which may be set some success in relieving temporarily the symptoms of Bright's disease and success in curing those forms of surgical nephritis known to be curable by nephropexy and nephrotomy. Whether decapsulation will prove of real value in parenchymatous nephritis or in commencing interstitial nephritis the future will decide.

[1] J. Am. Med. Ass'n, 1904, xlii, 580.
[2] N. Y. Med. J 1904, lxxix, 1078.

CHAPTER XLIV

OPERATIONS UPON THE KIDNEY—RENAL FISTULA

THE preliminary stage of renal surgery has passed. A surgeon is no longer justified in performing a nephrotomy or a nephrectomy according to his own whim. It is no longer proper to sacrifice a whole kidney when a part of it may be saved, nor to sacrifice any part of a kidney when the whole of it may be saved; nor is it proper to perform nephrectomy without the assurance that the opposite kidney is sound. Thus surgery of the kidney has begun to be conservative. It will doubtless progress further along the same lines. Exploratory nephrotomy is being more and more replaced by the X-ray and the ureteral catheter; and it is to be hoped that the day is not far distant when no operation shall be performed upon the kidney without a perfectly definite knowledge of the condition of that organ, so that the surgeon can make up his mind beforehand just what he intends to do, and, by the precision of his knowledge and the accuracy of his diagnosis, spare the patient that prolonged anesthesia which is so often fatal.

In the following paragraphs the more important operations upon the kidney are discussed. Special points of technic have been considered in the chapters relating to each special disease. Yet the surgeon must remember that in many cases it is impossible to perform a typical operation. One nephrorrhaphy is much the same as another, and in exploratory nephrotomy there are not many variations of technic. But when the surgeon undertakes nephrotomy or nephrectomy for the cure of the various suppurative, calculous, tubercular, and malignant diseases of the gland, his experience will suggest minor modifications proper to each case, modifications which it is impracticable and useless to enumerate. But they will all tend to the same ends—to obtain a wide operative field and, as far as possible, to save a kidney which may still be of some service.

Instruments Required.—Besides the clamps, scissors, knives, etc., necessary for any major operation, certain instruments are especially applicable to operations upon the kidney. It is well to have two broad, deep abdominal retractors in order to hold apart the edges of the wound in case the kidney cannot be readily loosened and brought out through the lumbar incision. It is also necessary to have a slender probe, 30 cm. long, to investigate the ureter. Moreover, one or more stone forceps (Fig. 114) may be required in calculous cases, cambric needles and fine silk for plastic work upon the pelvis, and chromicized catgut or kangaroo tendon for suturing the kidney tissue. It is always well to have a number of long artery clamps, a heavy pedicle clamp, an aneurysm needle, and some braided silk, any or all of these to be used on the renal pedicle if nephrectomy is to be performed.

Preparation of the Patient.—The patient should be prepared as usual for any operation upon the urinary tract. The bowels and stomach should be empty, the skin of the abdomen and back aseptic. Urotropin should be administered for two days before the operation, and during the same period it is well to have the patient on a fluid diet, drinking large quantities of water. All these precautions are employed in order to render the urine and the operative field as clean as possible and to avert post-operative suppression.

Choice of Incision.—Every operation upon the kidney and the ureter should be performed extraperitoneally, if possible. It is only in exceptional cases of difficult nephrectomy that the intraperitoneal route is to be preferred. The reasons for preferring the extraperitoneal incision are (1) the lessened danger from sepsis, for pus may be allowed to run all through the lumbar wound with impunity so long as sufficient drainage is maintained after operation; and (2) more satisfactory exposure of the kidney obtained through the lumbar incision; so that often those surgeons who attack the largest and most adherent malignant growths habitually do so through an extraperitoneal incision, although in such cases it is usually necessary to enter the peritoneal cavity first or last. For our present purposes, however, we shall consider only the lumbar or extraperitoneal incision.

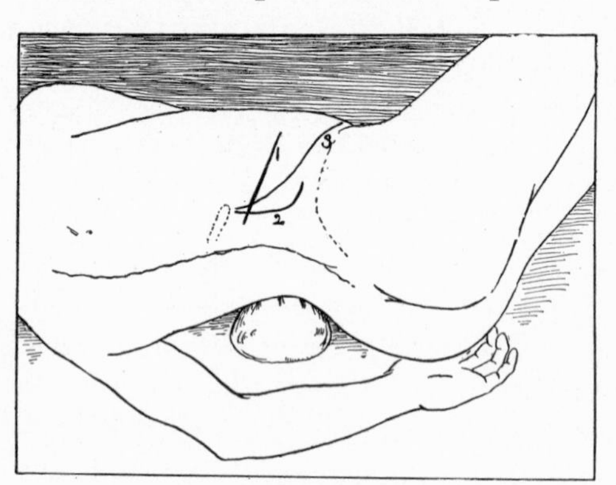

Fig. 153.—Position and Incisions for Renal Operation.

1, Transverse incision for nephrectomy; *2*, curved vertical incision for nephrotomy; *3*, oblique incision for nephrotomy or nephrectomy.

Position of the Patient.—The patient should lie upon the sound side in the Sims' position with hips and knees flexed, in order that the space between the ribs and the ilium may be as wide as possible. The opposite loin is forced upward by supporting it on a large pillow or on a kidney bag (Fig. 153).

NEPHROTOMY

The surgeon stands in front of the patient, who is in the Sims' position, as described above. It is best to have two assistants and at least one trained nurse, besides the anesthetist. My personal preferences on the subject of anesthesia have been suggested in a previous chapter (p. 511).

The Incision.—For simple nephropexy, exploratory nephrotomy, or nephrolithotomy, a vertical, a transverse, or an oblique incision may be employed. It often makes little difference which one is chosen, but, inasmuch as exploration of the renal pelvis and ureter may prove essential to the success of any operation, it is safer to employ an incision which may be readily extended down into the pelvis. For this purpose the oblique or curved lumbo-inguinal incision is always satisfactory, and on this account is generally employed. The surgeon feels for the extremity of the last rib and begins the incision a finger's breadth below and in front of its tip. This incision is carried obliquely downward and forward to within two fingers' breadth of the highest point of the crest of the ilium. The line of incision may be almost straight or markedly curved with its convexity backward (Fig. 153).

Having incised the skin and superficial fasciæ the external oblique muscle is exposed. This is divided in the line of its fibres. The internal oblique is then divided transversely, and the transversalis may be pulled forward and out of the way; if necessary the last dorsal nerve and vessels may be sacrificed. At this point in the operation pressure of the posterior flap backward reveals the thick rounded border of the quadratus lumborum muscle, while the bottom of the wound is closed by the glistening transversalis fascia. This is incised vertically, and immediately the perinephritic fascia presents itself. This structure resembles the subperitoneal fascia so closely as to mislead the inexperienced surgeon, and it may cause him to waste much valuable time in searching about for a means of discovering whether or not this is the peritoneum. The simplest guide is the border of the quadratus lumborum; the fascia underlying this is never peritoneal. Incision of this perinephritic fascia immediately permits the protrusion of the fatty capsule. With his fingers the surgeon enlarges this incision and proceeds to separate the fat by blunt dissection until he reaches the kidney, which can usually be felt high up under the ribs. Exceptionally this fatty capsule is so condensed by a fibro-lipomatous inflammation that it has to be incised. Ordinarily it is easily separated from the kidney. The remainder of the operation depends upon circumstances. For a nephropexy and some other operations it is not necessary to dislocate the kidney from its bed; but, as a rule, the organ can be handled more satisfactorily and explored more thoroughly if it be liberated and protruded through the lumbar incision.

Liberation of the Kidney.—The kidney is liberated by inserting the fingers behind it, sweeping them around the lower pole, then around the upper, and finally across the front of the organ, which, when thus freed from all its capsular attachments, may usually be drawn through the lumbar incision by gentle traction.

Several precautions must, however, be observed. An inflamed kidney may often defy all attempts at liberation by reason of its adhesions and its size. The *adhesions* which bind down a kidney must be respected. A considerable amount of force may be employed in separating the adhesions behind the kidney—so long as no great traction is made upon the organ—for in this region no damage can be done; but in working about the upper pole and in clearing the anterior surface great caution must be observed in order to avoid two accidents—viz., tearing the peritoneum and rupturing renal vessels. If the adhesions cannot be freed by a reasonable amount of force the kidney had best be explored *in situ*. In order to enlarge the field of operation for this purpose an accessory incision or the resection of a rib may be necessary (p. 641).

The second obstacle to liberation of a kidney is its size. A diseased kidney may be altogether too large to be extracted through the lumbar incision. If this be the case, rather than enlarge the incision it is better to force the kidney as near as possible to the surface of the body and explore it there. Inasmuch as these large kidneys are habitually pyonephrotic or hydronephrotic, incision of the organ may sufficiently reduce it in size to permit its extraction.

In all this work of liberating the kidney, or examining it *in situ*, the manipulations may be greatly aided by pressure of a fist upon the anterior abdominal wall. Properly applied, this pressure forces the kidney up into the wound better than does any form of traction.

It is especially necessary not to pull too hard on the kidney at any time. After its extraction from the loin it is customary to hold the organ by a long strip of gauze passed around its pedicle. The sudden tearing of the kidney from its attachments by undue traction upon this gauze sling is an evident example of how easily an accidental nephrectomy may be performed when the tissues about the hilum are rendered friable by prolonged suppuration or by malignant infiltration.

Nephrotomy and Pyelotomy.—From the large amount of clinical experience accumulated during the past two decades upon the relative merits of pyelotomy and nephrotomy it may be concluded that an incision in the pelvis of the kidney will heal about as well as one through the parenchyma. The earlier authors were convinced that pelvic incisions healed badly and in the majority of instances were followed by fistula; but the reason for this belief must have been the fact that the pelvis was incised only in conditions of renal retention, when fistula followed because the ureteral obstruction had not been removed. It is good surgery to incise the kidney or its pelvis, whichever presents in the field or affords the most appropriate access to the disease in the organ. Incisions in the parenchyma of the kidney should always be made along the convex border, and, if possible, should avoid the extreme tips, both upper and lower. Especially when exploring for stone, it is the practice of many surgeons to extract the kidney through the wound, to compress the renal artery, and then to split the kidney fairly into two halves. I have never seen the necessity for this operation, and, with the advances that have been made in X-ray diagnosis, it seems less and less essential. My favourite incision enters the convex border in the lower third of the organ and admits the finger into the lower portion of the sinus. If bimanual palpation with the finger in this position is not adequate to explore all the calices a supplementary incision may be made in the upper end of the organ. The hemorrhage that follows incision of the kidney is immediate and profuse; but if incisions are restricted to the posterior border, the gush is purely venous and may be readily controlled by pressure, and later by deep catgut sutures.

The incision of pyelotomy should radiate from the ureteral orifice towards the kidney tissue, in order that its two edges shall naturally fall together when the kidney is allowed to relapse into its place. The one precaution necessary in incising the pelvis of the kidney is to be sure that it is the pelvis which is incised. The renal vein and artery, subdivided into several large branches, run across the front of the pelvis and almost completely cover it, and since in some cases of dilated kidney only the front of the pelvis is accessible, the danger of opening one of these vessels will be readily understood.

Special Manipulations.—The various methods employed in resecting a portion of the kidney or in extracting a stone do not admit of any generalization. In performing a *resection* one has only to remember that any amount of kidney tissue may be sacrificed; but that if a large portion of the organ is to be removed, it is convenient to preface this operation by clamping that branch of the renal artery which supplies it. After resection the cut edges of the gap are to be united by deep catgut sutures. Large, branched *calculi*, fitting closely in the pelvis, are often very hard to remove. Rather than to struggle for an indefinite period in the effort to extricate such a stone it may be preferable to enlarge the parietal incision, to split the kidney from end to end, or even to remove it. But smaller stones are more easily handled: they may be picked from the pelvis or the calices by fingers or forceps, and in any case, whether the expected stone has been found or not, *the operation should never be considered complete until a probe has been passed from the pelvis of the kidney down into the bladder.*

Finally, the wound is irrigated according to the requirements of the case, and closed. An incision in the parenchyma of the kidney is best closed by one or two deep sutures of heavy catgut or chromicized gut. For incisions in the pelvis the finest silk is preferable, the sutures being inserted so as not to include the mucous membrane. But in the majority of cases the kidney is suppurating and requires to be drained. For this drainage a rubber tube is often more satisfactory than gauze, because of the very free flow of urine usually occurring during the first days after operation. This tube is inserted into the pelvis of the kidney, and drainage is also afforded by one or two strips of gauze leading to the dependent and pocketed portions of the wound. The external wound is sutured in its lower part, and the drain is left protruding from the upper end. No fear need be felt for the subsequent integrity of the abdominal wall. I have never seen hernia follow this operation, and I do not think it at all necessary to employ the incision suggested by Senn and others—namely, a muscle-splitting process comparable to the McBurney incision for appendicitis, the kidney being approached through the space between the abdominal muscles in front and the quadratus lumborum behind, or through the abdominal muscles themselves by splitting them along the line of their fibres.

NEPHRECTOMY

It may not be amiss to repeat in this place that, unless forced to it by immediate danger to the patient's life—such an excessive hemorrhage from the renal vessels—the kidney should never be removed unless the presence and functional capacity of the other kidney has been previously ascertained by the use of the ureteral catheter. It is even proper to defer nephrectomy until after nephrotomy shall have separated the urines—the urine from one kidney passing through the wound in the loin, that from the other issuing through the urethra. Nor should nephrectomy be contemplated, except for malignant disease, for tuberculosis, for inoperable obstruction of the ureter, or for such grade of renal disintegration by calculous or other suppuration as would make the organ a menace to its possessor. Nephrectomy is, immediately and remotely, a greater shock than nephrotomy. It involves longer anesthesia, inflicts greater traumatism, and lops off a large and important though damaged viscus. Hence it may be necessary to forego a contemplated nephrectomy and be satisfied with nephrotomy for any one of several reasons. First, the functional activity of the opposite kidney may not be known; second, the patient may be so weak that it is deemed inadvisable to expose him to the shock of the greater operation; and third, the suppuration may be so severe that it is thought prudent to drain the abscess for a few weeks, and then, after the suppuration shall have abated and the patient shall have rallied, to perform the radical procedure. In these cases the choice between primary and secondary nephrectomy is often entirely a matter of personal judgment. In any case, if a secondary nephrectomy is to be performed it should not be delayed many weeks, lest the kidney acquire adhesions to the surrounding parts that may many times multiply the difficulties of nephrectomy.

Lumbar Nephrectomy.—The kidney is reached by the oblique lumbar incision described above. Liberation of the organ is performed as in nephrotomy, but when dense adhesions are encountered the issue thus raised cannot be avoided: the kidney must be removed. In order to accomplish this one of several devices may be employed:

1. **Supplementary Incisions.**—The oblique incision may be enlarged by a transverse or a vertical incision from either extremity, or instead of the oblique incision a transverse cut one inch below and parallel to the last rib may be employed. A vertical incision dropped from the posterior extremity of this gives a very wide wound. Or it may seem preferable to use the combined incision of Morris, tying the pedicle, freeing the anterior and upper adhesions, and extracting the kidney through a vertical incision in the linea semilunaris after the lower and posterior adhesions have been freed through the lumbar wound.

2. **Resection of Ribs.**—Even in difficult cases of nephrotomy it is sometimes of the greatest assistance to enlarge the field of operation by extending the cutaneous incision up over the last two ribs and

by excising subperiosteally the outer half of these bones. Care must be taken to avoid wounding the pleura, which extends fully to the lower border of the twelfth rib and sometimes even lower. Excision of portions of these one or two lower ribs almost doubles the size of the operative field.

3. **Subcapsular Nephrectomy (Ollier) and Morcellation (Tuffier).**—When in spite of extending the incision the kidney still remains firmly adherent to its fatty capsule and to the surrounding tissue, the parenchyma may sometimes be stripped from under the fibrous capsule and the organ thus removed; but it is very difficult to control hemorrhage during this operation, and a procedure somewhat less troublesome is the morcellation of Tuffier. Even this operation requires plenty of light, plenty of time, and should not be undertaken unless the patient is in excellent condition. The lower extremity of the kidney is first attacked and usually can be quite readily separated from the surrounding strictures. One or two large, curved clamps are then fastened to the organ as high up as possible, and the lower third is removed.

The vascular pedicle is now sought for in front of the kidney, and when it has been recognised by the arterial pulsation it is clamped as near as possible to the kidney. This part of the operation is the most difficult and the most delicate. The middle third of the kidney is next attacked and its posterior surface freed from the parietes behind. The anterior surface is then somewhat liberated, another clamp applied, and the greater part of the middle third of the organ cut away. It may be of assistance to split the organ vertically at this juncture and remove the posterior half first. This done it is usually possible to separate the vascular pedicle completely and to clamp it satisfactorily, after which the upper third of the organ is shelled out bit by bit.

Treatment of the Pedicle.—If the kidney is readily separable the quickest way to remove it is to place a heavy clamp upon its pedicle as near as possible to the kidney tissue, to cut away the organ, and then, with plenty of space to work in, to ligate the artery and vein separately with heavy silk and to cut away the upper part of the ureter, ligating it as low down as possible. In those cases of malignant growth in which the kidney is not adherent, this procedure especially commends itself; although, if the tumour is large it is best to free the kidney without attempting to extract it from the wound, and to clamp the pedicle by the sense of touch only, after which the tumour may be morcellated or extracted whole. Israel insists upon the propriety of removing the cancerous kidney in one piece with its fatty capsule. Though this procedure commends itself it is not always practicable; but in any case it is not advisable to ligature the pedicle of an enlarged kidney before removing the organ. The slipping of ligatures has permitted fatal hemorrhage too often to leave any room for doubt upon this subject.

When the adherent kidney is to be removed piecemeal, or when the adhesions about the pelvis of a kidney make accurate identification of the vessels impossible, it is often necessary to grasp with clamps a mass of tissue containing the vessels, which may well be indistinguishable from the surrounding scar even after the kidney has been removed. In such an event it is safest to leave the clamps in place and to remove them at the end of the third or the fourth day.

Nephro-ureterectomy.—In tubercular or suppurative cases it is always proper and often essential to remove the ureter as low as the brim of the pelvis and there to ligate it, cauterizing the mucous membrane above the point of ligature. In tubercular cases it may be necessary to extend the parietal incision into the loin (parallel to and two fingers' breadth above Poupart's ligament) and to follow the ureter down into the pelvis, where it can be tied off almost at its point of entrance into the bladder.

Abdominal Nephrectomy. — In some cases, especially in very large adherent tumours, more space can be gained by boldly entering the peritoneal cavity through an incision in the linea semilunaris (Langenbuch) or in the linea alba, or by employing a transverse incision (Fig. 153). After entering the peritoneal cavity and pushing the intestines towards the median line, the outer layer of the mesocolon is incised (not the inner layer, for this implies division of the colic arteries and risks gangrene of the bowel). The peritoneum and colon are stripped up towards the median line, the vessels are secured, and the tumour removed. In tubercular or suppurative cases it is proper to fix the stump of the ureter into a hollow punched in the loin (Morris). The incision may be enlarged by transverse cuts at either extremity. The intraperitoneal incision has been employed for diagnosis and for the purpose of ligating or temporarily compressing the renal vessels in connection with extraperitoneal nephrectomy.

Closure of the Wound.—While the lumbar wound may be freely drained without fear of hernia, every effort should be made, if the peritoneum has been opened, to protect that cavity from infection by suture. The abdominal wall is usually sutured in layers.

OPERATIVE COMPLICATIONS

The immediate dangers of renal operations are injury to the peritoneum, the bowel, the pleura, and hemorrhage. If in removing an aseptic kidney the peritoneum is torn, it may be easily sutured and no harm is likely to result. Injury to the bowel is a more serious matter, for if the gut is opened upon a surface uncovered by peritoneum, as is usually the case, the resultant fecal fistula is likely to continue indefinitely. Injury to the pleura is rare and requires suture. Hemorrhage during operations upon the kidney is usually more alarming than dangerous. Every incision into the kidney evokes a gush of blood which may be controlled as readily as it is evoked. Exceptionally, however, alarming hemorrhage is encountered by reason of an inadvertent incision or tearing of one of the larger renal vessels, and this bleeding may require a hasty nephrectomy. Morris specifies a class of calculous cases in which the kidney is found filled with blood, and states that such cases are so prone to bleed upon section that they require immediate nephrectomy without any attempt to extract the stone.

The vena cava may be torn during nephrectomy, an accident which has been remedied by lateral clamping, but which, needless to state, is usually fatal. Pulmonary or cardiac embolism is an immediately fatal complication that may occur from thrombosis of the renal vein due to malignant growth.

Immediate Post-operative Complications

Shock, suppression, and sepsis are the three notable complications that occur immediately after operation. Shock may be associated with heart failure or it may be due simply to a severe and prolonged operation upon an enfeebled constitution. For this reason rapidity of operation and light anesthetization are especially desirable as preventives.

Shock.—The treatment of shock consists of the usual stimulants, saline infusion, and the external application of heat.

Suppression.—Suppression of urine, or uremia, with deficient urinary excretion, is doubtless due to congestion of the opposite kidney. This is obviously the case when suppression occurs after nephrotomy for calculous anuria. Therefore, if there is any question of surgical disease of the opposite kidney it is well to consider the propriety of a secondary rapid nephrotomy for the purpose of relieving congestion. Yet, practically speaking, the opportunities for such an operation are few. For if the patient becomes uremic after a nephrotomy, his vitality is likely to have sunk so low as not to withstand the shock of a second operative procedure. For this reason double nephrotomy is sometimes done simultaneously; and while I believe this treatment should almost always be adopted in cases of calculous anuria, the evidence thus far adduced is not sufficient to lead one to perform nephrotomy or to split the kidney capsule, as Sir Reginald Harrison and Edebohls would have us do, to relieve the tension alleged to exist in chronic nephritis.

In most cases, then, the treatment of suppression will be the administration of urotropin and diuretic fluids, catharsis, diaphoresis by the hot pack, and saline infusion (p. 373).

Sepsis.—Sepsis of an acute fulminating type sometimes follows nephrotomy for stone. It is very likely to carry the patient off in spite of the most vigorous stimulation and local antisepsis; but in most instances surgical wounds of the kidney drain well and are singularly free from septic complications. I have never known a clean lumbar incision to become infected, nor in my own practice have I ever had any difficulty in obtaining adequate drainage for whatever suppuration might exist in or about the kidney.

Secondary hemorrhage and hypostatic pneumonia are conditions that may follow any major operation.

RENAL FISTULA

Spontaneous Fistula.—Spontaneous renal fistula caused by the rupture of a perinephritic abscess is so rare in this surgical generation and post-operative fistula so common that it seems proper to classify renal fistula as the late complication of operations upon the kidney. Spontaneous fistula may be dismissed with a word. A pyonephrosis or a perinephritic abscess may burst through the loin into the stomach or bowel or into the pleura or lung. The occurrence of such a rupture is heralded by a sharp pain and followed by the passage of pus through the skin, from the bowel or from the bronchi, as the case may be. It is common knowledge that a large abscess bursting thus spontaneously will drain but poorly and should be submitted to prompt incision, even though the patient's condition is considered desperate; for, however ill he may be, the prolonged suppuration will only sap his strength, and his safety lies in adequate drainage.

Post-operative Fistula.—Post-operative fistula may be expected to remain patent for several weeks. In the first days the gush of urine through the wound is often considerable. In a case of calculous anuria which I operated upon on the seventh day, the kidney reacted so overwhelmingly that for twenty-four hours a bucket had to be kept under the patient's bed to catch the overflow which ran from the wound in his side. (Unhappily, the sequel was suppression and death.) In any case, this flow of urine will continue for a week or two, and probably longer after a pyelotomy than after an incision of the kidney substance. But all ordinary surgical wounds of the kidney may be expected to heal kindly unless foreign body, obstruction, disease, or a considerable loss of tissue impedes the natural process of repair.

Thus the causes of post-operative fistula may be grouped as follows:

1. Occlusion of the ureter.
2. Foreign body—e. g., stone, suture.
3. Inefficient drainage of suppurating pockets.
4. Tuberculosis or neoplasm.
5. Loss of substance of pelvis or ureter.
6. Low general vitality.
7. Lesion of the colon causing fecal fistula.

Occlusion of the ureter is probably the commonest cause of fistula after nephrotomy, and it is easily understood that so long as the ureter remains obstructed the urine will seek the right of way through the loin. In a certain number of cases the obstruction may be only comparative, the kidney being pouched and the ureter kinked. Such cases have been cured by the ureteral catheter *à demeure* (Albarran); but one cannot feel sure that a case so treated may not subsequently develop into a hydronephrosis.

The *symptoms* of a fistula are the discharge of urine or of urine mingled with pus, or, if the kidney be completely disorganized, of pure pus. In this last class of cases there is often a great deal of pocketing and marked sepsis.

Treatment.—The treatment of renal fistula is surgical. The manipulative treatment by ureteral catheter is rarely applicable. The removal of foreign bodies need not be insisted upon. For example, I have known a man to carry a tube in his loin for eight years because he feared to be without it, and to heal up in three weeks after it was extracted.

Of course local treatment by antiseptic and stimulating irrigations should be employed in conjunction with appropriate tonics and hygiene for a sufficient time before operative treatment of the fistula is considered. But if in spite of all such measures the discharge persists it can only be cured by operation. Before proceeding to cut down upon such a kidney the surgeon should familiarize himself with every detail of the patient's history and avail himself of every means of physical diagnosis in order to estimate the condition of the two kidneys. If, as is usually the case, all the urine of one kidney issues through the loin, the condition of the other is readily ascertained by examining the urine drawn from the bladder.

From the data thus obtained the surgeon should endeavour to

decide beforehand whether it is preferable to perform nephrotomy or nephrectomy. If the case is an old pyonephrosis and the opposite kidney is sound, nephrectomy usually offers the easier solution of the problem, although, under these circumstances, it is a difficult and dangerous operation. But if the kidney is comparatively sound every endeavour should be made by the use of the ureteral catheter and of any other device that may fit the case to save the kidney and to re-establish the ureteral right of way. All operations under these circumstances are complicated by the presence of masses of old fibrous scar. Hence the incision must be so planned as to reach the kidney after going through as little scar tissue as possible. In general it is preferable to make the external incision behind and below the line of the old scar (though this may not always be practicable), and to follow down behind it, guided by a finger or an instrument in the fistulous tract. The scar tissue leading down to the kidney had then best be completely excised, and the organ itself, lying embedded in a mass of fibrous tissue, dealt with as seems proper. It is in such cases as this that subcapsular nephrectomy and nephrectomy by *morcellement* are oftenest employed. Here the longest and most irregular incision and the resection of several ribs are quite justifiable procedures, while the surgeon will often save time by entering the peritoneum boldly at the beginning of the operation rather than to potter along and tear into it several times during the procedure.

PART II

DISEASES OF THE GENITAL ORGANS

CHAPTER I

DISEASES OF THE PENIS—ANATOMY—ANOMALIES—INJURIES—INFLAMMATIONS

ANATOMY

The penis is a genital organ. Its urinary function is purely secondary. It is conformed anatomically to subserve the genital function. In the adult it measures, when at rest, from the root of the scrotum to the meatus urinarius, from $2\frac{1}{2}$ to 4 inches; when erect, from 5 to 7 inches. It consists essentially of three segments—the two corpora cavernosa, lying together like the barrels of a gun, and the corpus spongiosum, like the ramrod, beneath them (Fig. 154, A), the whole surrounded by integument.

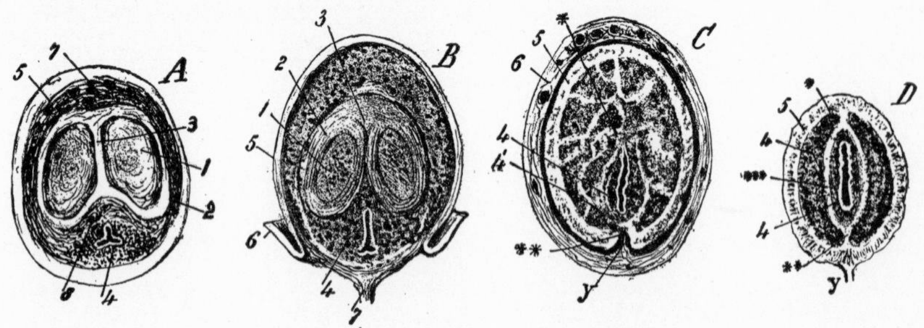

Fig. 154.—Cross-sections through the Penis (Henle).

A, through the penis just behind the glans; B, through the posterior border of the glans; C, through the middle of the same; D, just behind the meatus; *1*, corpus cavernosum; *2*, sheath of same; *3*, septum between the same; *4*, corpus spongiosum; *5*, skin of glans; *6*, prepuce; *7*, dorsal veins; *, connective tissue connecting frenum with sheath of corpus spongiosum; *y*, frenum.

The Corpora Cavernosa.—The corpora cavernosa arise on each side from the tuberosities and ascending rami of the ischium. They come together under the symphysis pubis, and continue side by side, forming the main bulk of the penis. They terminate anteriorly in a conical extremity, over which the glans penis (the terminal expansion of the corpus spongiosum) fits like a cap. There is no vascular communication between the corpora cavernosa and the glans penis, or the corpus spongiosum.

The corpora cavernosa are surrounded by fibrous sheaths which are so dense and strong that they will support the weight of the cadaver.[1] These sheaths are, however, plentifully supplied with elastic fibres, to allow for the variable size of the organ. The anterior portion of the partition between the corpora cavernosa is perforated by numerous apertures, to insure thorough and symmetrical erection. The tissue proper of the corpora cavernosa is known as spongy or erectile. During erection the areolæ of this tissue become distended with blood, as shown in Fig. 155.

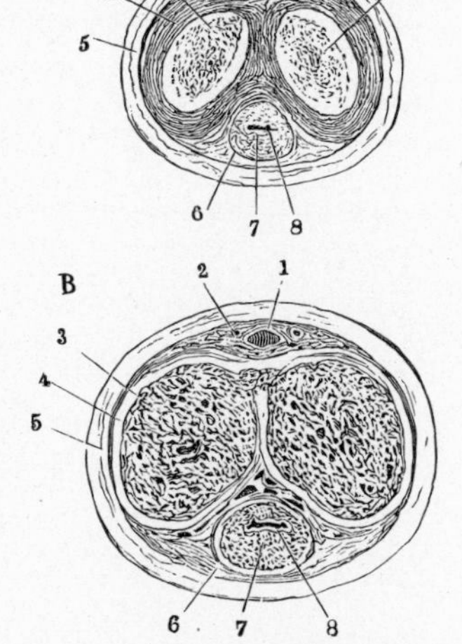

Fig. 155.—Transverse Sections of Penis (Cruveilhier).

A, flaccid. B, in erection. *1*, *2*, dorsal vein and artery; *3*, corpora cavernosa; *4*, tunica albuginea, *5*, integument; *6*, tunica albuginea of corpus spongiosum; *7*, erectile tissue; *8*, urethra.

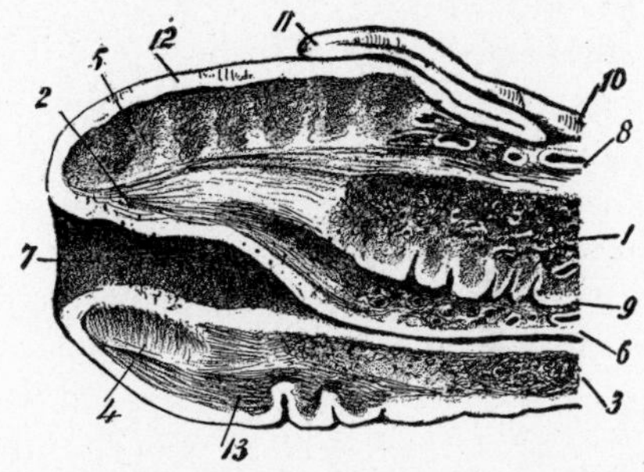

Fig. 156.—Median Section of the Glans Penis, etc. (Henle).

1, corpus cavernosum; *3*, corpus spongiosum; *5*, substance of glans; *7*, fossa navicularis; *8*, venous network of dorsum; *10*, skin; *11*, prepuce; *12*, epithelium of glans, *13*, frenum.

The Corpus Spongiosum.—The corpus spongiosum urethræ is also composed of erectile tissue. It surrounds all that portion of the urethra lying in front of the triangular ligament, anteriorly forming the glans penis which caps the conical extremity of the corpora cavernosa, posteriorly terminating in the bulb, which lies just in front of the triangular ligament in the angle of the converging corpora cavernosa.

The Glans.—The glans penis (Fig. 156) is covered by a semimucous membrane endowed with peculiar sensibility, especially

[1] Cruveilhier, Traité d'anatomie descriptive, Paris, 1865, ii, I, 386.

around the raised posterior border—the corona glandis. The epithelium covering the glans is fine, the papillæ minute (Home), the sebaceous glands (of Tyson) large and numerous, and most plentiful about the frenum. These glands secrete the white, badly smelling material (smegma) which collects behind the corona. The function of the glans penis is to furnish a soft-skinned expansion for the distribution of the terminal filaments of the nerves of sexual sensibility.

Muscular Action.—One important function of the corpus spongiosum is acquired through its bulb—namely, that of assisting in the expulsion of the last drops of urine or semen from the urethra. The prostate, the levator ani, and the deep urethral muscles—especially the compressor urethræ—contract upon the fluid remaining in the canal after micturition in that spasmodic effort called by the French *coup de piston.* This forces the last few drops beyond the bulb of the urethra. Now the fibres of the accelerator urinæ surrounding the bulb and adjacent portions of the corpus cavernosum contract, and forcibly drive the blood contained in the areolæ of the bulb forward along the corpus spongiosum, forcibly distending that body, and thus bringing the walls of the urethra more closely into contact in a progressive wave. This helps to explain, as shown by A. Guérin,[1] why in cases of organic stricture the last few drops of urine do not escape promptly but dribble away; for the scar tissue which constitutes stricture obliterates the areolæ of the erectile tissue and thus obstructs the free passage of the wave of blood along the corpus spongiosum.

Fascia.—The three erectile bodies which have been briefly described are surrounded by the fascial sheath of the penis—a membrane important in its pathological relations, and sometimes known as Buck's fascia, from the distinguished surgeon who first accurately described it.[2] This fascia arises from the symphysis pubis by a triangular bundle of fibres, the suspensory ligament of the penis, and from the pubic rami at the attachment of the anterior layer of the triangular ligament. Thence it runs forward, surrounding the corpora cavernosa and the corpus spongiosum in two separate compartments. The lower plane of this fascia is in its posterior part identical with the deep layer of the perineal fascia. The cavity of Buck's fascia is bounded anteriorly by the base of the glans penis and posteriorly by the triangular ligament. Hence periurethral cellulitis and extravasation are habitually confined within these limits

---

[1] Mém. de la Soc. de Chir., vol. iv, 1857.

[2] Trans. Am. Med. Ass'n, vol. i, p. 367.

for an indefinite time, unless at the root of the penis where the fascia blends with that covering the pubes, and leaves a loophole of escape into the areolar tissue of the abdominal wall.

Vessels.—The lymphatics and veins of the penis run along the dorsum, and receive in their course branches from the corpus spongiosum. The lymphatics lead mainly to glands lying along and above Poupart's ligament on each side. The arteries arise from the internal pudics.

Connective Tissue.—The connective tissue between the skin and Buck's fascia is very loose and elastic, and, like that of the eyelids, does not contain fat.

Skin.—The skin of the penis, except that it tends to become pigmented after puberty, does not differ essentially from ordinary integument. Over the glans penis it folds back upon itself, forming a non-adherent sheath for the glans (the prepuce), evidently intended to preserve the delicate sensibility of this portion of the member.

The Prepuce.—The prepuce is composed of two layers, a cutaneous (external) and a more delicate semi-mucous (internal). The point of junction of these two is called the orifice of the prepuce. Between these layers is a very loose and elastic connective tissue, without fat, which permits the two surfaces to be entirely separated from each other, and the prepuce effaced, by drawing back the integument of the penis until the glans is entirely uncovered. The mucous layer of the prepuce is supplied with glands (of Tyson). It is much less elastic than the cutaneous layer.

The prepuce is attached to the lower angle of the meatus urinarius by a triangular fold of mucous membrane called the frenum preputii—analogous to the frenum linguæ. The frenum contains a small artery which when cut or torn bleeds freely.

ANOMALIES OF THE PENIS

Deformities of the penis are constituted by abnormalities in some of its constituent parts. The most common examples will be mentioned in connection with these parts. As anomalies of the penis as a whole, two conditions demand special notice—double penis and absence of the organ. Anomalies in size occur, as when the penis is 9 or 10 inches long when at rest, or only a couple of inches long when erect; but these variations require no comment.

Double Penis.—Double penis is excessively rare. It is analogous to double uterus and vagina in the female, but by no means so common. Undoubtedly it is not so rare as the records of surgery imply, for the existence of this deformity is naturally accompanied by an excessive sensitiveness on the part of the patient which leads him to shun observation; and, as the defect is not necessarily accompanied by any injurious symptoms, the patient does not voluntarily subject himself to the inspection of a physician, and thus keeps himself out of the books. Hence the cases usually reported, such as those of Hart,[1] and Gorre,[2] accompany grosser malformations of fetal inclusion. The case reported in the first edition of this treatise [3] is a notable exception. Similar ones are reported by Drs. Alan P. Smith,[4] J. Lorthior,[5] and Carl Beck.[6]

Smith's patient had a stone in one of his bladders, was cut and cured. He could urinate from either bladder at will.

Torsion of the Penis.—With epispadias and hypospadias the penis may be more or less completely twisted upon itself. Jacobson [7] has collected a number of cases. In Caddy's [8] case the torsion was unaccompanied by any urethral defect.

Absence of Penis.—The various amputations of the penis, surgical, traumatic, or gangrenous, do not concern us here. The congenital deformity is a rare one, and usually unaccompanied by any faulty development of the testicles or of other parts of the body. The scrotum, however, is usually small and may be bifid. In either case the external genitals closely resemble those of a woman. In fact this is male pseudo-hermaphroditism. Harris,[9] in a recent review, emphasizes what he claims is an infallible sign of the sex of such a person if an adult. If a female, the upper border of the pubic hair forms a clearly cut transverse line across the hypogastrium, while the hair of the male rises up in a curved line towards the umbilicus.

The urethra opens in the median perineal raphe or on the anterior rectal wall. In the latter case there is danger of ascending infection, as actually occurred in Matthews's [10] case. This patient, in spite of his manifest impotence, was a married man. Harris collected 6 cases, including 1 of his own, omitting 2, Révolat's [11] and Wright's.[12] More recently Preston [13] has reported a case.

---

[1] Lancet, 1866, i, 71.

[2] Compt. rend. de l'Acad. des Sciences, 1844.

[3] Case I, p. 5.

[4] Trans. Med. and Chir., Faculty of Maryland, April, 1878.

[5] Centralbl. f. d. Krankh. d. Harn. u. Sex.-Org., 1901, xii, 381.

[6] Med. News, 1901, lxxix, 451.

[7] Diseases of the Male Organs of Generation, 1892, p. 612.

[8] Lancet, 1894, ii, 634.

[9] Phila. Med. J., 1898, i, 71.

[10] Amer. Practitioner and News, 1894, xvii, 27.

[11] J. de Sédillot, xxvii, 370, Demarquay, Maladies chir. du pénis, Paris, 1879, p. 538.

[12] Ashby and Wright, Diseases of Children, p. 531.

[13] Med. Record, 1898, liv, 315.

Apparent Absence of Penis.—Congenital dislocation or apparent absence of the penis exists when the penis, lacking its proper sheath of skin, lies buried beneath the integument of the abdomen, thigh, or scrotum. Boutelier [1] reports such a case. Under the skin above the scrotum a movable body was felt, liberated by incision, and discovered to be the penis. Another case, reported by J. Murphy,[2] would seem to be rather a penile adhesion to the hypogastrium, for the child could urinate through a hole in the lower part of the abdomen. The *treatment* of such a condition implies the immediate liberation of the incarcerated member to avoid urinary infiltration. In this emergency any method of covering the denuded penis with skin may be employed, the simpler the better, leaving until later years the task of affording a more satisfactory envelope to the organ.

Congenital incurvation of the penis and scrotal concealment of that organ occur as phenomena accessory to hypospadias, and will be considered as such in the proper place.

Hermaphroditism.—Accepting Klebs's definition of true hermaphroditism—viz., the existence of dissimilar genital glands (i. e., at least one testis and one ovary) in one individual—there is still some doubt whether any such individual has existed. Dr. Blacker and Mr. Lawrence [3] maintain the positive side of the question, and find in the literature foundation for their belief. However this may be, we may rest assured that in no case has it been recorded that the person was, functionally, both male and female, producing both spermatozoa and ova. On the contrary, as a general rule they are sexually neuter. These true hermaphrodites resemble clinically the pseudo-hermaphrodites—persons whose sex can with difficulty be determined—and they sometimes come to the surgeon asking him to make them distinctively male or female, whichever he may deem more appropriate. In deciding such a question, if the external genitals are quite indeterminate—as they often are—the chief characteristics to be considered are the shape of skeleton, the disposition of the superficial fat, the growth of hair, facial and pubic (see above), the voice and the shape of the larynx, and, finally, the sexual sentiments of the individual. The process of "making a man of him" or "a woman of her" may be long and tedious, but may prove successful, as in a case reported by Gruber,[4] in which amputa-

---

[1] Union méd. de la Seine infér., 1875, xi, 27.
[2] Brit. Med. J., 1885, ii, 62.
[3] Trans. Obstet. Soc., Lond., 1896, xxxviii, 265.
[4] Centralbl. f. d. ges. Therap., Wien, 1897, xv, 385.

tion of the hypertrophied clitoris, posterior colpotomy to enlarge the rudimentary vagina, and electric epilation of the facial hair sufficed to establish the external female characteristics.

ACCIDENTS TO THE PENIS AS A WHOLE

Wounds.—The penis is liable to be wounded by accident or by design. In the latter case insanity, or the melancholy depression produced by masturbation, usually induces the patient to mutilate himself; or the injury may be inflicted by a jealous woman.

Superficial cuts are unimportant, but wounds extending through the sheaths of the corpora cavernosa may give rise to troublesome, possibly fatal, hemorrhage, while the cicatrices left after healing may distort the penis and render erection imperfect and painful.

In a case of traumatic aneurysm of the penis due to a knife-cut, Malgaigne [1] had to tie the dorsal artery.

Treatment.—Cleanse the wound. If a large artery be spurting, tie it, but disregard the oozing points. Endeavour to obtain primary union by immediate suture. Introduce the sutures just deep enough to hold the fibrous sheath. Employ moderate pressure in dressing. Erections, which are sure to occur, since the local inflammation induces a flux of blood, always retard healing.

Even in cases seemingly desperate, where the penis has been almost wholly severed from the body, an attempt should be made to save it. A remarkable success in a case of this sort, where the whole penis was severed except a portion of one corpus cavernosum, is related by Artaud.[2] Erectile power is not regained after such a recovery.

Contusions.—The escape of blood under the skin after superficial contusions of the penis is often excessive, on account of the laxity of the connective tissue and the large size of the superficial veins. Deeper contusions give rise to localized swelling from circumscribed effusion of blood. This swelling fluctuates and deforms the penis more or less, sometimes causing it to deviate when erect. If the contusion be severe enough, inflammation of the corpora cavernosa results, ending in suppuration or gangrene. Severe contusions involving the urethra may lead to infiltration of urine and urethral fistula with loss of substance.

The introduction of the penis into a ring is a classical accident. The penis swells, the patient is ashamed to seek relief, and serious

---

[1] Revue Medico-Chir. de Paris, 1850, p. 52.

[2] Bull. de la Soc. de Chir., vii, p. 451.

inflammatory mischief—even gangrene, urinary fistula—may ensue. Guillot in such a case conceived the happy idea of dissolving the ring, which was of gold, in a bath of mercury. Demarquay [1] narrates many curious instances of a similar character.

Excessive subcutaneous hemorrhage may be controlled by the application of cold and pressure, with due regard for the possibility of sloughing if the treatment is overdone. Later, simple pressure to promote absorption will suffice, or the clots may be evacuated through an incision made under local anesthesia with the usual aseptic precautions. If gangrene occur, the penis should be kept absolutely dry and clean by applying a mildly antiseptic powder and a gauze dressing. The gangrenous tissue may be removed piecemeal, until it has all been cleared away, after which the gaps may be filled in by skin-grafting or by a plastic operation.

(For injuries involving the urethra, refer to diseases of that canal.)

Fracture of the Penis

When the fibrous sheaths of the corpora cavernosa are ruptured by sudden forcible flexion of the erect penis, a sort of fracture of the member is produced, with extensive extravasation of blood, sometimes amounting to traumatic aneurysm. Pain, generally present, is sometimes replaced by a sensation of heat, distention, and weight. Valentine Mott [2] reported 2 interesting cases of this accident, where the only treatment employed was rest and cold locally applied. Both recovered with a useful organ and no deformity. Demarquay has cited many others.

Treatment.—A stout woven catheter, strong enough to resist lateral compression, is passed into the bladder to insure the patulousness of the urethra. Upon this the penis may be bandaged and cold applied. If the pressure proves unbearable or if gangrene, extravasation or cellulitis threaten, the clots must be evacuated and the bleeding checked through an incision made with all aseptic precautions.

After recovery an indurated spot may remain permanently to mark the site of the injury, perhaps making erection imperfect or painful and interfering with sexual intercourse.

Fracture of the Corpus Spongiosum.—Fracture of the corpus spongiosum is generally occasioned by "breaking the chordee" in gonorrhea (p. 63). The inflamed tissue gives way, yielding urethral hemorrhage as an immediate and traumatic stricture as a remote result.

[1] Maladies chir. du pénis, Paris, 1877.
[2] Trans. of the N. Y. Acad. of Med., vol. i, Part I, 1851, p. 99.

The healthy corpus spongiosum may be fractured during erection. Dittel[1] gives one such case. I have seen another.[2]

Dislocation of the Penis

When the integument of the penis is violently dragged upon, as, for instance, when the clothes are caught and torn away upon a revolving wheel, the entire penis may be shot out of its investing cutaneous sheath and lodged in the scrotum, the perineum, the groin, or under the integument of the abdomen. In such cases, the semimucous membrane of the prepuce gives way either at the preputial orifice or just behind the corona. A number of instances of this curious luxation have been recorded.[3] The penile injury is usually not discovered until retention of urine or the passage of urine by some opening at a distance from the preputial orifice directs attention to the contused genitals, when the penis is found to be only a sheath of integument containing clotted blood. Sometimes it has been difficult to find the penis at all; but an intelligent search will always reveal it, and then the surgeon's obvious duty is to replace it in its sheath, incising the integument about the root of the sheath as far as may be necessary to attain the desired result.

In dislocation, the urethra is often ruptured low down, and, after the organ has been replaced in its sheath, external perineal section without a guide may be called for (p. 35). In this way the continuity of the canal is restored.

In one case, a six-year-old child, Nélaton reduced a dislocated penis through the preputial orifice by means of Cooper's aneurysm needle, assisting its hook action by external manipulation.

CUTANEOUS AND MUCO-CUTANEOUS AFFECTIONS OF THE PENIS

Many common skin diseases involve the skin of the penis as well as other integumentary parts. As a rule, they present no special characteristics and require no comment here. *Venereal sores*, true chancre and chancroid, are common, as also are soft venereal warts. These receive mention later. A rare disease is *scabies*, which, causing ulcerated spots and enlarged inguinal glands, may be mistaken for chancroid, from which it may be differentiated by the "burrows" and the accompanying interdigital lesions. Jacobson reports a case

---

[1] Wien. med. Blätter, 1885, Nr. 2.

[2] Van Buren and Keyes, 1st Ed., p. 7.

[3] *Cf.* Goldsmith, Lancet, 1898, ii, 387.

of epitheliomatous degeneration occurring in a patch of *eczema* which covered the root of the penis and the inner third of the groin. Hutchinson[1] circumcised a boy for *lupus* of the prepuce and obtained a perfect result. Rake, of Trinidad,[2] has performed circumcision on 16 *lepers*, and, even though the incision actually traversed a leprous patch, it always healed kindly.

Herpes Progenitalis.—This affection consists in the development of clusters of vesicles upon reddened patches on the mucous covering of the glans, or on either layer of the prepuce, or on other portions of the neighbouring skin, attended by a slight sensation of heat and tingling. When occurring on the cuticular layer, herpes runs its course as it does elsewhere on the body, but when vesicles develop within the preputial orifice the eruption is modified. Under these circumstances the epithelium of the vesicles is soaked off, little exulcerations result, more or less general inflammation is likely to arise from retention of the secretions, and balanitis, with posthitis, vegetations, and inflammatory phimosis, may be the ultimate result. In exceptional cases the ulcerations perhaps become deep and angry, and the diagnosis with chancroid difficult, while the glands in one groin or both may inflame and suppurate. These extreme results are rare.

When the affection has once occurred, it shows a marked tendency to recur. There is often a periodicity about the attacks. Tight prepuce and contact of irritating discharges act as predisposing causes.

Diagnosis.—Vesicles, usually in groups, always precede the ulcerations, while the latter are irregular in shape, superficial, and very rarely complicated by suppurating bubo. The pus is not auto-inoculable. Attention to these points will generally render diagnosis with chancroid easy; where grave doubts exist, auto-inoculation is the proper test.

Treatment.—The treatment is the same as for balanitis. Touching the tingling, congested patch before, or even just after, the commencement of vesiculation several times a day with eucalyptol, while it does not abort the attack seems to shorten it. As soon as the vesicles break a dry antiseptic powder is suitable (nosophen, bismuth). In relapsing cases circumcision or a long course of iron and arsenic internally often effects a permanent cure.

Herpes Zoster.—Zoster may occur upon the penis as elsewhere.

---

[1] Arch. of Surg., 1890, ii, 17.

[2] St. Louis Med. and Surg. J., 1893, lxiv, 221.

Balanoposthitis

Balanitis (*βάλανος, a gland*) is an inflammation of the surface of the glans penis. Posthitis (*πόσθη, the prepuce*) is an inflammation affecting the mucous surface of the prepuce chiefly. Neither can exist for any length of time without becoming more or less complicated by the other. For practical purposes they must be considered together.

Etiology.—Persons of irritable skin and gouty habit are predisposed to this disorder. A long and tight prepuce is always a predisposing cause. The exciting causes are mechanical irritation or uncleanliness from retention of smegma, or from prolonged contact with diabetic urine, gonorrheal, leukorrheal, menstrual, or other irritating fluids.

Symptoms.—The membrane at first becomes reddened, then mottled and moist; next the epithelium comes off in patches, leaving irregular excoriations which soon ulcerate and discharge a purulent fluid. The ulcerations are not preceded by vesicles. There is a burning soreness with itching at the end of the penis, usually scalding on urination. The entire substance of the prepuce may inflame, become intensely reddened around the orifice and infiltrated with serum, producing inflammatory phimosis, especially if the prepuce be naturally long or tight. The ulcerations rarely become deep, and the inguinal glands do not often suppurate, but they may grow somewhat large and tender. In chronic balanitis with phimosis, the mucous surface of the prepuce is granular and even condylomatous.

R. W. Taylor [1] has described a peculiar ringed affection of the prepuce and glans—narrow rings of reddened mucous membrane covered by a thin layer of epithelial scales. The inclosed area is normal, the rings vary from $\frac{1}{4}$ to $\frac{1}{2}$ inch in diameter. The affection is sometimes painful or itching. The rings remain stationary for a time. They may come out in successive crops. They get well without scar, slowly, under the use of arsenic internally. They should not be confounded with lichen planus of the glans penis.

Kaufmann [2] mentions a diphtheritic balanoposthitis occurring in the course of acute exanthems or by infection during circumcision. Taylor [3] has seen similar cases, some of them, when neglected, going on to gangrene and death.

Diabetic balanoposthitis is not uncommon. It is caused by con-

---

[1] Arch. of Med., 1884, vol. xii, No. 3.
[2] Billroth and Lücke, Deutsch. Chir., Part 50 a.
[3] Venereal Diseases, 1897, p. 393.

tact of the saccharine urine. In these cases German investigators have found a fungus which they regard as characteristic; Friedrich [1] even going so far as to diagnose diabetes from the presence of this fungus in the balanitic secretion, there being not enough sugar in the urine to respond to the copper test. Soundley [2] says: "Eczema of the genitals . . . is undoubtedly set up by the irritation produced by torulæ and other organisms which grow in the saccharine moisture remaining on the parts."

Although Hebrews are predisposed to diabetes, circumcision saves them from this complication.

Diagnosis.—Balanitis may be confounded with herpes, chancroid, chancre, or gonorrhea. At the ulcerative stage it cannot be distinguished from balanitis supervening upon herpes. If herpes be seen early its vesicular origin distinguishes it. Chancre is usually single and indurated. In chancroid the ulcerations are deeper and the pus auto-inoculable, yet both of these specific ulcers may be complicated by balanitis. Balanitis has been described under the name of external gonorrhea. It may be mistaken for actual gonorrhea if there be phimosis, under which circumstance it is very likely to complicate the main malady. When the meatus urinarius can be seen, however, it is easy to decide whether the pus comes from the urethra or not.

Prognosis.—While balanitis usually yields readily to appropriate treatment, diabetic cases are intractable as long as the exciting cause, glycosuria, persists, while the chronic balanitis of gouty individuals is as difficult to cure as the eczema from which they suffer.

Adhesions due to balanitis are uncommon after early childhood. In elderly persons, however, the possibility of epitheliomatous degeneration in a patch of chronic balanitis must be borne in mind.

Treatment.—If the prepuce can be easily retracted—without causing paraphimosis—simple balanitis may be speedily relieved. Cleanliness is of the first importance, but soap should not be used. Warm water, or sublimate solution (1: 5,000) will remove all the discharges. After washing, the parts should be dried by gently touching them with a soft cloth, and dusted (by the aid of a dry camel's-hair brush from which the powder may be evenly shaken) with bismuth and calomel, nosophen, or any fine stimulating powder. If the ulcerations are deep nosophen or deodorized iodoform is preferable. A piece of old linen, just large enough to cover the glans, and with a hole cut in its centre so that it may be slipped like a collar around the corona, is now to be moistened in a mild

[1] Virchow's Archiv, 1864, xxx, 476. [2] Allbutt's Sys. of Med., 1897, iv, 217.

antiseptic solution (sublimate 1:10,000, or acetate of aluminum 2%, or aromatic wine and water equal parts) and laid over the glans, leaving the meatus uncovered. The prepuce is then pulled forward to its natural position. In this way friction between the inflamed surfaces is avoided, all the discharges are absorbed, and a mildly stimulating fluid is kept in constant contact with the ulcerated or abraded surfaces. The dressing should be repeated 2 to 4 times daily, according to the discharge. After recovery a dry piece of linen should be kept between the glans and the prepuce for some weeks, renewed twice daily.

If the prepuce cannot be retracted, its *cul-de-sac* should be thoroughly washed out from 2 to 6 times a day, according to the severity of the inflammation, with peroxid of hydrogen; and each time after the cavity has been cleaned, enough of one of the lotions above mentioned to distend the prepuce should be gently thrown in, retained a moment, and then allowed to escape.

If the prepuce be much inflamed, rest, position, and wet antiseptic dressings locally should be used in addition to the other measures. If the inflammation run so high that sloughing of the prepuce seems imminent, it is better to take off the tension by slitting up the dorsum. If chancroid be present, however, the surgeon must remember that inoculation of the wound is inevitable. Yet chancroidal cases require operation most urgently in order to expose the sore, whose ravages (perhaps upon the glans penis) are progressing uncontrolled. A large chancroid exposed is better than a small one concealed. (See Circumcision.)

Circumcision.—In chronic and inveterate cases, or where insignificant causes produce constant relapse, circumcision affords a certain cure. All the unhealthy, thickened, inner layer of the prepuce should be removed. Where this is seriously objected to, which is rarely the case when there is much suffering, relapses may be rendered less frequent by the observance of the strictest cleanliness, and the use of a filtered solution of tannin and acetate of lead, or of tannic acid in glycerin (10%), or of alcohol (33%) kept up for a long time, followed by long use of a piece of dry linen to separate the mucous surfaces.

Circumcision in diabetics, while almost certain to prove curative, is no light matter. Diabetics bear any operative interference very ill, and several deaths from circumcision are recorded. Therefore, while trying the milder methods, special attention should be paid to the patient's general condition, in order that, if these methods prove unsuccessful, operation may be undertaken with the greatest possible chance of success.

ACUTE INFLAMMATORY AFFECTIONS OF THE PENIS

Superficial inflammation of the penis, while rare and usually mild, may require energetic treatment; for though the vascular supply is abundant the vessels, lying in a loose, cellular tissue, become occluded by slight inflammatory exudates whence gangrene or chronic edema results, and, moreover, the numerous lymphatics and the loose subcutaneous connective tissue encourage rapid dissemination of the inflammation.

The inflammation is rarely traumatic, usually venereal, and sometimes arises from the neighbouring parts.

The *varieties* of acute superficial inflammation are cellulitis, lymphangitis, and erysipelas.

Cellulitis.—Cellulitis arises from chancroids, balanoposthitis (especially if complicated by phimosis), traumatic infection, or gonorrheal periurethritis. The inflammation may spread to the abdomen, scrotum, or thighs, or it may involve the erectile bodies, thus adding the dangers of embolism, retention of urine, and urinary infiltration, and greatly increasing the tendency to gangrene.

Lymphangitis.—Lymphangitis is comparatively benign. A lymphangitis of the large dorsal lymphatic may be differentiated from phlebitis of the dorsal vein by the fact that the cord of induration extends outward, at the root of the penis, towards a group of enlarged glands, instead of disappearing beneath the symphysis pubis.

Erysipelas.—Erysipelas of the penis is rarely seen nowadays, though it was formerly not uncommon. It usually spreads to the penis from the adjoining regions, though it may originate in a local lesion. It is likely to be virulent and complicated by cellulitis (phlegmonous erysipelas).

Treatment.—Prophylaxis, by careful treatment of the causes of inflammation, is of the first importance. If the penis has already become inflamed it should be elevated, with the scrotum, by a T-bandage and wet dressings of sublimate (1:10,000) or aluminum acetate (2%) applied daily. Rest in bed, free purgation, and a light diet are essential in the more severe cases. Tension may be relieved by scarification or incision, abscesses must be opened and drained, and sloughs speedily removed.

In erysipelas, dressings of ichthyol (50% in glycerin and water, painted on) are especially valuable. A subsiding lymphangitis may leave a chronic induration behind it.

Cavernitis and Penitis (inflammation of the corpora cavernosa or of all three erectile bodies) arise from cellulitis or its causes, especially inflammation in the bulb of the corpus spongiosum.

Sexual excess (Demarquay) and iliac thrombosis have also been incriminated.

Course.—The course of the disease is that of an acute inflammation with constant priapism and edema added to the usual local symptoms. While the inflammation may be walled in by occlusion of the vascular spaces, pyemia is "a terribly frequent complication" (Jacobson).

Treatment.—The treatment should therefore be most energetic. Indurations in the erectile bodies should be freely incised, packed to check the hemorrhage, and irrigated frequently. This treatment and in doubtful cases the diagnosis, may require general anesthesia. Wet dressings should be employed.

Acute Gout of the Penis.—Sir J. Paget[1] reports a case in which penitis and urethritis alternated with and accompanied typical gouty symptoms. Sir Dyce Duckworth[2] chronicles a similar case. Priapism and retention were the chief symptoms.

OTHER DISEASES OF THE PENIS AS A WHOLE

Neuralgia of the Penis.—In some cases this might be classified as a gouty condition. The gouty diathesis, a neurotic temperament, and previous urethral disease are the chief etiological factors. The pain may be paroxysmal or continuous. It may be felt at the meatus, along the urethra, or throughout the organ. The first point in *treatment* is to insure the good health, physiological as well as anatomical, of the genito-urinary organs by appropriate treatment and insistence upon urethral and sexual hygiene. Following this the neurotic or gouty propensity must be combated. I have found the administration of large quantities of water, with alkalies or uric-acid solvents, peculiarly efficacious. Jacobson mentions a cure by colchicum.

Chronic Edema.—Chronic edema may be caused by a local obstruction to venous return, but is usually seen only as a feature of general anasarca. The swelling of the scrotum usually overshadows that of the penis and may be so great as practically to obliterate that organ. In the penis the edema is greatest in the prepuce and especially about the frenum. This edema may offer a mechanical impediment to urination, and the low vitality of the tissues renders them especially liable to become inflamed by contact with the urine that dribbles over them.

---

[1] *Op. cit.*, p. 684.
[2] Trans. Clin. Soc., Lond., 1891-92, xxv, 97.

Treatment.—The prepuce must be kept dry and dusted with a soothing powder. Multiple punctures or incisions may liberate the exudate sufficiently to keep the swelling within bounds, and, these failing, a dorsal incision will succeed. Light edema may be controlled by bandaging, elevation, and painting with collodion.

Dilatation of the Lymphatics.—This condition is secondary to trauma or inguinal adenitis. The dilated lymphatics appear as white, subcutaneous cords encircling the penis behind the corona or extending along the sides or dorsum, where I have seen them form a leathery patch an inch square. There are no subjective symptoms and the obstruction may be relieved spontaneously. For esthetic reasons multiple ligation or total excision may be resorted to, but a lymph fistula can result from such treatment.

Elephantiasis.—This condition is so rare in the penis alone that the whole subject receives more appropriate treatment with diseases of the scrotum.

Gangrene is usually the result of inflammation. It may, however, come on independent of any local inflammation. Spontaneous gangrene usually occurs in connection with the acute exanthems. Cases have been reported from typhoid, typhus, intermittent fever, and small-pox. Senile and diabetic gangrene also occur. Cases following prolonged priapism, iliac thrombosis, atheroma of the dorsal artery, exposure to cold, and acute alcoholism are also cited by Jacobson.

Treatment.—The prophylactic measure—incision of inflammatory and edematous areas—has already been noted. When gangrene has once declared itself, attention to the patient's general condition, the preservation of dryness, asepsis, and warmth locally, and the prompt removal of all frankly gangrenous tissue are the therapeutic indications. Later, plastic work may be required to cover areas left bare of integument. Cicatricial deformity of the erectile bodies can be remedied only by time and by such physiological rest or exercise as may suit each individual case.

Tuberculosis.—Tubercular urethritis apart, tubercular ulcers may appear upon the glans or result from infection during ritual circumcision. Senn[1] relates 2 cases illustrating the difficulty of differentiating the lesions of gumma, tubercle, and cancer. The diagnosis may depend upon the pathological examination of a snipping from the ulcer.

Treatment.—Poncet[2] advises internal remedies, aided by the curette or the cautery. This course has proved satisfactory at Senn's hands.

---

[1] Tuberculosis of the Genito-urinary Organs, 1898, p. 22.
[2] La médecine moderne, 1893, 750.

CHAPTER II

PHIMOSIS—CIRCUMCISION—PARAPHIMOSIS

Preputial Deformities.—Practically, the deformities of the foreskin (phimosis and atresia of the orifice excepted) are unimportant. The prepuce is sometimes bifid, enlarged into a pouch, redundant, projecting 1 cm. or more beyond the apex of the glans, or only rudimentary from arrest of development. Between the latter two limits it may be of any length, covering more or less of the glans. When the prepuce is deficient, the epithelium of the uncovered glans penis becomes hard and tough, more nearly resembling ordinary cuticle. Under these circumstances the sensibility of the part is diminished, but at the same time it is rendered less liable to become excoriated or inflamed. Hence, absence of the prepuce is not to be regretted, and the operation for its restoration (posthioplasty) need not be described. Dieffenbach performed it once on account of neuralgia of the glans penis.

PHIMOSIS

Phimosis (φιμοω, *I bind*) exists where the orifice of the prepuce is so small that the glans penis cannot be uncovered. The orifice of the prepuce may be congenitally absent (atresia preputii). Phimosis is congenital or acquired, simple or inflammatory, or complicated by other diseases or by adhesions.

In young children preputial redundancy is so common that it may be considered normal. The foreskin of an infant is developed out of all proportion to the rest of the penis, taking the member after puberty as a standard of comparison. This long prepuce is often a source of anxiety to young mothers, who fear that the condition may remain permanent. They may be assured that it will right itself as the child grows. Whenever the prepuce can be retracted sufficiently to permit the glans to be seen there need be no anxiety about the future; the preputial orifice will enlarge sufficiently before or at puberty.

A positive indication for operation upon a child does exist, however, where the preputial orifice is smaller than that of the urethra. This condition is evinced by ballooning of the prepuce during micturition, for the urine flows into the cavity more rapidly than it can escape from the orifice. In these cases the retention of a drop or two of urine in the cavity of the prepuce after each act of urination must, sooner or later, lead to inflammation of one or both of the mucous surfaces, and may give rise to severe suppurative inflammation, the growth of vegetations, adhesion of the prepuce to the glans, formation of preputial stone, or incrustation of the glans.

When the prepuce is tight in the adult, an operation may be called for as a prophylactic against future disease, although phimosis, strictly speaking, does not exist. For example, the collection of smegma, or repeated attacks of herpes, may give rise to an inflammation necessitating operation under unfavourable circumstances. Again, if an individual with tight prepuce gets chancre, chancroid, or gonorrhea, serious inflammatory complications are likely to arise.

Phimosis may be brought about secondarily through induration and inelasticity of the skin caused by frequent attacks of preputial inflammation. The meshes of the connective tissue, at first distended with serum, become secondarily thickened and hypertrophied, sometimes to an extent almost worthy of the name of elephantiasis. The serum is absorbed and its place supplied by a hyperplasia of connective tissue, leaving a thick, long, indurated, inelastic prepuce, interfering not only with sexual intercourse but sometimes even with urination.

Another common cause of acquired phimosis is the cicatrization of multiple chancroids around the orifice of the prepuce. Infrequently, diabetic eczema produces a phimosis. Circumcision under such circumstances is rather a serious matter, as several deaths have been put on record. Demarquay quotes a case, reported by Marx, where a passionate and jealous woman made her lover wear a gold padlock (sometimes two) with which she secured the preputial orifice, keeping the key herself. The victim of her charms carried his padlocks, which were replaced from time to time through new punctures, during four or five years, until such a degree of irritation had been set up that Petroz and Dupuytren, when consulted, diagnosticated cancer, and removed the prepuce. No relapse of the cancer is recorded.

Inflammatory Phimosis.—Inflammatory phimosis is a transient condition. It may leave true phimosis behind, as above detailed, but usually does not. Any variety of phimosis may be complicated by inflammation. It is better not to circumcise when the prepuce is inflamed, as the process of repair is slow and an ugly cicatrix may result. If the inflammation is caused by chancroid, however, circumcision is usually required to cure the disease, though the wound will probably become infected with the chancroidal virus.

Treatment.—Keep the patient in bed and elevate the penis over the hypogastrium. Astringent wet dressings must be employed locally, while the cavity of the prepuce is irrigated repeatedly by means of a syringe with a flat nozzle with some mildly stimulating lotion, such as dilute lead-water or carbolic acid (0.5%). If this fails, circumcise.

Remote Results of Phimosis.—Besides predisposing to local inflammatory disorders, leading to imperfect development of the glans penis, and acting as an obstacle to sexual intercourse, phimosis may occasion a variety of morbid conditions by reflex action. It may excite frequent desire to urinate (irritability of the bladder), even cystitis; but its disturbing influence in a reflex way upon the rest of the organism I believe has been very much overrated.

Dr. Sayre has published several cases of relaxation of the muscles of the back with curvature of the spine in children, caused by phimosis with adhesions, the local irritation being so great as to keep the little patient in a condition of almost constant priapism. Prolapsus ani and hernia not infrequently accompany phimosis in children, and symptoms resembling those of stone in the bladder are not uncommon from the same cause.

CIRCUMCISION

Excessive length of the prepuce may demand operative interference. Immoderate length alone, however, can hardly be said to constitute a defect, and may be left unmolested unless complicated by induration, thickening, or a contracted preputial orifice (phimosis), or unless it occasions and keeps up balanitis or herpes. Great length of the prepuce is sometimes the result of constant traction, as in children with stone.

Circumcision should be performed on uninflamed phimosis. The inconveniences and dangers likely to result from the phimosis when compared with the simplicity and innocuousness of the operation leave room for no exceptions.

Inflammatory phimosis should, as above noted, be treated by local applications until subsidence of the inflammation effects complete cure or permits the operation to be done without undue danger of infection. In some cases, however—notably the diabetic and chancroidal ones—operation may be indicated immediately.

Under such conditions the simpler procedure of dorsal incision (p. 670) recommends itself as being less of a shock to diabetics and presenting a smaller wound surface for auto-inoculation with the chancroidal virus. When the danger has passed, a secondary true circumcision will produce an esthetic result.

The Operation.—In the operation of circumcision the orifice of the prepuce, with more or less of its mucous and cutaneous layers, is cut away. According to Hebrew chronologists, circumcision was instituted as a religious rite by Abraham in the year of the world 2059—nineteen hundred and forty-one years before Christ. Several Eastern nations still practise it as a hygienic measure. The chosen people preserve the custom as a religious ceremony, performing it on the eighth day.

Few operations in surgery have received more modifications than this simple one of ablation of the prepuce. The indication is to remove the orifice of the prepuce and all redundant tissue, and to insure looseness of what is left. This may be accomplished as follows:

1. In the infant neither anesthetic nor sutures are essential, although one suture at the frenum is desirable. Older patients require general anesthesia if they are disposed to be nervous; otherwise local anesthesia may be satisfactorily employed. The cocain or eucain is injected in a circle around the penis just back of the proposed line of incision. The preputial cavity is then filled with a stronger (5%) solution, which is retained by pinching together the lips of the prepuce until anesthesia is complete—about five minutes should be allowed. Constriction of the penis is not essential.

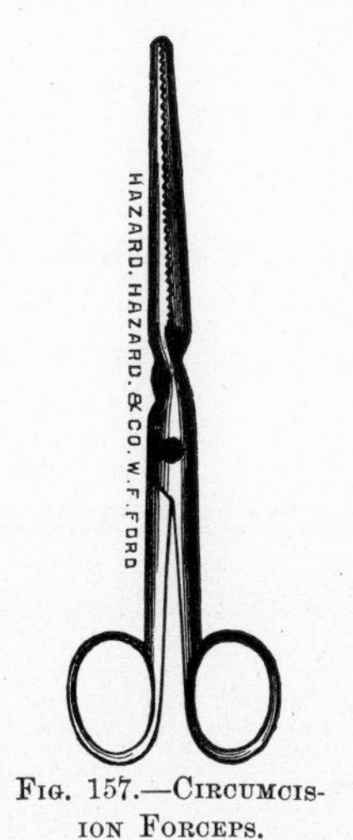

Fig. 157.—Circumcision Forceps.

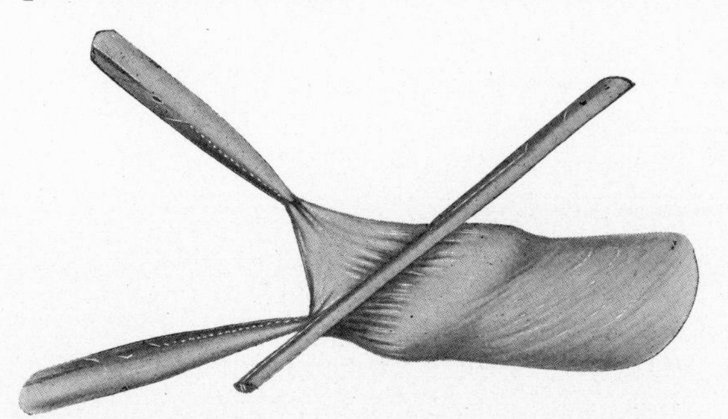
Fig. 158.—Method of applying Circumcision Forceps.

2. Insert a stout probe into the preputial *cul-de-sac*, and with it sweep the entire surface of the glans to detect adhesions, and break them up, if possible.

3. Then catch the prepuce at its muco-cutaneous junction above and below with artery clamps, and draw it forward as far as possible.

4. Now apply the circumcision forceps (Fig. 157). They are to be clamped on the foreskin at an angle of 60 degrees with the long axis of the penis. The point of the forceps should be just behind the lower artery clamp, and great care should be employed not to include any of the glans penis in the grasp of the instrument (Fig. 158).

5. While traction is kept up on the artery clamps, the redundant portion of the prepuce is cut away with scissors curved on the flat.

6. The forceps are now removed, and the skin slips back, exposing a raw surface, the bloody connective tissue overlying the mucous membrane which adheres closely to the glans. This is to be slit down to the corona upon the dorsum, or laterally, and trimmed away on each side up to the frenum, leaving only enough tissue to hold the sutures. Old adhesions may be torn or cut away.

7. Ligatures are rarely necessary. It is preferable to catch bleeding points in the sutures. Oozing vessels, detected by scraping away blood clots with the nail, may be twisted.

Rather coarse horse-hair has proved the best material with which to suture the cut edges. The first suture should be applied at the raphe, and then all the others are certain to fall naturally in place. They should be applied very close together, as many as 25 sutures being used when the wound is long. Each one should take in the least possible portion of integument on the one side and of mucous membrane on the other. The first knot is to be drawn very tightly to cut into the tissues, the second loosely, to avoid severing the first. The ends of each suture are to be cut off about 1 inch long. This prevents the wound from rolling in during the swelling of the first two days, and there are no short, sharp points left to prick the tissues during the displacement caused by swelling.

In the infant no suture (or one only at the frenum) is required. The parts coapt naturally, and healing is practically accomplished in a couple of days.

Variations.—This method of operating is as simple as any, is accurate, and is based on the fact that phimosis is caused by tightness of the inner layer of the prepuce, never by the outer one (unless it is inflamed). Hence the object is to remove as much of the inner layer as possible while preserving the skin to avoid the great danger of this as well as other amputations—namely, insufficient flaps. A circular skin incision might seem as satisfactory as this oval one; but inasmuch as the specialist is not infrequently called upon to relieve by operation a phimosis resulting from a former operation, the necessity for the oval incision is obvious, the size of which may be varied by adapting the inclination of the forceps to the requirements of the case. In any event a liberating incision may be made directly along the dorsum of the penis, and this is sometimes necessary in order to get a perfect result. The frenum is spared for esthetic reasons and to avoid hemorrhage from its artery.

Many different kinds of phimosis forceps have been devised. The ones figured are the simplest and therefore the best. Fenestration is unnecessary, as the sutures should not be introduced until the forceps have been removed and the mucous membrane trimmed down.

Light adhesions are to be broken with a sweep of a probe, stronger ones by peeling the mucous layer with the thumb-nail. It is the rarest exception only that calls for scissors or scalpel.

The *frenum* may be too short and require division.

After-treatment.—The member is now washed, dried, and may be inserted into a large roll made by tying up a towel with a string, and lashing this thick, perforated disk by cords passed about the thighs and body. Inside of this roll the penis rests, surrounded by loose sterile gauze to keep it from contact with the bed-clothing, and in the partially erect posture most suitable to prevent edema. It is not my custom to apply any snug dressing or any wrappings to the penis. For a child that wears a napkin I use the perforated piece of linen folded over the penis and well greased, simply to prevent adhesion of the wound to the diaper. Dispensary patients do fairly well with a light dressing wound around the penis.

No further attention surgically is required. The horse-hair sutures spontaneously cut out without suppuration, and come away in the scab. On the third day, as the swelling subsides, their long ends may be trimmed down close to the scab, to prevent their being pulled upon during the motions of the patient. Rest in bed, although not essential, is desirable, if prompt union is expected. Union by first intention may be expected, and the patient may go about practically well on the eighth day.

Other Operations.—The quality of any operation of circumcision—of which there are many—must be judged by the simplicity and certainty with which it insures, (1) a sufficiency of skin, (2) a large orifice, and (3) safety to the frenum.

No operation attains these ends more certainly than the one just detailed. Dilatation, divulsion, and elastic ligature are relics of the past, and most other operations err by superfluity of detail or by inaccuracy, putting it in the surgeon's power to make the incision transversely and to leave his patient still phimosed after recovery or to cut the skin flaps too short. Dressings about the penis induce erection and adhere, interfering with prompt repair. If the operation has been clean the wound never becomes infected.

Dorsal Incision.—When, however, from previous disease, specific cause, or otherwise, union by first intention is not to be expected, or when, as in diabetics, simplicity is of prime importance, the simple dorsal incision takes precedence. In the *infant* dorsal incision might as well always be employed because the prepuce, if cut well down behind the corona, does not grow with the development of the penis, and at adult age the result is quite the same as though circumcision had been performed. In the *adult* local anesthesia and the freeing of adhesions are obtained as above detailed. A grooved director is then introduced along the dorsum of the glans, and upon it the prepuce is cut entirely through with one stroke of the scissors, or (from within outward) with a sharp-pointed bistoury. This wound may be sutured unless infection threatens. Lateral and multiple incisions are advocated as preferable to the dorsal slit, but, while possessing the disadvantage of complicating an operation whose one advantage is its simplicity, they give but little better drainage of the preputial cavity and leave a foreskin that does not lend itself kindly to a secondary trimming, often desirable for esthetic reasons. But in certain chancroidal cases, complicated by inflammatory phimosis, the double lateral incision is better, as it lays open the preputial cavity more completely. Of course both incisions become infected.

Wound infections after circumcision, notably by tuberculosis and syphilis, have attracted the attention of many authors, and have been illustrated by many curious cases. But, except after ritual circumcision, they are practically unknown nowadays, and present no special features when they do occur. More remarkable is the occurrence of *implantation cysts* which has several times been noticed after this operation.

PARAPHIMOSIS

Paraphimosis (*παρα, outside; φιμοω, I bind*) exists when the prepuce gets behind the corona glandis and cannot be replaced.

Causes.—An unnaturally tight preputial orifice is a predisposing cause to paraphimosis. It sometimes happens that young boys, who retract the prepuce, perhaps for the first time, find themselves unable to replace it.

Inflammatory paraphimosis may depend upon balanitis, gonorrhea, herpes, chancroid, chancre, etc. The prepuce, already a little inflamed, is retracted for the cleansing of some ulceration concealed in its *cul-de-sac*, or is, perhaps, held back by bandage for convenience of dressing, or, if short, becoming inflamed and edematous, it may roll itself back. It soon inflames further, edema increases, and reduction becomes impossible.

Symptoms.—In paraphimosis the glans penis is swollen and livid. If the patient is seen at once there may be no inflammation either of the prepuce or of the glans; but in most cases—in all eventually, if unrelieved—both are inflamed to a greater or less extent, the glans even becoming gangrenous from arrest of circulation. Behind the corona, most marked below, rises a tense, shining, edematous belt of the mucous layer of the prepuce, the connective tissue of which is filled with serum. Behind this there is a deep sulcus or furrow, most marked above, often the seat of superficial ulceration. Here lies the stricture; behind it there rises another edematous fold, usually smaller than the one in front.

If the stricture of the prepuce is tight enough to arrest the circulation, it may finally cause the destruction by gangrene of all tissues lying in front of it.

Treatment.—The first point to decide in a case of paraphimosis is in regard to strangulation. If this exist, delay is inadmissible; if not, temporizing expedients may be resorted to, to reduce inflammation before appealing to forcible reduction or operation. The test is simple. In strangulation the glans penis is turgid, swollen, blue-black, cold, devoid of sensibility, and perhaps already showing points of commencing gangrene. If there be no strangulation, the glans may be normal, or, if swollen, is red—at least not black—warm, and by compression the blood may be driven out of it; sensibility is also preserved. A paraphimosed glans penis may be inflamed, but still not strangulated.

Paraphimosis with Strangulation.—In these cases general anesthesia should always be administered. Often under the relaxation of anesthesia reduction is accomplished with comparative ease. First ice should be used locally to produce shrinkage, and a few small punctures may be made to let out serum from the ridge in front of the stricture if the swelling be excessive. The following are the best methods of reduction: Seize the penis behind the strictured prepuce in the fork of the index and middle fingers of both hands, one placed on each side. This gives more even pressure forward than when one hand only is used. Now make pressure with the thumbs on both sides, in such a direction as to compress the glans laterally, rather than from before backward, and at the same time pull the strictured portion of the prepuce forward, the idea being to make the glans as small as possible by compression, and rather to pull the stricture over the glans than to push the glans through the stricture (Fig. 159).

In some cases it is preferable to encircle the penis with one hand, using the other for manipulation. Finally, Mercier's method may be tried. The surgeon stands on the patient's right, places the index and middle fingers of his right hand longitudinally along the lower surface of the penis, and the pulp of his thumb on the dorsum of the glans penis and the edematous ridge in front of the point of stricture. By firm pressure, crowding down the swollen mucous layer of the prepuce, he endeavours to insinuate the end of the thumb-nail under the stricture (Fig. 160). If he succeeds in this, grasping the penis and the two fingers of the right hand beneath in a circular manner with the left hand, he draws the strictured point up over the thumb-nail. Bardinet's [1] method—inserting the rounded end of a hair-pin under the stricture on each side, and with these making lateral pressure upon the glans while the prepuce is worked forward—is simple and often effective.

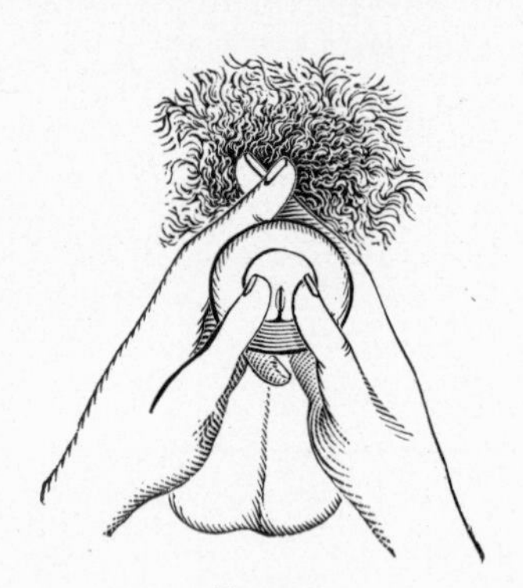

Fig. 159.

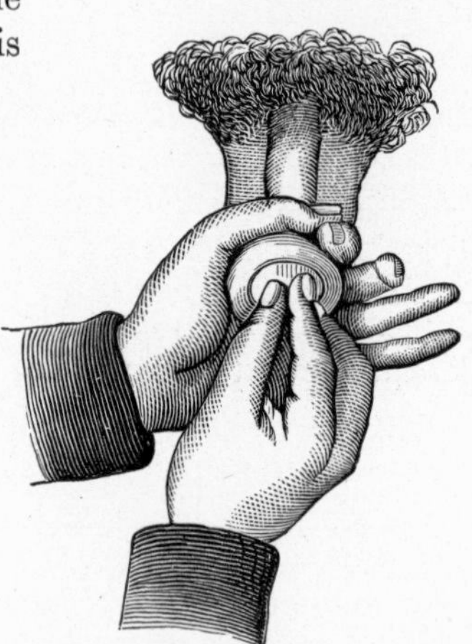

Fig. 160.—(Phillips.)

If a prolonged, careful attempt at reduction fails, the strictured point must be divided. To accomplish this subcutaneously, a tenotomy knife is introduced flatwise through an incision on the dorsum of the penis near its root, and slipped forward beneath the skin until its cutting edge is within the stricture. By simply turning the knife the stricture may then be nicked from within outward until all tension is relieved. Inflammatory consolidation of tissue may make it necessary to divide the stricture at several points. This subcutaneous incision presents the advantage over the usual open incision

[1] L'Union médicale, 1873, p. 900.

of being more easily insured against infection—a matter of no little moment in chancroidal cases.

After reduction, the treatment consists in position, rest, and cleanliness, and syringing the preputial cavity with a mild antiseptic solution. If any contagious ulcer has been the cause of paraphimosis, before commencing manipulation the surgeon should carefully examine his fingers for cracks or fissures. So much handling is required that infection is very likely to occur unless the epidermis of the hands is sound.

Paraphimosis without Strangulation.—If the case is recent, reduction must be effected or inflammation will surely set in and complicate the situation. Reduction may be accomplished as detailed above, or by subjecting the penis, prepuce, and glans together to strong continued pressure. Several narrow strips of adhesive plaster are applied longitudinally from the middle of the penis over the apex of the glans to the middle of the penis opposite the starting-point. The meatus urinarius is left uncovered. In this way the organ is surrounded and compressed by longitudinal strips. Over these, commencing just behind the orifice of the urethra, a narrow strip of plaster is wound spirally, using pretty firm pressure, until the penis is covered by its circular bandage up to the middle. The application is not painful. In twenty-four hours reduction may be accomplished. A thin rubber bandage is more simple in its application and more promptly effective.

In old or anemic patients having gonorrhea or an ulcer about the head of the penis, accompanied by lymphangitis, and where the prepuce is short, a large amount of serum may collect in the prepuce, roll it back, and render paraphimosis imminent. The best treatment here is a little rest, with elevation of the penis and application of a 4% solution of tannin, followed by free use of collodion as soon as the patient rises. Unlike the scrotum, the prepuce bears collodion well.

In the majority of cases, when complicating chancroid, herpetic, or other ulceration, paraphimosis is purely the result of inflammation and edema, and there is no strangulation. Here the main inflammatory condition must be treated, aided by position, pressure, puncture, evaporating and astringent lotions. These will usually be sufficient, but in severe cases a sharp watch should be kept for any evidences of commencing strangulation. Should it occur the point of stricture must straightway be relieved.

CHAPTER III

TUMOURS OF THE PENIS

Gumma.—Gumma occurs in the prepuce, the urethra (very rarely), and the corpora cavernosa. In the first two localities it may be mistaken for tuberculosis or cancer. The history, the influence of mixed treatment, and, if necessary, the examination of a section of the growth determine the diagnosis. In the corpora cavernosa it resembles circumscribed fibrosis, but is deeper, less cartilaginous, and almost always occurs in the posterior third of the organ (Zeissl). Gummata never increase in one direction while healing in another, and they are likely to break down and soften. The so-called relapsing chancre is a gummatous deposit in the scar of the initial lesion. The most important feature of preputial gummata is the frequency with which epithelioma originates in their scars.

BENIGN TUMOURS OF THE SKIN AND CONNECTIVE TISSUE

Cysts.—Mucous, implantation, and sebaceous spots occur. The last originate in the sebaceous glands of the skin or in Tyson's glands. Cysts occur almost always in the prepuce and are readily enucleated. (*Cf.* Gerulanos.[1])

Neoplasms

Lipoma, adenoma,[2] and angioma have been described. They are rare, and their removal is a question of judgment involving a recognition of the function of the penis as an intromittent organ, and the possible loss of this function from the formation of a cicatrix.

Papilloma.—More important because of their frequency are the papillomata (*warts or vegetations*) of the penis. They are commonly denominated *venereal warts.* This title, however, is not exact, since there is no necessary connection between them and any venereal

[1] Deutsche Zeitschr. f. Chir., 1900, lv, 326.
[2] Morrow's System, 1893, i, 58.

disease as a cause. They are nothing more nor less than papillary overgrowths, often highly vascular, and composed in large excess of epithelium. They may be prominent and pedunculated, or flat, and growing from a considerable surface. They are nearly always multiple. They are caused by the contact of irritating fluids with a membrane of naturally delicate texture, or simply by lack of cleanliness. Consequently the most favourable condition for their production exists in gonorrhea, in balanitis, or when mucous patches occupy the cavity of the prepuce. Their favourite seat is just behind the corona glandis, but they are also encountered anywhere within the cavity of the prepuce—at its orifice, upon its cutaneous surface—or even within the urethra. They are found also upon the scrotum, and frequently around the anus. They are, when numerous, bathed in a fetid, puriform secretion, and may grow large enough within the prepuce to cause phimosis. They occur upon young children, and are found in their greatest luxuriance within and around the vulvæ of pregnant women affected with irritating discharges—discharges not necessarily venereal in any sense. Implantation warts also occur after circumcision.

Diagnosis.—Warts should be differentiated from mucous patches and condylomata by the typical appearance of the syphilitic lesions and the accompanying symptoms of the disease.

From commencing epithelioma the diagnosis may be extremely difficult if the wart is a flat one and the base a little dense. When in doubt examine a snipping under the microscope, and if it appears benign, treat it as such, but remove it in any case. If it recur, and the patient is over fifty, it is safest to exsect it as though it were epitheliomatous, whatever the findings of the pathologist.

Prognosis.—Unless kept scrupulously clean, warts sometimes ulcerate, and they may even suppurate, light up suppurating buboes, and even cause gangrene of the penis. Simple cleanliness, on the other hand, often causes them to atrophy.

Epitheliomatous degeneration may take place, and is always to be feared. The implantation warts are especially liable to hypertrophy and become *horns.*

Treatment.—The observance of cleanliness alone often causes vegetations to shrink up and disappear. In any case this is the first essential to the success of any course. In case vegetations are complicated by balanitis, treatment of the latter will often at the same time triumph over the warts. Perhaps the most valuable local application is a 10% mixture of salicylic acid in acetic acid. This forms a chalk-and-water mixture of which the moist chalk is smeared over the warts. One or two applications cause the growths to wither away and drop off. Relapse does not seem to occur after this treatment. If they persist, however, or constitute the main disease, all the pedunculated growths may be removed with curved scissors, and the surface from which they grow cauterized with nitric acid or any other escharotic. The flat growths may be disposed of by the application of nitric acid, at intervals, until the base from which they spring has been destroyed. Where the number of vegetations is too great to allow of their treatment *seriatim*, attention to the general health, cleanliness, and local dusting with calomel is the proper course. This plan, so efficacious in treating condylomata and mucous patches about the anus, is particularly applicable if the vegetations are surrounded by an excess of moisture.

Horns.—Horny growths may spring from the glans or the integument. They begin as warts and are very prone to epitheliomatous change. Brinton,[1] of Philadelphia, has described a curious case and collected others from the literature. Baldwin [2] and Bruce Clark [3] mention others.

Benign Tumours of the Erectile Bodies

The benign tumours of the erectile bodies of the penis are four: *circumscribed fibrosis, enchondroma, osteoma, and calcification.* The first is comparatively rare, the others extremely so.

Circumscribed Fibrosis.—I have come to prefer this name for the malady heretofore usually known as *chronic circumscribed inflammation of the corpora cavernosa*, for the condition is a fibrosis, not an inflammation, and though it usually affects only the corpora cavernosa, the corpus spongiosum as well is sometimes involved. This malady was described in the first edition of this treatise upon a foundation of 5 typical cases which I had seen with Dr. Van Buren, and which were there detailed. Since that time I have seen at least 100 new cases, but I have learned few new features of the disease. I have but rarely seen a case become entirely well.

Though apparently observed by De Lapeyronie,[4] it was first accurately depicted by Kirby,[5] who concluded that gout was the efficient cause. Cruveilhier [6] first announced the affection to be a fibrous transformation of the erectile tissue. Marchal [7] and Verneuil [8] observed the disease in diabetics, and many others have reported individual cases.

---

[1] Med. News, 1887, li, 141. [2] *Ibid.*, 449. [3] Lancet, 1894, i, 219.
[4] Mem. de l'acad. de chir., 1743, i, 423.
[5] Dublin Med. Press, 1849, xxii, 210. [6] Anat. Path., iii, 594.
[7] De Calvi. Les accidents diabétiques, 1864, ii, 82.
[8] Bull. de la soc. de chir., 1883, viii, 826.

The affection comes on insidiously, without apparent cause, although the patient sometimes ascribes it to local injury. The first symptom is a bending or a slight pain at a certain point in the penis when the organ is erect. Examination detects a hard, flattened mass with sharply defined margins, occupying the substance of one or both corpora cavernosa near the surface, and feeling like cartilage —elastic, springy, not as bony as a calcareous plate. The corpus spongiosum rarely participates in the disease. The penis bends during erection at the affected point, and along the edge of the hardness a little pain is experienced. This indurated mass, which is usually irregularly oval in shape, with often a projecting line of hardness towards the root of the penis, may remain stationary for an indefinite period; or it may progress slowly backward or forward, sometimes retaining its size and shape, sometimes growing larger, sometimes smaller.

A slight tenderness is perhaps felt along the line of advancing induration, and moderate uneasiness is usually produced by pressing the induration between the fingers, the same feeling as that experienced during erection. The seat of election is the dorsum of the penis forward, the patch spreading equally around each corpus cavernosum, and being usually more blunt forward than posteriorly. Sometimes a single patch is found laterally in one corpus cavernosum, not reaching the dorsum, and there being no companion on the other side. The disease occurs after middle life. The patients are usually healthy, and certainly are not uniformly subject to any diathetic disease, although more patients are noticed as having had gout or rheumatism than any other malady. Gonorrhea, syphilis, stricture, bear no possible etiological relation to this malady, and treatment by mercury and iodid of potassium is absolutely negative. The integument of the penis is in no way involved. The malady appears to be a chronic thickening of the sheath and a portion of the underlying erectile tissue of the corpus cavernosum, which thickening appears to obliterate the meshes of the erectile tissue and prevent their distention with blood during erection of the rest of the organ.

Morbid Anatomy and Etiology.—Verneuil first suggested, correctly, I believe, that the condition was non-inflammatory and analogous to the contractions of the palmar and plantar aponeurosis encountered among gouty subjects. He thinks the cause is gout, and is interested in the fact that 3 out of 4 of his cases were also diabetic. Trélat, at the same meeting of the surgical society, reported that he had seen 2 cases, Monod 1, and Le Fort 3, none diabetic. I do not know that the urine was tested for sugar in the earlier cases seen by Dr. Van Buren and myself. None of the later cases examined was diabetic, so far as I know. Some of them had the gouty diathesis, but this cannot be affirmed of all. Tuffier,[1] in an exhaustive article, while omitting a number of cases of which I have record, has collected 35 cases, in which no diathesis is noted in 9, 15 were gouty, and 11 diabetic. The malady being far more common in advanced life than at any other time, he searched patiently among 2,500 old men at Bicêtre and Ivry without finding a single case, and mentions Cruveilhier and Ricord as having been equally unsuccessful in trying to find a case for dissection; but, after his article was finished, one of these nodosities was cut out by Verneuil (October 25, 1884), and Leloir reported that it was composed of a tissue analogous to that of keloids—embryonic cells in clusters tending to fibrous transformation, few vessels, with fibrous planes resembling cicatricial tissue.

Tuffier and Claude [2] report one specimen as a chondrofibroma of the sheath of the corpora cavernosa. Chetwood's case of osteoma of the penis proved to be in part fibroma, in part true osteoma.

From these scant records and the clinical data it may be definitely asserted that this condition is a fibrosis beginning in the sheath of the erectile bodies, tending to extend to the erectile tissue, and perhaps occasionally progressing to chondrification — very much more rarely to ossification. A distinction that may be made between these patches and true enchondroma and osteoma is that, while the former may diminish in size and disappear in one place while growing in another, the latter never undergo these retrograde changes.

Prognosis.—The prognosis is negatively good in that the fibrous mass never ulcerates or degenerates into anything malignant, may get spontaneously better, even possibly well, or may, and sometimes does, develop backward until it gets so low down towards the root of the penis that it no longer seriously interferes with upright erection. I have seen more than one patient who, at one time being debarred from sexual intercourse, has by a shifting of the position of the induration again become potent. I have met one person with a distinct softish plaque of some size, of which he had no knowledge whatever until I called his attention to it. The distinction between fibroma and enchondroma can only be made pathologically; clinically it is unimportant. The tendency to ossification manifests itself so rarely that it is a negligible quantity.

Treatment.—An effective treatment of this singular malady is yet to be discovered. Thus far time only has seemed to help it, while

[1] Guyon's Annales, 1885, July and August.

[2] *Ibid.*, 1894, xii, 838.

blisters, oleate of mercury, tincture of iodin, with mercury, the iodids, and electrolysis, have uniformly failed. Perhaps alkalin or anti-gouty remedies may have some beneficial effect. I always try them, and have thought they encouraged resolution in some cases. Yet in others they are absolutely inefficacious. Excision only replaces the fibrosis by scar tissue.

Calcification and Ossification.—Both of these conditions are usually, probably always, secondary to fibrosis, or enchondrosis of the erectile bodies. Calcification of small patches is quite rare, ossification is even more unusual. Cases of this latter condition have been reported by von Lenhossek,[1] Demarquay,[2] Porter,[3] Jacobson,[4] and Chetwood.[5] In Chetwood's specimen certain spots were simply fibrous, others were cartilaginous, while the bulk of the growth was true bone. Most of these specimens, whether calcified or ossified, if carefully examined, would probably show some trace of these different stages of development. To compare penile osteoma with the bony development normal in the penes of certain monkeys is scarcely logical.

Prognosis.—Calcification or ossification may cease after more or less of each corpus cavernosum has suffered, or it may involve the whole organ pretty generally. The hard masses can be distinctly felt. Sexual intercourse may be seriously interfered with, if not prevented altogether. Under these circumstances the patient is often driven to thoughts of suicide, urged on by that morbid depression, which, in the male, always accompanies a sense of sexual incapacity, be that incapacity fancied or real.

Treatment.—Medicine holds out no hope to the sufferer. If the disease has come to a standstill and the deposit is superficial and small, it may be removed with the knife—an operation which has been performed with success by Regnoli, MacClellan,[6] myself, and others.

MALIGNANT NEOPLASMS OF THE PENIS

The primary malignant new growths of the penis are *sarcoma* and *epithelioma.* The former is very rare. It arises from the erectile bodies, usually the corpora cavernosa. The latter, much more common, begins on the glans, on the prepuce, or in the urethra. Epithelioma of the urethra will be considered with the other diseases of that canal.

---

[1] Virchow's Archiv, 1874, lx, i.
[2] *Op. cit.*, p. 354.
[3] N. Y. Med. Record, 1882, 270.
[4] *Op. cit.*, p. 683.
[5] J. of Cut. and Gen.-Urin. Dis., 1899, xvii, 231.
[6] Velpeau. Nouveaux éléments de méd. opért., 1839, iv, 336.

Secondary new growths present no peculiar features. They either form part of a disseminated carcinosis or are mere extensions of the tumour from an adjoining region, usually the scrotum.

Sarcoma

With or without previous trauma a tumour appears in one of the erectile bodies. The fact that it is a distinct lump and not a flat indurated patch readily distinguishes it from the benign tumours of these structures. Moreover, sarcoma usually appears in early manhood and develops with characteristic rapidity and early involvement of the inguinal glands. Exceptionally, however, it grows slowly and the glandular involvement occurs late. Of the 13 cases recorded by Jacobson [1] some arose from the erectile tissue, some from the fibrous sheath, and one—a melanotic sarcoma—apparently originated in the urethral mucous membrane. The earlier cases were reported as fibroma or carcinoma. As the tumour grows it causes priapism by occluding the cavernous spaces, and may also occlude the urethra and so cause retention of urine. Early amputation of the penis is the only *treatment*. The *prognosis* is absolutely bad.

Epithelioma

Epithelioma of the penis (Fig. 161) begins on the prepuce or glans, both of which are usually involved when the patient presents himself for examination.

Etiology.—Though Freyer [2] has reported a case in a youth of seventeen, and Kaufmann places 6% of the cases in the third decade, here, as elsewhere, epithelioma is usually a disease of later life. One case developed in the scar of a horse-bite, others have arisen from the scars left by venereal sores, a few from urethral fistula; but warts and chronic balanitis are the most fruitful sources of epithelioma, the former especially if neglected and allowed to remain foul and moist. Indeed, 29 of the 33 cases collected by Kaufmann began as apparently benign warts. Finally, phimosis is a marked predisposing cause of epithelioma. By retention of the smegma and urine it predisposes the patient to balanitis, vegetations, and fissures of the foreskin, and these processes once set up are kept concealed and constantly bathed in an acrid and irritating fluid. Demarquay noted phimosis in 42 out of 59 cases, and it is claimed that the circumcised Jew is exempt from penile epithelioma. The question of inoculation from the cervix uteri is agitated from time to time, but the

---

[1] *Op. cit.*, p. 738.

[2] Brit. Med. J., 1891, i, 1173.

extreme rarity of the cases adduced indicates that they represent nothing more than a curious coincidence.

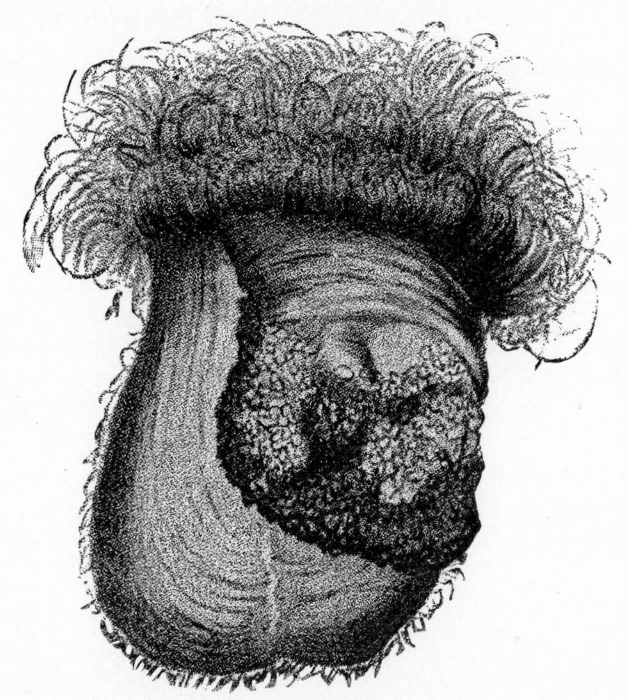

Fig. 161.—Epithelioma of the Penis.

Symptoms and Course.—Although epithelioma of the penis is not often seen until well under way and absolutely characteristic, the various aspects under which it first presents itself must be appreciated in order that intelligent radical treatment may be resorted to at once.

In about 5 out of 6 cases the disease begins as a wart situated on the glans or on the inner surface of the prepuce. This wart is intractable to ordinary methods of treatment, and recurs if cut or burned away. As it grows it assumes a lobulated, cauliflower appearance, and soon begins to ulcerate in places, and to exude the characteristic foul ichorous discharge. Then the base gradually takes on the hard induration of the epitheliomatous ulcer with everted edges. By this time the inguinal glands are probably involved and may be felt as shotty subcutaneous nodules in either groin. (For the lymphatics of the penis so anastomose that a so-called crossed bubo—the sore on the one side of the penis and the bubo in the opposite groin—occurs not infrequently.)

More rarely epithelioma begins as a raw spot or an indolent

ulcer, and still more rarely it appears first as a subcutaneous nodule or pimple which later ulcerates and assumes a warty growth.

In whatever way the disease begins, it comes after a time to the frankly cancerous stage. The ulcer advances, involving all the tissues in its path; the discharge is thin, sanious, fetid; the ulcer deep, irregular, unhealthy, its edges hard, livid, and coated. At the same time the exuberant warty growth progresses, either of these conditions predominating to make the case clinically a warty or an ulcerative lesion.

The inguinal glands now become prominent and partake of the pyogenic as well as of the cancerous infection, so that they become matted together, and may even go on to abscess formation, ulceration, and the production of an epitheliomatous ulcer in the groin.

Locally the growth may spread over quite a large superficial area without involving the corpora cavernosa, whose sheaths stoutly resist invasion, while it has frequently been noted that, though the entire glans may be involved in the disease, the corpus spongiosum is usually spared and urination is unimpeded. If, however, the canal does become obstructed, the urine usually manages to find its way through one or more fistulous openings in the floor of the urethra.

Lancinating pain is a prominent symptom only late in the disease. The chief inconveniences to the patient in the earlier stages are the presence of the growth, the foul discharge, and the tendency to annoying hemorrhage after the slightest abrasion. As the disease advances the strength of the patient fails. The tumour spreads up over the penis to the pubes, abdomen, and thighs, joining the ulcerated inguinal glands and extending down over the scrotum to the perineum, anus, and buttocks, until, finally, the patient dies of sepsis, cachexia, or hemorrhage. Curiously enough, lymphatic infection seems to stop for a long while at the inguinal glands, so that visceral metastases are the exception.

Diagnosis.—The diseases which may be confused with epithelioma of the penis are warts, chancre, chancroid, tubercular ulcers, and ulcers from chronic balanoposthitis.

As we have seen, the appearance of epithelioma is characteristic enough after its base has become indurated and the infection has begun to spread to the inguinal glands; but it is of the greatest importance that the diagnosis be made before that time, while the disease is yet eminently curable. To this end all growths or ulcers that prove intractable should be regarded with suspicion, and if that suspicion is confirmed by microscopical examination of a snipping from the diseased tissue, immediate operation should be insisted upon.

Prognosis.—Before the inguinal glands become involved the prognosis is good. Afterward it is bad, yet not absolutely so, for cures are reported in cases where unmistakable gland involvement had occurred. Thus Küttner[1] found a mortality of only 40.5% in 58 cases reported from three to twenty-nine years after operation. Indeed, in a few cases, slight glandular enlargements have been known to disappear permanently upon removal of the original focus of infection, as though the adenitis were purely inflammatory.

It is true the glands can and should be removed with the tumour, yet, in spite of the fact that infection is slow to pass them, the situation of these organs about the saphenous opening in the fascia lata, in close proximity to the great vessels, and the accompanying simple inflammation that usually mats the glands to one another and to the vessels themselves, render their removal an extremely delicate task and one of whose thoroughness the surgeon cannot always feel assured.

Treatment.—If the growth be seen before induration has occurred it may usually be removed by circumcision if on the prepuce, or by thorough cauterization if upon the glans. The patient should, however, be warned of the danger of recurrence, and should this appear, or should there be already some induration about the base of the tumour, the penis must be amputated behind the corona, and the inguinal glands of both sides extirpated, whether they are palpably enlarged or not, for the microscope has repeatedly shown these glands to be the seat of malignant deposits though their gross appearance was quite normal.

If the glans is extensively involved, the penis must be amputated close up to the pubes, or else extirpated entirely. Jacobson claims that simultaneous castration adds to the comfort of these patients, though most men refuse to part with their testicles even when their function has thus ceased.

Even though the disease has progressed still further, the ingenious surgeon will devise some irregular plastic operation which can be combined with complete extirpation to suit the exigencies of the case. The hope of cure may be slight indeed, but by vigorously attacking every outburst of the disease the surgeon may hope to prolong life for months or years and to render the sufferer at least fairly comfortable during that period. The various escharotics, the actual cautery, permanganate of potash and peroxid of hydrogen are of no small service in this terminal stage of the disease. Occasionally an actual cure may even be obtained, as in Taylor's case

---

[1] St. Louis Courier of Medicine, 1899, xxi, 72.

of removal of an epithelioma which had existed for six years. The patient died of intercurrent disease ten years after the operation, having shown no recurrence.

The type operations for removal of the penis which have been referred to in the preceding pages are, partial removal or amputation of the penis, and complete removal or extirpation of the penis. Amputation by cautery or écraseur need be mentioned only to be condemned.

Amputation of the Penis

The preparation for operation consists in the usual general and local preparation as for any aseptic procedure. General anesthesia is necessary. With the patient on the table a rubber catheter or tube is clamped about the root of the penis. Taylor suggests the use of hare-lip pins to retain it in place. Ample skin-flaps (see below) are then cut and dissected back a full inch, after which the knife is inserted between the corpus spongiosum and the corpora cavernosa, and these bodies separated and amputated, the former being left 2 cm. longer than the latter. The elastic ligature is now removed. This step will be followed by violent hemorrhage, but by the time spurting points have been caught and tied the oozing will be readily controllable by pressure. Hemostasis having been thus effected, the urethra is split into two or more short flaps (see below) and these sutured with fine catgut to the skin. The wound is then dressed aseptically with the stump of the penis erect, and provision made for the passage of the urine, either by a retained catheter, or by sealing the wound with absorbent cotton or gauze applied with iodoform collodion.

If the penis is to be amputated close to the pubes, elastic pressure may have to be dispensed with, and in such cases it is advisable to make a small buttonhole in the perineum, through which the urethra is isolated and sutured to the skin just in front of the anus.

Flaps.—A circular skin incision was used by early operators, but flap operations are now in vogue as giving more accurate apposition of the skin edges and cleaner healing. Senn and Jacobson both use long dorsal and short ventral flaps. Jacobson makes his so long that the urethra is sutured to a perforation in its lower part. Others prefer lateral flaps.

The end of the urethra is split in order to avoid a stricture at the new meatus. Guitéras [1] denies the necessity of this. Ordinarily it is split into two flaps to be sutured to the skin-flaps. Dr. Davis,[2] of

---

[1] J. of Cut. and Gen. Urin. Dis., 1898, xvi, 212.

[2] Univ. Med. Mag., 1896, ix, 264.

Philadelphia, suggests three urethral flaps, each cut to a point and sutured to the skin, divided circularly. Keller[1] advises that the stumps of the corpora cavernosa be sutured together end to end to prevent secondary hemorrhage. It would seem that subsequent erections might tear out these sutures, or at least give rise to considerable pain and tension.

After-treatment.—If the flaps are cut long, erections need not be feared. A light dressing held snugly in place by adhesive plaster should prevent oozing. Frequent change of dressing is necessary to prevent defilement of the wound by urine. The patient should be examined for stricture of the new meatus some weeks after healing is complete.

Extirpation of the Penis.—The patient is placed in the lithotomy position, and an elliptical incision is made around the base of the penis. The skin of the scrotum is incised along the entire length of the raphe. With the fingers and the handle of the scalpel the halves of the scrotum are then separated down to the corpus spongiosum, a full-sized sound is passed as far as the triangular ligament, and the knife inserted between the corpora cavernosa and the corpus spongiosum. The catheter having been withdrawn, the urethra is cut through just in front of the bulb and detached back to the triangular ligament. The suspensory ligament is then divided and the penis separated from the soft parts down to the attachments of the crura, and each crus separated from the pubic arch by means of a stout periosteal elevator. The edges of the incision in the scrotum are then brought together and the urethra split and stitched to the lower angle of the wound. Drainage is supplied by a tube placed deeply in the wound with its extremities protruding at the upper and lower angles. No catheter need be retained in the urethra. The operation is always protracted owing to the close and firm attachment of the crura to the bone and the excessive hemorrhage during their detachment. Four arteries—the two arteries of the corpora cavernosa and the two dorsal arteries—must be tied.

Total Emasculation.—The removal of the testicles adds little to the gravity of extirpation of the penis, and has been strongly urged as an essential part of that operation, on the ground that the testicles "remain ever after sad dumb witnesses of a function which is lost forever" (Montaz) or, in less poetical language, that castration in this case averts the hypochondriacal and maniacal tendency which in late years it has been said to cause when the operation is performed for the relief of prostatic hypertrophy. Pantalini[2] in

---

[1] Brüns, Beitrag zur. klin. Chir., iv, 235. [2] Arch. prov. de chir., 1898.

particular argues the case well, confronting the hysterical tendencies of those who have preserved their testicles with the clearheadedness of the emasculated, and the certified strength of mind of Oriental eunuchs. Whether this be generally true or not, it is not amiss to consult the patient's wishes in the matter.

The operation itself is simple enough. The cord with its vessels and the pampiniform plexus of veins are tied off by separate ligatures on each side at the external abdominal ring, and cord, vessels, and testicles are removed through the scrotal incision. Pantalini has collected 23 cases without operative mortality, 3 deaths by recurrence within a year, and 1 cure after three years. The remaining 15 were reported cured at shorter intervals.

Extirpation of the Inguinal Glands.—As has been already remarked, it is wise to remove the inguinal glands even if they appear normal. This may be readily done through oblique incisions in each groin, extending upward and outward from the upper angle of the peripenile incision. As the danger point in this operation is the saphenous opening and the vessels immediately beneath and below it, this should be laid bare at once and the dissection of the glands carried upward from this point.

After-treatment.—The most comfortable dressing after extirpation of the penis or total emasculation is a heavy pad of gauze held in place by a double spica of the thigh or by two pieces of adhesive plaster crossed. The dressing must be changed daily, and so arranged that its lower end is easily elevated to permit catheterization and urination.

CHAPTER IV

DIAGNOSTIC TABLE OF PENILE CHANCRE, CHANCROID, HERPES, AND SIMPLE ULCERATION

THE following table is intended to serve as a summary of the broad, classical characteristics of syphilitic chancre and chancroid, as well as for the differential diagnosis of syphilitic chancre, chancroid, herpes, and ulcerated abrasions; of the bubo of chancroid, and that of syphilis; and of the different forms of lymphangitis.

SYPHILITIC CHANCRE	CHANCROID	HERPES	ULCERATED (BALANITIC OR OTHER) ABRASION
1. *Nature.* — Always a constitutional affection.	1. Always a local disease.	1. Sometimes a local disease, sometimes a neurosis.	1. Always local.
2. *Cause.*—Sexual intercourse with a patient suffering from syphilitic chancre, or from some secondary syphilitic lesion of or near the genitals; vaccination with syphilitic blood; accidental or designed inoculation of any vehicle containing the syphilitic virus upon an abrasion of any portion of any tegumentary expansion.	2. Sexual intercourse with a patient suffering from chancroid of or near the genitals; accidental or designed inoculation with the secretion of chancroid or of virulent bubo. The specific bacillus may usually be isolated.	2. Mechanical irritation, friction, as in sexual intercourse; chemical irritation, as of acrid discharges. As a sequence of cold, fever, or as an essential neurosis.	2. All of the causes mentioned for herpes, except the last three.
3. *Situation.* — Usually upon or near the genitals, not very infrequent on the head, hands, or nipple.	3. Very rarely encountered except on or about the genitals.	3. Of very frequent occurrence upon the genitals.	3. Same.
4. *Incubation.* — Constant, not less than ten days, usually three weeks.	4. None after absorption of the poison. Ulcer usually fully formed on the second or third day; very rarely commences later than the seventh.	4. None.	4. None.

SYPHILITIC CHANCRE	CHANCROID	HERPES	ULCERATED (BALANITIC OR OTHER) ABRASION
5. *Commencement.* —Begins as an erosion or a papule, and remains an erosion or ulcerates.	5. Begins as a pustule or ulcer, and invariably remains as an ulcer.	5. Begins as a group of vesicles, rarely as a single vesicle, and becomes an ulcer.	5. Begins as an abrasion or fissure, and remains as an ulceration.
6. *Number.*—Usually unique or simultaneously multiple; never multiple by successive auto-inoculation; never confluent.	6. Usually multiple, both simultaneously and by successive auto-inoculation; often confluent.	6. Generally multiple, simultaneously and by successive crops of vesicles; sometimes confluent.	6. Generally multiple and confluent.
7. *Physiognomy.* —(*a*) Shape: round, oval, or symmetrically irregular.	7. (*a*) Shape: round, oval, or unsymmetrically irregular, with border described by segments of large circles.	7. (*a*) Shape: irregularly rounded, with borders described by segments of small circles left by the confluent vesicles.	7. Irregular, of any shape, otherwise resembling superficial chancroid ulcer.
(*b*) Lesion is habitually flat, capped by erosion or superficial ulceration; or scooped out; or a deep, funnel-shaped ulcer with sloping edges. Sometimes the papule is dry and scaly.	(*b*) Always a true ulcer, excavated, hollowed out.	(*b*) Ulcer usually superficial; sometimes in solitary herpes there is but one absolutely circular vesicle. There are usually neighbouring groups of vesicles to clear up the diagnosis. The general physiognomy of herpetic ulceration is similar to that of chancroid, but of less virulent aspect.	(*b*) Like herpes.
(*c*) Edges: sloping and adherent, sometimes prominently elevated.	(*c*) Edges: sharply cut, abrupt, often undermined.		
(*d*) Bottom: smooth, shining.	(*d*) Bottom: uneven, warty, irregular, without lustre.		
(*e*) Colour: sombre, darkish red, gray, or black; sometimes livid and scaly, occasionally scabbed.	(*e*) Colour: yellow, tawny, false-membranous - looking; sometimes bright.		

SYPHILITIC CHANCRE	CHANCROID	HERPES	ULCERATED (BALANITIC OR OTHER) ABRASION
(*f*) Secretion: slight, sero-sanguinolent, unless irritation provokes suppuration.	(*f*) Secretion: abundant and purulent.		
8. *History.*—Not found on patients who have had syphilis previously.	8. Found indifferently upon all.	8. Found by preference upon patients with long prepuce and tender balano-preputial mucous membrane, often showing a marked tendency to return at irregular intervals after lack of cleanliness, a carouse, or unusual sexual intercourse.	8. Found indifferently upon all. Most common on patients with long, tight prepuce, who are not cleanly in their habits.
9. *Inoculability.*—Not auto-inoculable unless secreting pus. Not hetero-inoculable on syphilitics.	9. Readily auto-inoculable, producing characteristic chancroid ulcer by the third day. Hetero-inoculable.	9. Sometimes auto-inoculable when secreting thick pus, producing abortive pustule, not characteristic chancroid ulcer.	9. Same.
10. *Course.*—Slowly progressive; cicatrization slow.	10. Rapidly progressive; cicatrization slow.	10. Does not usually get much larger than the size at which it started; limitation and cicatrization rapid.	10. Same.
11. *Sensibility.*—Rarely painful; almost insensitive to pressure.	11. Often painful; sensitive to pressure.	11. Stinging heat at commencement.	11. Usually painful.
12. *Induration.*—Constant, parchment-like, and very faint, or cartilaginous and extensive, terminating abruptly, not shading off into parts around, movable upon parts beneath the skin, and not adherent to the latter; may disappear in a few days, usually outlasts the sore, and may remain for years in the cicatrix.	12. Absent in typical cases. An induration may be caused by irritants or by inflammation. It is boggy, not elastic, shades off into surrounding tissues, is adherent to parts around, disappears promptly on healing of the sore, or before that time.	12. Inflammatory induration, capable of being produced by the same causes as in chancroid, and behaving in a precisely similar manner.	12. Same.

SYPHILITIC CHANCRE	CHANCROID	HERPES	ULCERATED (BALANITIC OR OTHER) ABRASION
13. *Phagedena.*—May occur rarely.	13. Much more common.	13. Very rare, if at all possible.	13. Same.
14. *Bubo.*—Syphilitic bubo constant.	14. In about two thirds of cases glands are unaffected, in the other third inflammatory or virulent bubo occurs.	14. Glands are very rarely involved. Inflammatory bubo may occur, virulent bubo is impossible.	14. Same.
15. *Lymphangitis.*—Syphilitic.	15. Inflammatory or virulent.	15. Inflammatory.	15. Same.
16. *Prognosis.*—For local consequences good, but syphilis follows.	16. For local consequences more serious; no after-effect.	16. Good in all respects; may recur.	16. Same.
17. *Treatment.*—Local treatment but slightly effective.	17. Local treatment curative.	17. Same.	17. Same.

SYPHILITIC BUBO	BUBO OF CHANCROID
1. *Nature.*—It is a specific affection, with peculiar characteristics.	1. It may be simple (inflammatory), such as might attend any inflammatory lesion, or virulent.
2. *Frequency.*—It is a constant symptom attending syphilitic chancre.	2. It is a complication occurring about once in three cases.
3. *Number of Glands Involved.*—In those regions where multiple glands are found, it is generally poly-ganglionic; these may be unilateral or bilateral in the groin, rarely matted together into one large mass, but, when so, the latter retains the characteristics of indolence, etc.	3. Usually consists of a single gland in any region of the body. In the groin it may be bilateral. It is never a group of small, movable glands.
4. *Date of Appearance.*—It develops during the first or second week of syphilitic chancre.	4. There is no fixed period of appearance.
5. *Size.*—The glands are usually only slightly enlarged.	5. The gland is greatly enlarged.
6. *Induration.*—The glands are specifically indurated, feeling like cartilage or wood.	6. No hardness except inflammatory.
7. *Evidence of Inflammation.*—None; the glands are freely movable among the tissue. The skin is neither adherent nor red, nor is there any pain. The most prominent feature of the swelling is its indolence.	7. Every appearance of inflammation. The gland becomes fixed (periadenitis), the skin adherent, the part feels hot, there is pain, the skin reddens, the prominent features are those of inflammation.
8. *Termination* always in resolution, except in occasional cases, where, from added simple or tubercular infection, suppuration ensues.	8. Inflammatory bubo may resolve or may suppurate. Virulent bubo invariably suppurates and becomes an open chancroid ulcer.

SYPHILITIC BUBO	BUBO OF CHANCROID
9. *Auto-inoculability.*—If suppuration occurs the pus is not auto-inoculable. The abscess does not become a chancre or a chancroid ulcer. It does not extend, and never becomes phagedenic.	9. The pus of inflammatory bubo is not auto-inoculable; the pus of virulent is readily auto-inoculable.
10. *Natural duration* in a few weeks or months.	10. Natural duration is a few weeks, or many months, as a chancroid; possibly years, if it becomes phagedenic.
11. *Prognosis* good as far as local results are concerned, but the patient invariably has syphilis.	11. Prognosis good for inflammatory, less so for virulent bubo, especially if it becomes phagedenic. In neither case does syphilis follow.
12. *Local treatment* ineffective, except for complications; general treatment of doubtful efficacy, but sometimes serviceable.	12. Local treatment useful and necessary to avert suppuration, to cure chancroid left by virulent bubo, and to lessen complications. Antisyphilitic treatment absolutely useless.

SYPHILITIC LYMPHANGITIS	LYMPHANGITIS OF CHANCROID
1. Occurs only in case of syphilis, and has peculiar characteristics.	1. Exists as simple inflammatory lymphangitis, or in virulent form; the former may complicate any inflammation, the latter found only with chancroid.
2. Feels hard, like the vas deferens, of the size of a knitting-needle or of a goose-quill; no pain on erection or on handling.	2. Some inflammatory hardness. Pain on erection and on handling.
3. Skin normal.	3. Skin red over inflamed vessel.
4. Termination by gradual resolution. Suppuration rare and adventitious; in such cases the pus is not auto-inoculable.	4. Termination by resolution or suppuration. Virulent lymphangitis invariably suppurates, the pus is auto-inoculable, and the openings become chancroids.
5. Treatment unnecessary and of little effect, except in case of inflammatory complication.	5. Local treatment advisable to quiet pain, to avert suppuration, or to limit extent and severity of chancroids.

CHAPTER V

DISEASES OF THE SCROTUM

ANATOMY

THE scrotum is a pouch formed of skin and of muscular and connective tissue. Its function is to contain and support the testicles. It is developed from lateral halves which unite centrally in the raphe (ῥάπτω, *I sew*), a raised line continuous with the raphe of the penis and that of the perineum.

The integument of the scrotum is delicate in structure, covered with a few hairs, and likely to become pigmented at puberty. The sebaceous glands are very large.

The dartos is a layer of unstriped muscle firmly attached to the integument, and reflected inward from the raphe, to form the septum scroti. Each testicle has thus a dartos of its own. On exposing the scrotum to the air, the vermicular contractions of this muscle can be readily seen. They occur under the influence of cold or fright, and during the venereal orgasm. In youth, especially in winter, the dartos is habitually contracted and holds the testicles well up under the pubes. The ancient sculptors did not fail to notice that contraction of the scrotum was a mark of general as well as of sexual vigour. In the aged and infirm, on the other hand, especially during summer, the muscle relaxes, allowing the testicles to hang low, supported mainly by the spermatic cords.

The septum scroti is pervious to fluids, so that serum or infiltrated urine can find its way readily from one side to the other. The lymphatics of the scrotum are large and numerous and lead to the inguinal glands.

The connective tissue within the scrotum, like that of the penis, is practically devoid of fat. The muscular dartos, described above, is the only layer of importance. The space between it and the testicle is filled with a loose mesh of fascia within which run the scattered fibres of the cremaster muscle, and beneath which the infundibuliform fascia, derived from the transversalis fascia, forms the investment of the spermatic cord.

ANOMALIES

The scrotum develops independently of the testicles, but if the latter fail to descend it remains rudimentary.

Failure of union between the lateral halves of the scrotum constitutes one of the features of pseudo-hermaphroditism.

CUTANEOUS DISEASES

The scrotum may be affected by most of the diseases of the skin. Only those that are modified by their position deserve notice.

Eczema.—Eczema attacking the scrotum and the surrounding parts is sometimes excessively obstinate and prone to relapse.

Intertrigo.—Intertrigo occurs in children and in fat men of rheumatic habit. Much can be done to prevent it by scrupulous cleanliness, and the use of a suspensory bandage to keep the cutaneous surfaces apart. To overcome the hyperemia, rest, cleanliness, and exposure of the parts to the air are speedily effective in mild cases. If the surface is moist and excoriated, it should be dusted with equal parts of finely powdered oxid of zinc, camphor, and starch, or it may be dressed with the oxid-of-zinc ointment or with a solution of sulphate of zinc. A strip of old thin linen should be used to sling up the scrotum and keep the cutaneous surfaces apart. Later, when the parts are dry, compound tincture of iodin, at first considerably diluted with water, locally, will hasten the cure. Avoidance of stimulating food and drink, to render the secretions less irritating, is advisable. Turkish baths avail much.

Pityriasis.—In men with a delicate skin, especially in summer, there is often a slightly brown discoloration of the thigh and the scrotum, where the two surfaces lie habitually in contact, caused by a vegetable parasite in the upper layers of the epidermis. It sometimes gives rise to a mild local erythema and considerable itching. A few applications of the compound tincture of iodin diluted to half strength, and painted on after the affected skin has been washed with soap and dried (to remove the fat from the scales and spores), will cure the discoloration and the itching. Sulphurous acid does well.

Eczema Marginatum.—This is another parasitic disease, affecting the scrotum, thighs, mons veneris, and buttocks. It is not an eczema, but a herpes tonsurans vesiculosus—a combination of herpes tonsurans and intertrigo, as proved by Pick.[1] The eruption commences in one or more small, round patches, red, elevated, and

[1] Archiv f. Derm. und Syph., 1, iii, 443.

itchy, just where the scrotum habitually lies in contact with the thigh. It spreads circumferentially, healing in the centre. The border of the eruption is sharply defined, and forms the distinctive feature of the disease. It is composed of papules, vesicles, excoriations, and crusts. The parts within this festooned border over which the disease has passed are left of a brown colour. Often, little heaps of dried-up scales lie here and there upon this surface. Patches of eruption break out in the neighbourhood or within the border, and behave exactly like the patches first constituting the disease. The affection is slow in getting well and tends to relapse. Friction and moisture of the parts, together with the parasite, are necessary for its production. Among the scales scraped from the margin, the microscope may detect the moniliform filaments and spores of the tricophyton of Malmster, the parasite of ordinary ringworm. In certain stages of the disease the parasite is difficult to find.

Treatment.—Dilute lead-water or oxid-of-zinc ointment may be used locally at first if there be much inflammation of the skin, to be followed by parasiticide lotions, or the latter may be commenced with at once. The best of these is a mild solution of corrosive sublimate in water (1: 2,000), which should be kept constantly applied. Sulphurous acid, pure, is an excellent parasiticide; tincture of iodin may be used, or an ointment of turpeth mineral (hydrarg. sulph. flav.) 2% to 4%. Treatment should be kept up for some time after apparent cure, as relapses are the rule, and can only be averted in this way.

Pruritus Genitalium.—This, like other purely pruriginous skin affections without eruption, is excessively obstinate, the sufferers are usually rheumatic or gouty subjects, and any dietetic or hygienic errors seem liable to induce or aggravate the disorder. After the exclusion of animal or vegetable parasites from the *rôle* of causality, the treatment consists in hygienic and dietetic precautions, with the internal exhibition of alkalies, and, if need be, tonics. Turkish and Russian baths are often very serviceable.

The following are among the most generally useful local measures, what is suitable for one case often having no effect upon another. Hygiene and change of air are sometimes the only really curative agents.

Hot water, tar, pure or in combination, yellow wash, chloral, camphor; or,

℞ Chloroform .... 2 gm.
Adipis .... 20 "
M. Keep corked in a wide-mouthed bottle.

Or,

℞	Acid. hydrocyanic. dil.	10 to 50 gm.
	Glycerini	15 gm.
	Aquæ q. s. ad	100 "
M.	Ft. lotio.	

Finally, local electricity, either the induced or the continued current, has moderate curative power over some cases.

Pediculi Pubis.—These parasites may be found upon the scrotum, as they may, in fact, upon any part of the body from which the hairs of puberty grow. They exist in greatest abundance, however, about the genitals, and particularly on the mons veneris. They are plainly visible to the naked eye, as are their eggs attached to the hairs (Fig. 162, *a*). They may be destroyed by sprinkling the parts with calomel, or by applying a 1:1,000 solution of corrosive sublimate in cologne-water, or a wash made of equal parts of tincture delphinii and water, or by the free local use of kerosene oil. When they infest the whole body, some few usually escape the ordinary application of lotions, and these soon breed a new crop. Care and patience, however, will always finally dislodge them. No treatment is better than the old-fashioned blue mercurial ointment, which may be rubbed into the hairy parts about the pubes and perineum and somewhat down the thighs, the patient going to bed in drawers and sleeping covered with the ointment all night. Two such applications, at a few days' interval, usually destroy the colony. The treatment is a very dirty one, and much soap and hot water form essential parts of it. Moursou,[1] a French naval surgeon, first pointed out the relation between certain blue spots on the skin and pediculi pubis, and Douguet confirmed the relationship by inserting a bruised pediculus under the skin and producing a spot. Mallet proved that the colouring matter resides in the salivary glands of the pediculus. In the early spring the spots are more abundant than in other months.

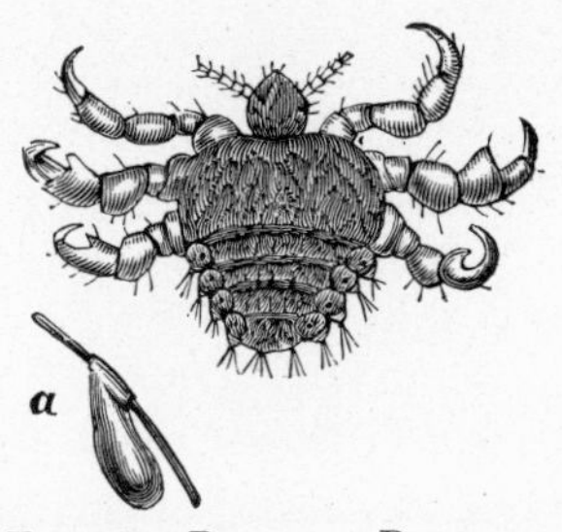

FIG. 162.—PEDICULUS PUBIS AND NIT.

INJURIES OF THE SCROTUM

Wounds.—Wounds of the scrotum, whether surgical or accidental, give rise to free bleeding. This must be entirely controlled

---

[2] Lancet, 1882, ii, 454.

by clamp and ligature before the wound is sutured, for in the lax scrotal tissues an insignificant oozing may give rise to an enormous hematoma extending to penis, thighs, and abdomen. Efficient hemostasis is therefore of prime importance. Every smallest clot adhering to the sides of the wound must be scraped away with the nail, and, if bleeding occurs beneath, it must be checked by torsion or ligature.

If the hemostasis is really efficient, the wound may be closed by a continuous suture with the points close together (since the dartos tends to separate the edges). As a further precaution, the scrotum may be compressed beneath a double hip spica and criss-cross bandage. I have recently employed an adhesive-plaster dressing suggested by Dr. W. Duff Bullard. An adhesive-plaster strap is laid tightly across the thighs beneath the scrotum, which rests upon it covered only by a light dressing. Compression is then obtained by passing a number of adhesive straps obliquely over the scrotum at various angles. The testicles are pushed up or down according to the requirements of the case. This dressing, if carefully applied, is light, snug, and comfortable.

Loss of Tissue.—When any considerable portion of the scrotum is destroyed by gangrene, accident, or the knife, the rapidity with which the defect covers in is little less than marvellous.

Castration need never be performed, however great the loss of integument. Kocher's[1] case, in which both testicles were practically covered over by skin in the short space of three weeks, shows what brilliant results may be obtained by expectant treatment. The surgeon need only help with tension sutures and aseptic dressings.

Hematoma and Hematocele.—Contusions of the scrotum give rise to extensive ecchymosis and edema quite comparable to the familiar black eye. If seen early the hemorrhage may be checked by adhesive-plaster compression and an ice-cap. Later heat promotes absorption, which is rapid. The hematoma need not be incised.

Scrotal or extra-vaginal hematocele (blood cyst of the scrotum) is a very rare result of scrotal hematoma. Jacobson[2] mentions two cases.

INFLAMMATIONS OF THE SCROTUM

Inflammatory Edema.—Extensive edema may complicate any inflammatory affection of the scrotum on account of the laxity of its tissue and its dependent position. Scrotal edema may also be

---

[1] Billroth and Lücke, Deutsche Chir., 1887, 1 (b), 8.

[2] Diseases of the Male Organ of Generation, 1893, 549.

due to any obstruction to the return of its blood, as occasionally to the hard inflammatory induration about an inguinal adenitis, or it may occur in connection with general anasarca.

Where edema is excessive, and the tension so great that injury to the skin seems imminent from pressure, a few punctures may be made on each side of the raphe, at the most dependent point of the scrotum. These punctures should be protected by a wet dressing to encourage oozing, to improve the circulation, and to prevent infection. In milder cases, strapping (p. 727) will quickly reduce the edema, if the cause has been removed and a suspensory bandage is applied.

Cellulitis and Abscess.—Cellulitis and abscess of the scrotum are encountered clinically as phenomena in the development of urinary infiltration (p. 233).

Cellulitis after operation reacts kindly to irrigation and drainage unless the patient is much debilitated, or unless some suture or other foreign body remains in the wound.

Erysipelas.—The peculiar virulence of scrotal erysipelas is in striking contrast with the milder inflammations of this region. It is most frequently observed in the aged and debilitated, and may be spontaneous or due to trauma.

The disease begins suddenly with a chill. A small red blotch upon the scrotum spreads until one side or both are involved in an intense phlegmonous inflammation. The scrotum is enormously swollen, covered with blebs, and mottled by subcutaneous hemorrhage. The pulse is rapid, the temperature septic. The patient usually fails rapidly, the scrotum becomes gangrenous, and death closes the scene.

In the beginning, the rapidity of invasion and the superficial nature of the lesion distinguish it from urinary infiltration. In the later stages the two closely resemble each other.

Treatment.—Multiple free incisions parallel to the raphe, and the lavish use of 1% carbolic-acid wet dressings and hot carbolic baths daily should be employed. Tonics and stimulants may not be neglected; notably, tincture ferri chlorid in large doses and alcoholic stimulants with strychnin.

Gangrene.—Gangrene of the scrotum, whether due to urinary infiltration, infection, or injury, usually involves the greater part of the scrotum, is accompanied by considerable constitutional disturbance, and often terminates fatally, especially in the aged and diabetic. The testicles are always spared and swing bare and bald. As already noted, the skin of the scrotum heals with such marvellous rapidity that plastic operations are rarely necessary.

Treatment.—Stimulation, free incisions, wet dressings, and excision of sloughs as fast as they form are the main lines of treatment. Castration is never indicated.

Diphtheria.—Le Clerc [1] has observed and collected a number of cases resembling, clinically, an acute erysipelas, and which he attributes to diphtheria, the Klebs-Loeffler bacillus having been cultivated, either pure or in mixed culture, from the wound discharges.

Emphysema.—This occurs with general subcutaneous emphysema and with scrotal gangrene.

Scrotal Fistula and Calculi.—See p. 235.

ELEPHANTIASIS, LYMPH SCROTUM, LYMPH VARIX

This disease is rare enough in our latitudes to warrant a superficial treatment here, especially as the usual cause of lymph scrotum, the filaria sanguinis hominis (Bancroftii), receives due notice in all the larger Systems of Medicine.

Elephantiasis is a condition of chronic distention of the lymph vessels of any part of the body, whereby the skin and subcutaneous tissues become thickened and indurated and the part often enlarges to an incredible size. It occurs usually in the lower extremity and in the penis and scrotum. With the last we are here interested.

Etiology.—The cause of elephantiasis is obstruction of the lymph channels. Thus I have seen scrotal elephantiasis following extirpation of the inguinal glands.[2] Severe chronic inguinal adenitis may have the same unhappy effect. But the enormous elephantiasis, so frequent in the tropics, is due almost always to the filaria sanguinis hominis. The fascinating life history of the filaria has been studied by Lewis,[3] Manson,[4] Le Dentu,[5] Mastin,[6] Lothrop and Pratt,[7] and many others. Born in some marsh or swamp, the embryo enters a man's alimentary canal in a sip of water. Thence it makes its way to the lymphatics, where, in some comfortable spot, it settles down for life and attains its full development. Here it is impregnated and pours into the blood-current an infinite stream of embryos. By night the blood is alive with them, by day not one can

---

[1] Guyon's Annales, 1898, xvi, 1102.

[2] *Cf.* Bull. soc. française de dermat. et syph., 1898, ix, 292.

[3] On a Hematozoön Inhabiting Human Blood, 1872, Calcutta.

[4] Med. Times and Gazette, 1875, ii, 542, 566; Trans. Path. Soc., 1881, xxxii, 285; Brit. Med. J., 1899, ii, 644.

[5] Revue de chir., 1898, xviii, 1.

[6] Ann. of Surg., 1888, viii, 321.

[7] Am. J. of Med. Sciences, 19, cxx, 525.

be found where, a few hours before, were myriads: where they hide no one knows. But in the human host they cannot develop. To reach maturity they must be sucked up by a mosquito—a night-prowling insect. The mosquito, gorged with blood, returns to deposit her eggs and die in his (or rather her) native swamp, where from her corpse arise the filariæ ready to develop, to infest the water, and again to be swallowed by some unsuspecting man.[1]

So much for the romance. The sorry fact is that these embryos, no larger than a leukocyte (or perhaps certain more corpulent ones—Manson), become impacted in the lymph glands or channels in such a way as slowly and progressively to obstruct the lymph flow. If this happens in the lower inguinal glands, elephantiasis of the lower extremity results; if in the upper chain, the scrotum and penis are affected; if in the iliac glands, *lymph varix* and *lymphadenoma* of the spermatic cord may result.

Chyluria (or hemato-chyluria) and *chylous hydrocele* are caused by rupture of a dilated lymphatic vessel into the cavity of the urinary tract or into the tunica vaginalis.

Symptoms.—Elephantiasis begins with recurring attacks of dermatitis and edema accompanied by fever. At first, there is between the attacks only a brawny patch upon the skin and a slight enlargement of the inguinal glands. As the disease progresses, the skin and subcutaneous tissues become thickened by an overgrowth of dense fibro-elastic tissue, and the vessels, especially the lymphatics, become enormously dilated. As the scrotum enlarges it drags down the skin of pubes and perineum and inverts the skin of the penis, leaving, finally, no trace of that organ, except a transverse slit on the anterior surface of the tumour. The tumour reaches incredible proportions. Wilkes removed a scrotum weighing 165 pounds, and Larrey mentions one weighing 200 pounds.

Treatment.—The *prophylaxis*, avoidance of unboiled drinking water in the tropics, need scarcely be insisted upon. *Curative* treatment is surgical. Though Flint [2] reports a cure of filarial chyluria by the use of methylene blue, I do not know that his experience has been repeated. Fortunately, ablation of the hypertrophied tissues is rarely followed by recurrence, though such an operation does not pretend to affect the mother worm or her ovulation. The chief danger of operation is the bleeding. This was successfully controlled in an operation for vulvar elephantiasis, at which I had the pleasure of

[1] Of late years there is a tendency to consider the mosquito the adequate intermediate host, as is the case in malaria. I have sketched the classic theory, although it will perhaps be proved incorrect.

[2] N. Y. Med. J., 1895, lxi, 737.

assisting, by Wyeth's hip pins and an Esmarch bandage.[1] It is essential to remove as much as possible of the indurated tissue, and yet to leave flaps to cover the testicles and penis. Radical cure of hernia may also be required. The strictest asepsis should be observed to avoid lymphatic absorption. In the smaller cases the inguinal glands may be removed.

TUMOURS OF THE SCROTUM

Cysts.—Small sebaceous cysts, shining white through the distended skin, occur on any part of the scrotum, but particularly on the raphe. They sometimes attain startling dimensions. Echinococcus cysts have been met with. A urinary pocket opening into the urethra behind a stricture has been mistaken for hydrocele. Jacobson [2] gives a detailed account of two cases of cystic disease of the scrotum, to which Tilden Brown [3] has added a third.

Multiple minute blood cysts, doubtless capillary dilatations, varying in size up to that of a large pinhead, and sprinkled abundantly over the entire scrotum, are sometimes found after middle life. They are of a dark-blue colour and give rise to no changes in the skin and to no symptoms whatsoever, excepting their appearance, which annoys the patient. They may be cured permanently by touching each one separately with an electro-cautery, or pricking it and touching the raw surface with a nitrate-of-silver point.

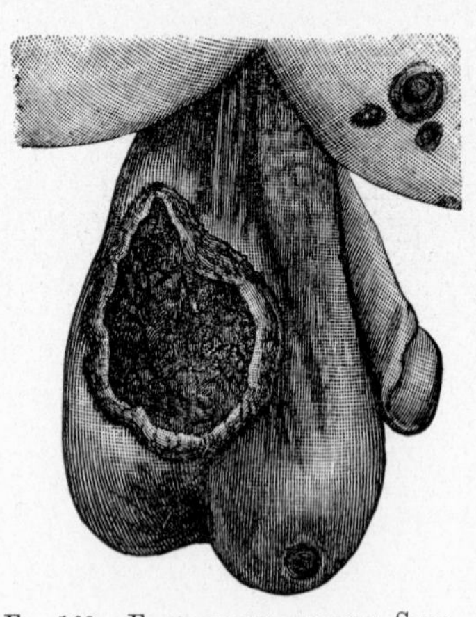

Fig. 163.—Epithelioma of the Scrotum in a Paraffin Worker.
Three ulcers covered with scabs can be seen on the right buttock.

Cases of *angioma*, *fibroma*, *lipoma*, *fibromyxoma*, *osteochondroma*, and *sarcoma* have been reported.

Epithelioma of the Scrotum (*Chimney-Sweeps' Cancer.*—Soot seems to be the exciting cause of scrotal epithelioma (Fig. 163) in England, although in other countries those whose occupation brings them into contact with this substance do not seem to suffer. Thus Warren [4] states that he has seen it a few times in this country, but never among chimney-sweeps.

---

[1] Bullard. Med. Record, 1899, lv, 128. [2] *Op. cit.*, p. 565.
[3] J. of Cut. and Gen.-Urin. Diseases, 1895, xiii, 33.
[4] Surgical Observations on Tumours, p. 329.

The disease begins as one or more small, soft warts or tubercles, usually at the lower forepart of the scrotum. These remain unchanged for a time, but finally indurate slightly, become excoriated, scab over, and ulcerate, the ulcer extending backward, and destroying, with more or less rapidity, the whole scrotum. Sometimes the testicles are involved, sometimes they escape. The ulcer is epitheliomatous. It has the hardened, irregular, purplish, everted, knotty borders; the hard, uneven, unhealthy looking base; the ichorous discharge, now sanguinolent, now purulent.

Death occurs by exhaustion, or by hemorrhage, if a large vessel be severed by the advancing ulceration. The disease continues local for some time. It is only tardily that the inguinal glands become involved.

Treatment.—Before the disease has assumed a malignant aspect it may be snipped or burned out. But when frankly cancerous an elliptical piece of the surrounding skin should be excised with the growth. If the testicle is involved, or if its integrity is doubtful, it had best be sacrificed. The inguinal glands, which enlarge late in the disease, should be treated according to the rules laid down for epithelioma of the penis (p. 686). The earlier the operation is undertaken the less the probability of relapse, though a second or third operation may succeed where the first has failed.

CHAPTER VI

ANATOMY, PHYSIOLOGY, EMBRYOLOGY, AND ANOMALIES OF THE TESTICLE

ANATOMY

THE testicles (Fig. 164), each suspended by its spermatic cord, lie loosely in the scrotum, surrounded by connective tissue. The left is usually slightly larger than the right and hangs lower, evidently for the purpose of permitting these important organs the more readily to elude violence. It has been observed, in transposition of the viscera, that the right testicle hangs the lower. The mean dimensions of the testicle, according to Curling, are $1\frac{3}{4}$ inches long, $1\frac{1}{4}$ inches antero-posteriorly, and 1 inch laterally. The average weight in the adult is about 6 drams. The dimensions, weight, and consistence vary considerably, according as the organ is in action or not. During venereal excitement it is turgescent, firm, and elastic; otherwise soft and yielding. Two of the envelopes of the cord, the cremaster muscle and the tunic vaginalis communis, also cover the testicle, while the remains of the gubernaculum testis attach it to the bottom of the scrotum.

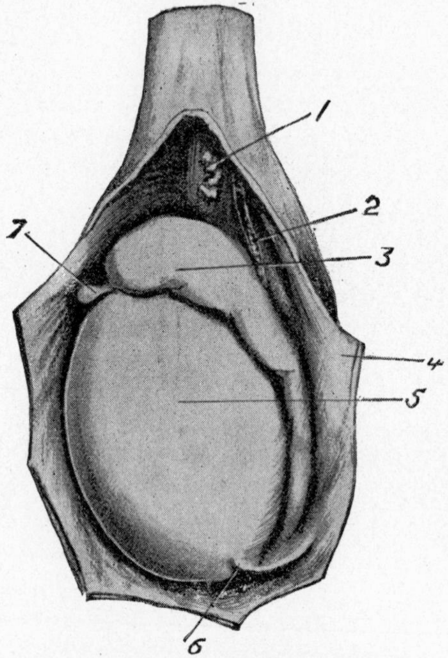

FIG. 164.—LEFT TUNICA VAGINALIS OPENED, SHOWING TESTIS, EPIDIDYMIS, ETC., FROM OUTER SIDE.
1, organ of Giraldès; *2*, vas deferens; *3*, globus major of epididymis; *4*, *6*, tunica vaginalis; *5*, testicle; *7*, hydatid of Morgagni (Quain).

Tunica Vaginalis.—The proper coverings of the testicle are two —the tunica vaginalis and the tunica albuginea. The former is a closed serous sac, investing all the secreting portion of the testicle, except where the epididymis is attached behind and the remains of the gubernaculum below. It dips down posteriorly, between the epididymis and the testicle, forming a *cul-de-sac*, at the bottom of which the sac on the two sides comes into close contact, and sometimes there is a communication at this point. On the outer side the tunica vaginalis covers and closely invests the epididymis. The reflected layer forms a closed sac, and extends up the cord to a greater or less extent.

The tunica vaginalis represents a portion of the peritoneum carried down by the testicle in its descent from the abdomen. Ordinarily, at birth, all connection between its cavity and that of the peritoneum is closed, a white, fibrous line (habenula) alone marking the original continuity of membrane. Sometimes, however, the opening persists, in which case congenital hernia is likely to occur; or the communication may be a narrow canal, open to the passage of fluid only; or again, partial obliteration may occur, isolated serous sacs being left along the cord; finally, it more often happens that the upper aperture is closed, and a considerable portion below remains unobliterated, so that the tunica vaginalis extends for some distance upward in front of the cord.

The cavity of the tunica vaginalis is lined by pavement epithelium, and normally contains only enough fluid to lubricate the surfaces. The function of the sac is to permit the testicle to slip away easily when in danger of being pinched.

Tunica Albuginea.—The tunica albuginea is the proper investing membrane of the secreting portion of the testicle. In its substance the branches of the spermatic artery ramify and break up, to be distributed to the seminal tubules within. It is composed of dense, white, fibrous tissue, is only slightly extensible (whence the pain in orchitis), and sends trabeculæ into the substance of the testicle to break it up into compartments (about 400 in each testicle) for the lodgment of the tubuli seminiferi. It forms the mediastinum (corpus Highmorianum) above and behind, where the vessels pass to and from the testicle, and where the straight tubes come out to form the coni vasculosi in the head of the epididymis.

Glandular Substance.—The glandular substance of the testicle consists of innumerable little tubes (tubuli seminiferi) closely packed in conical segments between the fine, fibrous septa thrown out by the tunica albuginea. The number of these cones is computed to be from 250 to about 500, and their combined length from 1,000 to

5,500 feet. The diameter of the tubules has been variously estimated at from $\frac{1}{18}$ of a line (Müller) to $\frac{1}{15}$ of a line (Lauth). Their mean length is estimated by Lauth at 25 inches.

The tubes anastomose frequently with their fellows of the same cone, and with those of neighbouring cones. They are much convoluted, and consist of a hyalin membrana propria, within which are several layers of epithelial cells, the outer ones polyhedral, those nearer the lumen spherical. These latter are known as spermatoblasts, and from them the spermatozoa are evolved. A section through a normal tubule shows the stages of this process by which the cells become pear-shaped, tailed, and finally full-fledged spermatozoa.

Issuing from the apices of the cones the tubes unite to form 20 or 30 tubes (vasa recta) which run straight into the fibrous mediastinum, and there form an irregular plexus of channels with no proper walls (rete testis). Issuing hence the ducts, now known as vasa efferentia, pierce the tunica albuginea to form the epididymis.

The Epididymis.—The epididymis (ἐπί, *upon*; δίδυμος, *testicle*) caps the testicle proper and skirts its posterior border. It begins above, where the vasa efferentia issue through the tunica albuginea. These canals immediately dilate and collect in convoluted cones (coni vasculosi), forming the broadest part of the epididymis, the head or *globus major*, which lies over the top of the testicle. The coni vasculosi all empty into one canal—the canal of the epididymis, which forms by its convolutions the central part or body of the epididymis. This body is separated from the testicle proper by the *cul-de-sac* of the tunica vaginalis already alluded to. Below, the canal of the epididymis exhibits further convolutions. At this point it is known as the *globus minor*, or the tail of the epididymis. Connective tissue unites it to the testicle at this point, and from here on the canal becomes more dense, and is known as the vas deferens.

The little supernumerary diverticulum (or there may be several), known as the *vas aberrans* of Haller, when present, usually empties into the canal of the epididymis at this point. The canal of the epididymis is furnished with ciliated epithelium whose cilia sweep its contents along towards the vas deferens.

There exist normally upon the head of the epididymis several little prominences, solid and cystic, known as the hydatid of Morgagni, or pediculated hydatid, the corpus innominatum of Giraldès, and the non-pediculated hydatids. They are the remains of the Wolffian body and of the duct of Müller.

The blood-supply of the testicle and epididymis is derived from the spermatic artery, a branch of the aorta. The lymphatics empty into the lumbar (not the inguinal) glands. There are nerve filaments from the lumbar plexus of the sympathetic.

PHYSIOLOGY

External Secretion.—The function of the testicle is to form spermatozoa, the male procreative seed. These micro-organisms are the result, not of a secretion, but of an evolution of the spermatoblasts of the seminal tubules. Thence they issue by force of their own motility to the epididymis, where their transit is hastened by the ciliated epithelium. From the vas deferens they are collected in the seminal vesicles, whence they are ejaculated during the sexual orgasm.

Internal Secretion.—The so-called internal secretion of the testicles—viz., the effect of the presence of the testicles upon the organism at large—has been studied anew of late years in connection with the discussion over the propriety of castration for hypertrophy of the prostate. It has long been known that the testicles are essential to a virile adolescence, since castration in infancy produces the recognised type of high-voiced effeminate eunuchs. The familiar contrast between ox and bull, horse and stallion, is equally to the point. As White [1] puts it: "The function of the testis, like that of the ovary, is twofold—the reproduction of the species and the development and preservation of the secondary sexual characteristics of the individual. The need for the exercise of the latter function—the one with which we are concerned—ceases when full adult life is reached." So much is universally conceded.

Whether, as White and many others believe, the testicle continues to influence the characteristics of the individual after puberty by some function distinct from its spermatogenesis; whether the "hypertrophies in closely allied organs, like the prostate and uterus," may occur as "the result of this misdirected energy," is not yet determined. While I am no believer in White's theory that the testicle produces hypertrophy of the prostate, and have failed to find documentary evidence of the alleged prostatic atrophy after castration,[2] I confess that congestion, hypertrophy, and carcinoma of the prostate, and contracture of the neck of the bladder are at present too hopelessly confused for any definite conclusion to be possible. I am inclined to accept the theory that the internal secretion of the testicle continues in adult life; but how much influence it has upon the characteristics, sexual or other, of the individual has

---

[1] Gen.-Urin. and Venereal Diseases, 1898, 995. [2] Med. Record, 1900, lviii, 81.

not been estimated. It is probably slight, for the mental and physical disturbances following castration, whether in the male or the female, are, in great part, attributable to the mental shock of knowing that those organs, about whose function so many see fit to centre their lives, are forever lost.

EMBRYOLOGY[1]

The two constituent parts of the testicle, which have been briefly described above, are developed separately in the fetus. Each receives its blood from a separate artery, although these arteries anastomose quite freely at their extremities. This peculiarity of vascular supply may account for the fact that one part of the organ is often diseased, the other part remaining sound. The epididymis is formed from the lower part of the Wolffian body, and its duct is a continuation of the Wolffian duct to the lower and back part of the bladder. The deferential artery, a branch of the hypogastric, supplies it. The secreting portion of the testicle, on the other hand, is formed from fetal tissue lying in front of, but seemingly independent of, the Wolffian body, and its artery, the spermatic, comes from the aorta just below the renal artery.

The Descent of the Testicle.—The descent of the testicle into the scrotum occurs during the last six months of intra-uterine life.[2] Indeed, in 10% or 20% of all children the testicles are still in the abdomen at the time of birth. In most of these the testicle descends during the following weeks, but in a small proportion of cases it is retained for years, or even permanently. The clinician need take no account of the position of the testicle during the first year, but if it is retained for longer than this the condition is definitely abnormal.

The testicle develops in front of the Wolffian body, resting upon the brim of the true pelvis near the site of the future inguinal canal, which at this period (fifth month) is represented by the *processus funiculo-vaginalis*, a pouch of peritoneum running into and terminating among the muscle fibres of the abdominal wall, through which it ultimately extends into the scrotum. This pouch offers a resting-place into which the testis tends to work its way, aided by the *gubernaculum testis*, a fibro-muscular cord attached above to the testis,

---

[1] *Cf.* Kocher, *op. cit.*, p. 547; Jacobson, *op. cit.*, p. 1; Curling, Diseases of the Testis, 4th Ed., 1878, p. 14; Monod and Terrillon, Traité d. mal. du testicule, 1889.

[2] Only mammals, and not all of them, have extra-abdominal testes, while some mammals retain the testes within the abdominal cavity, except during the rutting season, when they become congested and are extruded into the scrotum (*cf.* Griffiths, J. of Anat. and Phys., 1893–'94, xxvii, 209).

epididymis, and spermatic cord, below to the abdominal wall, the inner surface of the pubes, the bottom of the scrotum, the perineum, and by a few fibres to the thigh over the saphenous opening. Guided, or perhaps pulled—the point is disputed—by the gubernaculum, the testicle settles into the peritoneal pouch, and with it sinks gradually through the abdominal wall and into the scrotum. The stronger fibres of the gubernaculum, fastened to the bottom of the scrotum, persist in adult life as a fascial band, while the processus funiculo-vaginalis, inverted by the descent of the testis, becomes the tunica vaginalis. The part of the processus above the testis is obliterated by adhesion of its opposed surfaces, beginning at both ends, above at the internal abdominal ring, below quite near the testicle. When adhesion is complete only a fibrous cord, the *habenula*, remains.

ANOMALIES OF THE TESTICLE

Monod and Terrillon's classification of anomalies of the testicle is the following:

Anomalies in development	In number	In excess		Polyorchism.
		Deficient	Absence	Anorchism.
			Fusion	Synorchism.
	In size	In excess		Hypertrophy.
		Deficient		Atrophy.
Anomalies in migration	Undescended	Incomplete migration		Retention.
		Abnormal migration		Ectopia.
	Descended			Inversion.

I. **Anomalies of Development. — Polyorchism.** — Though many instances of supernumerary testis have been reported, and the condition is known to exist in the lower animals (Jacobson), the alleged instances in man have proved to be pedunculated tumours, encysted hydrocele, omental hernia, or have lacked the proof of a pathological examination, with the exception of the case reported by Arbuthnot Lane,[1] in which the diagnosis was confirmed by a microscopical examination of the supernumerary organ.

Anorchism.—The testicle may be lacking on one or both sides. With absence of the testicle is associated—

1. Usually absence of the epididymis and part of the vas, or
2. Exceptionally, entire absence of the seminal duct up to the vesicle, or
3. Still more rarely, the testis only is wanting, while
4. The testis may be present and the vesicle, epididymis, and vas absent (Jacobson).

---

[1] Brit. Med. J., 1894, ii, 1241.

During life anorchism cannot be differentiated from abdominal cryptorchism, except by operation.

Synorchism.—Jacobson cites the cases of Cruveilhier and Lockwood, the one in an adult, the other in a fetus, of intra-abdominal testicular fusion.

II. **Anomalies in Migration (Cryptorchism).**—*Cryptorchism* means absence of one or both testicles from the scrotum, and their presence elsewhere, in contradistinction to *anorchism*, mentioned above, meaning total absence. *Monorchism* is unilateral cryptorchism. A *retained testis* is one that has been arrested at some point in its normal descent. An *ectopic testis* is, strictly speaking, one that has lodged at some point out of its normal course. Ectopia testis is often used loosely as a synonym for cryptorchism.

Cryptorchism is an infrequent anomaly. Marshal found 11 cases among 10,800 English recruits, of which only 1 was bilateral. Rennes met with only 6 cases among 3,600 French recruits, of which none was bilateral.

Retention.—By obstruction to its progress or by traction from behind (peritoneal adhesions, shortness of the vas, etc.) the testis may be retained inside the abdomen, or it may be arrested at any point in its descent. Hence there may be: 1. *Abdominal retention*, the testis lying in the lumbar region, or floating attached by a "mesorchium," or resting in the false pelvis near the internal abdominal ring (iliac retention). 2. *Inguinal retention*, the most common variety, the testis lying at the internal abdominal ring (internal inguinal retention), in the canal (interstitial inguinal retention), or at the external ring (external inguinal retention). 3. *Pubo-scrotal retention*, the testis lying just under the pubic bone. 4. Rarely the testicle alone is retained, while the epididymis and vas are separated from it and descend normally into the scrotum.

Ectopia.—Abnormal tension of some of the accessory bands of the gubernaculum may drag the testis out of its normal course: (1) into the perineum, where it will lie beneath the deep fascia, in front of the anus; or (2) through the crural canal to the saphenous opening (very rare); or (3) into the opposite side of the scrotum (cases of Jordan [1] and von Lenhossek); or (4) to the front of the pubis at the base of the penis (2 cases of Popow's [2]).

Inversion.—The testicle may be turned upside down in the scrotum, or rotated so that its long axis is horizontal or abnormally attached to the epididymis (*cf.* Jacobson). The only clinical significance of these very rare anomalies is their bearing on puncture of

---

[1] Deutsch. med. Woch., 1895, xxi, 525. [2] Bull. de la soc. anat., 1888, v, ii, 653.

hydrocele, for the inverted testis often lies above and in front of instead of below and behind the tunica vaginalis.

Condition of the Testicle.—The retained testis is almost always found post mortem in a state of fatty or fibrous degeneration. In some cases the testicle may never have reached even an incomplete development on account of some congenital fault; but, as a rule, the testicle is normal at first, and its atrophy is rapid or slow in proportion to the pressure to which it is subjected. If both testes are retained in the abdomen they may atrophy so early in life as to leave the individual eunuchoid, practically asexual in both his mental and physical character; but, happily, the glands usually retain their physiological capacity long enough to endow their host with masculine attributes and even potency. The sterility of cryptorchids has been hotly debated. It is true that a great majority of double cryptorchids are sterile, and so general is the application of this rule that Curling,[1] after citing several cases of women married to cryptorchids bearing one or several children, felt compelled to doubt their paternity. But several similar cases have been reported since, a notable one by Milner Smyth,[2] whose patient begot five children, and the question is seemingly closed by the observations of Beigel[3] and of Valette.[4] The former found numerous spermatozoa in the semen of a double cryptorchid aged twenty-two. The latter found a few in the retained testicle removed from a man twenty-one years old.

In determining the sterility of any given patient several points must be taken into consideration.

1. The position of the testicles, since abdominal cryptorchids appear to be always sterile.
2. Freedom from previous or present inflammation.
3. The size, consistency, sensitiveness, and mobility of the testicles, and
4. The age of the patient. Bellingham Smith[5] observes that all the cryptorchids to whom children have been attributed were young men, and that, therefore, although cryptorchids may retain their virility until puberty, their period of possible paternity is not over five or ten years.
5. A definite conclusion is impossible, except from the microscopical examination of the semen for spermatozoa, obtained when possible by milking it from the seminal vesicles.

Complications of Cryptorchism.—Beyond the debatable point of the sterility of double cryptorchids, there are several very real com-

---

[1] *Op. cit.*, p. 467.
[2] Lancet, 1899, ii, 785.
[3] Virchow's Archiv, 1867, xxxviii, 144.
[4] Lyon méd., 1869, ii, 20.
[5] Guy's Hospital Reports, 896, liii, 215.

plications of retained or ectopic testicle. The remarks on this subject may be confined to inguinal retention, since this includes the vast majority of cases.

Neuralgia of the testicle is an early evidence that the surrounding muscles are exerting injurious pressure upon the gland. *Inflammation*, whether traumatic, gonorrheal, or tubercular, is not rare, and, if acute, is exquisitely painful. *Atrophy* follows. Hydrocele, gangrene, abscess, and fatal peritonitis are among the rarer consequences of inflammation.

Malignant growths are very frequent, especially sarcoma. The degenerated condition of the organ and the constant irritation to which it is subjected render it particularly liable to malignant changes. The frequency of these growths is the most weighty argument in favour of castration.

Hernia often accompanies inguinal retention, since the testicle keeps the canal patent. Absence of the testicle from the scrotum gives a clew to the differentiation between retained testis and hernia. When the testicle becomes strangulated by torsion of the cord it simulates strangulated hernia (p. 714).

Prognosis.—Spontaneous descent of the testicle may not be looked for after the first year in any large proportion of cases. A sudden muscular effort caused spontaneous descent of the testicles of a man thirty-three years old (Landouzy), but this is a most exceptional case. Ambrose Paré has left an amusing account of one Marie Germain who jumped a ditch in chasing her pigs when, feeling a sharp pain and "seeing her genitals develop" "s'en retourne larmoyant en la maison de sa mère disant que ses tripes lui estoient sorties hors du ventre," whereupon her true sex was recognised and she became a man, though doubtless not a very virile one.

In general the prognosis of retained testis is "atrophy, perhaps sarcoma."

Treatment.—During infancy every effort should be made by pad and truss to encourage the testicle to descend. I have succeeded in this endeavour several times, and success is possible up to the tenth year.

If mechanical treatment does not effect reduction, the testicle may be allowed to remain where it is, or operation may be performed to drag it down or to extirpate it. A great latitude is permissible in choosing a course of action, and, after all, the last word rests with the patient himself; but the ideal treatment is certainly reduction which, if successful, insures the patient against atrophy, malignant degeneration, and hernia, and, if unsuccessful, leaves him no worse off than before. If there is pain, frequent or severe, or hernia, this attempt should certainly be made and the testicle sacrificed if it cannot be brought down. Broca[1] has succeeded in bringing down 138 such testicles without a death. Of 79 cases observed for over a year 31 have apparently normal testicles, 35 have testicles normal in quality, but abnormal in position (near the external ring), while in only 13 had the gland atrophied. In 1 case the abdominal wall remained weak, and in no case was there any recurrence of pain. Only once was castration required. These brilliant results were obtained on young children, and form a striking contrast with the difficulty experienced in accomplishing anything with retained testis in the adult. The inference is obvious: operate in childhood.

Broca's method of operating is as follows: The inguinal canal is laid open and the hernial sac (if present) freed and tied off, as in Bassini's operation. The cremaster and any other restricting bands are then divided, the cord freed from the surrounding fascia (this must be done thoroughly), and the testicle placed as low as possible in a hole burrowed for it in the scrotum. The inguinal canal is then closed, as for the radical cure of hernia, and the fascia sutured snugly about the end (yet not so tightly as to strangulate it) so as to press down upon the testicle. After two or three weeks this pressure may be supplemented by a pad.

Wood's[2] device of freeing the vas from the globus major and then inverting the testis might be employed, and a suture anchoring the testis to the perineum may help.

When this operation fails, castration is, in most instances, preferable to abdominal reposition, an operation which has been several times performed, but which subjects the gland to the very dangers (except hernia) to be avoided.

---

[1] Gaz. Hebdom., 1899, iv, 289, and Gaz. des hôp., 1899, lxxii, 315.

[2] St. Louis Med. and Surg. J., June, 1884.

CHAPTER VII

DISEASES OF THE TESTICLE

LUXATION OF THE TESTICLE

Occasionally the testicle is dislocated. In 1 case reported,[1] the right testicle was suddenly and violently drawn up into the inguinal canal during masturbation, and did not come down again. Later in life, when the patient died, this testicle was found soft, atrophied, pulpy, about one fifth the size of its fellow. P. Brüns [2] records the case of a man run over while lying on his back. The right testicle was dislocated over the pubis at the root of the penis. It remained there and did not atrophy. He refers to other traumatic dislocations, one under the skin of the thigh (the testicle atrophied), and a number where the luxation was into the inguinal canal.

HYPERTROPHY AND ATROPHY

The testicle undergoes compensatory *hypertrophy* when its fellow is defective or wanting, and in certain lusty individuals the testicles are abnormally large.

Arrest of development is typical in the retained testis and may also affect the normally situated organ for no assignable cause.

True *atrophy* is caused by severe orchitis in any form, by pressure (hydrocele, elephantiasis), by section or obstruction of the spermatic artery, by contusion of the testicle, by severe varicocele, and by injuries to the nerves, spinal cord, and brain. It may occur spontaneously or during the course of a syphilis without gummy deposit; but it is never caused by the internal use of iodids, by injury to the vas deferens (unless the vessels are injured), or by continence. Sexual excess is alleged to have caused atrophy of the testicles. The physiological atrophy of old age has been studied by Desnos,[3] Griffiths,[4] and Pawloff.[5]

[1] Med. Times and Gazette, xviii, 67.
[2] Mittheilungen aus der chir. Klinik zu Tübingen, 1884, iii, 483.
[3] Guyon's Annales, 1886, iv, 72.
[4] J. of Anat. and Phys., 1893–'94, xxviii, 209.
[5] Guyon's Annales, 1894, xii, 291.

There are two forms of atrophy, the one *sclerotic*, the result of inflammation, the other *fatty*, the result of an obstruction to the circulation.

The orchitis of mumps is the most frequent cause of atrophy of the testicle.

Treatment.—For atrophy of the testicle but little can be done. The causes are usually beyond the surgeon's control. In certain cases the cause (neighbouring tumour, syphilis) may be removed.

CONTUSIONS OF THE TESTICLE

Owing to its peculiar anatomical surroundings contusions of the testicle are rare, notwithstanding its exposed position. In severe contusions there is ecchymosis, and perhaps hematocele or orchitis, and subsequent atrophy may result. One of the modes formerly adopted in the East for emasculating the attendants of the harem was that of squeezing the testis, and animals have been treated in this way in England and France (Curling). The inflammation after injury may be sufficiently severe to result in abscess or gangrene.

Kocher records 2 deaths from the shock of contusion of the testicle.

Treatment.—If the contusion be severe, the patient must be placed at once upon his back, with the testicle elevated and covered with a cooling application; if subsequent inflammation occur, it must be met appropriately (p. 733).

WOUNDS OF THE TESTICLE

Punctured wounds, if small, are of no importance. They give rise to no inconvenience and heal without trouble. Penetrating wounds of fair size, however, permit some of the tubular structure of the testis to escape. This, if projecting and covered with pus, is very likely to be mistaken for a slough, and to be pulled out as such. Malgaigne mentions a case where he saw the whole pulp of the organ pulled out in this way. Injuries to the testicle, whether contusions or wounds, are usually very painful, and give rise to faintness, nausea, vomiting, and even convulsions. The testis may atrophy as the result of the injury or of a subsequent orchitis.

Treatment.—If there is any hernia of the secreting substance, this should be reduced if possible, and retained by pressure, or by a suture through the tunica albuginea. If it cannot be reduced, it may be snipped off with the scissors, but should in no case be pulled upon. Large incisions should be cleaned, united by suture, and the parts carefully supported. Even if a large portion of the testicle has been destroyed by the accident, an effort should be made to preserve what is left. Dorsal decubitus must be maintained, and the testicle properly supported and dressed.

GANGRENE OF THE TESTICLE

Gangrene of the testicle is commonly due to **Torsion of the Spermatic Cord,** a condition not generally recognised until within a few years. Scudder [1] has collected 31 cases, to which he adds 1 of his own. Of the 32 cases, 17 occurred on the right side, 11 on the left. Seventy-five per cent of the cases occurred in patients under twenty-three, at an age, namely, when the individual is most exposed to traumatism, and yet the trouble was usually attributed to nothing more violent than hard work or some indefinite strain. Indeed, in several cases the attacks were recurrent; thus, Van der Poel's patient learned that untwisting the testicle relieved the pain. The only evident predisposing cause is malposition of the testicle. Ten times the affected gland was retained in the inguinal canal, 5 times close under the pubes. Hence Scudder infers that a long mesorchium is required to permit torsion of the testis.

Morbid Anatomy.—The pathological changes in the testicle are well known from the results of castration. The testicle is found congested, hemorrhagic, edematous, or gangrenous. There is usually vaginal hydrocele or hematocele. The cord is found twisted upon itself (outward in 7 cases, inward in 5) one half to two and one half turns, and strangulated at the point of torsion.

Symptoms.—The symptoms are those of strangulated hernia, for which it is commonly mistaken. The groin and scrotum swell rapidly and become exquisitely sensitive. The patient vomits and is feverish and faint. Chill and syncope may occur. If the testicle is normally situated it may unroll spontaneously, thus relieving all the symptoms; but with the testis in the inguinal canal this could scarcely happen.

It is probable that certain cases of acute spontaneous orchitis are due to slight or temporary torsion of the cord.

Diagnosis.—Torsion of the cord has been distinguished from strangulated hernia by the mildness of the systemic disturbance, after the first shock has passed, in contrast with the severity of the local symptoms. In case of doubt immediate operation solves the difficulty.

---

[1] Annals of Surgery, 1901, xxxiv, 234.

Treatment.—Recurrent torsion might be prevented by anchoring the testicle to the dartos.

In the emergency of an acute attack it may be possible to untwist the testicle, as was done by Nash an hour and a half after the onset of symptoms. (The testicle subsequently atrophied.) In the majority of cases, however, operation affords the only hope of relief. The operation has been performed 29 times with no deaths. Once the testicle was allowed to slough away through a simple incision. The cord was untwisted 5 times. This was followed twice by sloughing and thrice by atrophy. Twenty-three castrations were successful. Every case operated on, therefore, has been cured.

Injury to the Spermatic Cord.—While such injuries to the spermatic cord as totally shut off the blood-supply of the testicle are calculated to cause gangrene of the organ, the impunity with which the cord may be tied off is exemplified by numerous cases collected by Mauclaire.[1] This operation is, apparently, almost always followed by simple atrophy of the testicle, a fact explained by the blood supplied to the testicle from the surrounding fascia, which furnishes sufficient nutrition to prevent sphacelus.

IRRITABLE AND NEURALGIC TESTICLE

Irritable Testicle.—True irritability of the testicle consists in an extraordinary sensitiveness of the whole gland or of some particular part of it. Mere contact of the clothing may be exquisitely painful. In the recumbent posture with nothing in contact with the testicle, the pain usually disappears. Perhaps the organ is tense and engorged, but of full size, and seemingly normal. Again, it may be decidedly flabby, the scrotal tissues being soft and lax. Irritable testis occurs at all times, from early puberty to late middle life. It is met with chiefly in old bachelors and widowers. In other respects the patient may possess robust health; or he may be anemic, nervous, hypochondriacal, and dyspeptic.

The title has been inappropriately bestowed upon another condition, which may be briefly disposed of. When the sexual appetite has been kindled and kept excited for some time without being gratified, seminal fluid, which has been produced and is collected in the testicle, vas deferens, and seminal vesicles, will usually be discharged in an involuntary emission at night, and no inconvenience will be felt beyond slight aching and increase of size of the testicle. Sometimes, however, Nature fails to relieve herself, and then the testicle becomes

[1] Guyon's Annales, 1900, xviii, 356.

large, hot, and excessively tender, the epididymis is distended and knotty, the cord tender and tense, the suffering very considerable, and the testicle, apparently, about to become acutely inflamed. Such a condition is a mere sexual congestion. The origin of the mischief can always be ascertained. A cure follows natural discharge of the excess of semen, or may be brought about by rest, elevation of the testicle, and the application of ice.

Neuralgia of the Testicle.—An excessive irritability of the testicle constitutes neuralgia, a malady which sometimes attains horrible intensity, and assumes the paroxysmal tic douloureux type. In other cases the pain is constant, and perhaps quite mild, but increased by walking and standing so as to occasion great discomfort. The character of the pain is acute and darting, or heavy and dragging. The cremaster contracts spasmodically during severe paroxysms, forcibly retracting the testicle, and a cold sweat, with nausea and vomiting, is not a rare accompaniment. Between paroxysms the testicle is often entirely free from pain. Handling the organ may perhaps induce a paroxysm. The testis, sometimes swollen and tense, is usually unaltered. There is no febrile reaction. Neuralgia is usually confined to one testicle, unlike irritability which is frequently double.

Etiology.—Neuralgia of the testis, like that of the ovary, has been attributed to every possible reflex; but certainly its most potent cause is sexual excess or irregularity, frequently that unchaste continence which revels in the paraphernalia of indecency, lewd books, plays, tales, and thoughts, while seeking to hide beneath the cloak of physical propriety. Temporary irritable testis may be produced in a healthy person, at any time, by prolonged sexual excitement ungratified. Masturbators who have suddenly reformed, and those who have abused their sexual powers, are all liable to it. Add to these physical causes a neurotic disposition and the picture is complete.

The more severe forms of neuralgia may be symptomatic of renal or of vesical calculus. Neuralgia is often associated with a small varicocele, rarely with a large one. Sometimes prostatic congestion is the cause, and in isolated cases neuralgia has been caused by foreign bodies in the vaginalis, abscess of the testicle, and similar local conditions.

Symptoms.—Neuralgia due to the causes last mentioned is usually unassociated with any physical disturbance. Quite different is the condition of those who suffer from the ordinary irritable testicle. These patients are prone to become more and more self-centred and to look upon their condition as a pitiable one, ascribing it to loss of seminal fluid—perhaps to nocturnal emissions—to neither of which does it bear any relation. They often demand castration—a demand which should be acceded to on no account. Curling quotes from Romberg an interesting case bearing on this point: A young man acquired irritable testis after becoming engaged to be married. It distressed him so seriously that he demanded extirpation of the organ, and would not yield until at last the operation was reluctantly performed. Eight days afterward the pain reappeared in the other testicle. This being all he had left, the patient preferred to keep it. He married, and "very soon recovered completely."

Treatment.—Neuralgia dependent on disease of the urethra or testicle disappears with its cause. Yet in a notable proportion of cases of purely sexual origin, the gentle passage of a sound or the installation of nitrate of silver (p. 134) into the deep urethra will work wonders and start the patient on the road to a cure far more quickly than anything else. But too much dependence must not be placed on such methods. They are but palliative, and if not rapidly curative they soon lose their efficacy. The backbone of the cure is sexual reform. Sexual hygiene, which means strict purity of thought as well as action, must be insisted on. A strict celibacy is usually impossible to such patients, while a happy marriage affords them a natural antidote to the irritability of their sexual apparatus, and is therefore to be urged relentlessly. The wavering patient is usually most unwilling to assume the yoke, fearing to prove a laggard partner. But he must be made to understand that a happy marriage—not a marriage of convenience—is his surest guarantee. At the same time the regulation of physical hygiene, exercise, diet, fresh air, regular hours, all must be minutely arranged. Tonic preparations of hypophosphites, glycero-phosphates, bromid of gold and arsenic, Fowler's solution, strychnin, and belladonna may be prescribed according to the physician's experience. They answer the double purpose of steadying the patient through his first period of reform and of soothing his mind with the assurance that something is being done for him. Locally counter-irritants may be of service. Hammond has successfully used intermittent pressure on the cord. The actual cautery and electricity might be useful. I have effected a cure by the local application of ice. A daily rectal douche, hot or cold, is often very beneficial.

CHAPTER VIII

INFLAMMATIONS OF THE TESTICLE AND EPIDIDYMIS

Inflammation of the testicle may be limited to the epididymis (epididymitis), or may attack the secreting structure only (orchitis). Sometimes both parts inflame simultaneously—as after injury. The secreting structure may become secondarily involved by a simple inflammation commencing in the epididymis, but the latter rarely suffers in connection with primary, true orchitis. The tunica vaginalis, lying close to the epididymis, becomes inflamed in most cases of epididymitis, constituting acute hydrocele. On the other hand, hydrocele is rare with orchitis, since the dense tunica albuginea prevents an inflammation originating on one side of it from being readily transmitted to the other.

Etiology.—Inflammations of the testicle may arise by—

1. Infection passing along the seminal canals from the urethra.
2. Infection from the blood or the lymph.
3. Trauma.

1. To the first class belong simple inflammatory and gonorrheal infections; they involve the epididymis primarily, the testicle only secondarily.

2. To the second class belong tubercular and syphilitic inflammations (the former usually beginning in the epididymis, the latter in the testicle) and the orchitis of infectious diseases.

3. Inflammations of the third class (traumatic) implicate both testis and epididymis, but chiefly the former.

Omitting tuberculosis and syphilis, which require separate consideration, it may be observed that, while the inflammations of testicle and epididymis begin usually in the one (orchitis of infectious disease, orchitis of trauma) or the other (epididymitis of gonorrhea, epididymitis of urethritis) portion of the organ, no one of these inflammations is necessarily confined to either part alone. It is therefore proper to classify them under the title "epididymo-orchitis"; but in order to insist on the distinction, clinical as well as etiological, that exists between them, it is convenient to group the infections of urethral origin as epididymitis, the other varieties as orchitis.

EPIDIDYMITIS

Epididymitis is the most common of all the diseases of the testicle. It occurs at any age, most frequently during early adult life and middle age, since its chief cause—urethral inflammation or irritation—exists most commonly during these periods of life. It has an acute form, but is very prone to run into the chronic state, and may be subacute from the first. It habitually terminates in resolution, rarely in abscess. One attack predisposes to another. It is often double, but the two testicles are very rarely simultaneously involved; the inflammation of one usually precedes that of the other by a number of days or weeks, after which the disease sometimes returns to the testicle first invaded, chiefly in badly managed cases. Fournier [1] has never seen double simultaneous epididymitis. It is uncommon but does occur. I have encountered it twice.

Etiology

The prime cause of epididymitis is inflammation of the *posterior* urethra. The inflammation travels from the urethra up the ejaculatory duct and along the vas deferens, not by a microbic migration, but by an actual extension of the inflammation along the mucous membrane of these canals. This explanation has long been disputed; but three facts may be laid down to prove it:

1. No matter what the condition of the anterior urethra, epididymitis never occurs except from inflammation or trauma of the posterior urethra.

2. The prodromal symptoms usually point to inflammation of the vas before there is inflammation of the epididymis.

3. Vasectomy [2] has, in my experience, always cured the most inveterate cases of relapsing epididymitis, in 2 cases even bringing an acute attack to an abrupt termination.

Nearly all the causes enumerated as capable of producing orchitis may also exceptionally give rise to epididymitis. Gout, trauma, cold, and prolonged sexual excitement may cause it, but urethral inflammation or irritation is by far the most active cause. The most common form of this irritation is gonorrhea or urethritis, then stricture, finally, any prostatic or urethral irritation; the passage of instruments, especially through a urethra already affected by mild chronic inflammation or stricture, but occasionally where no appreciable disease exists; the use of the lithotrite; cutting operations for

---

[1] Art. Blennorrhagie, Dict. de méd. et de chir. prat., p. 211.
[2] *Cf.* Chetwood, J. of Cut. and Gen.-Urin. Diseases, 1900, xviii, 445.

stone; retention of a small calculus or stone fragment in the prostatic urethra—in short, any inflammatory affection of the prostatic sinus around the orifices of the ejaculatory ducts. In general it may be laid down that epididymitis is to be looked for mainly from the third to the eighth week of gonorrhea. A number of cases are on record in which it is alleged that epididymitis has preceded the gonorrheal outbreak (Fourneaux-Jordan, Sturgis, Stansbury, Castelnau, Vidal). In my opinion these are not true cases of new gonorrheal infection, but instances of relapsing gonorrhea, in which a prostate already damaged is kindled by sexual exercise into acute irritation, which first shows itself by producing swelled testicle, and only later manifests itself as a discharge at the urethral orifice.

Some individuals seem predisposed to epididymitis, so that notwithstanding the utmost care every attack of gonorrhea is invariably attended by swelled testicles; while others, regardless of all hygienic precautions, go around with a raging gonorrhea, employing perhaps no treatment, continuing sexual intercourse and the abuse of alcohol, not even supporting the testicles, and yet they escape. Indeed, the one patient who took more scrupulous care of himself than any other in my whole experience, who went to bed and stayed there, took no local treatment whatever, and lived on the lightest of diets, in due time developed a double epididymitis, which terminated in suppuration on both sides.

It may, however, be stated dogmatically, that while a gonorrhea of itself will sometimes, in spite of all precautions, occasion swelled testicle, yet this complication is not likely to ensue if the patient wear a suspensory bandage, abstain from violent or jolting exercise (horseback riding, dancing), and avoid bodily fatigue and efforts at lifting. Above all, sexual excitement or indulgence, and the use of alcohol in any shape, must be interdicted. The passage of instruments through a canal subject at the time to gonorrhea is a sufficient cause for epididymitis. The local, and especially the abortive methods of treatment are, therefore, peculiarly liable to occasion swelled testicle. Yet from an experience extending over several years, I am convinced that the modern, moderate local treatment, if promptly applied and properly administered, is the one way to prevent posterior urethritis, epididymitis, and all the other complications of gonorrhea.

The epididymitis of stricture and of prostatic hypertrophy is usually induced by instrumentation.

Morbid Anatomy

The inflammatory process is most acute at one or the other end of the *epididymis*, usually the globus minor. Here the inflamed ducts are thickened by the inflammation and dilated in places by the accumulated secretions, desquamated epithelium, and pus. The connective tissue between the tubules is infiltrated and edematous. Actual abscess formation is rare. The *testicle* is, in acute cases, soon invaded by the inflammation from the epididymis. The *tunica vaginalis* is also inflamed, and acute hydrocele occurs in one third of all cases (Jacobson). The *vas* suffers only a slight catarrhal inflammation. Perideferentitis, abscess, and fatal peritonitis have been noted, but these are to the last degree exceptional.

As the inflammation declines, the associated lesions clear up and the edema is absorbed, leaving only one or more hard lumps in the epididymis to mark where the inflammation centred. In these lumps the epididymal canal is found permanently damaged; dilated and catarrhal in some places, perhaps occluded in others. Occlusion of the epididymis is not the constant result of inflammation, but when it does occur is probably permanent. Hence spermatozoa can never again issue from that testicle, and if both testicles are involved the patient is sterile. But the testicle does not atrophy on this account, nor is the patient's potency or sexual appetite at all impaired. (See Prognosis.)

Symptoms

Epididymitis may come on in an acute or a subacute form, the latter where the epididymis has previously suffered from a similar attack. First attacks, like first attacks of gonorrhea, are usually the most severe. Epididymitis is ushered in by premonitory symptoms which precede the swelling by some hours. Usually the gonorrheal or gleety discharge is not visibly modified until after the testicle begins to swell. Then it diminishes, perhaps stops, to return again as soon as the inflammation of the epididymis is fairly on the decline.

Prodromes.—A vague uneasiness is felt in the testicle and along the cord up into the back, as if the cord were being pulled upon. Attentive patients will frequently aver that the pain was noticeable in the groin for some hours before any uneasiness was experienced in the testicle. This forerunning inguinal pain is rarely absent where the epididymitis is of urethral origin, except in hospital patients, who are unintelligent observers. There is usually only a slight painful tension in the groin, but sometimes it is very severe, extending around to the lumbar region and up the back. Sometimes there is a sense of weight in the perineum and frequent desire to urinate, with pain and difficulty in the act. Occasionally a chill will usher in the affection, but this is far more constant with orchitis.

Onset.—1. Whether any of the foregoing symptoms have attracted attention or not, the attack begins with pain in the testicle, attended by swelling. The amount of pain and swelling varies in different cases. In the *subacute*, non-gonorrheal form, the swelling is moderate, comes on rather slowly, and is confined almost exclusively to the epididymis, the testicle itself being unaffected as a rule. Periorchitis is absent usually. There is but little, if any, fluid in the tunica vaginalis. With such mild cases there are no constitutional symptoms and the pain is not excruciating. It is aggravated by the erect posture, but wholly disappears after the patient has been on his back for a few moments with the testicle elevated.

2. But the picture is a different one if the onset is *acute*. The swelling commences promptly and increases with rapidity. First it is localized posteriorly, but soon it spreads to the tunica vaginalis and to the testis: the former becomes filled with lymph, the latter first becomes congested and edematous, later inflamed. The scrotal tissues become edematous. Yet, even under all these disadvantageous surroundings, with an edematous scrotum and a tensely filled tunica vaginalis, careful examination will rarely fail to localize all the hardness and most of the pain in the epididymis. The inflamed mass rapidly reaches the size of the fist, but its shape is not so evenly oval as in orchitis. The cord becomes swollen and painful on pressure. Occasionally the cord becomes partly strangulated in the inguinal canal, since it is impossible for it to swell much there, surrounded as it is by firm fibrous structures. This gives rise to all the symptoms of strangulation (p. 714).

Pain.—Pain in acute epididymitis is great, increasing from the first proportionally to the swelling. The pain, however, is not so severe as in true orchitis. It is dragging, aching, and sickening, making the patient feel faint. Locomotion is almost impossible, the motions of the patient are very deliberate as he changes his position, and, if obliged to stand, he carefully supports and shields the swollen scrotum with his hand. While rest on the back with the testicle raised modifies, it does not allay, the pain, but in this position the torture is more bearable. If strangulation of the cord at the ring occurs, the pain is greatly intensified, resembling that of acute inflammatory true orchitis. If inflammation of the body of the testis exist, the pain will be proportionately heightened.

Course.—As the disease advances, pain increases in intensity for a day or two, remains stationary for several days after the organ has reached its full size, and finally begins to decrease, and, even in desperate cases, by the end of the second week has usually disappeared, or become reduced to the slight dragging uneasiness which constitutes the only pain of mild cases. This relief from pain is often experienced while the organ is yet large, the epididymis thickened, the scrotum edematous, and some fluid still left in the tunica vaginalis. For several days after the pain has ceased, a few moments in the erect posture, with the testicle hanging, will recall it.

The form and size of the swelling vary greatly. In the mildest cases the tail of the epididymis alone suffers. (Exceptionally the head alone is involved.) All the inflammation localizes itself there, forming a hard, sensitive lump, giving a little uneasiness unless supported. The head, together with the tail of the epididymis, may suffer, nothing else being involved; or the whole of the epididymis, while the testis proper may be felt normal in every respect in front of the inflamed mass. The vas deferens may also be involved even in mild chronic cases. In very acute attacks the whole cord is sensitive and hyperemic. The seminal vesicles are always inflamed (p. 100).

If the disease be at all acute, *the tunica vaginalis* is sure to be involved, the degree of its inflammation usually, but not invariably, coinciding with the intensity of the epididymitis. This hydrocele varies greatly. Fluid may be rapidly poured out, filling the sac to its utmost, giving rise to a tense swelling of considerable size, in which case it becomes impossible to distinguish the constituent parts of the testicle. This is often attended by excruciating pain which may be instantly relieved by puncture of the tunica vaginalis. Again, but little fluid may be effused. This, lying loosely in the sac, fluctuates freely, and does not in the least obscure the fact that the main disease is in the epididymis. The fluid may be absorbed speedily, permitting the plastic material effused with it to glue together the two surfaces of the vaginal tunic, or perhaps only to form numerous bridled adhesions. Some fluid may remain throughout—the nucleus of future hydrocele.

The constitutional symptoms, fever, loss of appetite, etc., are mild with epididymitis, do not occur at all in chronic and subacute cases, and, like the pain, vary in acute cases with the intensity of the inflammation. What fever there is disappears before the pain, and long before the swelling.

The gradual disappearance of the hardness from the epididymis may extend over many years, and in some cases is never entirely accomplished. The point first attacked is the last to resolve. The absorption starts rapidly, but progresses more and more slowly, until in some cases it seems to remain stationary. In such cases the little hard lump at the top or the bottom of the epididymis occasions the patient no uneasiness, is not sensitive to pressure, and is ignored. Suppuration is very rare in simple epididymitis; atrophy of the testis never occurs except from orchitis.

Chronic or Relapsing Epididymitis.—Epididymitis may be said to have a natural limit of about two weeks for its acute symptoms, but relapses are very common, and carelessness may prolong the trouble to as many months (p. 719). Relapses are habitually milder than first attacks. If the opposite testicle inflame before the first is well, the latter runs through its course more quickly.

Diagnosis

Nothing is easier than the diagnosis of an acute epididymitis occurring during a gonorrhea or provoked by urethral instrumentation. But chronic or subacute cases may be mistaken for tuberculosis. (See Diagnostic Table, p. 752.)

Acute orchitis is distinguished by its etiology, the more marked general symptoms, and the fact that the testis proper, and not the epididymis, is chiefly involved.

Prognosis

The prognosis may be summed up thus: there is no danger to life, to sexual potency, or to desire. Neuralgia or tuberculosis may follow acute epididymitis in subjects predisposed to these ills. Sterility (of the affected organ) and relapse are both possible results, but, contradictory as it may seem, the more liable the patient to relapses, the less likely is he to be sterile. This does not mean that the greater the number of attacks the less damage done. On the contrary, each attack doubtless leaves its mark and may obstruct an epididymis which previous attacks have left patent. Yet this very patency of the canal constitutes at once a liability to reinfection and an assurance of fertility; whence the apparent contradiction has evolved itself that persons who have had but one attack of epididymitis in both testicles are less likely to be fertile than those who have had several.

Yet even when a man is thus sterile, affairs are not so desperate. The patient is by no means impotent, his sexual power and appetite are unimpaired. He ejaculates semen resembling the healthy fluid in quantity, smell, and colour, but containing no spermatozoa, and consequently sterile.

Benzler's[1] investigations are interesting in this regard. By looking up the subsequent history of old soldiers who had had gonorrhea while in the German army, he found that among those who had been married three or more years 10.5% of those who had suffered gonorrhea without epididymitis were childless, against

[1] Archiv f. Derm. u. Syph., 1898, xlv, 33.

23.4% of those who had had single epididymitis and 41.7% of those who had had both organs inflamed.

On the other hand, traumatic epididymitis is far less likely than urethral epididymitis to lead to sterility, since the traumatic inflammation concerns the testicle and the surrounding tissue rather than the lumen of the canals. Thus Liégeois (Jacobson) found spermatozoa in the semen of only 7 out of 28 patients who had had double epididymitis, and of these, 5 cases were due to "local causes." Orchitis does not cause sterility unless the testicles atrophy. When in epididymitis the primary focus is in the globus major, it is conceivable that obstruction of one or more tubes would not entail sterility, since the excretory ducts in this region are numerous; but in the body and tail there is but one duct, the obstruction of which means the shutting off of the whole testicle.

Suppuration rarely occurs in the course of a gonorrheal epididymitis; but when recurrent swelled testicle complicates prostatic hypertrophy an abscess often forms, and this may give rise to a fatal pyemia.

Treatment

The prophylactic treatment of epididymitis is the use of a suspensory bandage during the existence of urethral disease, together with a strict observance of the hygiene of the urethra (p. 10). When, late in gonorrhea, or during treatment of stricture, complaint is made of a dragging, uneasy sensation in the groin or testicle, the patient should be immediately placed upon his back, with the testicle elevated and painted with guaiacol and thus the threatened attack may often be averted.

Elevation.—In mild cases, where rest on the back with elevation of the testicle is sufficient to quiet pain, these means alone will effect a cure, though it is always safe to apply guaiacol, followed by a poultice and a laxative. In a few days the patient can stand and, by supporting his testicle, walk without pain.

In acute cases the treatment must be more active. Rest on the back and elevation of the testicle over the abdomen are indispensable. A suspensory bandage does not suffice, since it permits the testicle to hang down; nor is it well to trust to pillows and compresses under the testicle, since they permit the patient no motion. Curling's method is an excellent one. It consists simply in a handkerchief or piece of bandage around the waist, and a large (preferably silk) handkerchief, folded in triangle. The base of the triangle is placed under the scrotum; one (acute) angle on each side is tied to the waistband, the other (right) angle is brought up over the testicles and penis, serving to retain dressings, and is pinned or tied to the waistband. If the swelling is slight or the patient restless the sling tends to slip up. This may be easily obviated by sewing a tape to that portion of the sling immediately under the scrotum, carrying it between the nates and attaching it at the back to the waistband. Some patients prefer a T-bandage, using for the perineal band a wide strip of cloth, or a towel folded lengthwise. A less efficient elevation may be obtained by resting the scrotum on a shelf of adhesive plaster passing from thigh to thigh.

Guaiacol.—Of no less importance than rest and suspension are the local measures used to lessen the pain and, if possible, to shorten the attack. The most efficacious application I know is guaiacol. I have employed it pure and in 50% and 10% solutions with glycerin. If seen before the testicle is much swollen, although there is considerable pain portending a sharp attack, a single application of pure guaiacol, laid on with a camel's-hair brush all over one half of the scrotum, may abort the attack. But this application is quite painful and cannot be renewed more than once or twice. I therefore prefer 50% guaiacol, which, if not so likely to abort the attack, can be used with more comfort and will, in almost every case seen before the swelling reaches its maximum, control the pain within three days and check the progress of the inflammation. Indeed, when the inflammation is at its height and any touch is agony, almost instantaneous relief may sometimes be obtained by this application. The weaker solutions I reserve for milder cases. The mixture may be applied once or twice a day. It dries almost immediately. The strong applications cause acute desquamation—a minor discomfort.

Nitrate of silver (10%) is preferred to guaiacol by some. It is usually applied but once. It often fails to relieve.

I have not tried Bettmann's salicylate of methyl (1 part, olive-oil, 2 parts). He employs it on cotton covered with gutta-percha tissue.

Heat.—Next in value to guaiacol stand the various poultices. As long as the patient remains in bed these may be advantageously employed with the guaiacol. In fact it sometimes seems as though after the first sharp attack had passed, the remaining inflammation resolves more quickly under poultices than under anything else. The old-fashioned tobacco poultice [1] still enjoys great vogue as a pain-killer,

---

[1] The poultice is made by mixing a paper of any fine-cut tobacco (1 ounce) in about 10 ounces of hot water, bringing the whole to a boil while stirring it briskly, and then adding ground flaxseed, with or without ground elm-bark, until the proper consistence of a poultice is obtained, stirring the tobacco well in with the meal. A poultice of this mass is made about a quarter of an inch thick, and large enough to envelop the whole testicle. A piece of fine muslin is put on the surface of the poul-

but in this it is excelled by the guaiacol, and, in the later stages, any poultice is equally efficient. Cold applications are not so good as hot ones. I have tried ice and abandoned it.

Strapping.—The patient is kept in bed and this treatment maintained until the pain has become bearable and the swelling remains at a standstill or begins to subside. This is the signal for strapping, at first lightly, then each day more tightly, until the edema is driven from the testicle. The strapping should be done so as to produce the maximum of pressure with the minimum of discomfort, and at no time should the testicle, which remains tender, be squeezed tightly enough to produce any lasting uneasiness. The method of strapping the testicle which I now employ is as far superior to the old way with overlying strips of adhesive plaster as guaiacol is to a tobacco poultice. A strip of light rubber (Martin) bandage, 15 or 20 cm. long and 10 cm. wide, and a piece of adhesive plaster, 1 cm. wide and 10 cm. long, constitute the apparatus. This adhesive strip for fastening is a most valuable addition and is due to the suggestion of Dr. Chetwood. It is stuck to one end of the bandage (Fig. 165) and all is ready. The scrotum is gently lifted and the uninflamed testicle pushed up out of the way.[1] The inflamed organ is then encircled with the rubber bandage as tightly as the patient can bear it (this is a matter of experience), and as the bandage is wrapped in place the adhesive plaster is brought around, and holds it fast (Fig. 166). Absolutely the only precaution necessary is to get the line of greatest pressure above the line of greatest swelling—i. e., to make the adhesive plaster encircle the organ above its equator, for otherwise it will promptly slip off. The advantages of this bandage need not be enumerated, but the chief one is that it may be removed daily or every other day to be put on more tightly. This it is expedient to do. Also it sweats the scrotum, acting like a poultice.

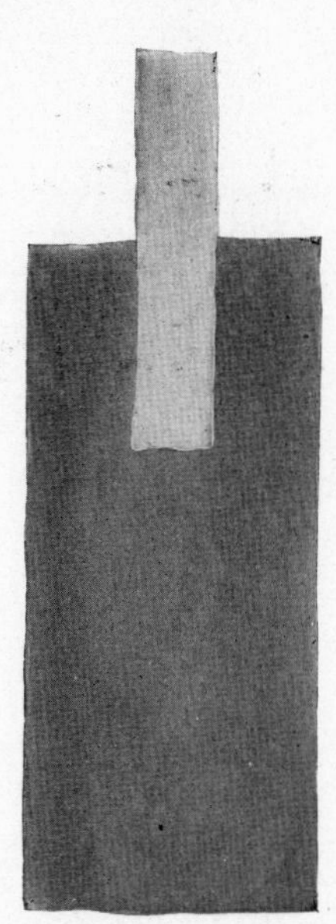

Fig. 165.—Rubber Bandage for Strapping.

---

tice, which is perhaps sprinkled with laudanum, and placed upon the testicle as hot as can be borne, the whole covered with a piece of oil-silk—for cleanliness' sake as well as to retain the heat—and supported in the handkerchief sling above described.

[1] To hold the testicle in place until the rubber can be snugly adjusted, it is occasionally necessary, as a preliminary step, to encircle the scrotum rather tightly above the testicle with a strip of gauze bandage.

Last, but not least, *no local treatment to the urethra* should be attempted during or after an attack of epididymitis. It will only harm the testicle without helping the canal. The length of time that must elapse before the urethra is again treated locally differs with every case. For some a few weeks suffice; others can never again take an instrument without more or less risk.

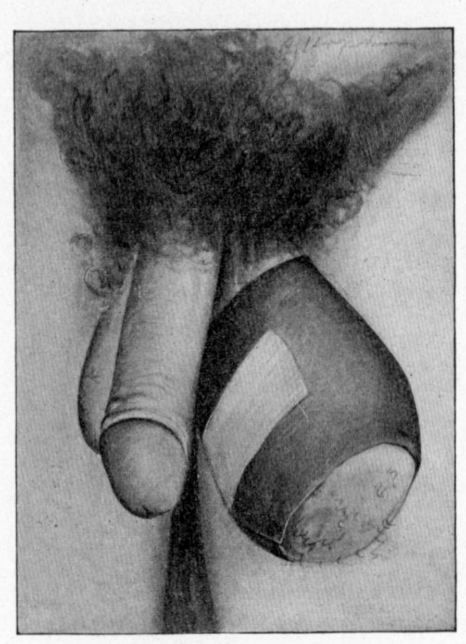

Fig. 166.—The Bandage Applied.

Leeches along the cord have been found useful, and puncture of the tunica vaginalis when it is extremely distended is sometimes followed by striking and immediate relief. Neither of these, however, should be employed as a routine measure.

Some patients refuse to go to bed, taking narcotics and wearing a poultice while they continue at their work. Such a course is certain to prolong the attack, and may result in chronic relapsing epididymitis. Then again, the impatience of restraint felt by a man lying on his back and suffering no pain, often induces him to leave his bed too soon, and sometimes a relapse is thus provoked. Patients anxious to be about should be advised from the start that they will save time and trouble, and perhaps avoid destroying the functional activity of the testicle, by yielding at once to the necessities of the case and going to bed. They may be assured that often four or five days are enough, and that not more than a week, or, in the worst cases, ten or twelve days in bed will be required, if they will lie absolutely quiet for that period.

A laxative and a light diet are in order while the patient is in bed. No internal medicine has any effect on the disease. I do not believe that iodid of potash aids resorption.

Recurrent Epididymitis.—Each attack of recurrent epididymitis may be treated by the measures detailed above; but between times preventive measures must be instituted to ward off future attacks. This prophylactic treatment may be directed towards the general health, the posterior urethra, and the testicle itself.

A strict hygiene, sexual and general, is essential in every case.

Aided by tonics, milk, fats, etc. (with perhaps a vacation and a change of climate), this alone may effect a cure.

The treatment of the posterior urethra depends upon its tolerance. If it will bear instrumentation, instillations, irrigations, and prostatic massage may well help; but in a certain proportion of cases such attempts only serve to stir up the testicle and make the patient worse. The hot rectal douche is here peculiarly applicable since it is absolutely harmless. Balsams, alkalies, and urinary antiseptics given by the mouth may be of service if not pushed to the point of straining the stomach.

The testicle itself should always be supported. I have known a man who could not for three months leave off a towel T-bandage which slung his testicles over his abdomen. No lesser support would prevent a recurrence of the attacks. Yet he is now permanently well. This case sufficiently exemplifies the principle involved.

If all these palliative measures fail, there is but one alternative. The patient must either get along with his testicle as well as he may, or submit to vasectomy. I hesitate to advocate this operation because it sacrifices the virility of a testicle which, from the very fact that recurrence of inflammation is possible, is probably able to produce spermatozoa, and because I confess it is hard to believe that this sacrifice will effect a cure in every case—and to sacrifice the testicle without curing the epididymitis would indeed be a grave error. But, on the other hand, in every one of 10 cases put to the test, the effect has been immediate, absolute, and permanent.[1] Not one died, not one relapsed, not one but was intensely gratified with the operation. I have watched one case for four years, others for a less time. Dr. Chetwood devised the operation, and the 10 cases mentioned are all his. This, at least, can be said of it: that the operation itself is quite insignificant, and that, like epididymitis, it never causes impotence, loss of desire, or atrophy of the testicle.

Vasectomy.—Under local or general anesthesia, and with the usual aseptic technic, the spermatic cord of the affected side is picked up by the surgeon and its various structures allowed to slip several times through his fingers. When he has identified the thickest and most cord-like structure of the group—which he finds behind and to the inner side of the others, one of the first to slip from his grasp—he brings it by a little dextrous manipulation close to the skin and quite free from the surrounding veins. A single small incision suffices to expose the tube with white fibrous walls, the vas defer-

[1] Chetwood, *loc. cit.* I have performed vasectomy once for this purpose and with an equally happy result.

ens, in fact. This is hooked out through the little incision, divided, each end ligated, and dropped back. A single suture closes the skin incision, and the operation is completed.

Only two points require emphasis. The incision is made near the raphe in front, and the vas should be freed as high up as possible and as completely as possible. If neatly performed there is no danger of hemorrhage after the operation. If there is any doubt, however, the adhesive plaster dressings may be applied (p. 727). The patient should remain in bed five days.

If the testicle is swollen at the time, it may be more convenient to seek the vas in the groin (p. 782).

ORCHITIS

Secondary orchitis—orchitis complicating epididymitis—is common. Primary orchitis—orchitis due to traumatism or to systemic disease—is rare. Exceptionally orchitis occurs without discoverable cause. Very rarely, true orchitis without epididymitis results from posterior urethritis, the epididymis being skipped by the inflammation.

Varieties

Several types of orchitis may be distinguished:

1. Traumatic orchitis. Testis and epididymis are both involved, and the malady runs a course quite comparable to that of acute epididymitis.

2. A low grade of orchitis, little more than a neuralgia. This attacks gouty or rheumatic individuals, and may be caused by a slight strain or by sexual excess.

3. Orchitis due to acute inflammations elsewhere. We are chiefly concerned with this form of the disease. It is a common complication of mumps, and has occasionally been met with during typhoid fever,[1] influenza, small-pox, tonsillitis, and rheumatism.[2] (*Cf.* Curling, Kocher, Jacobson.) The orchitis of mumps is a type of all these.

Traumatic Orchitis.—Severe contusion, commonly a kick or a blow inflicted by a missile, causes an acute inflammation of the testis and epididymis, which, though usually short-lived, may terminate in atrophy of the testis, abscess, or gangrene. Lesser bruises or strains cause an inflammation which habitually terminates in resolution only. Yet atrophy may follow a slight injury.[3]

---

[1] *Cf.* Kinnicutt, Med. Record, 1901, lix, 801. [2] Guyon's Annales, 1894, xii, 306.
[3] *Ibid.*, 1885, iii, 230.

Orchitis from strain has been attributed to spasm of the cremaster and to compression of the cord by the abdominal muscles (Velpeau).

Spontaneous Orchitis.—Delorme [1] cites cases of orchitis due to ungratified sexual excitement and excessive venery. A slight congestion with pain, tenderness, and a little swelling, is often met with from such causes.

The Orchitis of Mumps.—The orchitis of mumps is most frequent at about puberty. It is almost unknown in childhood. It comes on near the end of the first week of mumps, and is usually confined to a single testicle. The testicle may, however, become inflamed before the parotid, and the mumps may even be confined to the testicle. It occurs in at least 5% of cases of mumps in young adults. Indeed, Laveran [2] met with 156 cases of orchitis among 432 cases of mumps occurring in soldiers. The epididymis may or may not be involved. The affection runs a quick course of about a week or ten days, very rarely terminates in suppuration, may subside without leaving behind any impairment of the organ, but is often followed by atrophy. Thus atrophy occurred in 73 of Laveran's cases—an unusually large proportion. Abscess and gangrene are very rare terminations. This form of orchitis has been fancifully termed metastatic. It is, however, nothing more than an expression of the disease. The inflammation of the testicle is no more metastatic than is the inflammation of the parotid.

Symptoms

Local Symptoms.—In true orchitis the testis increases slowly in size, and seldom becomes very large until the affection has lasted several days. This is due to the unyielding nature of the albuginea, and to the fact that there is usually no effusion into the tunica vaginalis. The pain, which is often excruciating, and always out of proportion to the amount of swelling, is due to the tension of the albuginea. This pain has been compared to that of nephritic or hepatic colic. No position gives rest, and any handling of the organ may induce syncope. The irritated cremaster contracts upon the sensitive testis and draws it up towards the groin. The pain continues severe for several days, and then gradually becomes more bearable, or it may suddenly cease altogether. This last circumstance is gratifying to the patient only. The surgeon learns it with regret, for he knows that it may mean gangrene of the organ.

The shape of the testicle is rarely altered in orchitis; it is smooth-

---

[1] Thèse de Paris, 1877.

[2] Med. Times and Gazette, vi, July 20, 1878.

ly, regularly ovoid. The epididymis is not distinguishable from the rest of the tumour. The organ feels peculiarly indurated, the natural elastic feel having entirely disappeared. The scrotal tissues are often red, swollen, edematous, inflamed.

General Symptoms.—*The general symptoms* in true orchitis are marked, often severe: chills, high fever, anorexia, nausea, vomiting, hiccough, constipation, sleeplessness, anxiety, and great nervous irritation. The general symptoms have been compared to those of strangulated hernia, and, indeed, there is more or less strangulation of the testicle within its tight, fibrous sheath.

Termination.—The disease usually terminates by resolution. The testicle may then remain normal or it may go on to *atrophy*, this process requiring several weeks, at the end of which time nothing is left of the testicle but a small, insensitive mass. *Abscess* is a rare termination and gangrene still more rare. The former is often announced by the occurrence of chill. After the chill the testicle commences to enlarge more rapidly, the scrotal tissues adhere to its surface, and, after a longer or shorter period, according to the depth at which the pus forms, a soft, fluctuating spot surrounded by indurated borders clearly indicates the position of the purulent collection. After the pus has escaped, the severity of the symptoms abates, unless a second purulent collection exists in some other part of the gland. The flow of pus gradually diminishes. As it decreases the swelling subsides and partial or total atrophy of the testicle ensues. The resulting fistula may remain open for years. Sometimes exuberant granulations grow up out of the opening, forming a cauliflower excrescence (hernia testis), which may reach considerable size. Such a tumour growing from an enlarged, hardened testicle and accompanied by enlarged glands in the groin may well give rise to a suspicion of cancer, a suspicion which the history does not justify.

Sometimes in true orchitis an abscess forms centrally, and never comes to the surface. In such a case the symptoms run a despairingly slow course, but the hard and tender organ gradually diminishes in size and undergoes chronic inflammatory induration, while the purulent collection gradually becomes solidified and surrounded by a tough capsule. Such a condition may persist indefinitely, the function of the testicle being destroyed, unless the purulent collections have been very small. A somewhat similar state of affairs may succeed deep abscess which has discharged and remained fistulous for a considerable time. These testicles long remain the seat of chronic pain, and are liable to repeated outbreaks of inflammation.

The onset of *gangrene* is announced by a sudden cessation of the pain. Then, after adhesion to the scrotum, the slough makes its way through the skin, and is found not black, or brown and fetid, but yellowish, dry, and soft. It is a dry gangrene, a necrosis, and may be pulled away in long filaments.

Treatment

Treatment.—It is stated that the orchitis of mumps does not occur if the patient is kept in bed for eight days. Such a precaution is therefore a wise one for all young adults, though they cannot always be made to comply with it. The testicles should also be kept supported.

After the attack has once begun but little can be done beyond ameliorating the symptoms and endeavouring to prevent abscess or gangrene. The subsequent atrophy cannot be averted. The patient needs no urging to keep him in bed. Isham [1] refers to several reported cases which did well under jaborandi. I have used the drug and think well of it. Guaiacol and poultices may be employed to relieve pain. Early employment of these means gives the testicle its best chance. If in spite of them the symptoms fail to abate, on the slightest suspicion of impending gangrene, or in any case where the symptoms run very high, it is wise to resort without delay to subcutaneous section of the tunica albuginea in order to take off tension from the strangulated parts within. This simple operation is readily performed with a sharp tenotomy knife introduced through the skin, and then made to cut the tense fibrous capsule, while the testicle is steadied in the other hand. The incisions should be carried fairly through the tunica albuginea, three to six short cuts 5 to 10 cm. long being made at different points on the surface of the testicle. The pain will usually cease after the tension has been relieved. If abscess form, puncture should be made on the first appearance of fluctuation. For gangrene castration should be performed.

Nature and time are the chief agents in closing fistula of the testicle. All that art can do is to make the opening dependent, slit up sinuses, keep the parts clean, apply some stimulating lotion or injection to the sinus, and build up and maintain the patient's general health.

Benign fungus (hernia testis) may be cauterized, cut or tied off, subjected to pressure by adhesive straps, or, preferably, after other diseased conditions have been subdued, the edges of the wound may be incised, freshened, and united by suture after the fungus

---

[1] Am. J. of Med. Sci., 1878, lxxvi, 369.

has been replaced (Syme). Fungus should never be pulled upon for fear of drawing out the entire contents of the testicle.

In severe, long-standing cases, where a testicle is the seat of chronic induration full of fistulæ, or with a large, obstinate fungus, orchidectomy is advisable, sometimes necessary, in order to remove from the patient a source of physical irritation, and to save him from serious injury to the general health.

CHAPTER IX

TUBERCULOSIS OF THE TESTICLE

Tuberculosis affects the testicle in two ways:

1. Diffuse miliary tuberculosis, associated with general miliary tuberculosis, and of no interest to the surgeon.

2. Circumscribed tuberculosis, which concerns us here. This form of tubercle appears as localized deposits, one or more, usually beginning in the epididymis, and involving the testicle only secondarily.

Etiology

The *predisposing causes* of epididymal tuberculosis are three: 1. The tubercular diathesis. 2. The existence of a focus of tuberculosis elsewhere in the body. 3. Local trauma or inflammation (precedent or persistent).

Although the profession is by no means agreed in the matter, it has been my personal experience that, when there is tuberculosis in the testicle, tubercular lesions may invariably be discovered elsewhere in the body, the patient almost always has tubercular antecedents, and there is often some local disturbance to determine the localization of the tuberculosis.

The *efficient cause* is the tubercle bacillus.

Pathogenesis.—There are three theories concerning the genesis of genital tuberculosis:

1. That it is primary in the prostate or the seminal vesicles whence the epididymis is invaded secondarily, the inflammation extending along the vas, or, possibly, by way of the lymphatics (Kocher,[1] Lancereaux,[2] Guyon [3]).

2. That genital tuberculosis is primary in the epididymis, secondary in the prostate and seminal vesicles (Réclus,[4] Senn,[5] Councilman [6]).

---

[1] *Op. cit.*, p. 326.

[2] Guyon's Annales, 1883, i, 153.

[3] *Ibid.*, 1891, ix, 445.

[4] Du tubercule du testicule, Paris, 1876.

[5] Tuberculosis of the Gen.-Urin. Organs, 1897, p. 48.

[6] Dennis's Surgery, 1895, i, 246.

3. That the tuberculosis, whether occurring primarily in the one end of the seminal canals or in the other, may be due to inoculation during coitus (Verneuil, Jacobson,[1] Paladino-Blandini [2]).

Two questions, therefore, arise, Can the inoculation take place during coitus? Is the epididymis invaded primarily or secondarily?

As to infection during coitus, no one holds that such infection is at all frequent. The question is whether or not it ever occurs. Tubercle bacilli have been found in the healthy epididymis (Jani and Weigert [3]), and Paladino-Blandini has recently shown that all bacteria, tubercle bacilli among others, when deposited on the mucous membrane of the urethra near the meatus may reach the epididymis, but cause no inflammation there under ordinary conditions. Yet these experiments, though very interesting as showing that immobile bacteria can travel against the current, and thus giving experimental evidence of the propagation of disease along the vas, prove only that infection in coitus is barely possible, for the combination of circumstances postulated—viz., a massive urethral inoculation and a trauma to the testicle, would be, clinically, hard to find. Inoculation *per urethram* is, to say the least, improbable.

Is the testicle invaded primarily or secondarily? The highest authorities are divided on this point, and perhaps this division is founded on a diversity of cases, some primary, some secondary. There is no question here of the primary focus in the body, but only of the primary focus in the genital tract. Is it in the testicles, or is it in the prostate and vesicle? I cannot answer the question except by an array of facts, all of which seem to point towards the same conclusion: 1. I have examined the urine of every case of tubercular testis that I have seen in the last ten years, and in no case have I failed to find in the urine either shreds or pus indicative of a prostatic congestion, though there be no discharge whatever at the meatus. 2. I have often seen tubercular prostatitis and vesiculitis without any lesion of the testicle. 3. When, one testicle being already involved, the other one becomes implicated, I am confident that a tubercular prostate forms the bridge from one side to the other, and therefore the second testicle, at least, is not involved primarily.

To sum up: with a tubercular testis the prostate is never normal (though I confess that its congestion may possibly be similar to that seen about the mouth of the ureter in tubercular kidney) and is sometimes manifestly tubercular to rectal touch. On the other

---

[1] *Op. cit.*, p. 323. [2] Guyon's Annales, 1900, xviii, 1009.
[3] Virchow's Archiv, 1886, ciii, 522.

hand, with a tubercular prostate or vesicle the testicle is not necessarily involved. Involvement of the prostate precedes involvement of the second testicle. The migration of the bacteria in sufficient numbers to cause damage is rendered intelligible by Paladino-Blandini's experiments, referred to above, which, while they do not reproduce the conditions requisite for infection in coitus, do represent with sufficient accuracy the conditions of so-called ascending inflammation. All the weight of this evidence goes to show that, in many, if not in all cases, the prostate or vesicle is tubercular before the testicle becomes so.

The *age* at which tubercular inflammation is most common is between twenty and thirty. Fully half the cases occur between these years, and the disease is very rare before fifteen and after fifty.

By reason of its more sluggish circulation the left testicle is more often affected than the right.

Morbid Anatomy

Authorities differ as to whether the epithelium or the intertubular tissues of the *epididymis* are first involved, and on these differences build a support to their views upon the primary or secondary nature of the disease. Suffice it to know that the primary tubercles conglomerate to form the hard masses so typical of beginning tuberculosis. These go on usually to caseation, suppuration, and fistulization, or else cicatrize or calcify.

The Vas.—The vas is often lumpy with tubercular deposits, distended by the products of inflammation, and often involved in a perideferentitis throughout its length. When present this thickened, knobby vas is one of the characteristic features of the disease. The *vesicle* and *prostate* are usually tubercular.

The Testicle.—The testicle is often encroached upon by a tuberculoma or by an abscess. Though primary tuberculosis of this organ is rare, examinations by various authors of testes obtained by castration have almost always shown a more or less widely disseminated beginning tuberculosis of this gland. This discovery has usually been hailed as a startling proof of the advantage of total castration, it being very justly urged that the lesions in the testicle would be overlooked by the surgeon intent upon some conservative operation. It seems more than probable, however, that these lesions of the testicle are often present in cases treated by conservative operations, as well as in those not treated surgically, and that in most instances the testicle is able to overcome the infection if given an opportunity, although the occasional appearance of purely orchitic abscesses after epididymectomy is evidence that the enemy is not always repelled.

The Vaginalis.—The tunica vaginalis may be studded with tubercles, producing chronic hydrocele.

The Urinary Organs.—The urinary organs are often affected with the genital organs. Such cases form a picture of complete genito-urinary tuberculosis. Either the urinary or the genital tuberculosis may be primary (p. 598).

The Lungs.—The lungs are often enough spared. Thus Kocher among 451 autopsies on cases of urogenital tuberculosis found as many as 95 (21%) with normal lungs. During life the pulmonary involvement is often insignificant. On the other hand, Réclus found among 500 phthisical patients 64 with genito-urinary tuberculosis, 45 with involvement of the genital tract, and 19 with tubercular testes only.

Symptoms

The patient, a young man often with tubercular antecedents, comes complaining that one testicle is larger than the other. The swelling may have been spontaneous or it may have followed injury, or perhaps a previous gonorrheal epididymitis never got quite well and now has begun to swell again. Questioning may disclose a family or a personal history of tuberculosis, or an account of frequent and painful urination perhaps slight, previous, or still existing. The epididymal lesion is usually tender, rarely painful.

Less often the onset is acute. The testicle is greatly swollen and hard. There is considerable pain, and the vaginalis rapidly fills. This condition may subside, leaving a few nodules here and there, or it may go on to suppuration.

Upon examining such a testicle it is usually found somewhat enlarged throughout, with large, hard nodules at one end or the other of the epididymis, or throughout its length. There may be lumps in front in the testicle itself. The outline of the tumours may be obscured by fluid in the tunica vaginalis. The vas deferens is often knotty, enlarged, and hard, as far as it can be felt, and a finger in the rectum may detect the seminal vesicle similarly affected. Nodules may perhaps also be detected in the prostate and vesicles; the urine contains prostatic shreds and pus in small or large quantity, and there are, perhaps, symptoms referable to tuberculosis of prostate, bladder, or kidney. The lungs, too, may be involved. Until suppuration occurs the testicle is practically painless, testicular sensation is not materially reduced, and the opposite testicle is not usually affected. Sexual power and desire are influenced only by the fears of the patient. Later, if both testicles are destroyed potency may become impaired.

The malady advances slowly, sometimes remaining stationary for many months; finally, the nodules soften into abscess, the skin adheres, and the abscess bursts and discharges a thick, cheesy material. These abscesses remain fistulous for a long time, sometimes indefinitely, the fistulous tract being marked by great induration. New abscesses tend to form, pointing by old or by new routes. After abscess of the substance of the testis, hernia testis may come on. When the disease invades the scrotum the inguinal glands enlarge. Such a condition is often mistaken for cancer. A patient may have both testicles indurated, knotted, full of fistulæ for years, and still seem to enjoy excellent health, with the exception of more or less loss of sexual desire and power; but usually he is pale, thin, anemic, weak, perhaps with tubercular deposits in his lungs or elsewhere.

Course and Prognosis

The usual course of the disease has been described above. It is that of a local malady advancing slowly to a fatal termination. When, however, the patient's surroundings are unfavourable and his general health poor, he may succumb rapidly to the local disease. Indeed, we occasionally meet with a case which starts like an ordinary acute epididymitis, the *tuberculose galopante du testicule* of Duplay, and never remits its fury. In other cases, the chronic course of the disease is interrupted by acute exacerbations.

Although the testicular lesion is not always the most important feature of the disease, yet its progress affords a fair index for prognosis. If this can be controlled and the patient made to gain weight, the prognosis is good; if the testicle cannot be controlled and the patient loses weight, it is bad.

Under proper treatment I have known many patients to become and remain well. Others I have known to go on from one tubercular manifestation to another for an indefinite period. Thus, one patient whom I have seen recently has been ill since 1891, when the left epididymis and vesicle, and the left half of the prostate became manifestly tubercular. I removed his epididymis, and during the next two years twice cut down on and scraped a tubercular rib. In 1894 I scraped out an abscess in the opposite epididymis. At this time the right epididymis and right half of the prostate were most involved, and there was pain in the right loin, relieved by gushes of pus in the urine, showing that the disease had reached his right kidney. In 1898 he returned, his kidney still lame, but his general health unimpaired, and I incised and drained a tubercular tenosynovitis in his right wrist. At present both kidneys are, apparently, involved, but he still enjoys excellent health. The genitals are sound. So are wrist and rib. His lungs have never been touched by the disease. This result has been achieved by strict attention to hygiene and residence for several months during each year in a high dry climate. Other men I have known to conquer their disease while remaining here in New York amid highly unhygienic surroundings, and others again to fail in spite of all that surgery or medicine can do to help them. The more I see of tuberculosis the more I believe that, like syphilis, it can often be cured, but may relapse in the best of cases; that, again like syphilis, it is never a local disease and can never be lopped off; and that, once more like syphilis, the very best chance of a cure is obtained by a prolonged course of appropriate treatment in the early stages of the disease.

Death is usually due to tuberculosis of the kidneys or the lungs.

Diagnosis.—(See table on p. 752.)

Treatment

I believe that most surgeons in this country encourage immediate castration for every phase of tubercular testis, except, perhaps, the very earliest, or when bilateral disease is present. Thus Senn:[1] "Castration must therefore be regarded as the normal procedure in cases of uncomplicated, unilateral, tubercular epididymitis."

The more conservative views expressed by Bryson[2] ("Surgical measures should be held as a last resort"), Murphy,[3] and White, and Martin are, I believe, not received with any general favour.

It is impossible to review every phase of the question with impartiality, since no two surgeons exactly agree upon the indications for treatment. An excellent view of the subject may be obtained from the recent discussion before the Paris Surgical Society,[4] in which 16 of the leading French surgeons expressed their views on the subject. On only one point were all agreed—namely, that complete castration is rarely, if ever, permissible. Of the 16 only 2 stood out for immediate castration when the disease is unilateral, and only 2 others insisted upon complete removal of all local foci, with castration, if necessary to attain that end. Félizet employs castration for the virulent tubercular epididymo-orchitis of children when the child is cachectic and the testicle the only organ seriously diseased. He even sacrifices both testicles. Tuffier recognises only (1) hypertrophic tubercular orchitis (the hyperacute form) and (2) extensive suppuration as indications for castration. Bazy accepts only the latter.

---

[1] *Op. cit.*, p. 74. [2] Morrow's System, 1893, i, 873.

[3] J. of the Am. Med. Ass'n, 1900, xxxv, 1189, 1276, 1346, 1407, and 1478.

[4] *Cf.* also Longuet's exhaustive review, Revue de chir., 1900, xxi, 79; Guyon's Annales, 1900, xviii, 961, 1066.

I array myself among the most conservative. I believe that the removal of one testicle tends, if anything, to encourage recurrence on the opposite side. While I am not absolutely convinced as to the physical effect of removing one testicle, I know of few worse moral effects than that produced by relapse on the opposite side after such an operation. I have not seen any generalization of the disease immediately after operation, such as some surgeons have reported; but, nevertheless, I am perfectly confident that the knife never removes all the disease, even when the entire tubercular testis with its cord and vesicle is taken away. All that the knife can do is to remove the most active focus of the disease, and this is best accomplished by conservative surgery, not by radical measures. When the inflammation does not subside under hygienic treatment, the surgical requirements of the case may usually be met by epididymectomy or by incision of suppurating foci.

On the other hand, I have seen every form of tubercular disease bettered and permanently cured by hygienic and dietetic measures, and these should always be accorded precedence, if for no other reason, at least because of the uncertainty of the disease. No two cases act alike. I have seen a most violent *tuberculose galopante* become almost well after a six-months' course of creosote, and a carbolic-injection cure of hydrocele, although all the while the patient was pursuing his profession of dentistry through the hot summer months on the East Side of New York.

To speak practically, the patient with a tubercular testicle should wear a suspensory bandage. He should be encouraged to take every advantage of sunlight and climate that his station in life permits. He should be treated with general tonics and antitubercular remedies according to the surgeon's judgment. Local remedies are useless. The injection of an iodoform glycerin emulsion (Senn) or of a 10% chlorid-of-zinc solution (Lannelongue) has met with little favour.

Epididymectomy should be performed if the disease grows worse in spite of palliative treatment. When any of the tubercular lesions soften or begin to adhere to the skin they should be opened and scraped at once. The surgeon may take this opportunity to lay open other points of threatening suppuration, or he may shell off the entire epididymis from the testicle, dividing the vas at or near the external abdominal ring. If the vas is involved beyond this point, the incision may be prolonged upward and outward over the inguinal canal, and the vas freed and followed down to the vesicle, where it may be divided. (See Castration.) If the abscess involves the testicle I like to burn its walls with the Paquelin cautery.

I accept only two indications for castration, the destruction of the testicle by suppuration, and, in some cases, the hyperacute, galloping tubercular orchitis (usually due to a mixed infection).

All operations should be performed under general anesthesia, in order that the surgeon may have the opportunity to do his work thoroughly, unhampered by the patient's outcry. When epididymectomy is performed primary union may often be expected. Curetting and cauterizing operations should be terminated by drainage. Fungus may be amputated by the cautery, turned in and covered by the scrotum. If this operation fails castration is necessary. Pousson[1] has recently advocated ligature of the spermatic cord as a cure for tubercular testis. The suggestion is too new to receive calm judgment.

If the seminal vesicle is tubercular the question of operating upon it may arise (p. 788).

---

[1] Guyon's Annales, 1900, xviii, 356.

CHAPTER X

SYPHILIS OF THE TESTICLE—FUNGUS

There is no disease of the testicle so persistently misunderstood as syphilis. It is habitually mistaken for tubercle and cancer, and more than usually fortunate is that patient whose physician gives anti-syphilitic medication the opportunity of making the diagnosis for him. Yet the syphilitic testicle presents quite as characteristic a symptom-complex as does tubercle or cancer, and, while less common than the former, it occurs far more often than the latter.

There are two forms of syphilitic testis: an epididymitis of the secondary period, and an epididymo-orchitis of the tertiary period.

SECONDARY EPIDIDYMITIS

This affection is insignificant. It occurs in connection with other secondary symptoms, and, as it consists merely of a nodule often quite painless in one or both testicles—usually both—it is but rarely discovered. Dron [1] has left a classical account of it. The general coexistence of other secondary symptoms suggests its nature, and it reacts kindly to routine mercurial treatment.

TERTIARY LESIONS

The lesions of tertiary syphilis in the testicle are entitled orchitis. But the epididymis also may be implicated. This involvement has been noted in a desultory way by many authors; yet no one seems ever to have been struck by its frequency and its pathognomonic features. But of these anon.

Morbid Anatomy.—*a. The diffuse form*, like interstitial hepatitis, or nephritis, is an interstitial orchitis, a peculiar sort of chronic inflammation attacking the fibrous envelope and the septa of the organ. Ricord named it albuginitis. The process begins by hyperemia;

[1] Archiv. gén. de méd., 1863, ii, 513 and 724.

a new growth of connective tissue occurs in the stroma of the organ. This new tissue presses upon, and gradually causes atrophy of, the tubular structure. The tunica albuginea becomes thickened, as does also the tunica vaginalis. More or less fluid occupies the cavity of the latter, while many adhesions commonly take place between its free surfaces. In this way the organ reaches double its natural size, rarely more, unless there is a considerable collection of fluid in the tunica vaginalis. Often only a portion of the gland is involved in these changes. Both testicles may be affected, usually consecutively. After a time the newly formed connective tissue contracts, the septa between the lobes of seminal tubules become greatly thickened, composed of dense, fibrous tissue, showing white on section, while the intervening clusters of tubules, after first undergoing a brown pigmentation, become atrophied by pressure, and finally may disappear, lost in the general fibrous metamorphosis of the gland. The contraction may continue, much of the newly formed material being absorbed, and the process going on to wasting of the organ, until but a stump remains. If the gland has been only partially invaded, a depression may be left marking the site of the disease. In this form there is no tendency to suppuration, ulceration, or formation of fungus. This is the slower variety of disease.

b. The gummy form is marked by the formation of nodules, usually multiple, which seem often to take their origin in the external tunic of a vessel or in the wall of a spermatic tubule (Lancereaux). They may be found of all sizes up to that of an egg, and consist of an agglomeration of cells toughly united by fibrous elements into a lump, presenting, on section, a grayish-yellow or distinct dark-yellow colour. As they get larger these nodules tend to soften at the centre. They are surrounded by a grayish areola, traversed by vessels, and are often enveloped by a condensation of tissue somewhat resembling a capsule. These tumours may form near the surface or deep in the gland. They may occur in the epididymis. The latter, however, usually escapes, while the vas deferens is very rarely involved. The tunica vaginalis is usually more or less distended with fluid. In gummy orchitis the testicle may become very large.

The *epididymis* is not apparently involved in the diffuse orchitis; but with the more frequent gummatous process the epididymis is involved in a characteristic manner. I have never been able to obtain a pathological specimen showing this condition, but I have no doubt that the epididymitis as well as the orchitis is gummatous. The practical features I do know. The globus major is commonly involved, the globus minor less often. The inflamed portion of the epididymis forms a solid mass with a sharp edge which I have seen half as large as the palm of the hand. It caps the end of the testicle, separated from it by a distinct sulcus, so that the organ seems to be resting in a clam-shell. There are no nodules, as in tuberculosis, and the cord is uninflamed. The pathognomonic clam-shell is usually seen above the testicle, sometimes below it. At the same time the body of the testicle is usually implicated.

I have never seen double syphilitic epididymo-orchitis.

Symptoms.—True syphilitic orchitis rarely appears until after at least a year has elapsed from the date of chancre. Occasionally it may be more precocious. Ricord and Bumstead have seen it as early as the fourth or fifth month. It may coincide with iritis, with groups of tubercles, with ulcers, or with deeper lesions of bone or cartilage. Not infrequently, however, it comes on long after the patient has ceased to show any evidence of specific disease. The enlargement of the testis takes place gradually and without pain. It is usually first discovered by accident, already quite large, so that the patient affirms that the swelling came on very rapidly, in a day or so. There may, however, be some slight pain at first, especially along the cord and in the groin, with an uneasy sensation in the testicle itself. When first seen, the testicle is usually not more than twice or thrice its natural size. It may be perfectly smooth, and hard as wood, the epididymis not distinguishable. Sometimes the body of the testis is irregular and nodular and very hard, or there may be one or more prominent lumps of gummy exudation. Only a portion of the testicle may be involved, the rest being normal. In such a case the healthy portion may retain the natural testicular sensation. Often, however, the swelling is wholly insensitive, and may be squeezed at will without evoking the least uneasy feeling.

The outlines of the testicles may be obscured by a considerable collection of fluid in the tunica vaginalis. After drawing this off, the hard, nodular, uneven outline of the insensitive syphilitic testis becomes apparent. The vas deferens is nearly always healthy, and the characteristic clam-shell epididymis will be found in a certain proportion of cases.

The general health may appear excellent, but, if both testicles are involved, sexual appetite and power are almost invariably absent. The same impairment of sexual function exists in a less degree where one gland only is involved. There may be, very rarely, a syphilitic fungus, as described farther on. The glands in the groin are not affected.

Exceptionally the cord is involved. I have seen it thickened to the size of a lead-pencil, smooth, hard, painless. Fournier[1] records a similar case, and Després[2] another.

The course of the disease is infinitely slow. It may last thirty years, and commonly terminates in atrophy.

The *hereditary form* of the disease may appear up to the second or the third year. Fournier observed a case in the twenty-fourth year. The disease follows the type of diffuse orchitis in the adult. It is frequently bilateral and associated with hydrocele. It usually terminates in atrophy.

Prognosis.—The prognosis is good. The seminal tubules do not become occluded. They perish only by atrophy from pressure, and some of the canaliculi usually escape. The sooner treatment is commenced the better the prognosis. Under appropriate measures the gummy material melts away, liberating from pressure such of the tubules as have escaped atrophy, and, with a return of the organ to its natural size, erections and sexual appetite reappear. Gosselin has found spermatozoa in the semen of patients cured of double syphilitic orchitis. Relapse is always to be feared, especially if the treatment be not persisted in long enough, or if the testicle is injured.

Diagnosis.—(See Table, p. 752.)

Treatment.—All three forms of syphilitic testis are amenable to treatment. Early syphilitic epididymitis reacts promptly to mercury employed as for the earlier syphilids. Of the other two forms, the purely gummy may be more promptly relieved; but, in any case, the earlier an intelligent treatment is instituted the more speedily does the disease respond. Mixed treatment is most commonly applicable, but, as a general rule, the later the attack after the chancre the more reliance is to be placed upon the iodid and the less upon mercury. With distinct gummy tumours, with syphilitic fungus and in connection with other marked evidences of tertiary disease, the iodid should be used alone, carried rapidly to a high dose. A suspensory bandage should be worn and all hygienic means employed. Local treatment is useless.

Sometimes injections into the buttock of 1 gramme of a 10% solution of mercuric salicylate in benzoinol succeeds better than the iodid. The injections should be employed once or twice a week until the first signs of salivation appear or until the tumour subsides.

FUNGUS OF THE TESTICLE

The term fungus of the testicle is one of those which, though meaning nothing in particular—a relic of days when various patho-

---

[1] Sarcocèle syphilitique, Paris, 1875, p. 27. [2] Bull. de la soc. de chir., 1875, i, ii, 140.

logical conditions were classed as one—cannot yet be discarded. In its widest sense fungus of the testicle is protrusion of that organ, or of its contents, through the skin of the scrotum. Three kinds of fungi may be distinguished:

1. **Malignant Fungus.**—This is nothing else than malignant disease which has broken through the skin (p. 751).

2. **Hernia or Prolapse.**—In this form the entire testicle is protruded through a wound in the scrotum (p. 696).

3. **True Benign Fungus.**—Here the testicle is eviscerated, as it were, and its secreting structure, the seminal tubules, protrude through the tunica albuginea and the scrotum.

This true fungus is rarely seen nowadays. It results most frequently from the breaking down of a gumma, less often from the suppuration of a tubercular focus, rarely from trauma.

The syphilitic fungus is typical, and this only need be described.

The mechanism of its formation is as follows: The tunica albuginea undergoes gummatous degeneration, softens, and permits bulging of the contents of the testicle. The suprajacent skin now inflames and adheres, finally ulcerating and permitting the gummy growth to extrude through the opening, together with the tubular structure, which may be found in little clusters amid the yellow material. The fungus continues to grow, the dartos and skin contract about its peduncle, and the extruded mass becomes covered with granulation tissue and bathed in pus. These syphilitic fungi are rather firm in touch, painless, and do not bleed very easily. If cut off they continue to grow, or, if the disease be not arrested, the sprouting may continue until the whole tubular structure of the testis has been pushed out, after which it may wither and dry up, the testicle going on to complete atrophy. The seminal tubes in the fungus retain some of their activity, as shown by the fact that spermatozoa may be found in the discharge.

Réclus[1] claims that tubercular fungus arises only from lesions situated in the scrotum, not in the testicle itself.

Treatment.—The treatment of syphilitic fungus is primarily medical. Tubercular fungus commonly requires castration. When the fungus is not itself diseased, as in syphilis after a successful mercurial course has been carried out, or as in traumatic cases, every effort should be made to save the testicle. If the fungus is small, tight strapping, so as to turn in the edges of the wound after nitrate of silver has been applied, may succeed. If this

---

[1] Semaine méd., 1887, vii, 30.

fail, Syme's operation should be attempted. The fungus is gently scraped to freshen the granulations, the cicatricial collar about the neck of the growth divided, the skin dissected up, the tumour reduced, and the skin sewed over it. Asepsis and primary union are to be aimed at. If this operation fail the testicle must be removed.

CHAPTER XI

TUMOURS OF THE TESTICLE—DIAGNOSTIC TABLE—CASTRATION

Many kinds of morbid growths have been observed in the testicle, although no individual variety is at all frequent. In fact it is impossible clinically to distinguish between the various forms of tumour, and even the pathologists are not agreed. For most tumours of the testicle are mixed tumours, most of them are malignant, and "there's an end to 't," as far as the clinician is concerned. Therefore I shall not strain at giving every particular detail suspected as characteristic of some specific tumour, but, having described the morbid anatomy of each variety, I shall consider their symptoms, diagnosis, and treatment collectively.

Morbid Anatomy

Benign Tumours.—Enchondroma, fibroma, osteoma, and myoma [1] have been observed. If the tumour is small it is often not discovered until after death. If large it cannot be distinguished from beginning malignant disease.

In the *tunica vaginalis* lipoma (Roswell Park) and fibroma have been observed (Jacobson).

Cystic Growths —Three varieties of cysts are met with in the testicle—teratoma, benign cystic disease, and malignant cystic disease. Clinically they cannot be distinguished from one another.

Both simple *dermoid* cysts and more complex *teratomata* are met with in the testicle. In a personal case of teratoma the cyst contained a malformed mandible bearing several teeth. Teratoma is, doubtless, due to fetal inclusion (Saint-Hilaire), while dermoid cysts probably are merely epithelial inclusions. Lébert accounted for the relative frequency of teratoma of the testis and the ovary by a sort of hermaphroditism, by virtue of which the sexual gland impregnates itself in an imperfect manner, and so evolves certain "odds and

[1] *Cf.* Becker, Virchow's Archiv, 1901, clxiii, 244.

ends" of a fetus. It is not clear whether teratoma is developed sometimes within the testis or always alongside of it.

Cystic Disease.—Cystic disease (cystic degeneration) is a general term embracing a large class of mixed tumours which have this striking characteristic in common, that they are riddled with cysts, large and small. Benign cystic disease is a cystic fibroma (Eve). Malignant cystic disease is sarcomatous, fibro-myxo-sarcomatous, myxomatous, carcinomatous, enchondromatous. Sturgis[1] has recently given a detailed expression of the views of various authors on this subject, and has collected 40 cases.

The pathogenesis of these tumours is still disputed. Sir Astley Cooper believed that the cysts are derived from dilated canaliculi. Curling alleged that this, like most other tumours of the testis, originates in the mediastinum. Later, Malassez introduced the theory that it is produced in the intertubular connective tissue. Finally, Eve concluded that the cysts probably grow from certain epithelial nests derived from the Wolffian body included in the mediastinum. For him, therefore, cystic disease is a teratoma.

Malignant Tumours.—**Carcinoma.**—Carcinoma and sarcoma have been confused to some extent, owing to the mixed and cystic nature of many of the malignant tumours, and the obscurity which, as we have just seen, still shrouds the pathogenesis of these cystic growths. Carcinoma is not so common as sarcoma. Pure medullary carcinoma is the most common variety. Cystic and chondro-carcinoma have been described. Nepveu alone asserts the existence of scirrhus.

Sarcoma.—Kober[2] has recently collected 114 cases of sarcoma of the testicle. Seventy-one per cent occurred between the ages of twenty and fifty. There was a history of trauma in 43%. The round-celled, small round-celled, and mixed (round and spindle-celled) varieties afforded 65.2% of the 75 cases examined microscopically; 28.9% of the others were of the cystic, alveolar, and spindle-celled varieties.

Lymphadenoma.—The existence of lymphadenoma has been affirmed by the French, notably Malassez, Trélat, and Monod and Terrillon. Morestin and Milian[3] have recently reported a case. The Germans, led by Birch-Hirschfeld and Kocher, class these tumours with small round-celled sarcoma.

Jacobson cites 3 cases of pure *myxoma*.

Sarcoma originating in the *tunica vaginalis* has been observed 4

[1] Am. Med. Quart., 1899–1900, i, 110. [2] Am. J. of Med. Sci., 1899, cxvii, 535.
[3] Guyon's Annales, 1900, xviii, 311.

times (Jacobson). Rockwell[1] has reported an alleged bilateral cancer of the *epididymis*.

Symptoms

Since malignant tumours of the testicle often appear benign at the outset, and since benign tumours may, at any time, become malignant, it is quite impossible to say of any given tumour of the testicle at any given time that it does or does not menace its possessor's life. The tumour is not usually noticed until it has involved the entire organ. Carcinoma, apparently, grows more rapidly than sarcoma, and the benign cystic disease may attain a certain size and retain it for many years, although there is no sign to indicate the change which may ultimately alter it into a malignant growth. Thus in one of Conché's cases (Sturgis) the tumour began to grow after having been quiescent for five years. On the other hand, in a case recorded by Socin, in six months the tumour attained the size of a man's head, and Sturgis's case of sarcoma grew in a year to the size of a child's head. Kocher collected 32 cases of carcinoma, 25 of which came under observation within a year and a half of the beginning of the disease, and of which only 1 had lasted six years—an average of one year and four months; while 83 of Kober's sarcoma cases show an average of two years and eight months from the beginning of the disease to the time of operation. As the tumour is commonly accompanied by hydrocele, the absorption of this fluid sometimes causes an apparent recession in the size of the tumour which the surgeon should not allow to mislead him. The pain is often slight throughout, though it may well become severe in the later stages. Testicular sensation is lost.

The oval shape of the testicle is preserved. As the tumour grows it becomes uneven on its surface, nodular, elastic in places, perhaps fluctuating when there are large cysts or a flaccid hydrocele. Finally, the scrotal veins enlarge, the iliac and lumbar glands can be felt by deep abdominal palpation, and, ultimately, the tunica albuginea gives way and elastic masses can be felt projecting through it. Thence the fascia and skin are involved and the tumour eats its way through the tense integument, forming the malignant fungus, the fungus hematoides of the testicle. This occurred only once in Kober's 114 cases of sarcoma, but it is more frequent in the rapidly growing carcinoma. The inguinal glands do not enlarge until the scrotum becomes invaded by the growth, for the lymphatics from the testicle run directly up the cord to the iliac and lumbar glands.

---

[1] Annals of Surgery, 1888, viii, 446.

Diagnosis

The diagnosis of one new growth of the testicle from another is usually impossible, always unnecessary. The diagnosis between the various chronic diseases of the testicle is given below. Unless the case is absolutely clear-cut, the aspirator (p. 760) and antisyphilitic remedies should be allowed a share in the diagnosis. It is well to remember that every neoplasm of the testicle is possibly syphilitic until the contrary is proved. A short, sharp course of mixed treatment with iodids in excess will decide.

Diagnostic Table

	Simple chronic epididymitis.	Tuberculosis.	Syphilis.	Tumour.
History	Gonorrhea, stricture, or hypertrophy of the prostate.	Tuberculosis, family or personal.	Syphilis, inherited or acquired.	Perhaps trauma.
Frequency	Uncommon.	Frequent.	Frequent.	Rare.
Size	Small between attacks.	Does not reach any great size.	Does not reach any great size.	May reach any size.
Sensitive	Yes.	Yes.	No.	No.
Shape	Between attacks testis normal, epididymis nodular.	Epididymis nodular. Testis not involved unless acute or ancient.	Testis evenly enlarged, slightly nodular. "Clam-shell" epididymis.	Testis considerably enlarged. No characteristic involvement of epididymis.
Cord	May be slightly thickened.	Usually enlarged and nodular.	Free.	Free. Veins dilate in later stages.
Seminal vesicles	Usually distended	Tubercular.	Uninfluenced.	Uninfluenced.
Prostate	Posterior urethra congested or inflamed.	Congested. May be tubercular.	Uninfluenced.	Uninfluenced.
Urine	Cloudy.	Cloudy. May contain bacilli.	Clear.	Clear.
Hydrocele	Unusual.	Often.	Nearly always.	Unusual.
Onset	Usually acute.	Usually chronic.	Chronic.	Chronic.
Course	Recurrent acute attacks.	Usually chronic.	Chronic.	Fairly rapid.
Opposite testicle	Often involved simultaneously.	Usually involved subsequently.	Free.	Free.
Abscess	Unusual.	Common.	Rare.	None.
Potency	Unimpaired.	Somewhat impaired.	Somewhat impaired.	Unimpaired.
Atrophy of testis	Rare.	Rare.	Common.	Never.

At the end, as at the beginning, the iodids with mercury, and the aspirator.

CASTRATION

The treatment of tumour of the testicle is castration.

Preparation.—The usual preparation for an aseptic operation must be rigorously adhered to. But as the skin of the scrotum is very tender the soap poultice should not be left on more than three hours. I prefer general to local anesthesia.

The Incision.—An incision may be made over the testicle in front, or a perineo-scrotal incision behind (Félizet), or the incision may be made just below the groin, so that the testicle requires to be pulled up in order to be extruded through it. Both testicles may be removed through a single incision in the raphe. The incision may be modified to excise fistulæ, or carried up over the inguinal canal to trace the cord or to perform radical cure of hernia.

The Orchidectomy.—The fascia is torn through down to the testicle. When the albuginea has been laid bare, testicle, epididymis, and vaginalis may be shelled out by cutting the remains of the gubernaculum running from the lower end of the testicle to the bottom of the scrotum. If there is the slightest doubt about the nature of the growth it should be incised, for not a few hydroceles and hematoceles have been removed for cancer. A clamp is then put upon the cord, which is severed below it.

Treatment of the Cord.—If the operation is performed for tubercle or tumour the cord should be tied off as high as possible. To do this the inguinal canal may be opened, the vessels tied and divided at the internal ring, and the vas followed by stripping up the peritoneum almost or quite to the seminal vesicle. Or vas and vessels may be tied and divided at the external abdominal ring. If there is any possibility of recurrent tuberculosis in the stump of the vas, absorbable ligatures must be employed, and the stump fastened close to the skin incision so as to avoid a burrowing sinus. Under no circumstances should the vas be torn by brute force from the pelvis. I consider it unwise to search for enlarged iliac glands. If deemed advisable the end of the vas may be cauterized.

Termination of the Operation.—The scrotum should be turned inside out on the finger and every point carefully scraped with the finger-nail and scrutinized for bleeding vessels, all of which must be tied off. If the inguinal canal has been opened it is then closed, the wound sutured, and a compressing bandage (p. 696) applied.

Replacing the testicle by a celluloid substitute is an operation suggested by Weir,[1] and successfully practised by him and others.

The only special post-operative complication is hemorrhage, which may require the reopening and repacking of the wound.

---

[1] Med. Record, 1894, xlvi, 164.

It has been alleged that post-operative insanity is especially common after double castration. If true, this is doubtless due to the mental shock upon an individual who attributes an exaggerated importance to this gland. I do not believe it due to the withdrawal of the internal secretion of the testicle.

CHAPTER XII

HYDROCELE AND HEMATOCELE

Hydrocele is usually defined as an accumulation of serous fluid in the tunica vaginalis. This definition covers the ordinary cases; but hydrocele may also occur in the funicular process of the peritoneum (encysted hydrocele of the cord) or in the form of a number of cysts about the head of the epididymis or along the cord (encysted hydrocele). The fluid may be bloody (hematocele), milky (chylocele), or filled with spermatozoa (spermatocele). These varieties will be discussed in the next chapter. Serous hydrocele of the tunica vaginalis alone concerns us here.

Varieties.—Hydrocele may be idiopathic or symptomatic. It may be acute or chronic. While all idiopathic cases are chronic, not all symptomatic cases are acute, therefore the terms are not quite interchangeable.

SYMPTOMATIC HYDROCELE

As its name suggests, symptomatic hydrocele occurs only as a symptom of disease in the testicle and epididymis. It is often acute, and is especially common with acute epididymitis, syphilis, and the more acute forms of tuberculosis. Indeed, according to certain French writers, the acute tuberculosis of the testicle often begins as a tuberculosis of the tunica vaginalis. Hydrocele also accompanies quite frequently all other diseases of the testicle and epididymis. A *fibrous vaginalitis* has been identified post mortem or after castration. It gives no clinical symptoms. The *serous vaginalitis*, as symptomatic hydrocele is sometimes called, rises and falls with the disease of which it is a complication. It is acute with acute disease, chronic with chronic disease. Injections into the vaginalis may cause an acute hydrocele (p. 761).

Treatment.—The treatment of symptomatic hydrocele is, in some degree, comparable to the treatment of serous pleurisy. If the primary disease is acute and the hydrocele insignificant, it may be disregarded and allowed to be absorbed as the acute disease abates. If large and tense, or its absorption too slow, it may be aspirated one or several times, after which it will disappear in due course. But if the primary disease is chronic, while aspiration may hold the hydrocele in check some more radical procedure is often demanded. The treatment by injection, which is so habitually successful in idiopathic hydrocele (p. 761), may be tried, but it often fails. The need of a more radical procedure may prove the surgeon's opportunity to induce the patient to submit to an operation upon his testicle from which he otherwise would shrink.

IDIOPATHIC HYDROCELE

Most French writers maintain that there is no such thing as idiopathic hydrocele, that every *vaginalite séreuse* is symptomatic. This theory I cannot accept, since it does not explain why idiopathic hydrocele is so common in the tropics; why idiopathic hydrocele does not follow acute epididymitis, a disease which leaves far greater changes in the epididymis than those alleged as cause of idiopathic hydrocele; why idiopathic hydrocele, is, in all its clinical features, marked out as a clinical entity, while symptomatic hydrocele is so manifestly dependent upon neighbouring inflammation. The clinic at least teaches that idiopathic hydrocele is a distinct malady, not a dropsy, but a definite disease of the tunica vaginalis, known only by its effects, and hence deserving the title of confessed ignorance —viz., idiopathic.

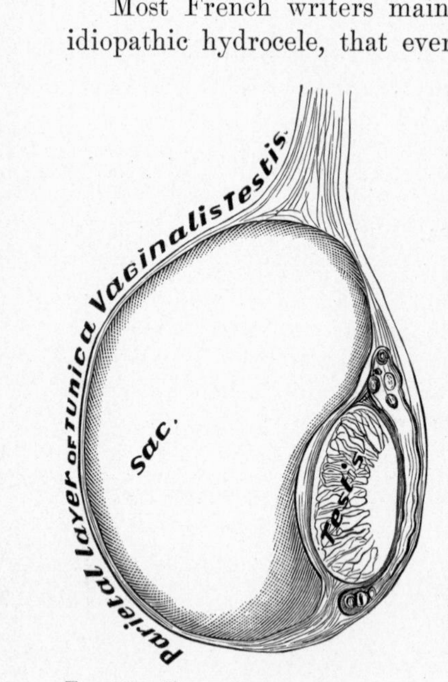

Fig. 167.—Usual Form of Hydrocele.

Varieties.—Hydrocele is usually confined to the tunica vaginalis (Fig. 167). In infants, however, it may occur before the funicular process has begun to close (*congenital hydrocele*), so that the cavity of the hydrocele communicates with the peritoneal cavity, yet by such a small opening that there is often no hernia and the fluid does not spontaneously drain off into the abdomen (Fig. 169). A more frequent variety is *infantile hydrocele*, occurring when the funicular process has quite closed at its upper end, so that the fluid distends both vaginalis and funicular process (Fig. 170). Hydrocele occurring in a retained testis is termed *inguinal hydrocele*. These and other varieties mentioned above will be dealt with in the next chapter.

Etiology

Hydrocele does not occur as a dropsical phenomenon, and it has already been distinguished from inflammatory or symptomatic vaginalitis. It is possible that certain cases are due to the bursting of an epididymal cyst into the tunica vaginalis,[1] but beyond this we are quite in the dark as to its cause.

Hydrocele is most common in the middle-aged. In the tropics it is said to afflict one man in ten. It is far less common in temperate climes.

Morbid Anatomy

The Character of the Fluid.—The fluid of hydrocele is viscid, odourless, straw-coloured, clear or opalescent. It looks like blood serum. Its specific gravity is about 1.024. It contains about 6% of organic matter, notably fibrinogen, to which it owes its property of coagulating blood serum. The alkalin carbonates and sodium chlorid are present in some quantity. The reaction is neutral. The presence of fibrinogen and inorganic salts distinguishes it from ascitic fluid. It may contain a few flakes and strings resembling urethral shreds. It is sometimes full of bacteria, sometimes brown from the admixture of blood. These bacteria and this blood are usually the result of previous punctures. The microscope reveals blood and epithelial cells and leukocytes. Cholesterin crystals are usually present, not often in any numbers. Suppuration is rare.

The Quantity of Fluid.—A good-sized hydrocele contains about a pint of fluid. Mr. Cline removed 6 quarts from the scrotum of Gibbon the historian. Breisson, after removing 16 litres on one occasion, drew 26 litres from the same patient ten months later. It takes from three months to a year for a good-sized hydrocele to refill after tapping. The largest hydrocele I have tapped held 2 quarts.

The Tunica Vaginalis.—The sac of a hydrocele may remain normal in structure even after the disease has existed for some time. Support to the testicle and systematic tapping may prolong this condition indefinitely. But if the scrotum is not supported, the slight bruising which the tumour continually suffers may produce a chronic thickening in the tunica vaginalis. In such instances the surface loses its gloss and becomes wrinkled and irregular, while the vaginalis becomes thick and leathery. Here and there warty growths may pro-

---

[1] Lancet, 1885, i, 748.

ject, and there may be cysts in the epididymis. Adhesions and masses of fibrin result from inflammation and are features of inflammatory, but rare in idiopathic, hydrocele. Obliteration of some part of the sac may subdivide it, causing the rare *multilocular hydrocele.* I have once met with *calcification of the vaginalis*, a very rare condition, which has been exhaustively described by Roswell Park.[1]

The Testicle and Epididymis.—Unless inverted or displaced by adhesions, the testicle lies below and behind the hydrocele. In mild cases the testicle remains normal, but after evacuation of the fluid one or more areas of induration may commonly be found in the epididymis. These are points of intertubular edema due to the interference with circulation. In old and inflamed cases of hydrocele, both testis and epididymis may be quite sclerosed and so atrophied as to be scarcely recognisable in the sac wall. Sometimes the tunica vaginalis forces its way between the testicle and epididymis, forming quite a pouch there.[2]

Multilocular Hydrocele.—Multilocular hydrocele is quite rare. It may be produced in one of three ways:

1. Several varieties of hydrocele exist simultaneously (e. g., hydrocele of the vaginalis and hydrocele of the cord).
2. The sac becomes subdivided by adhesions.
3. There is hernia of the sac between testis and epididymis.

Fibrous Bodies.—The so-called fibrous bodies occasionally met with upon opening a hydrocele are concretions of earthy phosphates or carbonates covered with fibrin. Probably they are for the most part due to a deposition of the hydrocele salts upon some warty growth, followed by atrophy of the little nucleus, after which the concretion breaks free. Wendlung met with concretions 6 times in 109 operations (Péraire[3]). They do not exceed the size of a pea—though Chassaignac met with one 2 cm. long and 12 mm. wide—and are usually single.

Symptoms

Idiopathic hydrocele is always chronic. The effusion takes place slowly and painlessly, and the swelling is only discovered after it has attained some size, for which reason the patient fancies it has appeared suddenly. The accumulation of fluid is slow and interrupted, but continues indefinitely. After tapping, the reaccumulation is at first rapid and then slow until the tumour reaches its original size, usually several months after tapping. Thus I have a patient who, refusing any radical measures, has returned once or twice a year since

---

[1] J. of Cut. and Gen.-Urin. Diseases, 1895, xiii, 361. [2] *Cf.* Jacobson, *op. cit.*, p. 134.
[3] Bull. de la soc. anat., 1899.

1895 to be tapped, having, for a number of years previous to that date, visited other surgeons for the same purpose.

There are no subjective symptoms attached to hydrocele, except the sensation of dragging felt in the loin and groin from the weight of the tumour.

Signs.—Hydrocele is usually pear-shaped, larger below than above; or it may be oval, and, if very large, almost spherical. It cannot be reduced by pressure. Fluctuation can usually be made out. The tumour is generally very tense, the scrotum often stretched and shining. The cord, of natural size and feel, can be grasped above the tumour. The testicle is usually situated behind, a little below the centre (Fig. 167), and pressure on this point gives rise to the peculiar sensation experienced when the testicle is squeezed. Occasionally the testicle is found below and in front, more rarely in the centre, in front, from plastic adhesion. Its position should always be ascertained before operating on a hydrocele. Dupuytren mentions several cases where this precaution was overlooked, the testicle wounded, and the diagnosis unconfirmed. As a rule no serious inflammation results if the testicle be punctured. Pressure on a hydrocele does not produce pain; there is no heat or redness of the skin unless the tumour be large enough to keep it constantly on the stretch. There is flatness on percussion. There is no impulse on coughing. Exceptionally a large hydrocele extends into the inguinal canal and so exhibits a slight cough impulse.

The weight of the tumour is a criterion that has been much depended upon to distinguish solid from fluid tumours. It is absolutely unreliable.

Varicocele and hernia may complicate hydrocele, and the pressure on the testicle may render it sterile. But if the hydrocele is cured the testicle will resume its functions unless it has become atrophied.

Suppuration and transformation into hematocele (p. 770) are rare. Spontaneous cures have been recorded after an infectious disease (Monod and Terrillon), sloughing of the scrotum (Cooper), rupture, and epididymitis. Such spontaneous cures are most unusual, except in the young. Curling cites the case of a Spaniard who had ruptured his hydrocele 30 times by horseback riding and other violent exercises; yet the swelling always returned after a few months. Infants often get well spontaneously, and expectant treatment is therefore most suitable for them.

Treatment

Palliative Treatment.—This is appropriate to symptomatic hydrocele, for children—for whom it is often curative—and for patients refusing radical measures. Before undertaking any operation for hydrocele the testicle must be accurately located by the testicular sensation or the light test.

Tapping.—This is best performed with the aspirator (using needle No. 2, Dieulafoy). The skin is made tense, and the needle plunged into the anterior part of the tumour, a little above the centre. The testicle should be carefully avoided (Fig. 168).

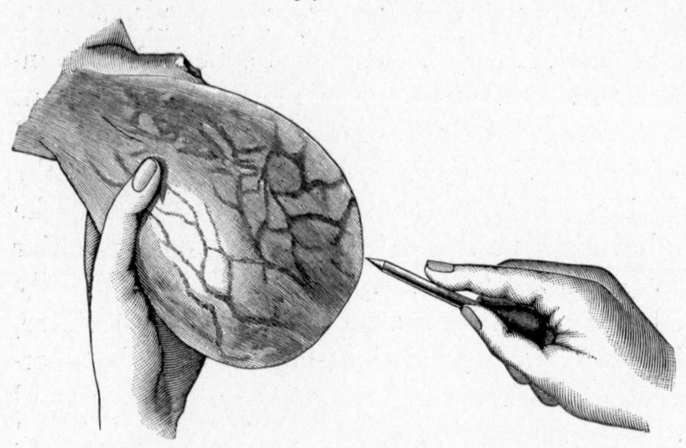

Fig. 168.—The Tapping of a Hydrocele of Tunica Vaginalis. Showing finger resting on instrument and tumour compressed by hand.

This simple operation will always efface the tumour at once, but in the majority of instances the sac will begin to refill in a few days, and after some weeks, or at most months, will have regained its previous size. Sometimes the tumour never refills, and the palliative eperation thus becomes radical. This rarely occurs, except in children.

Sir Astley Cooper mentions 2 cases of inflammation with sloughing, followed by death, in old men who took a long walk immediately after the operation. If the collection of fluid is very large, especially if the patient is old, it is well not to draw it all off at one sitting.

If the testicle has been wounded, the patient will complain of some pain, and blood will flow after the serum has been evacuated. To prevent the further effusion of blood into the sac it is advisable to strap the testicle immediately after the operation. Collodion is recommended by some authors to compress the testicle in this and other conditions, but its application to the thin and sensitive integument of the scrotum sometimes gives rise to exquisite and prolonged torture.

Acupuncture.—This consists in making the skin tense over the tumour, and penetrating the sac rapidly a number of times with a needle, which should be rotated as it is withdrawn. The serum, in cases so operated upon, gradually escapes into the scrotum (in twenty-four to forty-eight hours), where it does no harm, and whence it is absorbed.

Hydrocele in the adult will usually fill up after this operation, as it will after tapping, but in children acupuncture often suffices, especially if the internal surface of the sac be scratched. If the cyst wall be thick and the tumour not translucent, neither tapping nor acupuncture will ever effect a cure. Healthy young patients can put on a suspensory bandage and resume work at once after tapping or acupuncture.

Galvano-puncture is useless.

Radical Treatment.—Of the many methods of treating hydrocele only two need be detailed—namely, injection and incision—including excision of the tunica vaginalis.

Injection.—All simple hydroceles which are translucent, no matter what their age or how great their size, are amenable to treatment and cure by injection. Injection is not applicable to cases where the contents of the tumour are sero-purulent or sero-sanguinolent, or where the tunica vaginalis is extensively thickened, with or without calcareous deposit. In such cases incision or excision should be resorted to. Hydrocele complicating syphilitic or tubercular testis should be let alone or treated by palliative tapping, as it is but rarely curable by carbolic injection. Generally the hydrocele accompanying syphilitic testicle disappears spontaneously as the testicle improves under internal medication.

Celsus alluded to the injection method of treating hydrocele, but Munro, of Scotland, Sir James Earle, and Sir James Ranald Martin, of England, are the names most prominently connected with it. Inflation with air has been employed, and the most varied substances used in injections, from distilled water to the strongest acids. Many substances have been employed successfully, such as spirits of wine, port wine, solutions of alum or sulphate of zinc, air, chlorin gas, lime-water (Curling), chlorid of zinc, bichlorid of mercury, tincture of iodin (Martin), and last and best carbolic acid. When the tumour is very large, it is best first to reduce its size by one or more tappings, and finally to inject when the surface has become contracted by being relieved from prolonged tension.

If the hydrocele is found to contain more or less blood, injection should be postponed until some future tapping yields a comparatively limpid fluid. I have used many substances in injection for the radical cure of hydrocele, and have finally come to rely wholly upon pure carbolic acid. It is more certain, more speedy, less painful, and less dangerous than any substance I have ever used. To R. J. Levis,[1] of Philadelphia, belongs the credit of having introduced this substance to the profession as a proper injection in cases of simple hydrocele. I have adopted the suggestion with thanks, but think I have improved

[1] Trans. of the Med. Soc. of the State of Pennsylvania, 1881

the method. I have applied it with entire success to simple hydrocele, and to encysted hydrocele of the cord.

I have operated upon a child two months old and an old man past eighty, always successfully thus far, and in many instances I have effected a cure after the previous use of iodin by another surgeon had failed. In no case has any complication or serious reaction occurred at my hands. Pain is uniformly moderate. No symptoms of carbolic-acid poisoning have occurred. Upon one occasion I injected with entire success 2½ drams into three separate cysts in the cords of an old gentleman over sixty. He was confined to the house only a few days. I have operated at the hospital clinic, and had the patient get up from the table and walk down smiling to the wards —an impossibility if iodin had been used. I have operated in New York and sent the patient home to Brooklyn in a carriage. The number of my operations I do not know, but they count by scores. I look upon the injection as entirely innocuous and harmless, but I usually ask my patient to remain in bed one day. If, at the end of that time, he can get up and go about, he may; if pain and swelling prevent, as they sometimes do, he must remain in bed until motion is possible, using a poultice and taking an anodyne if necessary. When the patient goes about he should wear a suspensory bandage. The tunica vaginalis always refills after the operation, and the testicle is generally quite tense and hot for a few days, though sometimes it remains cool and flabby and the patient suffers no pain from beginning to end of the treatment. If the fluid reaccumulates in any amount, a simple tapping between the third and the eighth day completes the cure. When this secondary tapping is performed it is cheering to note how the fresh adhesions creak under the finger after the fluid has been withdrawn.

My operative method is very simple. The instruments are a glass syringe holding 100 minims, having an ordinary hypodermic point (rather large and about 2 inches long)—this, and an aspirator. I fill the 100-minim syringe with pure carbolic-acid crystals deliquesced by heating. I plunge into the hydrocele the needle of this syringe detached, and watch for the oozing out of a drop of clear serum to announce the fact that the tip of this needle is well within the cavity of the tunica vaginalis. I now insert the aspirating needle and rapidly exhaust the hydrocele, *if possible to its last drop,* an important measure, that the carbolic acid may not be diluted. Meantime the hypodermic needle first introduced has not been disturbed. When all the serum has been removed by the aspirator, I screw upon the hypodermic needle first introduced the 100-minim syringe, and rapidly inject from 10 to 100 minims of the pure acid, according to the size of the hydrocele, immediately withdrawing the needle, and leaving the acid within the cavity of the tunica vaginalis. This little operation is clean, almost painless, absolutely bloodless. No anesthetic is required. The testicle is manipulated a moment to insure the diffusion of the acid, an anodyne is left to be taken if required, and next day, if there is only moderate pain and swelling, the patient gets up and continues about. If the reaction has been considerable, he remains in bed for a few days with the testicle supported, and using such anodyne or local soothing measures as his surgeon thinks it proper to order. If the tension is great secondary aspiration gives relief.

The advantages of injection over any form of incision are manifest if only success may be anticipated. The failures so frequently reported are due to three causes—viz.:

1. Application of injection to cases incurable by this method —i. e.: *a.* Most symptomatic hydroceles.
    b. Some spermatoceles.
    c. Hydroceles with inflamed, indurated, or calcareous walls.
    d. Hematoceles and chyloceles.
2. Errors of technic, notably—
    a. Endeavouring to cure too large a hydrocele. If the sac contains more than 8 ounces its contents must be reduced by one or more preliminary tappings.
    b. Incomplete evacuation. This I believe to be the most frequent cause of failure. To insure success the last drop must be squeezed from the vaginalis.
    c. Injection of the carbolic acid into the cellular tissue. I need scarcely insist upon this point.
    d. Failure to perform the secondary aspiration which is sometimes part of the cure.
3. The use of iodin instead of carbolic acid. The iodin injection is painful and uncertain, while the carbolic acid, being a local anesthetic, produces only a momentary tingling and, at my hands, has been a certain cure.

The Open Operation.—This operation is indicated when there is any possibility of hernia, when the case is not suitable to injection, or when injection has failed. Three forms of operation are employed—viz., incision, excision, and eversion.

Incision (*Volkmann's Operation*).—The sac is incised vertically after the position of the testicle has been ascertained, and its cut edges are sutured to the skin. The surface of the sac is swabbed with pure carbolic acid and drained. The healing of the wound requires an interminable time, and the operation has been dropped in favour of

Excision (*Bergmann's Operation*).—The skin and fascia are divided down to the surface of the tunica vaginalis and dissected back from it, great care being taken not to injure the sac (Horwitz[1]). The sac is then opened, its contents allowed to drain away and the entire parietal layer snipped off. The visceral layer (the part adherent to the testicle) is swabbed over with pure carbolic acid and the incision closed over a drainage-tube. Complete dissection of the parietal layer is a tedious procedure, and yet recurrence has followed the operation on account of inattention to this detail. A simpler operation therefore is

Eversion of the Sac.—The sac is bared and opened as in Bergmann's operation, and all the parietal layer of the vaginalis that can be readily freed is excised. The testicle is then completely extruded from the scrotum, and the tunica, thus turned inside out, is held so by a few sutures passed behind the testis. The cavity of the vaginalis having thus been obliterated beyond peradventure, the testicle is replaced and the wound closed without drainage. Unless traumatic orchitis ensues the cure should be complete within ten days.

CONGENITAL HYDROCELE

In congenital hydrocele there has been no obliteration of the peritoneal prolongation (funicular process), and, instead of the usual solid, thin, fibro-cellular cord (Scarpa's habenula), there is an open canal making the cavity of the tunica vaginalis continuous with that of the peritoneum (Fig. 169). Congenital hydrocele is idiopathic, traumatic, or perhaps due to gravitation into the sac of an excess of the peritoneal fluid. It occurs in infancy.

Diagnosis.—The diagnosis is usually easy, but in certain cases there is some danger of confusion with hernia.

CONGENITAL HYDROCELE	HERNIAL TUMOUR
1. Appears soon after birth.	1. May appear at any time.
2. Tumour continues into inguinal canal.	2. Same.
3. Impulse on coughing.	3. Same.
4. Flatness on percussion.	4. Resonance on percussion.
5. Always reducible at an even rate, more or less rapidly according to size of opening; no jerk; no gurgle.	5. If reducible, goes back suddenly, with a gurgling sound.
6. Testicle, entirely obscured by the tumour, reappears on the reduction of the latter.	6. Testicle can usually be made out as a distinct lump.
7. Feel soft, not doughy; no gurgling.	7. Doughy feel—perhaps gurgling—on manipulation.
8. Always translucent.	8. Never translucent.

[1] J. of Cut. and Gen.-Urin. Diseases, 1896, xiv, 343.

A simple hydrocele may coexist with hernia at any time of life, and it is not uncommon for congenital hydrocele to be complicated by congenital hernia. Congenital hydrocele may be found in adults, but is rare. Horwitz met with it once in 110 cases, but Kocher estimates that it occurs 4 times in every 100.

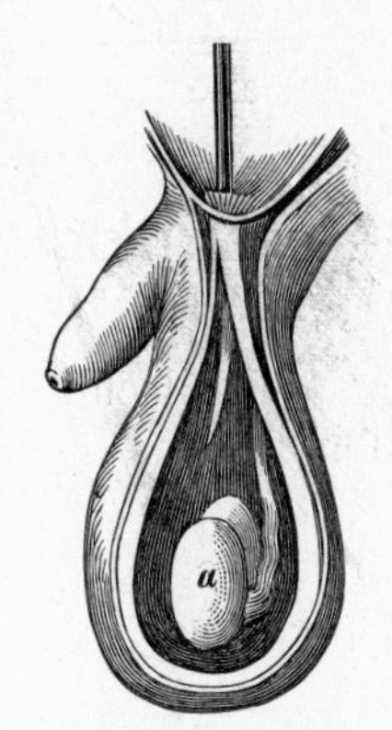

Fig. 169.—Congenital Hydrocele.

Treatment.—A well-fitting truss must be applied, which will usually obliterate the neck of the sac and is Nature's cure. The fluid should be absorbed in from two to eight months after closure of the neck of the sac. If not, the case may be treated as infantile hydrocele. Complication with hernia does not call for any modification of treatment. Congenital hydrocele should never be injected. Desault and Dupuytren did inject congenital hydrocele with a stimulating fluid, at the same time making firm pressure at the ring. This treatment, though sometimes successful, has always been followed by fatal peritonitis. If the neck of the sac cannot be closed the case may be submitted to herniotomy in later life.

INFANTILE HYDROCELE

Infantile hydrocele is far more common than the congenital variety. Horwitz met with 22 cases. The hydrocele occupies the tunica vaginalis and the funicular process up to the inguinal canal, where it is shut off from the general peritoneal cavity (Fig. 170). It resembles a congenital hydrocele, but is quite irreducible.

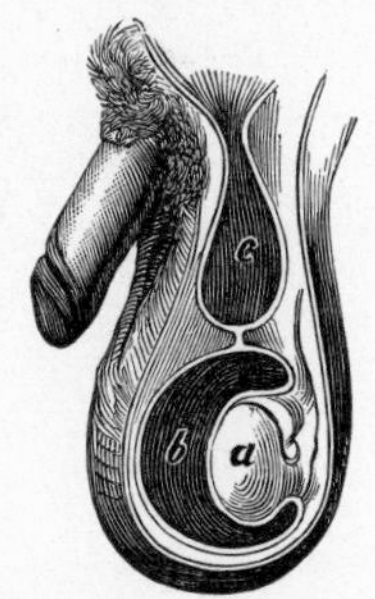

Fig. 170.—Infantile Hydrocele.

Treatment.—These hydroceles may get well spontaneously, and applications of iodin, methyl salicylate, or 50% guaiacol encourage resorption. Acupuncture or tapping repeated once or twice usually cures. Carbolic injection is a difficult operation on an infant, though it insures a cure. It is best performed by injecting the carbolic (0.5 gramme) through the same hypodermic needle used to withdraw the fluid. Incision is quite uncalled for.

Abdominal Hydrocele (*Bilocular hydrocele, hydrocèle en bissac*).—This is a very rare variety of infantile hydrocele, in which the hydrocele is partly in the scrotum, partly in the abdomen. The abdominal portion, which may grow to an enormous size, usually lies between the general peritoneal cavity and the anterior abdominal wall. Cures have been reported from simple drainage, injection, and incision, and the choice of treatment would depend upon the features of each individual case. Villeneuve[1] has collected 18 cases and Jacobson records several others.

MULTILOCULAR HYDROCELE OF THE SPERMATIC CORD

Multilocular hydrocele of the cord was first described by Pott and Scarpa as diffuse hydrocele of the cord, and most authors retain that title. The pathogenesis of this rare affection is habitually misunderstood. Kocher,[2] however, after a critical survey of the literature, concludes that an actual diffuse hydrocele can be due only to a rupture of some hydrocele or spermatocele, a temporary accumulation of fluid in the connective tissue about the cord. All other cases he classifies under five heads, viz.:

1. Echinococcus cyst.
2. Spermatocele.
3. Encysted hydrocele of the cord subdivided into loculi by adhesive inflammation.
4. Cysts of fetal remains (Müller's Duct, Wolffian Body, Organ of Giraldès).
5. Cystic lymphangioma.

He cites several examples. This classification certainly merits further investigation.

Symptoms.—The symptoms are characteristic, whatever the nature of the disease. The tumour extends about the cord from the testis up or into the spermatic canal. It is smooth, rounded, translucent, and boggy rather than fluctuating, though a difference in this regard may be made out in different parts of the tumour. It may be partly reducible. There is a slight impulse on coughing.

Diagnosis.—The diagnosis from encysted hydrocele of the cord is established by the boggy feel and the irregular, indistinct outlines of the tumour. In fact it resembles an incarcerated omental hernia in everything but its translucency and its fluctuation in places. Incision may be required to establish the diagnosis.

Treatment.—The tumour may safely be let alone. To cure it multiple puncture and carbolic-acid injection may be tried, unless it is a lymphangioma. Incision has usually been employed. Pott's classical case of lymphangioma died of lymphorrhagia after incision.

---

[1] Mercredi méd., 1890.

[2] *Op. cit.*, pp. 170, 180.

ENCYSTED HYDROCELE OF THE CORD

There are three conditions commonly grouped as encysted hydrocele of the cord, viz.:

1. Hydrocele of the processus funicularis.
2. Pedunculated cysts of the epididymis.
3. Hydrocele of an old hernial sac.

1. **Hydrocele of the Processus Funicularis.**—The sac is shut off below from the tunica vaginalis, above from the peritoneum. The hydrocele may be single or multiple (*hydrocèle en chapelet*). Usually single, it presents the features of a hydrocele of the tunica vaginalis, but is situated above the testicle and about the vas. Sometimes it may be reduced into the inguinal canal, but never into the abdomen. Although it usually occurs in children, I have twice seen it in the adult.

2. (See below.)

3. **Hydrocele of an Old Hernial Sac.**—This occurs in the process of peritoneum left behind by a hernia which has been reduced and the neck of the sac closed, either spontaneously or by the use of the injection cure for hernia. The hydrocele is usually mistaken for a recurrence of the hernia, but is translucent unless its walls are thickened.

Treatment.—For large encysted hydrocele of the cord injection is the best treatment. For small cysts, as well as for multiple and multilocular cysts, incision is the best treatment, care being taken to avoid wounding the constituents of the cord. Incision is indispensable for cysts situated within the inguinal canal or where there is any doubt as to hernia.

Hematocele.—Hematocele of the cord is rare, but may occur in the same way as hematocele of the tunica vaginalis, usually after injury. Indications for treatment are the same.

INGUINAL HYDROCELE

Hydrocele about a retained testis is one of the indications for operation upon that organ (p. 708).

CYSTS OF THE EPIDIDYMIS—SPERMATOCELE

This condition, commonly known as spermatocele or encysted hydrocele of the testicle, is a collection of fluid "contained in a cyst or cysts, distinct from but close to the cavity of the tunica vaginalis" (Jacobson). These cysts are developed in and about the epididymis, very exceptionally in the testicle itself, and should be classified as epididymal cysts. Two classes may be recognised.

1. Small cysts developing (usually) about the epididymis.
2. Large cysts originating within the epididymis.

1. The *small cysts* are rarely encountered before middle age, while they are very common in later life. They usually project more or less distinctly from the head of the epididymis, often into the tunica vaginalis, where their rupture is among the possible causes of hydrocele, and their detachment the origin, perhaps, of calculi (p. 758). They do not attain any notable size; they rarely contain spermatozoa—in short, they have little clinical significance.

2. The *large cysts* are found in the epididymis rather than projecting from it. They usually appear before middle age and commonly contain spermatozoa. They are often multiple and grow between the epididymis and the testicle, separating them and unravelling the former. Thus they form irregular fluid tumours about the top of the gland. Exceptionally, the cysts are pedunculated and grow upward, simulating hydrocele of the cord. They rarely contain more than 4 ounces, though Curling drew off 32 ounces from one individual and 40 ounces from another. Jacobson mentions a case from whose right side 49 ounces were drawn, and 58 from the left. Frost's[1] case yielded 52 ounces. The nature of these large cysts is identified by the fact that the fluid is milky and swarming with spermatozoa.

Pathogenesis.—Since the smaller cysts are met with later in life than the larger, and less frequently contain spermatozoa, many authors attribute the larger cysts to persistent fetal remains, such as the vasa aberrantia, the hydatid of Morgagni, or the paradidymis (Organ of Giraldès), and the smaller cysts to dilatations of the seminal canals. The recent tendency, however, has been to discredit the claims of the fetal elements, and to attribute the earlier and larger cysts to dilatation of the vasa efferentia or of the epididymis itself behind an obstacle more or less impervious,[2] and the later, smaller tumours to a cystic enlargement of the tubules due to senile changes after the organ has passed the height of its activity.

The presence of spermatozoa in the cysts is explained by those who cling to the theory of embryonal rests upon the ground that the

---

[1] Lancet, 1878, ii, 483.

[2] Griffiths (J. of Anat. and Phys., 1893-94, xxviii, 107) maintains that, like hydronephrosis, these dilatations are caused by partial obstruction due, in this case, to catarrhal inflammation. He also maintains that the hydatid of Morgagni is always a solid body, never cystic, and that there is no evidence that embryonal remains are in any way connected with spermatocele.

cyst has burst into the epididymal canal. *The absence of spermatic elements* is explained by those of the opposite camp on the ground that the cysts become occluded from the main channel and their seminal elements gradually disintegrate. The communication between a cyst and a seminal duct has been observed a number of times.

Symptoms.—The *small cysts* are occasionally met with in older men. They produce no symptoms.

The *large cysts* have peculiar features. Usually a slight uneasy sensation is experienced near the head of the epididymis, not amounting to pain, often entirely unnoticed, or at least forgotten by a patient who may afterward find the little tumour by accident. If seen early, an undefined sense of thickening, with extra resistance, is distinguishable by the finger in the region of the top of the testicle. This goes on increasing, usually at so slow a rate that the patient soothes himself with the idea that it will become no larger. It grows constantly, however, and may attain a large size. There is no pain, except a slight dragging on the cord. The cyst keeps its position at the upper end of the testicle, and becomes gradually heart-shaped, the testicle lying below the cyst which is notched above. The walls are usually thin and tense, so that fluctuation cannot always be distinguished, but translucency is usually present. The fluid may be dark-coloured or very milky, somewhat masking translucency. The patient is prone to become hypochondriacal, and to imagine that his sexual appetite and power are failing.

The cyst tends to increase in size indefinitely. It may coexist with hydrocele and be masked by it. It may be broken into the vaginalis by accident, and, continuing to secrete, form spermatic hydrocele, or it may be punctured when a supposed simple hydrocele is tapped.

Diagnosis.—The heart shape of the cyst, though pathognomonic when present, is not constant. The diagnosis is usually made by the irregular shape and position (above and behind the testicle) of the tumour and the presence of fluctuation over irregular areas. Aspiration usually completes the diagnosis by withdrawing a milky fluid full of spermatozoa. If the fluid is limpid it may be distinguished from hydrocele fluid by its neutral reaction, its low specific gravity (less than 1.010), and its low percentage of albumin (about $\frac{1}{2}\%$ against 4% to 7% in hydrocele). When hydrocele and spermatocele coexist the latter is not discovered until the former is tapped.

Treatment.—A cure usually results from aspiration and injection of carbolic acid through the same needle. If this fails the cyst should be excised. There is no object in disturbing small cysts.

HEMATOCELE

The term *hematoma* is applied to a tumour caused by the effusion of blood into the tissues, whether of the testis or the scrotum. If the effusion becomes encysted, or if it occurs within a cyst or the serous tunic of testicle or cord, *hematocele* results (Fig. 171).

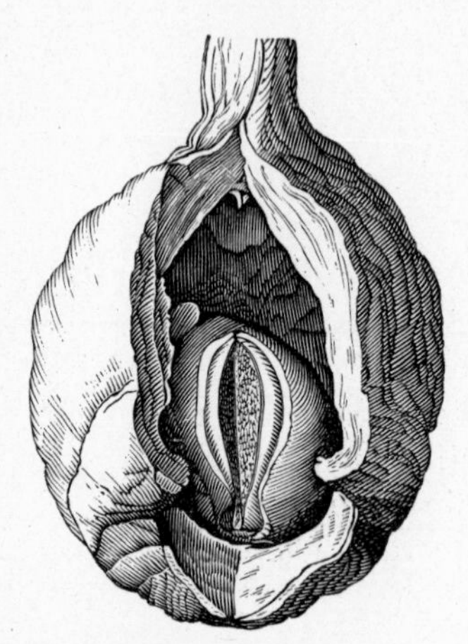

FIG. 171.—HEMATOCELE.

Etiology.—The most common cause is a crushing injury. Any operation upon the testis may result in hematocele.

Scrotal hematocele and testicular hematocele are always traumatic. Vaginal hematocele is usually traumatic but, exceptionally, may have a spontaneous origin from active or passive hyperemia; or, rarely, from a hemorrhagic secretion in scorbutic individuals. Sir Benjamin Brodie mentions as a cause a diseased (calcareous) condition of the arteries of the tunica albuginea, similar to the degeneration of the arteries of the brain which often precedes apoplexy. One of them may rupture into the tunica vaginalis.

Symptoms.—There are consequently two varieties. The one comes on rapidly after injury and is attended by scrotal hematocele. If there has been a pre-existing cyst or hydrocele this becomes suddenly larger, more tense, and painful. There is more or less fever, and suppuration may ensue.

In the other, or spontaneous variety, the tumour increases slowly in size and simulates hydrocele, except in regard to translucency.

The blood in hematocele may be found red and fluid, but is usually black or brown, and it may be mixed with pus if severe inflammation has followed its effusion. The walls of the cyst may be coated with layers of fibrin as in aneurysm, and they tend to thicken and become adherent to the surrounding connective tissue, while the inner surface becomes rough and uneven, resembling anything but a serous surface.

Diagnosis.—The diagnosis of hematocele of the second or spontaneous variety presents many difficulties. Here there is no guide in the history nor any local signs of injury. The records of surgery possess many cases where perfectly healthy testes, surrounded by a hematocele inside of a thickened tunica vaginalis, have been extirpated as cancerous. Often the diagnosis cannot be made without an exploratory incision. There are, however, characteristics of hematocele which may serve to distinguish it from hydrocele and from malignant growths.

The pyriform shape of hydrocele exists, but the tumour is not translucent. This, however, would also be the case in an old hydrocele with thickened walls. If it has been attentively watched, it will be found to have decreased a little in size at some period of its growth, which does not occur in malignant disease. The peculiar sensation produced by pressure on the testicle can often be evoked by pressing upon the mass behind at about the middle portion. In a doubtful case an exploratory aspiration or incision is demanded.

In the traumatic variety, the diagnosis is made at once from the history. It is unimportant, often impossible to distinguish between traumatic hematocele of testis, vaginalis, and scrotum.

Treatment.—For *hematoma* all that can be done is to keep the patient upon his back, with the testicle supported and covered with cold lotions, administering perhaps an occasional laxative and an anodyne if the pain be severe. If the quantity of blood effused is not too great, the pain will soon begin to subside, and the patient may be allowed to go about with a suspensory bandage. The blood will gradually be absorbed.

If, in spite of these means, *which will rarely be found to fail*, blood continues to be poured out into the cavity of the vaginalis so that the pain becomes excessive, and the tension of the parts very great, a trocar may be introduced to draw off the blood, and cold and pressure applied to prevent refilling of the sac. If it fills again, a second tapping, delayed as long as possible, will probably afford a more serous fluid than the first, and a third, a fluid still less tinged, after which the cyst will probably disappear.

Incision is required when inflammation is imminent or when the blood is so clotted that it will not flow through the needle. The cavity should be freely opened, irrigated, and drained.

Long-standing *hematocele* requires treatment by the knife. The sac must be opened, its contents evacuated, and as much as possible of the thickened wall cut away.

If the testicle is disorganized it should be removed. When the disease is spontaneous the possibility of hemophilia must be borne in mind.

CHYLOCELE

Chylocele (fatty, milky, chylous hydrocele, galactocele) is an accumulation in the tunica vaginalis of chyle or fatty lymph. It is a common feature of lymph scrotum (p. 698) and is caused by the rupture of a dilated lymph vessel into the tunica vaginalis. Filarial embryos have been seen in the fluid by Martin[1] and Davies.[2] Chylocele may also be due to traumatic rupture of a lymphatic into the tunica vaginalis. False chylocele is due to a fat- or cholesterin-producing degeneration in the fluid or in the epithelium of a hydrocele.

Chylocele when occurring without lymph scrotum resembles hematocele. The treatment is the same.

---

[1] Annals of Surgery, 1888, viii, 321.

[2] Brit. Med. J., 1885, i, 1245.

CHAPTER XIII

DISEASES OF THE VAS DEFERENS AND SPERMATIC CORD

ANATOMY

THE *cord* is made up of the vas deferens, the habenula or remains of the funicular process of the peritoneum, and certain vessels and nerves, all held together by meshes of connective tissue containing unstriped muscular fibre (internal cremaster of Henle). Surrounding these is a continuous layer of connective tissue (tunica vaginalis communis) adherent to the tunica vaginalis below and continuous with the fascia transversalis above. Outside of this the cremaster muscle lies in loops, some of them embracing the testicle in a fan shape, others extending only a short distance down the cord.

The *arteries* are, the spermatic from the aorta, the deferential from the superior vesical, and the cremasteric from the epigastric. The *veins* from the testicle and epididymis unite in the *pampiniform plexus* which constitutes the bulk of the cord. The larger veins have valves; they usually unite to form one large trunk, which empties, on the left side into the renal vein, on the right side into the ascending cava. The spermatic plexus of *nerves* is derived from the renal, the aortic, the superior mesenteric, the hypogastric, and the lumbar plexuses of the sympathetic, the genital branch of genito-crural nerve supplying the cremaster and the inguinal branch of ilio-inguinal.

The *cremaster* muscle varies in size and power in different subjects; it is a voluntary muscle; most persons can exercise it on both sides simultaneously, drawing up and holding the testicles against the abdomen; occasionally the muscles can be exercised separately, one testicle being elevated while the other is lowered. The function of the muscle is to assist in sustaining the testicle by its tonic contraction, and to compress the organ during the sexual orgasm. The muscle is subject to painful spasmodic contraction in kidney colic, in neuralgia of the testicle, and sometimes in connection with prostatic or urethral irritation. The *cremasteric reflex* is the retraction of the testicle caused by irritation of the adjoining portion of the thigh.

The Vas.—The vas deferens is the excretory duct of the testicle. It runs upward from the tail of the epididymis to form one of the chief constituents of the spermatic cord. It lies in the inner and posterior portion of the cord, where it may be identified as a rigid tube, the only element of the cord that does not slip almost insensibly from between the examining fingers. After passing through the inguinal canal the vas curves obliquely downward and backward over the base of the bladder, crosses behind the ureter and runs to the inner side of that duct, separated from it by the seminal vesicle. At this point it becomes markedly sacculated, then narrows to its original dimensions, and is joined by the duct of the seminal vesicle to form the *ejaculatory duct*, which pierces the prostate and opens into the posterior urethra just in front and to one side of the verumontanum.

The vas deferens is lined throughout with columnar epithelium. Its muscular coat consists of two layers, the inner circular, the outer longitudinal. Surrounding all is a dense fibrous tissue.

Relations.—The chief relations of the vas have been described above. In the scrotum it is closely surrounded by its own artery and one or two small veins. These vessels and the nerves run near it, and, except for a few veins to the inner side, the whole pampiniform plexus lies to its outer side.

ANOMALIES

Curling[1] relates a number of cases reported by various authors, in which the vas deferens was absent wholly or in part, on one or both sides. When the testicular end is missing the epididymis seems always to be wanting.

INJURIES

Wounds.—Wounds of the cord may cause profuse hemorrhage and rupture of the vas. The hemorrhage may be checked readily enough. If the vas is cut it should be united by Van Hook's method of ureteral anastomosis (p. 491). If some such operation is not performed, the duct becomes occluded, and, although this does not cause atrophy of the testicle, yet it shuts off the spermatozoa of that side from the urethra.

Complete division of the cord causes atrophy or gangrene of the testicle. Division of the pampiniform plexus causes only a temporary edema.

Torsion of the Cord.—(See p. 714.)

---

[1] Diseases of the Testis, 4th Ed., 1878, p. 7.

INFLAMMATION

Inflammation of the vas is usually incident to gonorrheal or tubercular epididymitis. It is rarely of any importance, unless an abscess forms. If this occurs in the scrotal portion of the duct it may be incised, if in the pelvic portion its existence is unsuspected, and it has been known to result in a fatal peritonitis.

Hydrocele and Hematocele.—(See p. 766.)

VARICOCELE

Varicocele may be either symptomatic or spontaneous.

Symptomatic Varicocele

Symptomatic varicocele is rare. This is caused by the pressure of some intra-abdominal growth obstructing the spermatic veins. The tumour is usually of renal origin and malignant. As Guyon, the original observer, remarks, the varicocele does not develop until the tumour of the kidney has become plainly palpable, so that symptomatic varicocele is not a very early sign of new growths of the kidney. Indeed Legueu [1] has shown that the veins are obstructed, not by the tumour itself, but by the enlarged glands along the renal vessels. Hence the varicocele is symptomatic of glandular enlargement, which argues ill for the ultimate results of any operation. Legrain [2] has once observed a varicocele symptomatic of gumma of the kidney.

Diagnosis.—Symptomatic varicocele cannot be mistaken for spontaneous varicocele. It develops very rapidly, late in life, on either side; is painless, attains a large size, and is always associated with a palpable abdominal tumour, against which the treatment should be directed.

Spontaneous Varicocele

Varicocele is a varicose enlargement of the pampiniform plexus and veins of the spermatic cord (Fig. 173). In a mild form, it is perhaps the most common affection of the genital organs. It has been estimated that about 10% of males have slight varicocele.[3] It occurs almost invariably on the left side; when very marked on this side it may exist slightly on the right, but varicocele of the right side is almost unknown. Pott met with it only once on both sides. Breschet,

---

[1] La presse méd., 1895, iii, 321; J. des practiciens, 1897, xi, 731.

[2] Guyon's Annales, 1898, xvi, 1155.

[3] Bennett estimates 7%, while Senn states that among 9,815 recruits 2,075 were affected with varicocele.

in 120 operations, operated only once on the right side. I have operated on both sides several times.

Slight turgescence of the veins of the cord does not deserve to be called a disease. The chief factor in its production is ungratified sexual desire, unrelieved erotic fancies, or, less often, the opposite condition, abuse of the sexual powers, by which the veins are kept constantly engorged. Most slight varicoceles are encountered in young unmarried men; the affection rarely commences after twenty-five; it is unusual to find it in a married man whose sexual relations are satisfactory. The slight turgescence of the veins constituting varicocele in a young bachelor and often causing him incessant and needless alarm, disappears after marriage, together with the uneasy sensations which accompanied it.

Old men whose testicles are inactive rarely have varicocele, though their legs show many tortuous veins and their tissues be degenerating. This fact is of the utmost importance, and is dwelt upon thus early in the consideration of the disease in order that attention may be specially directed to it. The idea that slight varicocele is often a sexual derangement, a functional disorder depending upon vicious sexual hygiene, is not emphasized by text-books, and is rarely appreciated by practitioners. In many cases young men distress themselves unceasingly, and importune their surgeons for an operation to cure a disorder which would be more speedily and effectually removed by marriage.

The degree of varicocele alluded to above may be dismissed briefly. It is found upon the left side; the vessels are a little full, the cord loose, feeling like a small bundle of earthworms, no one vessel being exceptionally large; the testicle is perhaps oversensitive (irritable), and there is usually a slight dragging sensation in the groin, but beyond this nothing except the fancied ills and the hypochondriacal complainings of the young man who is cheating Nature or abusing her gifts. The proper treatment of such cases is found in the employment of all hygienic and tonic measures. The patient's mind must be diverted, he must be dissuaded from an operation, told to wear a snugly fitting suspensory bandage, and if possible to forget his sex until marriage affords him an opportunity to get well. The free local application of cold water daily is a very useful adjuvant.

Yet varicocele serious enough to constitute a disease and to demand active surgical measures for its relief does occur. It is an exaggeration of the milder form; it comes on in early manhood, and has no connection with varices of the legs or anus (hemorrhoids). It is found on the left side, rarely on the right.

Pathogenesis.—Any theory to be adequate must explain the prevalence of the disease among the adolescent and its occurrence, almost entirely, upon the left side.

Many authors look for an anatomical predisposing cause. Thus certain French writers invoke a pre-existing phlebitis. Bennett [1] and Spenser [2] suppose a congenital anomaly of the veins. Such predisposing causes are not generally accepted. Sufficient anatomical predisposition is found in the position of the veins, dependent, unsupported, surrounded by the loosest kind of a fascial envelope. To this add the continual congestion set up by the untamed and pampered passions of youth, and no further predisposing cause is necessary.

But why should the varicocele occur upon the left side? To answer this question an infinite variety of theories has been proposed. There is space to enumerate only the more important ones. The left testis hangs lower than the right, and the left renal vein is higher than the opening in the cava which receives the right spermatic vein, hence the left vein is longer than the right. To this add the fact that the left spermatic vein, entering the renal vein at right angles, is not affected by suction as is the right vein which enters the cava at an acute angle. So far we are on safe anatomical ground; beyond all is theory. Perhaps, as has been alleged, right-handed men transmit the force of their exertions to the left foot by means of the abdominal muscles of the left side. But I have seen left-handed men with varicocele, always on the left side. Perhaps the sigmoid flexure, overloaded with feces, presses upon the veins. But this is as rare in youth when varicocele is common, as it is common in old age when varicocele does not occur. Curiously enough the ovarian veins are very rarely varicose, except on the left side.

A violent strain may induce acute varicocele.

Morbid Anatomy.—In mild cases the veins are merely tortuous and dilated. But in a full-formed varicocele the vessels are elongated, their valves broken down, their walls affected by fatty atrophy, and thickened, as is also the surrounding connective tissue. The veins sometimes contain phleboliths.

Symptoms.—I have seen a number of cases of *acute varicocele* resulting from straining, or coming on spontaneously. I have never seen it terminate otherwise than in recovery, under a suspensory bandage, a mild anodyne and a laxative. I have seen it last a number of weeks, and occasionally leave slight permanent enlargement of the veins of the cord.

---

[1] On Varicocele, London, 1891.

[2] St. Barthol. Hosp Rep., 1887, p. 137.

Except in acute cases, such as those just detailed, *varicocele comes on gradually*, and is discovered by accident. The amount of *pain* complained of varies greatly; a very large varicocele is often attended by absolutely no pain, while a very slight enlargement of the veins may give rise to considerable uneasiness extending up the back and down the thigh, perhaps amounting to neuralgia of the testis. Landouzy has noticed that the symptoms are markedly relieved during and immediately after coition, but become worse on the following day.

The only *general symptoms* in varicocele besides pain are those of hypochondria and defective *morale*, so common in all affections of the genital organs. The impotence often alleged by gentlemen of an incredible "years' experience" to result from varicocele is the veriest fiction. When impotence and varicocele coexist they are due to the same causes; but neither is the impotence due to the varicocele nor the varicocele to the impotence.

The *local conditions* are typical. The left testicle hangs considerably lower than the right, borne down, and perhaps completely surrounded by the mass of dilated veins. The mass feels soft, like a bunch of earthworms. In bad cases the testicular scrotal veins may be similarly affected. The scrotum is thin and relaxed, the dartos powerless. In long-standing cases of severe varicocele the testis gradually atrophies because of the interference to its circulation. This result is in no way due to the weight of the mass of veins.

The course of the disease is not progressive. Of the many men who have slight varicocele, only the smallest percentage fails to get well under the regulated sexual exercise of married life. Exceptionally, however, the veins do grow and enlarge indefinitely.

Diagnosis.—There are few diseases more readily recognisable than varicocele; the peculiar appearance and wormy feel of large tortuous veins can scarcely be confounded with anything else, except, possibly, omental hernia. However, a simple test will remove all doubt. If the patient lies down the swelling may be readily reduced. The fingers are now placed at the abdominal ring, and the patient told to rise; hernia will be retained, the swelling of varicocele will return, the vessels filling from below. If the pressure be sufficiently strong to occlude the arteries as well as the veins the tumour will not reappear. Varicocele, complicated by large hydrocele or by hernia, is more difficult of diagnosis.

Treatment.—If the varicocele be small and its symptoms inconsiderable, the palliative treatment already recommended for simple cases will suffice. Varicocele never compromises life, rarely deteriorates health, and, when it only causes moderate inconvenience, may be overcome by mechanical means. If these fail, or if the patient insists upon more radical measures, surgical treatment must be employed. The operations for the cure of varicocele are three: injection, subcutaneous ligature, and the open operation; this last including ligature, excision of the veins, and ablation of the scrotum. I consider subcutaneous ligature the operation of choice in almost every case.

Injection.—Englisch[1] has recently revived the injection treatment of varicocele. He employs from 2 to 6 hypodermic injections of alcohol into the bundle of veins. His statement that the treatment requires one or two months and is available only in the mildest cases is quite sufficient to condemn the method.

Subcutaneous Ligature.—Though the open operation for varicocele, as well as for hydrocele and stone in the bladder, will always appeal to the general surgeon, I can now heartily reiterate my opinion announced in presenting this as a perfected operation to the profession fifteen years ago[2]—time and experience having but fortified my belief—that subcutaneous ligature of varicocele is a simple operation, and, if properly done, perfectly safe and absolutely curative.

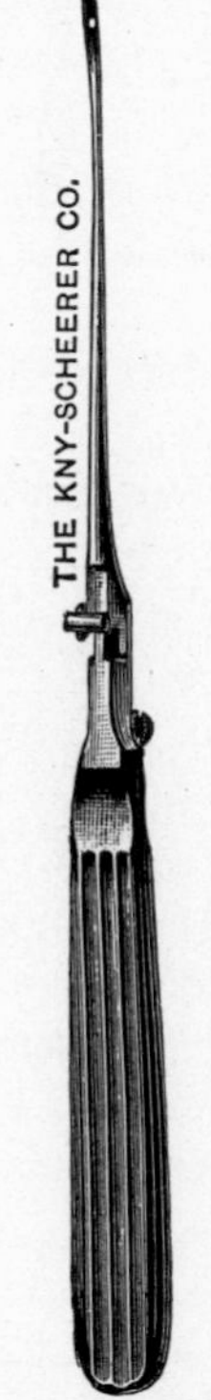

Fig. 172.—Needle for Subcutaneous Ligature of Varicocele.

The instruments required are: (1) a rather large straight needle in a solid handle, the eye of which is closed on the Reverdin principle, and kept closed by a spring in the handle (Fig. 172), and (2) a spool of heavy (No. 12) twisted white silk. The patient is prepared in the usual manner. The surgeon's hands and instruments are sterilized. By means of a 1% solution of cocain an area 1 cm. in diameter is anesthetized in a place selected in the upper part of the front of the scrotum, and a similar area in the back. The needle is then armed with a strand of silk 25 cm. long; its eye keeps closed by the automatic action of the spring. With the patient standing beside the bed and the surgeon seated on a low stool facing him, the operation now begins.

The surgeon grasps the scrotum with the thumb and index finger of his left hand. By drawing the fingers slowly towards the patient's

[1] Allgem. Wien. med. Zeitung, 1897, xlii, 233, 243, 255, 267.

[2] N. Y. Med. Record, February 20, 1886, September 18, 1886, and November 26, 1887.

right side the spermatic cord is allowed to slip piecemeal from the grasp. First the flabby veins of the plexus slip through in a worm-like bundle, then, after a slight interval, the solitary thick vas, followed perhaps by one or two more veins. This maneuvre is repeated once or twice until the surgeon is absolutely sure that he has identified the interval between the vas and the plexus. Then, holding the veins well to the outer side, and pinching the scrotum tightly to be sure that no veins elude his grasp, the needle is plunged into the anesthetized area close to the tip of the thumb. If the skin in front and behind has been anesthetized this maneuvre is quite painless. When the needle emerges from the back of the scrotum (Fig. 173), its eye is opened by retracting the button in the handle, the silk loop disengaged from it, and *one end* of the silk pulled through and out of the scrotum posteriorly. Now the scrotum is traversed independently by the needle and a single strand of silk.

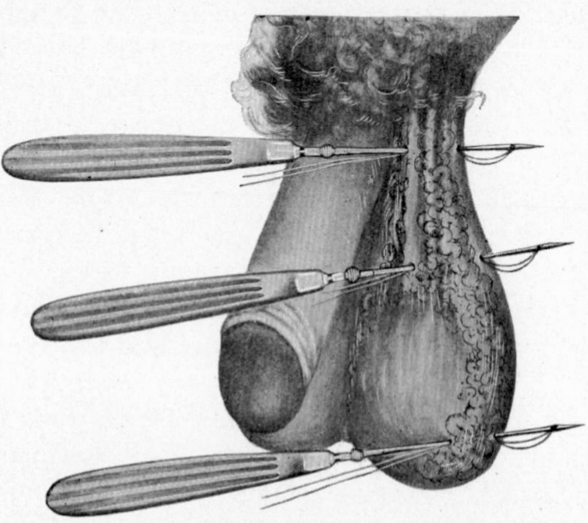

Fig. 173.—Subcutaneous Ligature of Varicocele.

At this juncture the patient usually feels faint, and he may be allowed to lie upon the bed. The remainder of the operation may be performed under general anesthesia if the patient so elects.

The needle, with its eye tightly closed but empty of thread, is now withdrawn partly, but not from the point of anterior puncture, and the veins are allowed to slip back towards the vas. As soon as this occurs the needle, which has not been withdrawn entirely, is again advanced outside of the veins close under the dartos and carefully made to emerge behind at the exact point from which the silk is protruding. The bundle of veins now lies between the strand of silk and the needle. The eye of the latter is again opened, the silk engaged in it and drawn through the scrotum and out of the anterior opening. A little piece of dartos will always be included in the silk at the point of posterior puncture. This is torn away by pulling the scrotum backward while making strong traction upon the loop of silk. The veins only are thus caught in a loop of silk, which is tied firmly and tightly in a triple knot. The ends are cut short and the knot allowed to recede into the scrotum. A drop of collodion upon each puncture completes the operation.

This single ligature suffices for most cases. I also often tie the veins just above and, exceptionally, below the testis, and, in a few cases, I have applied the ligature to dilated veins on the inner as well as on the outer side of the vas. I have never introduced more than 3 ligatures in any one case. Like the first, each ligature must be introduced on a separate needle before the patient is permitted to lie down; after which the second puncture may be made for each needle and then the strands of silk tied consecutively. The veins below the testicle are especially hard to separate from that gland.

In a few recent instances I have performed the entire operation with the patient anesthetized and recumbent; but, although the cases have all progressed satisfactorily, I am not yet prepared to sanction this method, since the possibility of puncturing a vein is far greater with the patient recumbent than when he is standing and the veins are dilated.

For *after-treatment* the patient is kept in bed with the testicle supported for forty-eight hours. The pain is insignificant and may be soothed by a hot-water bag. A certain amount of edema persists for two weeks, during which time perfect comfort is insured by a suspensory bandage. After this edema disappears the ligature may be distinctly felt, and usually remains unabsorbed for years. I have found it in place six and seven years after the operation. Rarely the ligature works its way out at the end of several months. This does not incapacitate the patient since it is accompanied by no active suppuration.

To insure the success of this little operation several points must be insisted upon:

1. Cleanliness, to prevent suppuration.
2. Careful exclusion of the vas deferens from the ligatures.
3. Careful inclusion of all the varicose veins. If all are not included the varicocele may not be cured, or a vein may be punctured.
4. Tying the first knot tightly. If the first knot is not tied with all the surgeon's strength he cannot feel assured that all the veins are obliterated. The tying of this first knot causes considerable pain and faintness.
5. Tying the veins internal to the side of the vas if they are varicose.

If precautions 3, 4, and 5 are observed there can be no recurrence so long as non-absorbable ligatures are employed. With catgut relapse is certain, with silk practically impossible. I have seen relapses and once atrophy of the testis after operations by others, but have not known either of these accidents to occur in any of my cases since I began to use silk fourteen years ago. An abscess formed about the ligature after one of my first operations, when the eye of the needle caught in the fascia and tore the tissues considerably. The patient left the hospital as usual on the third day, but returned a week later with an abscess, which was opened and continued to discharge until the fourth week, when the suture came away and the wound promptly healed. During this time the patient was able to continue his work without any inconvenience beyond wearing a suspensory bandage and keeping the wound dressed and clean. At the end of the fifth week after operation he was entirely well, and the cure has been permanent. This case is in striking contrast to the bad results so often seen from the open operation, after which I have known a case to drag along for two months and a half, with recurring abscesses.

The Open Operation.—The open operation for varicocele is calculated to appeal to the general surgeon. Excellent results may be obtained by this method at the cost of a little extra trouble, a little more time in bed, and a little more danger of prolonged suppuration. Yet the ultimate results are quite as good as those obtained by the subcutaneous method, and there is no danger to life in either case. I have seen complete atrophy of the testicle from an open operation performed by one of New York's best surgeons.

It is best to make the incision where the scrotum joins the groin, so that the veins are exposed just below the external inguinal ring. By operating in this region the danger of scrotal hematoma is materially lessened and the veins are encountered above their point of varicosity and tortuosity and can be conveniently handled. The vas, with its accompanying vessels, is separated from the bundle of veins and drawn to one side. The veins are then divided between two ligatures, or else the bundle of veins is drawn up out of the scrotum, an inch or so excised between ligatures, and the ends of the ligatures left long and tied together. By this means the cord is shortened and the testicle hoisted to its proper position alongside of its partner. Oozing is then checked and the wound closed. The operation may be performed under local anesthesia.

Ablation of the scrotum may be employed when it has been greatly stretched, but I do not believe the distensible scrotal skin can ever be depended upon to support the testicle so as to cure varicocele, and therefore I see no purpose in reefing the scrotum, except to remove redundant tissue. To elevate the testicle the veins must be shortened. Ablation of the scrotum may be performed with a curved scissors. Special clamps have been devised for the purpose, but a long, springy, curved pedicle clamp, such as the older gynecologists used, is as good an instrument as any to mark off the quantity of tissue to be excised.

Choice of Operation.—I employ the subcutaneous operation for all varicoceles except those enormous ones in which the scrotum is much distended and elongated. For these incision and resection of the veins is the operation of choice.

TUMOURS OF THE CORD

Cystic Tumours.—See Hydrocele of the Cord (p. 766).

Solid Tumours.—Solid tumours of the cord are rare. Fibroma, fibro-myoma, and sarcoma, all of the vas deferens, have been observed in isolated instances. Gumma is very rare (Goldenberg).[1] The only tumour of clinical importance is lipoma of the cord. The frequency of lipoma of a hernial sac lends colour to the theory that lipoma of the cord is secondary to hernial lipoma. In structure the tumour may be a pure lipoma, a fibro-lipoma, or a myxolipoma.

These tumours are usually small and reducible into the inguinal canal, stimulating epiplocele, from which they are only differentiated by operation, unless they can be drawn entirely out of the canal. Exceptionally, however, they attain an extraordinary size. Nové-Josserand [2] reports a specimen weighing 6½ kilos, and cites two others weighing respectively 20 and 15 pounds.

---

[1] J. of Cut. and Gen.-Urin. Diseases, 1901, xix, 113.

[2] Lyon méd., 1897, lxxxiv, 237.

CHAPTER XIV

DISEASES OF THE SEMINAL VESICLE

ANATOMY

The seminal vesicle (Fig. 174) is a reservoir connected with the vas deferens. Each vesicle lies to the outer side of its vas, its apex buried in the prostate, where it joins the vas at an acute angle to form the ejaculatory duct. The body of the vesicle is directed obliquely upward and outward, lying along the upper border of the prostate and projecting beyond it laterally. The fundus of the vesicle lies just external to the termination of the ureter in the bladder. Each vesicle is bound close to the bladder and prostate by a dense fascial envelope containing many unstriped muscular fibres. Within this fascia ramify numerous large branches of the prostatic plexus of veins. The relation of the vesicles to the peritoneum is variable. The recto-vesical pouch always dips sufficiently to touch the fundus of each vesicle, and when the bladder is full there is usually a small triangular space between the vesicles, just above the prostate, where a trocar may be passed from rectum to bladder without invading the peritoneum. But sometimes the peritoneal pouch fills even this triangle, a fact which adds weight to the obvious objections to recto-vesical puncture, and which explains the occasional extension of inflammation from the vesicle to the peritoneum.

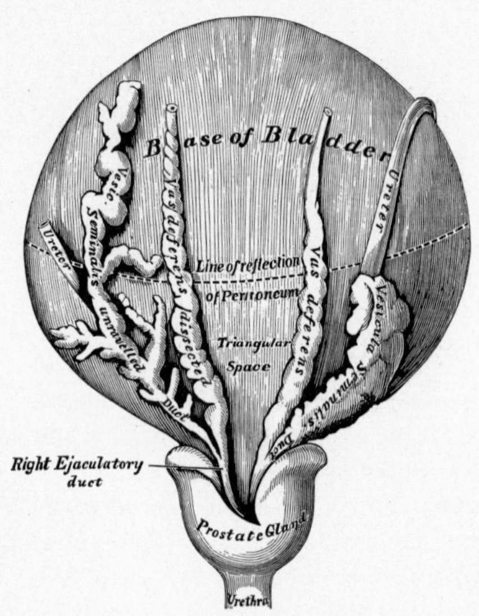

FIG. 174.—SEMINAL VESICLE (Gray).

The vesicle is elliptical in shape, flattened antero-posteriorly. Guelliot[1] gives 49, 18.5 and 10 mm. as its average length, breadth,

[1] Des vésicules séminales, Paris, 1883, p. 27.

and thickness. The lumpy surface of the vesicle has been compared to the convolutions of varicose veins or of the intestine. By a tedious and delicate dissection the vesicle may be unravelled. It is a single canal 10 to 15 cm. long. From this canal spring numerous small diverticula, one of which, originating near the orifice of the organ, may be almost as long as the vesicle itself. The blind end of the vesicular tube may be doubled back, so that the tube actually terminates near the orifice of the vesicle, and the fundus represents the middle part of the tube.

The tube is quite as irregular within as without. Here and there the orifices of diverticula loophole the tortuous wall, while the mucous membrane is thrown into folds extending in various directions.

The vesicle is made up of three coats: a thin outer fibrous coat, a thick middle layer of circular and longitudinal muscular fibres, and a mucous membrane. The latter contains many elastic fibres. Its epithelium is cylindrical in youth, cuboidal or flattened in old age. The epithelial cells often contain granules of brownish pigment, masses of which are occasionally found in the semen. Guelliot denies the existence of special glands in the vesicle, and affirms that the epithelium is identical throughout the organ. Rehfisch recognises vesicular glands.

The *arteries* of the vesicle are derived from the inferior vesicle and the middle hemorrhoidal. The *veins* join the prostatic and lateral vesical plexus. The *lymphatics* empty into the pelvic ganglia. The *nerves* are derived from the hypogastric plexus of the sympathetic.

The *ejaculatory ducts* begin at the junction of the vas deferens and seminal vesicle. Becoming smaller and of even calibre these ducts run obliquely forward and upward through the prostate, approaching each other until they nearly touch in the median line. Yet they are quite separate to their openings on the lips of the prostatic utricle. They are closely surrounded by a dense elastic tissue and contain a few straggling muscle fibres derived from the longitudinal muscle of the vesicle.

PHYSIOLOGY

The functions of the vesicle are three:

1. To store the secretion of the testis.
2. To dilute it.
3. To expel it into the prostatic sinus just before ejaculation.

1. Rehfisch,[1] in a detailed study of the comparative anatomy and physiology of the seminal vesicles, showed that in rats, guinea-

[1] Deutsche med. Wochenschr., 1896.

pigs, and other mammals, the vesicles empty by a separate duct into the urogenital sinus and at no time contain spermatozoa. But he confirmed on man De Graaf's experiment of injecting the vas deferens, showing that the vesicle fills with fluid before the ejaculatory duct is forced open. Hence it is fair to assume that the vesicle, as well as the ampulla of the vas, is a place of storage for the spermatozoa.

2. The *secretion* of the seminal vesicle dilutes the semen and probably has some obscure function of stimulating the vitality of the spermatozoa. This secretion is albuminous, alkaline, and odourless. It contains a large proportion of mucin. Besides blood-cells, leukocytes, and epithelia, the fluid contains many little hyalin pellets rarely visible to the naked eye. These bodies (sympexions, globulin körner) appear under the microscope as hyalin spheroids showing radiating lines of cleavage. They may contain masses of spermatozoa or pigment granules, and may attain a size sufficient to obstruct the ejaculatory duct (p. 790).

3. The vesicle becomes distended with fluid by the accumulation of its own secretion and the influx of testicular fluid. Unless there is spermatorrhea (p. 103) little or none of this fluid escapes, except during the sexual orgasm. This act occurs as follows: after a period of sexual excitement, varying in duration according to the nervous calibre of the individual, the muscular coat of the vesicle and the ampulla of the vas contract peristaltically, driving the fluid into the ejaculatory duct, which, very probably, is relieved of the elastic pressure that usually occludes it by a simultaneous muscular contraction of the prostate. The semen is thus ejaculated into the prostatic sinus, where it mingles with the prostatic secretion. The congested verumontanum blocks the way into the bladder and the prostatic and urethral muscles project the fluid forward by jets. I think the function of the verumontanum in preventing regurgitation is overestimated, for it is a matter of daily experience that the few drops of fluid left in the prostatic urethra at the end of urination are ejaculated by the urethral muscles, though the verumontanum is not at all congested.

Science and experience agree that the seminal vesicles are not emptied by a single orgasm.

ANOMALIES

Anomalies of the seminal vesicles are usually part of some general genital malformation. Guelliot has analyzed and refused to accept the alleged cases of multiple seminal vesicles. When the vesicle is absent the corresponding testicle may yet be present. Extreme dilatation of the vesicles is probably always acquired.

The ejaculatory ducts may empty into one of the ureters instead of on the edge of the prostatic utricle. In a few cases they have been found to continue forward alongside of the urethra the whole length of that canal to the meatus.

WOUNDS OF THE VESICLE

Guelliot recognises only one case of undoubted accidental wound of the vesicle. The patient had suffered a fracture of the ischium.

Operative wounds of the ejaculatory ducts are very frequent. The patency of the ducts is imperilled by all perineal cystotomies and prostatotomies, including lithotomy, Bottini's operation, and prostatectomy. Two results follow: inflammation (acute vesiculitis and epididymitis) possibly, obstruction probably. If the obstruction is partial, dyspermia results; if total on both sides, sterility. Therefore it is proper when operating upon a young adult, to whom the power to procreate is of some importance, to perform suprapubic, rather than perineal cystotomy, thus sacrificing the patency of one duct but not imperilling both.

Fistulæ of the spermatic duct have resulted from the old-fashioned lateral lithotomy operations. The resultant spermatic fistula heals kindly unless the parts are cancerous or tubercular.

EXAMINATION AND INFLAMMATION

The simple inflammations of the seminal vesicle are so bound up with the subject of gonorrhea that they have been described under that caption (p. 99).

The vesicle is examined by rectal touch. The methods of examination and of stripping are described elsewhere (p. 143).

TUBERCULOSIS

Tuberculosis of the vesicle is always at first unilateral. Before both vesicles are affected the prostate must become inflamed. Whether tuberculosis is usually primary in the prostate or in the vesicle is not clear (p. 244).

The lesions of localized tuberculosis—tuberculization, caseation, and suppuration terminating in fistula or atrophy—appear first near the mouth of the organ, where they may remain localized or whence they may be disseminated throughout its length.

Symptoms.—Commonly there are no symptoms directly referable to the vesicle. Hemospermia, abscess, fistula, increase or decrease in the sexual appetite—all these are rare. In most cases there is simply evidence of a tuberculosis of the prostate or of the epididymis, and examination reveals the condition of the vesicle. Simmonds[1] examined 25 cases of tubercular vesiculitis post mortem and only 6 of these were found to be sterile.

Diagnosis.—When the prostate or epididymis is known to be tubercular and the vesicle is found dilated or tender it may be assumed to be tubercular as well.

On the other hand, when there is doubt as to the nature of the prostatic inflammation an examination of the vesicles may sometimes throw some light upon the subject. If typical hard nodular areas of tubercularization are encountered they at once establish a diagnosis. But more often the organ is merely dilated in a manner suggestive of simple inflammation. If, in such a case, the urinary and physical examinations fail to indicate the nature of the disease, the latter may declare itself in a characteristic but disagreeable fashion by an outburst of tubercular epididymitis directly referable to the examination of the vesicle. Hence the rule: *never massage or examine a suspected vesicle except with the lightest possible touch.*

Treatment.—All local treatment of a palliative sort must be studiously avoided. Massage and douching do not benefit the vesicle, but endanger the testicle. Here as elsewhere the general hygienic treatment of tuberculosis is of prime importance.

It is but recently that the vesicle has come fairly within the reach of the scalpel, and many vesicles are sacrificed to celebrate this new triumph of surgery. The circumscribed lesions of tuberculosis have proved especially tempting. Even those who believe that the disease is primary in the testicle or epididymis may feel justified in extirpating the vesicle, either when known to be diseased, or in all cases, as a routine precaution. I am not ready to accept either alternative. Of the large number of cases in which the vesicle is known to be tubercular, only the smallest percentage shows grave symptoms of this lesion. Whether the vesicular inflammation be primary or not it is usually amenable to hygienic treatment. Yet exceptional cases with extensive caseation, suppuration, or fistulization, demand operative relief, and to these it should be accorded, but to no others.

Three varieties of operations are performed upon the vesicle:

1. Puncture—perineal or rectal.
2. Incision—perineal or rectal.
3. Excision—perineal, sacral, or inguinal.

Puncture may be summarily dismissed. It is always dangerous, never permissible.

---

[1] Deutsch. Archiv f. klin. Med., 1898, lxi, 412.

Incision is appropriate to simple non-tubercular abscesses that may be expected to heal. Incision through the anterior rectal wall is allowable, and may be performed with a tenotomy knife guided and protected by the finger. Perineal incision—a more formidable operation requiring general anesthesia and considerable surgical skill —is a more safe and thorough procedure at the hands of an experienced operator (see Excision). In tubercular conditions, however, incision is never more than palliative. It changes an abscess into a permanent fistula and should therefore be performed by the perineal route.

Perineal excision is the operation of choice for a tubercular vesicle. The operation is performed through a curved incision extending in front of the anus from tuberosity to tuberosity and carried on the affected side around to the coccyx (Guelliot [1]), thus encircling the anus on three sides (*EFG*, Fig. 60, p. 204).

Keeping a full ½ inch away from the bowel, and with the finger in that viscus and a sound in the urethra as guides, the perineal muscles are divided. The levator ani is thus revealed. Its anterior fibres (levator prostatæ) are severed, and the prostate, with the vesicles above it, is thus brought into the field. The wound is deep and the hemorrhage profuse, but efficient retraction, hemostasis, and a well-directed artificial light render the operation methodical and comparatively simple. With the prostate once well exposed and hooked gently but firmly downward by volsella, the distended vesicle is brought well into view. The surgeon first endeavours to hook his finger above the vesicle and thus to free its anterior surface and fundus from the peritoneum. This is the delicate part of the operation, and during this procedure the peritoneum must be respected. Happily, however, the vesicle, inflamed as it is, usually shells out readily. If the fundus is adherent the dense fascial envelope of the testicle may be divided close above the prostate and an intracapsular enucleation attempted. When enucleation succeeds, the vesicle alone or the vesicle with part of the vas may be removed. If the testicle has already been cut away the remainder of the vas may be drawn down and out through the perineal wound. When enucleation does not succeed, the best that can be done is to incise and scrape the abscess cavity and pack it tightly with iodoform gauze. In any case plentiful drainage must be provided for.

Sacral excision is preferred by many. A Kraske or Rydygier resection of the sacrum is performed upon the affected side. The rectum is drawn away and the vesicle exposed. A sound in the blad-

---

[1] Presse méd., 1898, i, 193.

der is of assistance as a guide. This operation exposes one vesicle much better than does the perineal route; but the opposite organ can not be reached. My preference remains for the perineal route, because the greater shock and the prolonged convalescence unavoidable after a sacral operation are handicaps to which no tubercular patient should be required to submit.

Inguinal excision was suggested by Villeneuve as a fitting complement to castration. It has led to disastrous failure even at the hands of competent surgeons, but has recently been performed successfully by Young.[1]

CYSTS

Prolonged inflammation sometimes causes gradual dilatation of the vesicles until they become two or three times their normal size and even overlap in the median line. Such cysts have only a pathological significance. Occlusion of the ejaculatory duct does not cause the vesicle to dilatate.

Several examples of echinococcus cysts occurring between rectum and bladder have been attributed, without convincing proof, to the vesicle.

CONCRETIONS AND CALCULI

While it is not unusual to find a number of concretions or small calculi in the vesicles of the aged, they have, as a rule, no clinical symptoms. It is only very rarely that they give rise to spermatic colic.

Symptoms.—Spermatic colic was first described, in 1879, by Réliquet. The colic occurs at the moment of ejaculation, during coitus, or during a nocturnal emission. The pain is very sharp, colicky in fact, and nauseating. It is centralized about an inch up the rectum, or at the neck of the bladder, and thence radiates up the posterior wall of the pelvis or to the testicles. The pain is caused by the impaction of a concretion or a mass of inspissated semen in the duct. The obstruction may be forced, and a painful and deficient emission ensue after a few moments of colic, or, if the occlusion is complete, emission may fail and the pain continue from fifteen to thirty minutes.

Treatment.—The treatment is palliative and curative. I have found the hot rectal douche (p. 131) an excellent remedy to relieve the pain and to shorten the attack. Many persons who are subject to mild attacks of spermatic colic obtain relief by introducing a finger into the rectum and pressing upon the offending organ.

[1] Annals of Surgery, 1900, xxxii, 557 and *ibid.*, 1901, xxxiv, 601.

If the attack has been severe, after it has passed off massage of the prostate and vesicle against a full-sized sound in the urethra should be employed. The concretion may thus be either disintegrated or expelled. This failing, incision of the vesicle might be employed.

MALIGNANT GROWTHS

Guelliot recorded but one authentic case of primary carcinoma of the seminal vesicle. Secondary involvement occurs from the prostate, bladder, or rectum.

CHAPTER XV

MALADIES INVOLVING THE GENITAL FUNCTION

IMPOTENCE

Impotence is usually a symptom of some physical morbid condition entailing inability to accomplish the sexual act. It is a complaint not infrequently submitted to the surgeon; not always frankly and openly as such, but often by implication, as though it should be recognised and inquired about in answer to remote indications which the patient has scantily furnished. Indeed, the surgeon who would meet the daily wants of his fellow-men in reference to troubles of this sort, must possess an accurate knowledge of the physiology of the sexual function and of its various derangements, and be ready to anticipate the reticence of patients; otherwise he will fail to sound many of the depths of human nature where suffering lurks—which suffering is for the most part preventable or relievable.

Impotence signifies that an individual cannot beget children because he cannot perform the sexual act properly, no matter what the obstacle may be, whether he have spermatozoa or not. The term must be carefully distinguished from sterility, which signifies inability to beget offspring on account of defect in the semen, whether the individual can have sexual intercourse properly or not. Undoubtedly the two are often associated in the same individual, but they may be totally distinct, as the following examples will illustrate. Thus, in the East, there are two methods of making eunuchs: either the penis is removed together with the testicles (and such a eunuch is necessarily both impotent and sterile), or the testicles alone are removed (and such a eunuch, though sterile, may be still partly potent), and does not bring so high a price as the eunuch who has no penis. It is a well-known fact that both animals and men, from whom the testicles have been removed after puberty, still retain sexual desires, and may have intercourse, with venereal orgasm and ejaculation of prostatic mucus, during a period of many years. A cryptorchid is rarely impotent, but is very apt to be sterile, and such is the case of many patients after double gonorrheal epididymitis; while, as causes of impotence without sterility, may be mentioned deformities preventing sexual intercourse, though the spermatic fluid is normal, such as exstrophy of the bladder, and extreme incurvation of the penis, with or without hypospadias.

The distinction between impotence and sterility being now clear, a few words regarding each of these complaints will perhaps serve to dispel the mists of uncertainty which often envelop them.

Impotence may be true or false.

True Impotence

This is exceedingly rare in the male. Any one who can perform the sexual act is potent. This act implies two conditions, namely, sufficient erection to make intromission possible, and a mucous fluid leaving the body by ejaculation.

That lack of desire before the act and pleasure during its accomplishment are not absolute essentials to sexual intercourse is exemplified by the two conditions, priapism from cantharides, in which there is no desire, and yet intercourse is possible with perfect intromission and ejaculation, and certain diseases of the cord attended by more or less paraplegia, where intercourse followed by conception may take place, and yet there be no pleasure in the act of ejaculation, the patient being unconscious at what moment it occurs.

Conditions involving True Impotence.—1. Absence of penis (p. 652). In such cases, if there are healthy testicles, the patient cannot be called sterile.

2. Minute size of penis may involve impotence. That small size is only relatively a cause of impotence is evident, and that it by no means involves sterility is shown by Orfila, in a case where an action for rape was brought against a man with only the stump of a glans in place of the entire penis, by a woman who was impregnated by him. Orfila decides that impregnation may take place under these circumstances, but only through the consent of the woman, and that consequently rape is impossible. The numerous cases on record where impregnation has taken place without rupture of the hymen show that a deposit of semen within the ostium vaginæ may fertilize an ovum, and such a deposit of semen *might* be accomplished by the smallest possible penis. Intromission and ejaculation might take place, and impotence, though possible, is not essential. The patient is not sterile.

3. Extreme size of the penis is a relative cause of impotence.

4. Extreme epispadias and hypospadias, with or without incurvation and exstrophy of the bladder, likewise involve impotence, without sterility; for though copulation might be possible with

exstrophy, yet intromission of semen would not take place, and impotence would be inevitable. The female with exstrophy is neither impotent nor sterile. Slight hypospadias may, but does not necessarily, involve impotence. The semen is not properly ejaculated into the upper part of the vagina, and impregnation sometimes fails to take place on this account. A very short frenum may have a similar effect.

5. Large size of the prepuce, or excessively tight and narrow orifice of the same, may involve impotence, as may also any tumours or growths upon or about the penis, elephantiasis, fatty tumour, hydrocele; or neighbouring deformity, as faulty position of the thigh from ankylosis of hip, excess of abdominal fat, etc., all of which may mechanically interfere with copulation without in the least implying sterility.

6. Very tight stricture of the urethra, especially if there be large and multiple fistulæ behind it, may involve impotence if the semen does not escape by ejaculation, but dribbles away after erection subsides. A similar cause of impotence exists in a vicious direction of the orifices of the ejaculatory ducts, by which during ejaculation the semen is turned backward into the bladder and escapes afterward with the urine. According to Grimaud de Caux, such a condition of things may be caused by the action of a certain class of Parisian prostitutes, who, fearing pregnancy, watch for the moment of ejaculation, and then press forcibly upon the urethra of their partner just in front of the prostate, by inserting a finger into his rectum, thus causing the semen to be ejaculated into the bladder. A similar condition has been known to result from prolonged posterior urethritis. When, from these or any other causes, there is no ejaculation, the condition is known as *aspermatism*.

7. Imperfect, irregular, or bent erections, due to inflammation, injury or tumour of one of the erectile cylinders of the penis, may sometimes prevent intromission and entail impotence.

8. Eunuchs, and those having atrophy of both testicles, are usually impotent, always sterile.

9. Injuries or diseases of the central nervous system sometimes cause impotence by interfering with either erection or ejaculation.

10. Impotence may be *symptomatic*—not to speak of the physiological impotence of childhood and old age—and then is only conditional or temporary, and usually disappears with the removal of its cause. Critically speaking, impotence depending upon most of the conditions already enumerated is symptomatic; but the term "symptomatic" is used to make a class apart. A single example will illustrate the point: A has double syphilitic orchitis; has no desire, no

erections—has, in short, impotence symptomatic of syphilis. Prompt treatment is employed; his testicles regain their normal state, his erections reappear, and he is well. B has the same condition of the testicles, the same impotence, but he employs no treatment; both testicles go on to atrophy, and he passes from a condition of symptomatic into one of true impotence, with sterility as well.

In symptomatic impotence there is always lack of erection, and often also temporary sterility. Such impotence is always associated with severe acute febrile diseases and with conditions of lowered vitality, whether due to wasting disease, to shock, or to other causes. Long-continued sexual excess, whether by masturbation or otherwise, produces impotence, though this is commonly a false impotence, an inability of the jaded body to keep pace with the lecherous mind. Finally, all drug habits—opium, tobacco, cocain, etc.—tend to produce impotence; and above all may be placed alcoholism. When a man is thoroughly drunk he is impotent; when a steady drinker, his sexual powers are always diminished, sometimes lost. Partial erection, attended by rapid ejaculation, is a common variety of impotence, due usually to sexual overexcitement, etc., and observed in animals as well as in men. In such cases a neuralgic condition of the prostatic sinus usually exists, and the most effective treatment is that for neuralgia of the vesical neck, with instillations of nitrate of silver, the cold sound, local external applications of cold water, and general hygienic measures.

The alleged efficacy of stripping the vesicles I have not been able to verify, but the hot rectal douche is useful. These means, aided by the confidence with which a physician should inspire his patient, and the counsel to be deliberate in the sexual act, and to practise it in the early morning rather than in the evening, or even to trust to a second effort, rather than to place all hope on the first, will often overcome this variety of impotence in time. Circumcision is sometimes useful to diminish hyperesthesia of the glans penis.

False Impotence

False impotence is an affection which the practical physician is often called upon to treat. True impotence calls for treatment of the physical irregularity, deformity, disease, cachexia, etc., giving rise to it. False impotence requires treatment of the individual, and not of any disease. In false impotence the cause is a nervous, or, it may be, a moral one; and there is no impotence whatever except in the mind of the patient. Here the surgeon requires all his delicacy, all his sympathy, in order to obtain the confidence of his patient, to overcome his suspicions, and to lead him gently to a cure, which is always possible if only the patient have faith.

Among the causes of false impotence may be mentioned sexual indifference, either temporary and spontaneous or more or less prolonged, as a result of sudden shock, grief, excessive joy, fright, repugnance, or lack of affection for the individual with whom copulation is attempted. Under the last two circumstances, the patient can sometimes think of another person than the one with whom he is lying, and thus maintain erection and effect ejaculation. The sudden flooding of the vagina with warm mucus will sometimes cause erection to cease at once. Roubaud mentions a curious case where impotence came on with an indigestion, and remained long after its cause had disappeared. He speaks of another man who became impotent on drawing a prize of 30,000 francs in a lottery. The various forms of sexual perversion afford numerous examples of false impotence.

Treatment.—This form of moral impotence requires special attention to all the agencies which may act as causes, and the exercise of tact and sympathy to acquire and retain the patient's confidence, a point of treatment most essential to success. The surrounding hygienic conditions must be made favourable, the advantages derived from change employed, and all indications of deviation from health in any respect appropriately met. It is necessary to arouse the moral sentiment of carnal desire, as well as the power of the organs to respond. The first is attained by favourable relations to the sex—opera, theatre, etc. The second, by general dry frictions of the whole body, by massage and flesh-brush, cold bath, sea-bathing, generous diet, and the internal use of tonic medication; the mineral acids, strychnin, ergot, and especially phosphorus and cantharides, or the two combined, commencing at a fair dose, $\frac{1}{40}$ of a grain of the former to 10 drops of the tincture of the latter, three or four hours before the desired erection, and increasing the dose carefully. Cantharides produces erection without desire; phosphorus and damiana directly increase desire. Cold and heat, by the douche, electricity, and local applications of mustard, are sometimes serviceable in recalling erection. In such cases the opportunity of the quack and the charlatan is unlimited. If he can, by whatever preposterous claims, once drive the obsession from the patient's brain, cure is assured. The regular physician cannot debase his self-respect by lies and trickery, but he can and must marshal all the strength of truth and virtue that lies in him to impress upon the patient's mind a respect for himself and his personal decency, as well as an appreciation of the subjective character of his defect.

Nervous Impotence

In a sense, all false impotence is nervous impotence; but there is a distinct and very common class of sufferers conveniently grouped under this heading. These are mostly young men who, from one cause or another, have got into the habit of acting abnormally in sexual congress. They get either no erection or a very slight one. Emission is absent, or premature, or without any sensation of pleasure. Each case has some peculiarity fondly alluded to by its possessor as proof that he is quite unique. Indeed, the patient's sole desire sometimes seems to be to persuade the physician that he has never before seen a case quite like this one. No possible classification of such cases can be satisfactorily minute, but the following may suffice:

1. The individual's potency is quite normal, but not what the patient thinks it ought to be.

2. The potency has been diminished by some early impression or by excesses.

3. The potency is congenitally slight.

1. The first class may be passed over lightly. Unhappily, there will always be among us a class of men, of splendid physique and infinite endurance, who elect to spend their lives in ignoble homage to Venus. And such men have their followers, their admirers—puny, dyspeptic, rabbit-eyed creatures—whose sole ambition is to flog their bodies on to wondrous feats of venery and bestiality. And since Nature never cast them in this mould, they come crying out because their bellies are not so big as their appetites, instead of thanking God for it.

2. Here is lost manhood! What a picture it recalls of errors of youth, thirty years' experience, electric belts, and what not! Here is the man of fifty, sixty, seventy, whose habits have him in their clutch. "Just once more!" "Days of my boyhood!" Here is where the moral lecture is the most deserved and does the most good. Or it may be the young man with premature ejaculations, weak erections, or nocturnal emissions. He has masturbated more or less, and has nocturnal pollutions. He has usually plentiful evidences of virile power. His desires may be excessive. He awakes with erections. He can provoke erection, or even emission, at will; but, in presence of a woman, and when he desires to have sexual intercourse, his organs will not respond; or, if erection comes on, it lacks energy, and is liable to fail at any moment during the act. In short, the patient can do anything he wishes, except rely upon an erection at the critical moment.

This form of impotence is the result of unnatural excitement of the sexual functions. It may come from prolonged ungratified desire or excessive erotic excitement at the moment. It is not infrequently accompanied by involuntary emissions during sleep, and by urethrorrhea, especially after the matutinal erection and defecation. Encouraged by the flaming advertisements of the omnipresent quack, the patient's fevered fancy pictures his condition as one of incurable gleet or wasting spermatorrhea. Probably the entire train of mental association can be traced back to some occasion, perhaps his first attempt at coitus, perhaps his last, when things went wrong through some external circumstance. He was frightened; he tried again, with worse result than before. Immediately his mind reverted to his youthful experiences. He had masturbated either too much or too little. He lays the blame of his condition upon his unusual chastity or his abnormal passions. He broods over his hopeless lot. False promises of a cure often tempt him to a trial, and their failure relegate him, more than ever deeply despondent, to the surgeon.

Treatment.—The treatment is threefold:

1. *The Patient's Sexual Coefficient must be Discovered.*—By the sexual coefficient I mean the amount of sexual power with which he is endowed by Nature. Mankind at large is possessed of the notion that, although men's noses and digestions need not all be cut of the same pattern, it is to be expected that the sexual capacity of every one should be all-embracing. Thus, while it is no disgrace to be dyspeptic about the stomach, it is to the last degree shameful to be dyspeptic about the genitals. Theoretically, such a distinction is absurd; but practically, no man is willing to brand himself a sexual laggard. In some way, by dint of enumerating emissions, copulations, masturbations, the physician must learn what ideal he can set before the patient. If a man's natural capacity for sexual congress is only once a month, it is hopeless to try and tune him up to three times a night.

2. *The Patient must be Encouraged.*—The first point of encouragement must be to depress him by bidding him look for a protracted and relapsing convalescence. Then he must be made to understand that his sexual possibilities are just so great and no greater; and that, however well he may get, overstepping his allotted bounds will call down swift retribution upon him. Finally, he must really be encouraged to feel that his malady is a functional disorder, a dyspepsia, which, like other dyspepsias, is curable, but only at the cost of a prolonged fast. He must abstain from coitus, from masturbation, from lewd companions, from obscene thoughts and things. The more thoroughly he abstains, the more certain his cure. Usually

he will try to adopt half-way measures, caring more for his "pot of ale" than for body and soul together. But such a course may not be countenanced. The ideal of absolute purity must be forever set before him and, as it were, hammered into him.

3. *He must be Assisted Physically.*—When possible, an entire change of scene presents the best opportunity for a man to get out of his old rut. Nothing could be better than a hunting or fishing trip. But if this is impossible, tonics may be given him, and sounds, nitrate-of-silver instillations, rectal douches, according to the choice of the physician. To some hyperesthetic individuals, massage of the vesicles is so nearly a suggestion of the sexual act that I fear it is quite as likely to do harm as good. If a strong moral influence, as that of father, brother, or priest, can be brought to bear, so much the better.

But all these measures are frankly palliative. When a man has once got into the habit of concentrating his whole mind upon his sexual organs, it is not to be expected that he should be entirely diverted to higher things. Chastity all can aim at, but celibacy is beyond the reach, beyond even the understanding of the many. Hence the proper cure for such a man, if he can be got into such a condition that he has an erection ever so rarely, is to instruct him in sexual physiology and hygiene, to acquire his confidence by sympathy, and to get him married, with the advice to attempt no intercourse, to be entirely frank and honest with his wife (who will more than equal him in timidity and ignorance), and, awaiting some morning when awaking with a vigorous erection, to accomplish coitus promptly, without delay, as a matter of imperious duty. The act once accomplished, the charm is broken. He knows he is a man and his confidence in himself returns.

STERILITY

The consideration of sterility is so interwoven with that of impotence that but little remains to be said. Sterility is an inability to beget children on account of absence or imperfection of the semen. In many cases there is impotence as well. All eunuchs are sterile. When both testicles are degenerated or destroyed by disease or atrophy sterility results.

The spermatic fluid, though ejaculated, may contain no spermatozoa (*azoöspermia*). This condition results from any obstruction to the formation of spermatozoa, any obstruction to their passage from the testicles to the meatus, or any inflammation in the seminal canals of sufficient intensity to destroy the spermatozoa. Without enumerating all the possible causes of azoöspermia, three may be especially designated:

1. Obliteration of both epididymes or both vasa deferentia by (gonorrheal) inflammation.

2. Debilitating diseases and, above all, alcoholism. Simmonds[1] estimates that 61% of alcoholics are sterile.

3. Inflammation of the prostate or vesicles. If the inflammation is severe the spermatozoa may be killed *in transitu;* but only a mild catarrh is required so to alter the quality of these secretions as to deprive them of the property of nourishing the spermatozoa.

Aspermatism, absence of ejaculation, is another less frequent form of sterility. It may be idiopathic, associated with anesthesia of the prostatic urethra, and due to the loss of some link in the nervous chain connecting ejaculation and sexual intercourse. More frequently it is due to operations upon the bladder and prostate that obliterate the seminal ducts. Such cases are not often encountered nowadays, but in former times, perineal lithotomy and Lallemand's porte-caustique made many a man sterile. Grimaux de Caux remarked of the latter that it made more eunuchs than did the demands of all the harems of the East.

Treatment.—Sterility from obstruction is incurable. Sterility from inflammation or from systemic disease is usually as curable as its cause.

SELF-ABUSE

Self-abuse is the production upon one's self of the venereal orgasm. The term masturbation signifies that an orgasm is produced by means of friction with the hand. Masturbation is not a malady. It does not necessarily produce disease unless carried to excess. Its practice is not confined to man. Monkeys are often masturbators; bears have the same habit; goats, making use of the mouth, indulge in it; turkeys sometimes practise it. In the human being it is practised by both sexes at all ages, females being much less addicted to it than males. The majority of women have very little passion, and suffer the first approaches of a lover or husband largely as a matter of complaisance. Undoubtedly there are numerous exceptions to this rule, but still a rule it is that the female, naturally modest, retiring, refined, learns what passion is only as the result of experience. With the male it is different. His passion is natural. He often has erections while yet a child, and has sexual yearnings long before puberty. Planque mentions two children four years old whose sexual organs were so developed that they could have sexual inter-

[1] Deutsch. Archiv f. klin. Med., 1898, lxi, 412.

course. Rarely does a boy escape initiation into forbidden pleasures by his school-fellows or his elders, and, though he escapes these, he is still very likely, when handling himself during erection, to find the sensation agreeable, and to go on, really ignorant of what he is doing, until he becomes a confirmed masturbator. Male babies are sometimes handled by their nurses to keep them quiet, a practice which is certain to beget the habit even in the earliest years of life. Stone in the bladder, irritation of the prepuce from retained smegma, traumatic stricture and bladder disease, ascarides, etc., lead a child to handle himself, and end in masturbation, if long continued; indeed, there are so many causes, natural and unnatural, why a boy should masturbate that few escape. But the most common cause is undoubtedly instruction, and this is usually received from other boys at school.

It may be safely assumed that a large proportion of mankind have masturbated more or less at some period in their lives, and it is equally safe to assert that at least 90% of such masturbators are not physically injured by the habit. If carried to excess, sexual indulgence in the natural way will produce evil effects, yet sexual intercourse is not only harmless, but even beneficial in moderation, as it can be only in the married state. It is not the loss of seminal fluid which is of the first importance in producing disease from sexual excess, but the nervous shock of the oft-repeated orgasm. Babies and young children lose no seminal fluid, women have none to lose, yet, in all of these, evil results follow excess as certainly as they do in the male after puberty. It is probable that any succession of nervous shocks as sharp and decisive as the sexual orgasm, even although purely intellectual, such as joy or fear, would shatter the vitality and nervous tone of an individual as much as masturbation.

Such writers as Lallemand, Acton, Belliol, certainly make too much of the solitary vice, while quacks find here the largest and most lucrative field for their nostrums. These men scatter their books and circulars broadcast over the land, and often, under alluring titles, thrust them within the eager grasp of the young, the inexperienced, the hypochondriacal, the nervous, overworked, unmarried youth, whose sexual needs, stimulated by his impure thoughts, find no adequate relief. Their tenets find ample faith and ready acceptance in the ingenuous mind, and errors are implanted which years of sober after-thought and experience, aided by the surgeon's careful and conscientious advice, are scarcely able to eradicate. Self-abuse is not confined to youth; middle and old age are not free from it. The numerous foreign bodies found in the urethra and bladder attest the tendency that men of all ages have to meddle with their genitals.

The use of tobacco, alcohol, and, it might be added, tea, is as widespread as the habit of masturbation; and each of these, or certainly the first two habits, probably inflicts as much injury upon the human race as does the secret vice. Yet who would affirm that every man who smoked would have headache, dyspepsia, heartburn, neuralgia, intermitting pulse, or would become thin, depressed, nervous, sleepless—all of which effects may be produced by an excess of tobacco; or that another who drank liquor would necessarily have delirium tremens, cirrhosis of the liver, fatty kidney, and die with ascites and Bright's disease? As with whisky and tobacco, so it is with masturbation carried to excess. Masturbation is capable of producing the most serious results, among which idiocy, insanity, epilepsy, dementia, physical prostration, hypochondria, impotence, and sterility are prominent, but these are practically extremely rare, and even in these rare cases it will often be found that some other cause, such as a blow on the head, congenital degeneracy, or abuse of stimulants has acted in conjunction with the masturbation. Hence it is evident that, while the intelligent physician must recognise the possible physical evils produced by masturbation, he should boldly oppose himself to that sickly sentimentality which shrouds in mystery one of the failings of our physical nature because it involves the sexual function, and should try to look the subject honestly in the face and to handle it as if it were a problem in mathematics.

The majority of mankind who indulge in masturbation do so just before and after puberty. At first most of them are ignorant that they are harming themselves, but they soon find it out by one means or another, and then sooner or later give it up. The longer and the more frequently they yield to the vicious habit the stronger does its hold become, so that in case they escape the mental and physical disorders to which excessive venery in extreme cases may give rise, still they may pay the penalty of excess by some diminution of vigour in after-life, by upsetting their sexual hygiene, and by establishing sexual necessities which they find it difficult to satisfy; and, finally, they may continue on through life victims to a perverted sexual sense, shunning women, from whom they aver that they derive no pleasure, totally wrecked as to their *morale*, often hypochondriacs, and suffering from all sorts of functional distress, physical and intellectual, real and fancied.

The chief reason why so much is said of venereal excess by masturbation, and so little of sexual excess in the natural way is, that the former is so much more common, and not that the act itself is physically more harmful. The solitary vice, as it is aptly styled, may be practised on all occasions, even in company, by the hand in the pocket, or by friction against some prominent object. In schools, not infrequently, boys practise it upon one another; but, generally, masturbation is performed in bed and in solitary places where there is no possibility of disturbance. Hence, in some cases, the frequency of its performance is very great and the effects of often-repeated nervous shock more pronounced. On the other hand, sexual intercourse requires the consent of two individuals and opportunities which are comparatively hard to find. Moreover, a man's moral sense will often keep him from committing excess with a woman, when nothing will restrain him while alone. In married life, excess is the exception; sexual hygiene is more apt to be correct, man is in his natural condition, other emotions enter largely into his daily life, and it is rare that the surgeon encounters a man happily married complaining of any disorder of the genito-urinary system, except those of a purely physical nature. On the other hand, the old rounder, who flatters himself upon the number of women he has ruined, but lays the blame upon Dame Nature, is usually a masturbator and, not infrequently, a pervert.

Symptoms.—A young child who has been taught to masturbate will be seen constantly at work at his genitals, and observed to have erections with unnatural frequency. No further signs are needed. Such children become fretful, peevish, thin, nervous, excitable. They sleep badly, have a haggard look, seem prone to convulsions, and, it is said, are apt to have epilepsy.

Boys who masturbate to excess usually have a long prepuce (they may have none, for Jews masturbate); they get a sallow look, have a sheepish, hang-dog expression; their eyes are deep-set, they incline to melancholy broodings, to staying apart and reading rather than to joining their companions at play. They become absent-minded, and their memory seems defective. Their palms are apt to be cold and moist. They lose the innocent frankness of youth.

The young man is overshy, unambitious, he shrinks from a steady gaze, blushes readily, and seems to be conscious of having done something unmanly and little.

Adult masturbators often show no sign of the habit, though they are apt to be cowardly, mean-spirited, poor specimens of humanity. But it is rare for adults to practise masturbation to great excess, and, if they suffer from any of the supposed evil consequences of the habit, it is either on account of excess in earlier life, of imperfect sexual hygiene, or of irregularly gratified sexual desire. Their symptoms assume a multiplicity of expression, and are generally hypochondriacal, and manifestly not entirely dependent upon masturbation; for the same symptoms may be relieved by marriage and are very common in patients who do not masturbate, who, indeed, are perfectly continent. As to atrophy of the genitals, varicocele, etc., these are not due to masturbation; and although this vicious habit may be the most important cause in a given case of chorea, insanity, etc., and should always be sought for, and if possible corrected, yet some other cause is usually to blame for the masturbation as well as for the idiocy or the epilepsy.

Castration has been employed in the vain hope of checking the vice. It is quite useless.

The foregoing remarks are not intended to palliate in the least degree the baseness of the practice of self-abuse, or to deny that lack of physical and sexual vigour, spermatorrhea, neuralgia of the urethra, etc., may be caused by its excessive indulgence; but they are intended to combat the idea, seemingly so prevalent, that very few men indulge in the secret vice, and that all who do so suffer; and they are also intended to advance the proposition that in the vast majority of instances masturbation does little harm to the individual, except in regard to his *morale*. It unmans him, makes him untrue to himself, and cowardly; and most sensible boys find this out before a great while, and give up the practice, which they feel to be sapping their manhood and self-esteem.

Treatment.—It is infinitely better that a boy should never masturbate if he can be prevented. Prophylactic treatment may save him. In the case of babies who do not do well, nurses should be watched and discharged if they are found handling the child. If the infant have already acquired the habit, his hands must be tied when he sleeps, and at all other times he must be watched until he grows out of the habit. Boys should always be made to sleep alone, never allowed to consort habitually with any other boy, especially older ones. All close intimacies between boys of different ages should be broken up, and, on the appearance of any of the signs of masturbation, a close watch should be maintained.

In most cases it is not good policy to ask a boy if he fingers his privates. He will be pretty sure to say no, and then to tell other lies to substantiate the first. To assume the fact after a careful study of the case is the safest course, and the boy, thrown off his guard by the statement that he does masturbate, will rarely deny it, or will do so in such a lame manner or with such overpositiveness as to convict himself. Finally, when the patient has confessed his folly, it is not wise to try to terrify him out of his habit by brilliant and exaggerated statements of the possible misery he may bring upon himself if he does not desist. This is appealing to a base motive, and, although sometimes successful, it is often inadequate to the proposed end, for a healthy boy cannot realize what it means to be sick; he cannot understand it, and consequently is not afraid of it. The method of treatment that is most effective, but requires the most force to carry out, is to elevate the boy out of his bad habit, to shame him, to make a man of him, to reason with him, and to talk to him honestly and openly, without reserve or mysticism; to sympathize with him, not to wound him; to study him and treat him morally. This course will succeed with the greatest number, provided only sufficient time and attention be given to it.

When a man comes complaining of the results of masturbation, an attentive study of the symptoms will prove his disease to be hypochondria, and his malady ungratified sexual desire, often with neuralgia of the vesical neck (p. 314). His training should consist in encouragement and continence, with absolute purity of thought, and subsequently marriage, to regulate his sexual hygiene. After marriage we hear no further complaint from these cases, always provided there is really nothing more than functional derangement at the bottom of the patient's complaint, as is the case in the vast majority of instances.

As for medicines, they are of little or no value; camphor, bromid of potassium, or lupulin may be given as placebos, but it is doubtful if they have any efficacy. Cold sponge-baths, outdoor sports, physical fatigue, sleeping in a cool room on a hard bed with a light covering are all useful; eating lightly at night, not retiring until very sleepy and rising immediately on waking in the morning, are powerful assistants in breaking up the habit; but all will be of no avail unless the *morale* of the patient be elevated, unless he keep his thoughts pure, and desire, for the manliness of it alone, to be rid of his bad habits.

POLLUTION

Pollution is a term applied to involuntary emissions of semen in ejaculation, attended by a more or less marked venereal orgasm. Pollutions are nocturnal or diurnal.

Nocturnal Pollutions.—Nocturnal pollutions are exceedingly common. They usually accompany an erotic dream, and the patient wakes just as the ejaculation is occurring. Sometimes, when sleep is profound, the patient does not wake, or, if he does, he forgets his dream, so that the sensation of pleasure accompanying ejaculation is faint and forgotten. Occasional nocturnal emissions are entirely natural and by no means a sign of disease. Their frequency compatible with health varies with the purity of mind and the sexual vigour of the patient. A man who is happily married rarely has nocturnal emissions while living with his wife, but, if he leaves her for several weeks, it is natural that there should be a formation and collection of semen which, distending the seminal vesicles, excites erotic fancies and, in the relaxed condition between sleeping and waking, escapes at the conclusion of a dream. Any man suffering from ungratified sexual desire is normally in a condition demanding relief for his overdistended seminal vesicles and, if that relief be not afforded in some way, it comes spontaneously during sleep. This is all the more certain to be the case if he has established a habit of rapid formation of semen by excessive sexual intercourse, or by habitual masturbation; and especially if, when natural or unnatural gratification is given up, lascivious thoughts are indulged in and impure associations continued. Occasionally nocturnal emissions may be overfrequent, and indicate a condition of irritation in the deep urethra—some modification of neuralgia of the prostatic urethra which requires treatment.

Treatment.—When emissions do not exceed three a week they should be disregarded, and attempts made only to purify the patient's thoughts, to elevate his tone, and if possible to get him happily married. When they occur as frequently as once or several times a night for a considerable time, certain special attempts to correct the habit are advisable, besides the employment of all known tonic and hygienic means and the measures detailed above. The patient should exercise and develop his muscular system. He should endeavour to tire himself out by physical work so as to sleep soundly. Locally, cold baths and cold douches are useful. He should sleep on a hard bed, lightly covered. The stomach should not be full on retiring. Most patients have involuntary emissions towards morning, and waking, find themselves lying on their backs. This position, with the bladder somewhat distended, tends to beget erection, and, by avoiding it, pollution may be escaped. This is accomplished by tying a towel round the waist on retiring, with a hard knot in the back over the spine. When the patient lies upon this knot it awakens him. Besides these means (among which purity of thought comes first), bromid of potassium, camphor, and lupulin may be given internally, with strychnin and a mineral acid, or such tonic as the physical conditions seem to call for. Decided advantage may be derived from the gentle use of the steel sound, and instillations of nitrate of silver.

From time to time different mechanical devices appear for treating pollution, their object being either to prevent the patient from handling himself during sleep or to awaken him before emission when he gets an erection. I believe them valueless and as likely to do harm as good, by keeping the patient's mind concentrated upon his malady and leading him to attach too much importance to the physical act of emission. I have used one which started a battery and gave an electric shock in the back when erection occurred. Verneuil used a similar instrument, which caused a bell to ring when erection came on, and he reports a successful case, as does also Tillaux. There is another machine, a ring, which encircles the penis lightly, but when distended by erection causes pain and awakens the sleeper. I think these mechanical means bad, and unsatisfactory in their result. They attack one symptom only and neglect the real malady.

Diurnal Pollution.—Diurnal pollution is rare. Some impressionable patients acquire so intense a prostatic irritability from venereal excess that the sight or thought of certain women or the lightest friction upon the glans penis will produce ejaculation. Such injuries to the spine as are caused by the garrote, the guillotine, and the gallows commonly cause ejaculation; and sexual perverts find in shoes, hats, odours, and various abominations sufficient cause for pollution.

Treatment.—The treatment of diurnal pollution is by steel sounds and local astringents to the prostate, together with most of the means detailed for nocturnal emissions. Circumcision should be performed if the glans penis is sensitive.

PRIAPISM

Priapism is more or less continuous erection without desire. With some forms of priapism intercourse with ejaculation may take place. The connection between injuries of the cerebellum and spinal cord and erection has long been observed. Roubaud quotes Serres in stating that out of 11 cases of cerebellar hemorrhage erection of the penis was noted 6 times. Death by hanging is often accompanied by partial erection. After injuries to the spine, and in some diseases of the cord producing paraplegia, erections are often absent, returning as the paralysis improves. On the other hand, certain diseases and injuries of the cord are notably attended by priapism, disappearing as the paraplegia gets well.

The effect of large doses of cantharides in producing erection without desire is well known.

Prolonged mental exertion, overanxiety, and other causes capable of reducing the tone of the nervous system are sometimes attended by priapism, which also occurs in the early stages of prostatic hypertrophy and as an evidence of leukemia.

Priapism in children is often due to stone in the bladder, tight prepuce, worms in the rectum, etc. Extreme cases are on record where priapism has terminated in gangrene of the penis.

Treatment.—Priapism usually gets well under hygienic and symptomatic treatment, beyond which no special measures can be suggested, except irritating the lower part of the spine, blistering the perineum, an india-rubber seton at the nucha, possibly the use of electricity, and strychnin, ergot, bromid of potassium tentatively, notably in cantharidal priapism. Iodid of potassium has been successfully used.

LIST OF AUTHORS QUOTED

INDEX